Handbook of Systemic Autoimmune Diseases, Volume 14

The Heart in Systemic Autoimmune Diseases

Handbook of Systemic Autoimmune Diseases

Series Editor: F. Atzeni and P. Sarzi-Puttini

Volume 1 The Heart in Systemic Autoimmune Diseases
Edited by: Andrea Doria and Paolo Pauletto

Volume 2 Pulmonary Involvement in Systemic Autoimmune Diseases
Edited by: Athol U. Wells and Christopher P. Denton

Volume 3 Neurologic Involvement in Systemic Autoimmune Diseases
Edited by: Doruk Erkan and Steven R. Levine

Volume 4 Reproductive and Hormonal Aspects of Systemic Autoimmune Diseases
Edited by: Michael Lockshin and Ware Branch

Volume 5 The Skin in Systemic Autoimmune Diseases
Edited by: Piercarlo Sarzi-Puttini, Andrea Doria, Giampiero Girolomoni and Annegret Kuhn

Volume 6 Pediatrics in Systemic Autoimmune Diseases
Edited by: Rolando Cimaz and Thomas Lehman

Volume 7 The Kidney in Systemic Autoimmune Diseases
Edited by: Justin C. Mason and Charles D. Pusey

Volume 8 Digestive Involvement in Systemic Autoimmune Diseases
Edited by: Josep Font, Manuel Ramos-Casals and Juan Rodés

Volume 9 Endocrine Manifestations of Systemic Autoimmune Diseases
Edited by: Sara E. Walker and Luis J. Jara

Volume 10 Antiphospholipid Syndrome in Systemic Autoimmune Diseases
Edited by: Ricard Cervera, Joan Carles Reverter and Munther Khamashta

Volume 11 Pediatrics in Systemic Autoimmune Diseases, Second Edition
Edited by: Rolando Cimaz and Thomas Lehman

Volume 12 Antiphospholipid Syndrome in Systemic Autoimmune Diseases, Second Edition
Edited by: Ricard Cervera, Gerard Espinosa and Munther Khamashta

Volume 13 The Digestive Involvement in Systemic Autoimmune Diseases, Second Edition
Edited by: Manuel Ramos-Casals, Munther Khamashta, Pilar Brito-Zerón, Fabiola Atzeni and Joan Rodés Teixidor

Volume 14 The Heart in Systemic Autoimmune Diseases, Second Edition
Edited by: Fabiola Atzeni, Andrea Doria, Michael Nurmohamed and Paolo Pauletto

Handbook of Systemic Autoimmune Diseases, Volume 14

The Heart in Systemic Autoimmune Diseases

SECOND EDITION

Edited by

Fabiola Atzeni
Rheumatology Unit, L. Sacco University Hospital, Milan, Italy

Andrea Doria
Department of Medicine and Rheumatology Unit, University of Padova Medical School, Padova, Italy

Michael Nurmohamed
Amsterdam Rheumatology and immunology Center,
Departments of Rheumatology Reade & VU University Medical Center
Amsterdam, The Netherlands

Paolo Pauletto
University of Padova Medical School, Department of Internal Medicine
Treviso, Italy

ELSEVIER

elsevier.com

Elsevier
Radarweg 29, PO Box 211, 1000 AE Amsterdam, Netherlands
The Boulevard, Langford Lane, Kidlington, Oxford OX5 1GB, United Kingdom
50 Hampshire Street, 5th Floor, Cambridge, MA 02139, United States

Library of Congress Cataloging-in-Publication Data
A catalog record for this book is available from the Library of Congress

British Library Cataloguing-in-Publication Data
A catalogue record for this book is available from the British Library

ISBN: 978-0-12-803997-7
ISSN: 1571-5078

Publisher: Sara Tenney
Acquisition Editor: Linda Versteeg-Buschmann
Editorial Project Manager: Halima Williams
Production Project Manager: Edward Taylor
Designer: Victoria Pearson

Typeset by TNQ Books and Journals

Dedication

Fabiola would like to thank her family and all of her friends for their incredible support and help during one of the most difficult periods of her life.

We would also like to thank **Linda Versteeg-Buschman, Halima Williams,** and their staff at Elsevier for their hard work. It has been a great pleasure to work with them on this second edition.

The Editors

Contents

6. Inflammasomes and Inflammatory Cytokines in Early Atherosclerosis

E. Matsuura, X.W. Tan, L.H. Shen, N.U. Azmi, L.R. Lopez

7. Treatment of Lipid Metabolism Disturbances in Autoimmune Diseases

N. Ronda, P.L. Meroni

8. Cardiac Imaging Techniques in Systemic Autoimmune Diseases

M. Turiel, L. Gianturco, F. Atzeni, P. Sarzi-Puttini, M. Porcu, M. Corda

11. Cardiac Involvement in Systemic Lupus Erythematosus

L. Iaccarino, M. Gatto, M. Zen, A. Doria

12. Cardiac Involvement in the Antiphospholipid Syndrome

I. Rodriguez-Pintó, G. Espinosa, R. Cervera

14. Cardiac Involvement in Systemic Vasculitis

M. Sebastiani, A. Manfredi, C. Ferri

15. Cardiovascular Involvement in Ankylosing Spondylitis

I. Sari, N. Haroon

List of Contributors

M. Afanasyeva, Johns Hopkins Medical Institutions, Baltimore, MD, United States

R. Agca, Amsterdam Rheumatology and Immunology Center and Reade, Amsterdam, The Netherlands

F. Atzeni, IRCCS Galeazzi Orthopedic Institute, Milan, Italy; Rheumatology Unit, L. Sacco University Hospital, Milan, Italy

N.U. Azmi, Collaborative Research Center for Okayama Medical Innovation Center (OMIC) and Department of Cell Chemistry, Okayama University Graduate School of Medicine, Dentistry, and Pharmaceutical Sciences, Okayama, Japan

P. Brito-Zerón, Hospital CIMA-Sanitas, Barcelona, Spain; Laboratory of Autoimmune Diseases Josep Font, CELLEX-IDIBAPS, Department of Autoimmune Diseases, ICMiD, Hospital Clínic, Barcelona, Spain

A. Brucato, Internal Medicine, Ospedale Papa Giovanni XXIII, Bergamo, Italy

J.P. Buyon, Hospital for Joint Diseases, New York University School of Medicine, New York, NY, United States

A.L.P. Caforio, Division of Cardiology, Department of Cardiological Thoracic and Vascular Sciences, Centro 'V. Gallucci', University of Padova-Policlinico, Padova, Italy

F. Caso, Rheumatology Unit, Department of Clinical Medicine and Surgery, University Federico II, Naples, Italy

R. Cervera, Department of Autoimmune Diseases, Hospital Clínic, Barcelona, Spain

R. Clancy, Hospital for Joint Diseases, New York University School of Medicine, New York, NY, United States

J.G. Coghlan, Royal Free Hospital, London, United Kingdom

M. Corda, Cardiology Unit, Brotzu Hospital, Cagliari, Italy

A. Courties, Department of Rheumatology, DHU i2B, Saint-Antoine hospital, Assistance Publique–Hôpitaux de Paris (AP-HP), Paris, France; Sorbonnes Universités UPMC, Paris, France

C.P. Denton, Royal Free and University College Medical School, London, United Kingdom

A. Doria, University of Padova Medical School, Padova, Italy

G. Espinosa, Department of Autoimmune Diseases, Hospital Clínic, Barcelona, Spain

D. Lisa Fairweather, Johns Hopkins Medical Institutions, Baltimore, MD, United States

C. Ferri, Rheumatology Unit, Azienda Policlinico of Modena, Department of Medical and Surgical Sciences, University of Modena and Reggio Emilia, Modena, Italy

M. Gatto, Division of Rheumatology, University of Padova, Padova, Italy

M. Gerritsen, Amsterdam Rheumatology and Immunology Center and Reade, Amsterdam, The Netherlands

L. Gianturco, Cardiology Unit, IRCCS Galeazzi Orthopedic Institute, Milan, Italy

N. Haroon, Division of Rheumatology, University Health Network, Toronto, ON, Canada; University of Toronto, Toronto, ON, Canada; Krembil Research Institute, Toronto, ON, Canada

M. Heslinga, Amsterdam Rheumatology and Immunology Center and Reade, Amsterdam, The Netherlands

L. Iaccarino, Division of Rheumatology, University of Padova, Padova, Italy

S. Iliceto, Division of Cardiology, Department of Cardiological Thoracic and Vascular Sciences, Centro 'V. Gallucci', University of Padova-Policlinico, Padova, Italy

L.R. Lopez, Corgenix/Orgentec, Broomfield, CO, United States

G. Malipiero, Hematology and Clinical Immunology, University of Padova, Padova, Italy

A. Manfredi, Rheumatology Unit, Azienda Policlinico of Modena, Department of Medical and Surgical Sciences, University of Modena and Reggio Emilia, Modena, Italy

R. Marcolongo, Hematology and Clinical Immunology, University of Padova, Padova, Italy

I.F. Masala, Santissima Trinità Hospital, Cagliari, Italy

E. Matsuura, Collaborative Research Center for Okayama Medical Innovation Center (OMIC) and Department of Cell Chemistry, Okayama University Graduate School of Medicine, Dentistry, and Pharmaceutical Sciences, Okayama, Japan

M. Meroni, Internal Medicine, Ospedale Papa Giovanni XXIII, Bergamo, Italy

P.L. Meroni, University of Milan, Milan, Italy; IRCCS Istituto Auxologico Italiano, ASST G. Pini, Milan, Italy

C. Nardin, Department of Medicine – DIMED, University of Padova Medical School and Medicina Interna 1, University Hospital Cà Foncello, Treviso, Italy

M. Nurmohamed, Amsterdam Rheumatology and Immunology Center and Reade, Amsterdam, The Netherlands

P. Pauletto, Department of Medicine – DIMED, University of Padova Medical School and Medicina Interna 1, University Hospital Cà Foncello, Treviso, Italy

R. Pérez-Álvarez, Department of Internal Medicine, Hospital Alvaro Cunqueiro, Vigo, Spain

M. Pérez-de-Lis, Department of Internal Medicine, Hospital Alvaro Cunqueiro, Vigo, Spain

C. Perricone, Rheumatology, Department of Internal Medicine and Medical Speciality, University of la Sapienza Rome, Rome, Italy

M. Porcu, Cardiology Unit, Brotzu Hospital, Cagliari, Italy

M. Ramos-Casals, Sjögren Syndrome Research Group (AGAUR), Laboratory of Autoimmune Diseases Josep Font, CELLEX-IDIBAPS, Department of Autoimmune Diseases, ICMiD, University of Barcelona, Hospital Clínic, Barcelona, Spain

M. Rattazzi, Department of Medicine – DIMED, University of Padova Medical School and Medicina Interna 1, University Hospital Cà Foncello, Treviso, Italy

I. Rodriguez-Pintó, Department of Autoimmune Diseases, Hospital Clínic, Barcelona, Spain

N. Ronda, Department of Pharmacy, University of Parma, Parma, Italy

N.R. Rose, Department of Molecular Microbiology and Immunology, Johns Hopkins Medical Institutions, Baltimore, MD, United States

I. Sánchez Berná, Department of Internal Medicine, Hospital Virgen de las Nieves, Granada, Spain

I. Sari, Division of Rheumatology, University Health Network, Toronto, ON, Canada; Division of Rheumatology, Department of Internal Medicine, Dokuz Eylul University, Izmir, Turkey; University of Toronto, Toronto, ON, Canada

P. Sarzi-Puttini, Rheumatology Unit, L. Sacco University Hospital, Milan, Italy

M. Sebastiani, Rheumatology Unit, Azienda Policlinico of Modena, Department of Medical and Surgical Sciences, University of Modena and Reggio Emilia, Modena, Italy

J. Sellam, Department of Rheumatology, DHU i2B, Saint-Antoine hospital, Assistance Publique–Hôpitaux de Paris (AP-HP), Paris, France; Sorbonnes Universités UPMC, Paris, France

L.H. Shen, Collaborative Research Center for Okayama Medical Innovation Center (OMIC) and Department of Cell Chemistry, Okayama University Graduate School of Medicine, Dentistry, and Pharmaceutical Sciences, Okayama, Japan

Y. Shoenfeld, Zabludowicz Center for Autoimmune Diseases, Sheba Medical Center, (Affiliated to Tel-Aviv University), Tel-Hashomer, Israel

A. Sisó-Almirall, Consorci d'Atenció Primària de Salut Barcelona Esquerre (CAPS-BE). Transversal Group for Research in Primary Care. Institut d'Investigacions Biomèdiques August Pi i Sunyer, (IDIBAPS) Barcelona, Spain; University of Barcelona, Barcelona, Spain

F.R. Spinelli, Rheumatology, Department of Internal Medicine and Medical Speciality, University of la Sapienza Rome, Rome, Italy

Z. Szekanecz, Department of Rheumatology, Faculty of Medicine, University of Debrecen, Debrecen, Hungary

X.W. Tan, Collaborative Research Center for Okayama Medical Innovation Center (OMIC) and Department of Cell Chemistry, Okayama University Graduate School of Medicine, Dentistry, and Pharmaceutical Sciences, Okayama, Japan

M. Turiel, Cardiology Unit, IRCCS Galeazzi Orthopedic Institute, Milan, Italy

M. Zen, Division of Rheumatology, University of Padova, Padova, Italy

Preface

This second edition of *The Heart in Systemic Autoimmune Diseases* details the current state-of-the-art of cardiovascular disorders in patients with systemic and organ-specific autoimmune diseases.

The first chapters deal with general aspects, i.e., the role of immunity and autoimmunity in the etiology and pathogenesis of cardiac manifestations as well as the use of cardiovascular imaging in defining cardiovascular features.

The following chapters focus on clinical aspects, including identification, diagnosis, and treatment of cardiovascular involvement in organ-specific and rheumatic autoimmune diseases, spondyloarthropathies, vasculitis, and gout.

The last chapter reviews the cardiovascular complications associated with antirheumatic drugs, synthetics, and biologics used in everyday clinical practice.

We hope that you will find this book interesting and useful.

The Editors

Chapter 1

Cellular Immunity: A Role for Cytokines

D. Lisa Fairweather,* M. Afanasyeva* and N.R. Rose§
*Johns Hopkins Medical Institutions, Baltimore, MD, United States; §Department of Molecular Microbiology and Immunology, Johns Hopkins Medical Institutions, Baltimore, MD, United States

The chapter has been revised and updated by Francesco Caso, Rossella Talotta, and Fabiola Atzeni for the 2016 edition.

Key Points

- Myocarditis is a process characterized by an inflammatory infiltrate of the myocardium with necrosis and/or degeneration of adjacent myocytes not typical of the ischemic damage associated with coronary artery disease.
- The development of autoimmune heart disease following viral infection involves the production of key cytokines by immune cells such as macrophages and natural killer cells.
- Environmental or genetic factors allow overproduction of proinflammatory cytokines, then progression to chronic autoimmune myocarditis may follow.

1. INTRODUCTION

The heart is a remarkably durable and efficient pump that provides all cells of the body with nutrients and removes waste products. If cardiac dysfunction occurs for any reason, it can have devastating results. Consequently, heart disease accounts for the majority of illness and death in Western populations (Schoen, 1999). Myocarditis or inflammation of the heart muscle is a significant contributor to heart disease, especially in infants, children, and young adults, and its treatment remains problematic (Drory et al., 1991; Rose and Afanasyeva, 2003). Importantly, myocarditis often precedes the development of dilated cardiomyopathy (DC), which can lead to heart failure and the need for cardiac transplantation.

The Heart in Systemic Autoimmune Diseases.

Myocardial inflammation is a major diagnostic characteristic of myocarditis. According to the current histologic definition based on the Dallas criteria, myocarditis is a "process characterized by an inflammatory infiltrate of the myocardium with necrosis and/or degeneration of adjacent myocytes not typical of the ischemic damage associated with coronary artery disease" (Aretz, 1987). Although inflammation can also occur as a result of ischemic injury, in myocarditis the inflammatory infiltrate plays a primary role in causing the myocardial damage.

The true incidence of myocarditis in the human population is unknown, but up to 10% of routine post-mortem examinations show histological evidence of myocardial inflammation (Gore and Saphir, 1947; Gravanis and Sternby, 1991). Because myocarditis is often difficult to diagnose with standard cardiologic tests, a definitive diagnosis depends on an endomyocardial biopsy, a relatively insensitive procedure due to the focal nature of the inflammation. Histologically defined disease has been confirmed in only approximately 30% of the patients with clinically suspected myocarditis, and in 30−60% of patients with DC (Marboe and Fenoglio, 1988; Peters and Poole-Wilson, 1991). The wide range in the rate of detection of myocarditis in biopsy specimens probably reflects local differences in diagnostic criteria and patient selection as well as the insensitivity of biopsy in general.

To further complicate diagnosis, myocarditis can be induced from many different agents including infections, immune-mediated reactions, or drugs (Table 1.1). Viral infections, such as Coxsackievirus B3 (CVB3) and cytomegalovirus (CMV), are widespread in the population, and most individuals in Western populations will be infected with one or both of these two viruses at some point, although acute viral myocarditis may occur frequently without clinical detection (Forbes, 1989; Grist and Reid, 1993). Advances in molecular techniques, such as genomic hybridization and the polymerase chain reaction (PCR), have confirmed the presence of infectious agents like CVB3 in the hearts of some myocarditis and DC patients, but the high prevalence of these infections in the population makes it difficult to relate infection with disease. Because these viruses are so common, diagnostic tests based on detection of viral antibody tend to be overly sensitive and the viral infection has usually cleared from the blood stream by the time heart disease occurs. Hence, a better understanding of the pathogenesis of disease is needed in order to find measures that both confirm diagnosis and determine whether the disease is at an early viral or later immune-mediated stage. When viruses directly damage myocytes or initiate immune-mediated damage is often unclear (Huber, 1997; Fairweather et al., 2001).

A number of infectious agents other than viruses are associated with myocarditis. Parasites such as Trypanosoma cruzi (the causative agent of Chagas disease) are the primary cause of myocarditis in Latin American populations where parasites are estimated to infect 16 to 18 million people (Table 1.1) (Cunha-Neto et al., 1996). Chagas disease can afflict nearly 50% of

TABLE 1.1 Major Causes of Clinical Myocarditis

Infections
Viruses (e.g., Coxsackievirus, CMV, influenza)
Bacteria (e.g., streptococci, Borrelia burgdorferi (Lyme disease), *chlamydia*)
Protozoa (e.g., Trypanosoma cruzi (Chagas disease))
Immune-mediated reactions
Post-viral
Post-streptococcal (rheumatic fever)
Systemic lupus erythematosus
Drug hypersensitivity (e.g., sulfonamides)
Transplant rejection
Chemical
Drugs (e.g., adriamycin, cocaine, lead)
Physical
Radiation
Hyperpyrexia
Exercise stress
Unknown
Sarcoidosis

Modified from Huber, S.A., 1997. Autoimmunity in myocarditis: relevance of animal models. Clin. Immunol. Immunopathol. 83, 93 and Schoen, F.J., 1999. The heart. Cotran, R.S., Kumar, V., Collins, T. (Eds.), Robbins Pathologic Basis of Disease. W.B. Saunders Co., Philadelphia, pp. 544.

endemic populations with 80% of infected individuals developing myocarditis (Schoen, 1999). Likewise, bacterial infection with Streptococcus pyogenes may result in rheumatic heart disease, which remains a major cause of heart disease in many developing countries. Myocarditis has also been associated with systemic autoimmune diseases such as systemic lupus erythematosus and polymyositis.

2. AUTOIMMUNITY IN MYOCARDITIS

Soon after autoimmune diseases were first recognized more than a century ago, researchers began to associate them with infectious organisms. The basic task of the immune system is to recognize the myriad of foreign molecules that enter the body from the environment and to avoid harming self (Rose, 2002).

Despite such protective mechanisms, autoimmune diseases are common in industrialized societies. Although autoimmune diseases present differently in different organs, they share many common mechanisms.

In order to better understand the relationship between infection and autoimmune disease, we established a mouse model of myocarditis induced by CVB3 (Fairweather et al., 2001). Coxsackievirus is believed to account for the majority of cases of myocarditis in North America and Europe (Fujioka et al., 1996; Friman and Fohlman, 1997), and the same virus is capable of inducing myocarditis in humans and mice. Following CVB3 infection, BALB/c mice develop an acute, focal inflammatory myocarditis with a mixed cellular infiltrate peaking around day 12 after infection (Fig. 1.1). Infectious virus can be detected in the heart during this time, but viral levels do not correlate with the severity of inflammation (Fairweather et al., 2001, 2003). Inflammation subsides by day 21 after infection, when heart sections look relatively normal under the microscope. A similar course also occurs following murine CMV (MCMV) infection of BALB/c mice (Fairweather et al., 2001). We surmise that a parallel sequence of events occurs in humans infected with diverse types of viruses such as CVB3 (a small, nonenveloped RNA virus) or CMV (a large, enveloped DNA virus). That is, individuals typically develop acute but self-limiting viral myocarditis that heals without residual lesions. In some individuals, as in susceptible mouse strains, the disease develops a chronic phase associated with inflammation and fibrosis accompanied by an autoimmune response to cardiac myosin and other cardiac antigens. The pathogenic process sometimes progresses to DC.

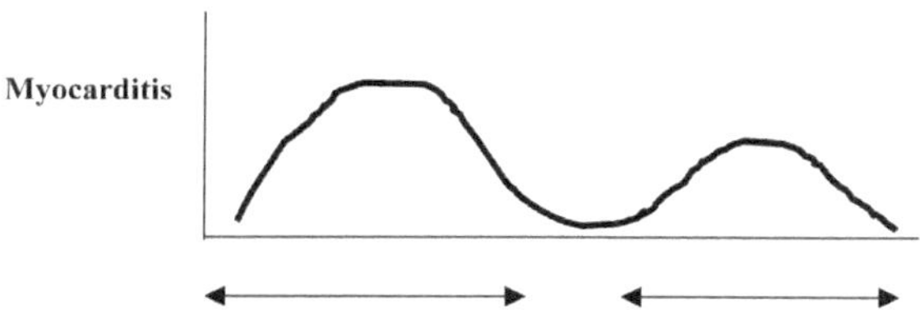

	Acute, Viral	**Chronic, Autoimmune**
Course	day 7 to 14	day 28 to 56
Peak	day 12	day 35
Inflammation	focal, mixed infiltrate	diffuse monocytic infiltrate, necrosis, fibrosis
DC	rare	present

FIGURE 1.1 Progression to autoimmune myocarditis following Coxsackievirus B3 (CVB3) infection of BALB/c mice. Infection of BALB/c mice with CVB3 results in the development of acute, viral myocarditis. During this time, infectious virus can be detected in the heart, but does not correlate with the level of inflammation. The acute inflammatory infiltrate in CVB3 infection is comprised predominantly of macrophages, $CD4^+$ T cells, $CD8^+$ T cells, and B cells. The inflammation subsides by day 21 after infection. In BALB/c mice, the chronic, autoimmune stage of the disease emerges around day 28 after infection. Acute myocarditis is characterized by a mixed cellular infiltrate but very little necrosis or fibrosis, in contrast to the autoimmune chronic phase where the lymphocytic infiltrate is associated with large regions of fibrosis and necrosis that may be followed by the development of dilated cardiomyopathy (DC).

We propose that certain cytokines released in response to viral infection are key in driving the progression to chronic, autoimmune heart disease in mice. We have studied the influence of the immune response to the virus on the subsequent development of myocarditis using mice deficient in immune cells or cytokines due to antibody treatment or genetic manipulation. This chapter will focus on the role of these cells and cytokines in the pathogenesis of myocarditis in mice.

3. PATHOGENESIS: THE ROLE OF CELLS AND CYTOKINES

Although a number of animal species (such as primate, pig, dog, rabbit, guinea pig, and rat) have been used in myocarditis research, most animal investigations utilize mice (Huber, 1997). A number of experimental mouse models of myocarditis and DC have been developed, which closely reflect the course of human disease. These include immunization of animals with antigens, such as cardiac myosin, or the use of infectious agents such as viruses. The viruses most often studied in animal models include reovirus, encephalomyocarditis virus, MCMV, and CVB3.

Animal models have provided valuable information on factors important for susceptibility to viral infection, such as age, sex, nutritional status, pregnancy, and genetic background (Khatib et al., 1980; Huber et al., 1981; Wolfgram et al., 1986; Fairweather et al., 2001). Infants are more susceptible to Coxsackievirus infections than are young children or adults (Kaplan, 1988), and similarly, susceptibility in mice decreases with increasing age (Khatib et al., 1980). Furthermore, individuals in the human population respond differently to the same infectious agent, with similar observations reported with different mouse strains. Studies to determine the genetic predisposition for myocarditis involved infecting many types of inbred mouse strains with CVB3 (Wolfgram et al., 1986). Susceptibility to autoimmune myocarditis, whether inoculating with CVB3, MCMV, or cardiac myosin plus adjuvant, is under strict genetic control (Rose et al., 1988; Lawson et al., 1990; Fairweather et al., 2001; Rose and Afanasyeva, 2003). For example, A/J mice are highly susceptible, BALB/c mice are intermediate, and C57BL/6 mice are resistant to the development of the chronic, autoimmune phase of myocarditis (Fig. 1.1). Surprisingly, this susceptibility is due primarily to genes that are not part of the major histocompatibility complex (MHC) (Rose and Afanasyeva, 2003).

Key in our understanding of the control of susceptibility to autoimmune disease was the finding that inoculation with bacterial lipopolysaccharide (LPS), interleukin (IL)-1β, or tumor necrosis factor (TNF)-α after viral infection resulted in the development of the chronic, autoimmune phase of disease in resistant strains of mice (Lane et al., 1991, 1992; Lenzo et al., 2002). Moreover, when genetically susceptible A/J mice are treated with agents that block IL-1 or TNF, they fail to develop myocarditis induced by cardiac myosin (Neumann et al., 1993). From this series of experiments, we conclude that inflammatory mediators are critical for the development of a pathogenic autoimmune response following viral infection. The production of key cytokines following infection may vary depending on the virus, the mouse strain, the conditions surrounding the infectious process, or the interplay of these and other genetic and environmental factors.

3.1 Viral Mouse Model

Infection of BALB/c mice with CVB3 results in the development of acute myocarditis from day 7–14 after infection (Fig. 1.1). During this time, infectious virus can be detected in the heart, but does not correlate with the level of inflammation (Fairweather et al., 2003). The inflammatory infiltrate in CVB3 infection is comprised predominantly of macrophages, natural killer (NK) cells, $CD8^+$ T cells, and $CD4^+$ T cells, B cells and neutrophils (Godeny and Gauntt, 1986, 1987a,b; Henke et al., 1995; Fairweather et al., 2001). The inflammation in the heart subsides by day 21 after infection, when heart sections look relatively normal under the microscope. In BALB/c mice, the chronic, autoimmune stage of the disease emerges around day 28 after infection and can be detected at least until day 56 (Fairweather et al., 2001). Acute myocarditis following viral infection is characterized by a focal, mixed cellular infiltrate but very little necrosis or fibrosis, in contrast to the autoimmune chronic phase where a diffuse lymphocytic infiltrate is associated with large regions of fibrosis and necrosis that may be followed by the development of DC (Fig. 1.1).

It is important to note that many of the studies of virally induced myocarditis used high doses of virus that resulted in death during the acute phase of myocarditis (Huber, 1997; Horwitz et al., 2000; Fong, 2003). In these models, necrosis of myocytes and fibrosis can be observed during acute myocarditis with few animals surviving to the chronic phase. In contrast, a low dose of virus results in virtually no deaths, allowing 100% of mice to survive to develop chronic myocarditis and DC (Fairweather et al., 2001). Since young adults rarely die from acute Coxsackievirus infections (Schoen, 1999), we feel that the low-dose model more closely resembles the disease as it occurs in human populations. Interestingly, inoculation of higher doses of CVB3 actually results in lower levels of inflammation in the heart than inoculation of low doses (D. Fairweather, unpublished observations).

A study investigating the global expression profile of proinflammatory genes induced by acute and persistent CVB3 infection in human fibroblast cell cultures found the rapid induction of a typical spectrum of various inflammation-related genes including IL-1β, IL-6, IL-8, and a number of metalloproteases (MMP-1, MMP-3, and MMP-15), thus suggesting that IL-1 plays an essential autocrine role. Neutralization experiments confirmed that IL-1α and IL-1β were key factors for the induction of inflammation-related genes during CVB3 infection (Rehren et al., 2013).

Baldeviano et al. showed that the immunization of mice with myocarditogenic peptide in complete Freund adjuvant induced the infiltration of IL-17A–producing Th17 cells into the inflamed heart. However, the incidence and severity of myocarditis was similar in the IL-17A–deficient and wild-type mice (Baldeviano et al., 2010).

Treatment of BALB/c mice with anti-IL-17A monoclonal antibody administered after the onset of myocarditis abrogates myocarditis-induced cardiac fibrosis and preserves ventricular function (Baldeviano et al., 2010).

Further, IL-17A deficiency does not improve the myocarditis of interferon (IFN)-gamma–deficient mice, thus showing that IL-17A plays a minimal role during acute myocarditis. On the other hand, IL-17A–deficient mice are associated with reduced interstitial myocardial fibrosis and the absence of the development of post-myocarditis remodeling and progression to dilated cardiomyopathy (Baldeviano et al., 2010).

The use of a recent experimental autoimmune myocarditis (EAM) mouse model has shown that IL-17 promotes B cell autophagy and facilitates myocarditis severity (Yuan et al., 2014).

Savvatis et al. have recently investigated whether treatment with anti-IL-6 receptor antibody improves cardiac dysfunction and left ventricular (LV) remodeling in experimental CVB3-induced myocarditis. IL-6 receptor blockade shifted the immune response in a Th1 direction and significantly reduced viral load (Savvatis et al., 2014).

Recent evidence has shown that IL-17 contributes to cardiac fibrosis following experimental autoimmune myocarditis by means of a PKCβ/Erk1/2/NF-κB–dependent signaling pathway (Liu et al., 2012).

The increased frequency of IL-22–producing Th22 cells may play an important role in the pathogenesis of acute CVB3-induced mouse viral myocarditis, and IL-22 may act as a myocardium-protective cytokine via the IL-22-IL-22R pathway (Kong et al., 2012).

IL-35 is a member of the IL-12 cytokine family that plays a suppressive and antiinflammatory role in autoimmunity and the immune response to infectious agents (Hu et al., 2014). It also protects the myocardium from the pathogenesis of CVB3-induced viral myocarditis, possibly as a result of reduced Th17 production (Hu et al., 2014).

It has been shown that the autoreactive T-cell repertoire derived from mice infected with CVB3 includes frequent IL-17-producing cells capable of inducing myocarditis in naïve recipients. This demonstrates that CVB3 can primarily infect the heart, lead to autoreactive T cells, and contribute to cardiac pathology (Gangaplara et al., 2012).

3.2 Cardiac Myosin Mouse Model

Cardiac myosin is the major target of the autoimmune response in many cases of myocarditis in humans and mice (Neu et al., 1987; Caforio et al., 1996;

Wang et al., 1999; Lauer et al., 2000). Evidence that persistent viral infection is not required for the development of myocarditis comes from the demonstration that inoculation of BALB/c mice with cardiac myosin, emulsified in complete Freund adjuvant, induces an experimental autoimmune myocarditis (EAM) that closely resembles the myocarditis associated with CVB3 infection (Fig. 1.1) (Neu et al., 1987; Lawson et al., 1992; Rose, 1996). Twenty-one days after immunization, the disease is characterized by a predominantly mononuclear infiltration of the myocardium and some cardiomyocyte death and replacement fibrosis (Fig. 1.1). The myocardial infiltrate contains many macrophages, $CD4^+$ T cell and some $CD8^+$ T cells, and $B220^+$ B cells (Pummerer et al., 1991; Wang et al., 1999). Among the infiltrating cells are eosinophils and occasional giant cells, both of which are more prominent in severe myocarditis as often occurs in highly susceptible A/J mice (Afanasyeva et al., 2001a). At later time points, inflammation recedes and myocardial fibrosis becomes the hallmark of disease, similar to the late chronic phase of myocarditis after viral infection (Fig. 1.1). Extensive myocardial damage eventually leads to the development of DC and congestive heart failure (Afanasyeva and Rose, 2002).

After the injection of cardiac myosin peptide emulsified in complete Freund adjuvant, IL-6 plays a key role in EAM pathogenesis (Eriksson et al., 2003).

IL-6−deficient mice show a reduction in innate and adaptive immune responses including the expression of adhesion molecules, inflammatory responses, and autoantibody levels, and the expansion of autoimmune $CD4^+$ T cells, possibly due to the upregulation of complement C3 (Eriksson et al., 2003).

There are increasing data concerning the role of antagonists of P2X7 receptors (which are involved in the pathophysiology of cardiovascular inflammation) in suppressing the development of EAM (Zempo et al., 2015). In a recent study in which mice with experimental autoimmune myocarditis were treated with the P2X7 receptor antagonist A740003 ($n = 10$) or not ($n = 11$), the hearts harvested on day 21 showed that the antagonist improved myocardial contraction by suppressing the infiltration of $CD4^+$ T cells and macrophages. Further, the mRNA expression of IL-1 β, the P2X7 receptor, and NADPH oxidase 2/4 was lower in the heart of the P2X7 receptor antagonist-treated group (Zempo et al., 2015).

3.3 Role of Cells

Myocarditis may be the result of myocardial infection (i.e., *Trypanosoma cruzii* or Coxsackievirus) or sterile inflammation induced by various causes (cardiac surgery, allergic reactions, excessive stress) in a genetically predisposed subject. In both situations, microbial or endogenous products may trigger the immune response.

Both cellular and humoral autoimmunity are involved in the pathogenesis of CVB3-induced myocarditis in susceptible mice, but distinct pathogenic mechanisms may function in different strains of mice. For example, CBV3 infection in DBA/2 mice has an exclusively humoral pathogenesis, whereas BALB/c mice develop primarily cell-mediated disease, and the pathogenesis of disease in A/J mice involves both autoimmune T cells and autoantibodies (Huber and Lodge, 1986; Lodge et al., 1987).

Various cell populations belonging to the immune system or of cardiac origin are presumably involved in the pathogenesis of myocardial inflammation. Both may have proinflammatory or antiinflammatory properties, and cells belonging to the immune system can give rise to innate and adaptive responses.

The innate immune response to pathogens has recently aroused considerable interest. It used to be thought that innate immunity only provides rapid (but incomplete) antimicrobial host defense before the development of the slower, more definite acquired immune response (Fearon and Lockley, 1996; Parish and O'Neill, 1997; Hoffmann et al., 1999), but recent research indicates that innate immunity critically affects the subsequent development of the adaptive immune response and autoimmunity (Carroll and Prodeus, 1998; Seder and Gazzinelli, 1999; Kadowski et al., 2000; Kaya et al., 2001). How innate immunity controls the initiation of an adaptive response and the development of autoimmune disease is not clear, but is likely to involve the innate immune cell release of proinflammatory cytokines.

Innate responses involve neutrophils, macrophages, monocytes, and innate lymphoid cells.

Neutrophils are the first cells recruited in the case of cardiac injury. During myocardiocyte necrosis, mitochondrial DNA and formylated peptides, which have a similar molecular structure to that of bacterial products, may attract and activate neutrophils by interacting with toll-like receptors (TLRs) or formyl-peptide receptor-1, and the release of cytokines such as IL-1, IL-6, and TNFα further promotes the recruitment of neutrophils at the site of injury. IL-6 may be released by injured cardiomyocytes, monocytes, macrophages and, in an autocrine manner, by neutrophils themselves. IL-17, another cytokine that strongly recruits and activates neutrophils, is produced by mononuclear cells and its production decreases following neutrophil apoptosis, thus establishing negative feedback. Neutrophils sustain inflammation by secreting proteases and reactive oxygen species.

Monocytes and resident macrophages may also contribute to inflammation and tissue repair. Circulating monocytes are induced to adhere to cardiac vessels in order to reach the damaged tissues. Different pools of circulating monocytes may account for different pathogenic roles mouse models: e.g., Ly6c^{Hi} monocytes are recruited in the case of ischemic or hypertensive cardiac damage, whereas Ly6c^{Low} monocytes are not (Epelman et al., 2015).

Resident macrophages can be divided into three subsets on the basis of the expression of major histocompatibility class II and C–C chemokine receptor 2 markers (CCR2). The pool of $CCR2^+$ macrophages, which are mainly derived from circulating monocytes, expands after an inflammatory stimulus, and may activate the NLPR3 inflammasome pathway in response to ischemic, hypertrophic, or hypertensive diseases, thus generating large amounts of IL-1. Conversely, CCR2-resident macrophages are indispensable for myocardial tissue remodeling, scar healing, and repair. Macrophages are also involved in the phagocytosis of apoptotic cells, including neutrophils, and impaired clearance (possibly due to local inflammation and an imbalance of regulatory and proinflammatory cytokines) may amplify the inflammatory burden.

Cells belonging to the innate immune response, may recognize microbial and endogenous peptides [pathogen-associated molecular patterns and damage-associated molecular patterns (DAMPs)] via the TLR pathway, and generate a cascade of intracellular signals culminating in the nuclear translocation of NFkB and the final transcription of various genes coding for the cytokines and other molecules involved in the inflammatory response. MyD88 or IL-1 receptor–associated kinase 4 (IRAK4) knock-out mice infected with CVB3 show a more favorable disease course related to the reduced nuclear translocation of NFkB and the higher production of protective type I interferons.

NK lymphocytes anticipate the adaptive response by secreting large amounts of IFNγ after encountering the antigen. A recent study of murine EAM has shown that NK lymphocytes may prevent the infiltration of the eosinophils finally responsible for myocardium fibrosis directly (by inducing apoptosis) or indirectly by inhibiting the release of chemokines (Ong et al., 2015).

NK cells are an important first line of defense against viral infections as they efficiently limit the replication of CVB3 and MCMV (Godeny and Gauntt, 1987a; Bancroft, 1993; Tay et al., 1998). When antigen-presenting cells detect a viral infection of host tissue, they release cytokines and chemokines that attract NK cells to the site of infection. The ability of NK cells to produce IFNγ rapidly after infiltrating infected tissues and before the clonal expansion of T cells is critical for an effective innate immune response (Fairweather and Rose, 2002). Depleting NK cells by means of anti-asialo GM_1 (a pan-NK marker) increases myocarditis in outbred CD-1 mice with CVB3 infection (Godeny and Gauntt, 1986), thus suggesting that NK cells primarily protect against myocarditis by inhibiting viral replication. In order to examine the role of NK cells in the development of acute MCMV-induced myocarditis, $NK1.1^+$ cells have been depleted from normal C57BL/6 or BALB.B6-Cmv1^r mice using antibodies against NK1.1 (Table 1.2) (Fairweather et al., 2001). BALB.B6-Cmv1^r is a congenic mouse strain that carries the NK cell gene complex found in B10 mice (i.e., NK1.1) on a BALB/c genetic background (Scalzo et al., 1995). As BALB/c mice do not have NK1.1 cells, they primarily clear MCMV infection by means of the cytolytic activity of $CD8^+$ T cells (Lathbury et al., 1996). Depleting $NK1.1^+$ cells from C57BL/

TABLE 1.2 Role of Immune Cells in Murine Cytomegalovirus-Induced Myocarditis

Genetic Background[a]	Depletion[b]	Myocarditis	p
BALB/c (no NK1.1)	Control	24±	
	Anti-NK1.1	15±	<0.05
	Anti-CD4	14±	<0.05
	Anti-CD8	7±	<0.01
	Anti-CD4/8	5±	<0.01
BALB.B6 congenic (BALB/c $^+$ NK1.1)	Control	5±	
	Anti-NK1.1	23±	<0.01
C57BL/6 (NK1.1)	Control	5±	
	Anti-NK1.1	19±	<0.01

[a]*BALB/c (do not have NK1.1$^+$ cells), BALB.B6-^{r}Cmv1 (BALB.B6 congenic) (have NK1.1$^+$ cells on a BALB/c genetic background), and C57BL/6 mice (have NK1.1$^+$ cells on a C57BL/6 genetic background) were infected with MCMV intraperitoneally.*
[b]*Mice were also treated with antibodies that deplete NK1.1$^+$ cells, CD4$^+$ T cells, CD8$^+$ T cells, both CD4$^+$ and CD8$^+$ T cells, or saline control. Successful cell depletions were confirmed by FACS analysis (data not shown).*
Modified from Fairweather, D., Kaya, Z., Shellam G.R., 2001. From infection to autoimmunity. J. Autoimmun. 16, 175.

6 or BALB.B6-Cmv1^r mice significantly increases myocarditis to levels found in BALB/c control mice (Table 1.2). The role of NK cells in NK1.1$^-$ BALB/c mice is not yet clear, but these findings indicate that the protection mediated by NK cells during acute myocarditis is more important in reducing myocarditis than other traits in the BALB/c genetic background as the only difference between congenic and regular BALB/c mice is the NK-cell gene complex.

Cells belonging to the adaptive immune system include dendritic cells and T and B lymphocytes. Dendritic cells (DCs) can recognize antigenic peptides and present them to T lymphocytes, thus further guiding their differentiation. In response to different TLR stimulation, these cells may secrete IL-23, IL-12, or IL-4, thus promoting the differentiation of autoreactive T helper cells. On the contrary, following other specific molecular pathways such as the production of nitric oxide, DCs may counteract the expansion of T effector cells and favor the expansion of the T regulatory pool (Kania et al., 2013). The survival and activation of DCs seem to be related to a paracrine loop that intertwines these cells with cardiac fibroblasts.

The involvement of autoimmune T cells in the pathogenesis of CVB3-induced myocarditis was first inferred from the observation that T-cell depleted mice have less severe disease than normal mice (Woodruff and

Woodruff, 1974). It has been shown that T cells play a decisive role in disease pathogenesis in models of both CVB3- and MCMV-induced myocarditis (Lawson et al., 1989; Schwimmbeck et al., 1997). Athymic nude mice also develop less severe disease after CBV3 or MCMV infection (Hashimoto and Komatsu, 1978; Lawson et al., 1989). Furthermore, myocarditis can be transferred by inoculating autoimmune $CD4^+$ T cells from virally infected mice to uninfected recipients (Guthrie et al., 1984; Huber, 1997). The infection of mice depleted of T cell subsets or genetically altered to the same effect leads to less severe myocarditis (Henke et al., 1995; Schwimmbeck et al., 1997; Fairweather et al., 2001). Table 1.2 shows the important role T cells (particularly $CD8^+$ T cells) play in the development of acute MCMV-induced myocarditis in BALB/c mice (Fairweather et al., 2001). Although depleting $CD4^+$ T cells from MCMV-infected BALB/c mice reduces myocardial inflammation, the reduction is far more dramatic if $CD8^+$ T cells are removed, alone or together with $CD4^+$ T cells. Furthermore, acute myocarditis is more severe in CD4 C57BL/6 knockout (KO) mice ($CD4^+$ T cells are absent due to gene deletion) following CVB3 infection (Henke et al., 1995). These studies confirm that the development of myocarditis, although requiring a virus to initiate the process, also needs components of adaptive immunity for disease progression.

Autoreactive T cells and autoantibodies are also present in myosin-induced EAM (Neu and Ploier, 1991; Pummerer et al., 1995). T cells are necessary for the development of disease in this model, with myosin-stimulated T cells capable of transferring myocarditis into immunodeficient severe combined immunodeficient mice (Smith and Allen, 1991, 1993; Pummerer et al., 1995). Depleting $CD4^+$ or $CD8^+$ T cells in myosin-immunized susceptible mice diminishes myocarditis, thus suggesting that both cell types are important in the pathogenesis of EAM, as well as virally induced models (Pummerer et al., 1991; Smith and Allen, 1991, 1993; Penninger et al., 1993). However, CD4 KO mice have reduced inflammation, but myocarditis is exacerbated in immunized CD8 KO mice (Penninger et al., 1993; Pummerer et al., 1995), which indicates that $CD8^+$ T cells sometimes suppress the disease in this model. $CD4^+$ T cells are involved in the pathogenesis of EAM as they recognize the antigens presented by MHC class II (Smith and Allen, 1992a; Donermeyer et al., 1995), which may be important regulatory molecules for the induction of autoimmunity (Todd et al., 1988; Nepom, 1993). An understanding of the cell mechanisms driving the autoimmune response in EAM may help to distinguish the role of the cellular response to viral infection from that directed against cardiac myosin.

$CD4^+$ T helper lymphocytes may differentiate into various subsets depending on the cytokine milieu. Th1 lymphocytes are the main producers of IFNγ and IL-2. IFNγ activates macrophages by increasing the expression of MCP-1 (the data concerning fibroblast activation are uncertain), whereas Th2 cells mainly producing IL-4, IL-5, and IL-13 are responsible for the phenotypic transition of fibroblasts into myofibroblasts and the inhibition of extracellular matrix degradation.

By secreting IL-17, Th17 lymphocytes induce the downstream production of IL-1, IL-6, TNFα, chemokines, and granulocyte colony-stimulating factors, which have multiple effects on the inflammatory cascade. Th17 lymphocytes induce the production of autoantibodies and may simultaneously favor and inhibit heart fibrosis (Machino-Ohtsuka et al., 2014), whereas recent studies have highlighted the protective role of Th22 lymphocytes in both infective and autoimmune myocarditis (Amoah et al., 2015). Similarly, T regulatory cells have antiinflammatory and antifibrotic effects by secreting IL-10. It has been reported that a genetically determined imbalance between Th17/Th1 and T regulatory lymphocytes is related to a higher risk of developing autoimmune myocarditis in mice models (Chen et al., 2012).

Cardiac remodeling is the final step of the inflammatory process occurring during myocarditis and may lead to dilated cardiomyopathy. This is due to a complex interplay between innate and adaptive immune cells, cardiac cells, and fibroblasts. Cardiac fibroblasts are responsible for the homeostasis of the extracellular matrix (ECM) and also preside over mechanical and electrical functioning. They represent 60–70% of all cardiac cells and may arise from a local embryonic pool, or endothelial, or bone marrow cells recruited under inflammatory conditions. Cardiac fibroblasts may change from a contractile α-smooth muscle actin to an active-secreting phenotype. In addition to producing collagen and other components of the ECM, they may also synthesize and respond to many cytokines, hormones, and growth factors. TLRs are found on cardiac fibroblasts and may induce the deposition of collagen types I and III, thus leading to cardiac fibrosis. The production of the ECM is controlled by macrophages through the release of metalloproteases and tissue growth factor-β (TGFβ), which respectively have antifibrotic and profibrotic effects.

In conclusion, the cell network of myocarditis embraces a wide spectrum of effectors, ranging from professional cells belonging to the immune system to resident stromal cells. The cytokine *milieu les* at the basis of cell differentiation and activation and may favor or antagonize the inflammatory cascade.

3.4 Role of Cytokines

Many of the mediators associated with the innate immune response, particularly cytokines, can act in a long-range endocrine manner so that antigen-presenting cells far removed from the site of infection are activated to present either viral or autoantigens to T and B cells (Parish and O'Neill, 1997; Carnaud et al., 1999; Kadowski et al., 2000). Moreover, recent evidence suggests that a bidirectional relationship exists between innate and adaptive immunity (Rose, 2011).

IFN-α production following viral infection stimulates an effective NK cell response. The type 1 IFNs belong to a multigene family that include multiple IFN-α subtypes and IFN-β (Bellardelli, 1995). IFNs also provide an important link between the innate and adaptive immune responses (Kadowski et al., 2000). Previous studies have shown that administration of IFN-α subtypes or IFN-β to MCMV-infected BALB/c mice not only reduces viral replication, but also decreases acute and chronic myocarditis (Table 1.3) (Lawson et al., 1997; Yeow et al., 1998; Fairweather et al., 2001). These results emphasize the role of innate cytokines in modulating the adaptive immune response and autoimmune disease.

As pointed out previously, cytokines can determine whether mice develop autoimmune myocarditis. For example, administration of IL-1 or IL-2 augments disease in CVB3-infected susceptible mice (Table 1.3) (Huber et al., 1994), while blocking these receptors inhibits the development of myocarditis (Neumann et al., 1993). On the other hand, C57BL/6 mice, which are resistant to the development of chronic myocarditis following CVB3 or MCMV infection, can be induced to develop chronic myocarditis by administration of LPS (a generator of several proinflammatory cytokines), IL-1β, or TNF-α with the virus (Table 1.3) (Lane et al., 1991, 1992; Lenzo et al., 2001). Cytokines may play a number of different roles. They may provide second signals after viral infection that stimulates an effective protective immune response or a deleterious response in individuals susceptible to autoimmune disease (Fairweather et al., 2001). Thus, certain cytokines can influence whether chronic autoimmune disease develops in response to viral infection, bridging the gap between the innate and adaptive immune response.

LPS and TNF-α are also important in the development of cardiac myosin-induced myocarditis. Neutralization of TNF-α effectively inhibits the initiation of EAM, although neutralization is not beneficial in suppressing ongoing disease (Table 1.4) (Smith and Allen, 1992b). TNF-α is believed to be necessary for upregulating MHC class II binding of self-reactive peptides on antigen-presenting cells in EAM, since upregulation of MHC and accessory molecules fails to occur in TNF-deficient mice (Smith and Allen, 1992a). Furthermore, myocarditis can be transferred by injection of cardiac myosin-specific T cells into mice pretreated with LPS or TNF-α (Penninger et al., 1997). Thus, the primary role of virus or adjuvant, in the EAM model, may be to provide an optimal cytokine environment (i.e., increased IL-1β and TNF-α) in the context of self-antigen thereby allowing an autoimmune response to occur.

According to the current dogma, inflammatory autoimmune diseases are primarily attributable to Th1 responses, of which IFN-γ is the prototypic cytokine, while Th2 responses, where IL-4 predominates, should reduce autoimmunity (Cunningham, 2001). Th1-mediated immune responses have been implicated in the pathogenesis of a number of autoimmune diseases including inflammatory bowel disease, type I diabetes, multiple sclerosis, and

TABLE 1.3 Role of Cytokines and Cytokine Signaling in Virus-Induced Myocarditis

Cytokine	Method Studied[a]	Effect on Myocarditis	References
Promotes Myocarditis			
LPS	CB3 + LPS (using BL/6 mice)	Develop chronic myocarditis by increasing IL-I and TNF	Lane et al. (1991), Lenzo et al. (2001)
TLR4	TLR4 KO	Reduces myocarditis, IL-1, and IL-18	Fairweather et al. (2003)
TNF-α	CB3 + TNF-α (using BL/6 mice)	Develop chronic myocarditis	Lane et al. (1992), Lenzo et al. (2001)
IL- 1β	CB3	IL-1 levels correlate with increased myocarditis	Fairweather et al. (2003)
	IL-1 administration	Increases myocarditis	Huber et al. (1994)
	CB3 + IL- 1β (using BL/6 mice)	Develop chronic myocarditis	Lane et al. (1992)
IL-12Rβ1	IL-12Rβ1 KO (signaling for IL-12p70 and IL-23)	Decreases myocarditis, IL-1, and IL-18	Fairweather et al. (2003)
IL- 18	CB3	IL-18 levels correlate with increased myocarditis	Fairweather et al. (2003)
Reduces Myocarditis			
IFN-α	IFN-α administration	Decreases viral replication	Fairweather et al. (2001)
IL-12p35	IL-12p35 KO (effect of IL-12p70)	Decreases viral replication, no effect on acute myocarditis	Unpublished
IL-12p40	IL-12p40 KO (effect of IL-12p70, $p40_2$, IL-23)	Increases acute myocarditis, IL-1, and IL-18	Unpublished
STAT4	STAT4 KO	Decreases viral replication, no effect on myocarditis	Unpublished

Continued

TABLE 1.3 Role of Cytokines and Cytokine Signaling in Virus-Induced Myocarditis—cont'd

Cytokine	Method Studied[a]	Effect on Myocarditis	References
IFN-γ	IFN-γ KO	Decreases viral replication, increases chronic myocarditis, fibrosis, and DC	Unpublished
IL-4	IL-4 KO	Increases myocarditis	Unpublished
STAT6	STAT6 KO	Increases myocarditis	Unpublished

BL/6, C57BL/6; *CB3*, Coxsackievirus B3; *DC*, dilated cardiomyopathy; *IFN-α/γ*, interferon-α/γ; *IL*, interleukin; *KO*, knockout; *LPS*, lipopolysaccharide; *p40₂*, p40 homodimer*R*, receptor; *STAT*, signal transducer and activator of transcription; *TLR4*, toll-like receptor 4; *TNF*, tumor necrosis factor.
[a]*BALB/c mice are used unless otherwise stated.*

TABLE 1.4 Role of Cytokines and Cytokine Signaling in Cardiac Myosin-Induced Myocarditis

Cytokine	Method Studied[a]	Effect on Myocarditis	References
Promotes Myocarditis			
TNF-α	Blocking Ab	Prevents EAM	Smith and Allen (1992a,b)
TNFRp55	TNFRp55 KO	Reduces EAM	Bachmaier et al. (1997)
IL-12p40	IL-12p40 KO (effect of IL-12p70, $p40_2$, IL-23)	Reduces EAM	Eriksson et al. (200la,b)
IL-12p70	IL-12p70 administration	Exacerbates EAM	Afanasyeva et al. (2001b)
IL-l2Rβ1	IL-12Rβ1 KO (signaling for IL-12p70 and IL-23)	Prevents EAM	Afanasyeva et al. (2001b)
STAT4	STAT4 KO	Reduces EAM	Afanasyeva et al. (2001b)
IL-4	Blocking Ab	Reduces EAM	Afanasyeva et al. (2001a)
Reduces Myocarditis			
IFN-γ	Blocking Ab	Increases EAM and DC	Afanasyeva et al. (2001a,b)
	IFN-γ KO	Increases EAM and DC	Afanasyeva et al. (2001b), Eriksson et al. (2001a), Kurrer et al. (2002)
IFN-γ R	IFN-γ R KO	Increases EAM and DC	Eriksson et al. (2001b)
IL-10	Blocking Ab	Increases EAM	Kaya et al. (2002)

Ab, Antibody; *EAM*, experimental autoimmune myocarditis; *IFN-α/γ*, interferon-α/γ, *BL/6*, C57BL/6; *IL*, interleukin; *KO*, knockout; *$p40_2$*, p40 homodimer; *R*, receptor; *STAT*, signal transducer and activator of transcription; *TNF*, tumor necrosis factor.
[a]*Using A/J or BALB/c mouse strains.*

rheumatoid arthritis (O'Garra, 1998). IFN-γ stimulates Th1-cell development, activates macrophages, induces MHC class I and II expression, promotes delayed-type hypersensitivity reactions, induces certain immunoglobulin class switching, recruits Th1 cells to the site of inflammation, and is important for clearing intracellular bacteria, parasites, and viral infections (Boehm et al., 1997). IL-4, on the other hand, stimulates Th2-cell development, activates B cells, induces MHC class II expression on B cells, promotes allergic reactions, induces immunoglobulin class switching to immunoglobulin (Ig) G1 and IgE, recruits eosinophils and Th2 cells to the site of inflammation, and is important for clearing parasites (Nelms et al., 1999). Thus, determining whether a predominantly Th1 or Th2 immune response occurs to virus or cardiac myosin immunization may promote understanding the pathogenesis of autoimmune heart disease.

It has been demonstrated that CD4($^{+}$) Th17 cells and Th17-produced cytokines play a critical role in inflammation-induced cardiac remodeling and the progression to dilated cardiomyopathy. It has been hypothesized that blocking IL-17A may be therapeutic option for inflammatory cardiomyopathy (Baldeviano et al., 2010; Myers et al., 2016) as it plays a key role in the myocardial upregulation of IL-6, TNFα, and IL-1β, and the recruitment of CD11b($^{+}$) monocytes and Gr1($^{+}$) granulocytes in the heart (Baldeviano et al., 2010). Furthermore, it has been found that IL-17A can induce cardiomyocyte apoptosis through the p38 mitogen-activated protein kinase (MAPK)-p53-Bax signaling pathway, and promotes both early- and late-phase post-myocardial infarction (MI) ventricular remodeling (Zhou et al., 2014).

It has also been shown that a Th17-cell immunophenotype is linked with the effects of cardiac myosin, which acts as an autoantigen arising from damaged myocardiocytes on CD14($^{+}$) monocytes and TLR2 and heart failure.

High levels of IL-17—producing T cells and IL-17—promoting cytokines cells are associated with persistent heart failure, and it has been shown that the myocarditis/dilated cardiomyopathy phenotype contains low percentages of FOXP3($^{+}$) Tregs that contribute to disease severity. TLR2 peptide ligands from human cardiac myosin can stimulate exaggerated Th17-related cytokines such as TGFβ, IL-6, and IL-23 from myocarditic CD14($^{+}$) monocytes in vitro (Myers et al., 2016).

It has been reported that the myeloid differentiation factor (MyD)88/IL-1 axis in the bone marrow compartment plays a critical role in post-inflammatory cardiac fibrosis and heart failure (Blyszczuk et al , 2009).

IL-12 is produced by phagocytic and antigen-presenting cells. Produced during the early phase of an infection, IL-12 promotes the differentiation of T cells to a Th1 phenotype with IFN-γ production, which in turn supports cell-mediated immunity, cytotoxic T-cell generation, activation of phagocytic cells, and eventual eradication of intracellular pathogens (Ma and Trinchieri, 2001). IL-12 is a heterodimer composed of IL-12p35 and IL-12p40 subunits bound via disulfide bonds and secreted as a biologically active IL-12p70 molecule.

IL-12 receptors (R) are primarily expressed on activated NK and T cells, and signaling requires coexpression of the IL-12Rβ1 and IL-12R β2 chains for the generation of high-affinity IL-12p70 binding and maximal IFN-γ production. In the mouse, IL-12R signaling activates the signal transducer and activator of transcription (STAT)1, STAT3, and STAT4, with STAT4 being responsible for most of the biological activities of IL-12 through the production of IFN-γ (O'Garra, 1998; Moser and Murphy, 2000). IL-12p40 is also produced as a monomer and homodimer ($p40_2$) in great excess over IL-12p70. The IL-12p40 homodimer has been found to antagonize IL-12p70 activity by competitively binding the IL-12R (Mattner et al., 1993).

IL-18 has emerged as an important cytokine along with IL-12 for increasing IFN-γ production from immune cells. The synergistic effect is mediated through the induction of IL-18R-α by IL-12 and the upregulation of IL-12Rβ2 by IL-18 on naï ve T cells (Yoshimoto et al., 1998). In contrast, NK cells constitutively express IL-18R and IL-12R β2 and are able to immediately respond to these cytokines (Nakanishi et al., 2001). The IL-18R has been identified as a member of the IL-1R/TLR superfamily and shares a common signal transduction pathway with IL-1R (O'Neill and Dinarello, 2000). Importantly, IL-18 can also stimulate IFN-γ production through STAT-independent pathways (O'Neill and Dinarello, 2000; Nakanishi et al., 2001). IL-18 is produced by a wide range of immune and nonimmune cells as a biologically inactive precursor that is activated in the same manner as IL-1 by cleavage with caspase-1. Likewise, caspase-1 undergoes proteolytic cleavage to produce its active form after stimulation through TLR4 (Akira et al., 2001). Respiratory syncytial virus was discovered to be a ligand for TLR4, along with LPS, suggesting that activation of TLR may be involved in protecting the host from viral infections (Kurt-Jones et al., 2000).

It has also been shown that the DAMPs released by necrotic myocardial cells induce fibroblast activation in vitro and myocardial inflammation and fibrosis in vivo, at least partially as a result of TLR4-dependent signaling (Zhang et al., 2015).

How MI induces the initiating mechanisms of the sterile inflammatory response that contributes to adverse cardiac remodeling is still unknown, but Lugrin et al. have recently found that necrotic cardiomyocytes release a heat-labile proinflammatory signal by activating MAPKs and NF-κB in cardiac fibroblasts, with the secondary production of cytokines. This response was abolished in Myd88(−/−) fibroblasts but was unaffected in NLRP3-deficient fibroblasts, thus showing that IL-1α is a crucial early danger signal triggering post-MI inflammation (Lugrin et al., 2015).

Recently, we examined the role of IL-12—induced IFN-γ on the development of CVB3-induced myocarditis using mice deficient in IL-12p35 (lacking IL-12p70), IL-12p40 (lacking IL-12p70, IL-23, and $p40_2$), IL-12Rβ1 (lacking signaling induced by IL-12p70 and IL-23), STAT4, IFN-γ, or TLR4 (Fairweather et al., 2003). We found that decreased levels of IL-1β and

IL-18 in the heart following CVB3 infection of IL-12Rβ1 or TLR4-deficient mice was directly associated with decreased myocardial inflammation (Table 1.3). Unexpectedly, deficiency of either of these two receptors also decreased viral replication in the heart. These results suggest that IL-12Rβ1 and TLR4 share common downstream pathways that directly influence IL-1β and IL-18 production and viral replication. Examination of IL-12p35 (IL-12p70), IFN-γ, or STAT4-deficient mice confirmed that IFN-γ protects against viral replication in the heart but did not affect acute myocardial inflammation, indicating that the role of the IL-12R in exacerbating acute myocarditis is not via IFN-γ production (Table 1.3) (D. Fairweather, unpublished results). Furthermore, we found evidence that IL-12p40 (probably the p40 homodimer) protects against acute CVB3 myocarditis by reducing the level of IL-1β and IL-18 in the heart. In contrast, IL-12p70 facilitates viral clearance by increasing IFN-γ levels.

IRAK4, a major nodal signal transducer in innate immunity, exacerbates viral myocarditis by inhibiting interferon production and reducing the mobilization of protective CCR5($^+$) monocytes/macrophages to the heart (Valaperti et al., 2013).

A good candidate to explain the increased production of IL-1β and IL-18, and the myocardial inflammation observed in wild-type BALB/c mice following CVB3 infection is IL-23, which has been shown to be released following viral infection (Oppmann et al., 2000; Pirhonen et al., 2002). IL-23 is a heterodimer composed of IL-12p40 and a p19 subunit. The IL-12p40 subunit binds to IL-12Rβ1 and the p19 subunit binds to a recently identified IL-23R (Parham et al., 2002). Although IL-23 can activate STAT4, STAT3 is believed to be the primary transcription factor activated following IL-23R ligation (Parham et al., 2002; Lankford and Frucht, 2003). Interestingly, transgenic mice that ubiquitously express the p19 subunit of IL-23 develop severe multiorgan inflammation and elevated levels of TNF-α and IL-1 (Wiekowski et al., 2001). Recently, IL-23, rather than IL-12p70, was discovered to be primarily responsible for exacerbating EAE (Cua et al., 2003; Zhang et al., 2003); IL-12p70 has been considered the key cytokine mediating EAE and many other autoimmune diseases (Caspi, 1998; Watford and O'Shea, 2003). Our findings corroborate and extend the studies by Cua et al. and Zhang et al. demonstrating that IL-12p70 is not responsible for increasing IL-1β/IL-18 levels or inflammation in the heart. However, IL-23 does not account for the increased inflammation and IL-1β/IL-18 levels in IL-12p40–deficient hearts since this cytokine is absent. In this case, signaling via TLR4, perhaps exacerbated by other molecules such as Epstein-Barr virus–induced gene 3 (EBI3)/IL-12p35, can lead to increased IL-1β/IL-18 levels and myocarditis (Fairweather et al., 2003).

In the EAM model, IL-12Rβ1–deficient mice do not develop myocarditis, suggesting a role for this receptor in increasing inflammation (Table 1.4) (Afanasyeva et al., 2001b). In the absence of IL-12Rβ1, IL-1β production from splenocyte cultures was also significantly reduced (Afanasyeva et al., 2001b), further suggesting an important role for this cytokine in the development of autoimmune heart disease. While STAT4 deficiency has no effect on inflammation in CVB3-induced myocarditis (Table 1.3), inflammation is reduced in STAT4–deficient mice in the EAM model. IL-23 is also a likely candidate for the increased disease that is mediated via IL-12Rβ1 and STAT4 in the EAM model. In contrast to CVB3-induced myocarditis, IL-12p40–deficient mice do not develop EAM (Eriksson et al., 2001a,b). It may be that IL-1β levels are regulated by different mechanisms in the EAM model.

In contrast to the role for IL-12Rβ1 and STAT4 in exacerbating EAM, IFN-γ plays a protective role in both EAM- and CVB3-induced myocarditis. Mice genetically deficient in either IFN-γ or IFN-γ R or mice treated with IFN-γ neutralizing antibody develop severe EAM with large, dilated hearts and some mice even developed congestive heart failure (Table 1.4) (Afanasyeva et al., 2001a,b; Eriksson et al., 2001b; Rose and Afanasyeva, 2003). The role for IFN-γ in mediating Th1-mediated autoimmune responses has been attributed to its ability to expand autoreactive $CD4^+$ T cells. However, the simplistic distinction between Th1 and Th2 responses and autoimmune disease requires reevaluation in light of these findings (Gor et al., 2003; Rose and Afanasyeva, 2003). The mechanisms whereby IFN-γ protects against EAM and the chronic phase of CVB3 myocarditis remain to be understood.

Conflicting data exist regarding the role of IL-4 and a Th2-mediated immune response in autoimmune myocarditis. Blocking IL-4 with neutralizing antibody reduces the severity of EAM (Table 1.4) and produces a shift from a Th2- to a Th1-like response indicated by increased IFN-γ and decreased IL-4, IL-5, and IL-13 production from splenocyte cultures (Afanasyeva et al., 2001a). However, IL-4 and IL-4 receptor KO mice are not protected from the development of EAM (Table 1.4) (Eriksson et al., 2001a; Kurrer et al., 2002). These contrasting findings may be due to the differential effect of antibody administration versus complete lack of the molecule and other factors such as the dose of cytokine, timing of administration, or difference in the strain of mice (A/J mice used in antibody blocking experiments versus genetically deficient BALB/c mice). Eosinophils and multinucleated giant cells are prominent in EAM (Afanasyeva et al., 2001a). Eosinophils are known to be associated with Th2 type cytokines such as IL-4, IL-5, IL-10, and IgE antibodies (Cunningham, 2001). Although IL-4 can also lead to the formation of multinucleated giant cells, these cells have long been associated with the granulomatous lesions formed in response to intracellular bacterial infections such as mycobacterium tuberculosis, which is a component of the adjuvant used in the EAM model (Cunningham, 2001). Thus it appears that components of both Th1 and Th2 responses contribute to severe autoimmune myocarditis. In CVB3-induced myocarditis, however, infection of IL-4 and STAT6 KO mice (STAT6 mediates signaling through the IL-4 receptor) results in increased acute and chronic myocarditis indicating a protective role for IL-4 in virally induced autoimmune myocarditis. These findings suggest that a delicate balance of key cytokines determines whether an autoimmune response occurs following viral infection or cardiac myosin and adjuvant inoculation (Fairweather et al., 2001; Rose and Afanasyeva, 2003). A better understanding of the individual cytokines involved in mediating the immune response, particularly the early innate response that determines the profile of key cytokines, will be necessary in order to develop therapies for human autoimmune heart disease.

3.5 Summary of Pathogenic Mechanisms

The development of autoimmune heart disease following viral infection involves the production of key cytokines by immune cells such as macrophages and NK cells. Activation of TLRs by virus (Fig. 1.2A) or the bacterial component of complete Freund adjuvant (Fig. 1.2B) leads to the production of

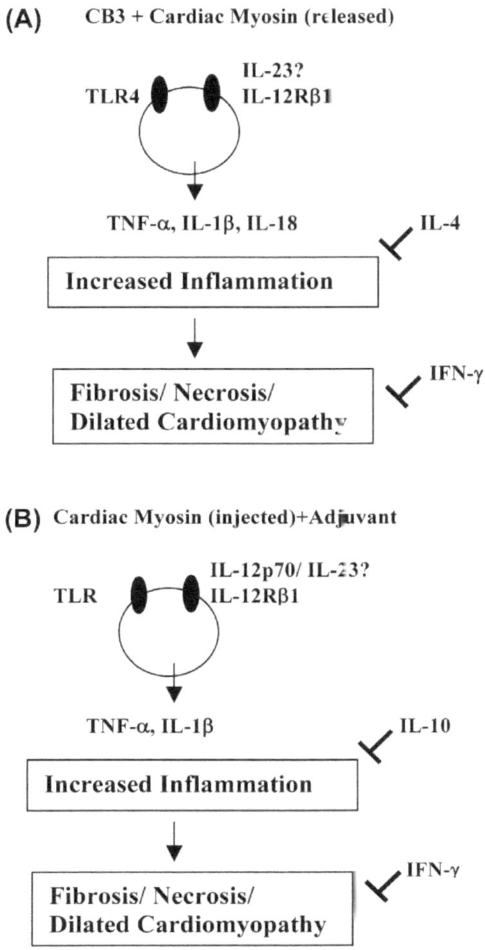

FIGURE 1.2 Activation of toll-like receptors by virus (A). The bacterial component of complete Freund's adjuvant (B).

IL-1β and TNF-α. Overproduction of these proinflammatory cytokines increases the inflammatory infiltrate in the heart. Regulatory cytokines such as IL-10, and possibly the IL-12p40 homodimer, decrease the severity of inflammation in the heart. However, if environmental or genetic factors allow overproduction of proinflammatory cytokines, then progression to chronic autoimmune myocarditis may follow.

REFERENCES

Afanasyeva, M., Rose, N.R., 2002. Immune mediators in inflammatory heart disease: insights from a mouse model. Eur. Heart J. Suppl. 4 (Suppl. I), I31.

Afanasyeva, M., Wang, Y., Kaya, Z., Park, S., Zilliox, M.J., Schofield, B.H., Hill, S.L., Rose, N.R., 2001a. Experimental autoimmune myocarditis in A/J mice is an interleukin-4-dependent disease with a Th2 phenotype. Am. J. Pathol. 159, 193.

Afanasyeva, M., Wang, Y., Kaya, Z., 2001b. Interleukin-12 receptor/STAT4 signaling is required for the development of autoimmune myocarditis in mice by an interferon-γ-independent pathway. Circulation 104, 3145.

Akira, S.A., Takeda, K., Kaisho, T., 2001. Toll-like receptors: critical proteins linking innate and acquired immunity. Nat. Immunol. 2, 675.

Amoah, B.P., Yang, H., Zhang, P., Su, Z., Xu, H., 2015. Immunopathogenesis of myocarditis: the interplay between cardiac fibroblast cells, dendritic cells, macrophages and $CD4^+$ T cells. Scand. J. Immunol. 82, 1–9.

Aretz, H.T., 1987. Myocarditis: the Dallas criteria. Hum. Pathol. 18, 619.

Bachmaier, K., Pummerer, C., Kozieradzki, I., 1997. Low-molecular-weight tumor necrosis factor receptor p55 controls induction of autoimmune heart disease. Circulation 95, 655.

Baldeviano, G.C., Barin, J.G., Talor, M.V., Srinivasan, S., Bedja, D., Zheng, D., Gabrielson, K., Iwakura, Y., Rose, N.R., Cihakova, D., 2010. Interleukin-17A is dispensable for myocarditis but essential for the progression to dilated cardiomyopathy. Circ. Res. 106, 1646–1655.

Bancroft, G.J., 1993. The role of natural killer cells in innate resistance to infection. Curr. Opin. Immunol. 5, 503.

Bellardelli, F., 1995. Role of interferons and other cytokines in the regulation of the immune response. APMIS 103, 161.

Blyszczuk, P., Kania, G., Dieterle, T., Marty, R.R., Valaperti, A., Berthonneche, C., Pedrazzini, T., Berger, C.T., Dirnhofer, S., Matter, C.M., Penninger, J.M., Lüscher, T.F., Eriksson, U., 2009. Myeloid differentiation factor-88/interleukin-1 signaling controls cardiac fibrosis and heart failure progression in inflammatory dilated cardiomyopathy. Circ. Res. 105, 912.

Boehm, U., Klamp, T., Groot, M., 1997. Cellular responses to interferon-γ. Annu. Rev. Immunol. 15, 749.

Caforio, A.L., Goldman, J.H., Haven, A.J., 1996. Evidence for autoimmunity to myosin and other heart-specific autoantigens in patients with dilated cardiomyopathy and their relatives. Int. J. Cardiol. 54, 157.

Carnaud, C., Lee, D., Donnars, O., 1999. Cutting edge: cross-talk between cells of the innate immune system: NKT cells rapidly activate NK cells. J. Immunol. 163, 4647.

Carroll, M.C., Prodeus, A.P., 1998. Linkages of innate and adaptive immunity. Curr. Opin. Immunol. 10, 36.

Caspi, R.R., 1998. IL-12 in autoimmunity. Clin. Immunol. Immunopathol. 88, 4.

Chen, P., Baldeviano, G.C., Ligons, D.L., Talor, M.V., Barin, J.G., Rose, N.R., Cihakova, D., 2012. Susceptibility to autoimmune myocarditis is associated with intrinsic differences in CD4($^{+}$) T cells. Clin. Exp. Immunol. 169, 79–88.
Cua, D.J., Sherlock, J., Chen, Y., 2003. Interleukin-23 rather than interleukin-12 is the critical cytokine for autoimmune inflammation of the brain. Nature 421, 744.
Cunha-Neto, E., Coelho, V., Guilherme, L., 1996. Autoimmunity in Chagas' disease: identification of cardiac myosin-B13 Trypanosoma cruzi protein crossreactive T cell clones in heart lesions of a chronic Chagas' cardiomyopathy patient. J. Clin. Invest. 98, 1709.
Cunningham, M.W., 2001. Cardiac myosin and the Th1/Th2 paradigm in autoimmune myocarditis. Am. J. Pathol. 159, 5.
Donermeyer, D.L., Beisel, K.W., Allen, P.M., 1995. Myocarditis-inducing epitope of myosin binds constitutively and stably to I-A^{k} on antigen presenting cells in the heart. J. Exp. Med. 182, 1291.
Drory, Y., Turetz, Y., Hiss, Y., 1991. Sudden unexpected death in persons less than 40 years of age. Am. J. Cardiol. 68, 1388.
Epelman, S., Liu, P.P., Mann, D.L., 2015. Role of innate and adaptive immunity in cardiac injury and repair. Nat. Rev. Immunol. 15, 117–129.
Eriksson, U., Kurrer, M.O., Sebald, W., 2001a. Dual role of the IL-12/IFN-γ axis in the development of autoimmune myocarditis: induction by IL-12 and protection by IFN-γ. J. Immunol. 167, 5464.
Eriksson, U., Kurrer, M.O., Bissinger, R., 2001b. Lethal autoimmune myocarditis in interferon-γ receptor-deficient mice: enhanced disease severity by impaired inducible nitric oxide synthase function. Circulation 103, 18.
Eriksson, U., Kurrer, M.O., Schmitz, N., Marsch, S.C., Fontana, A., Eugster, H.P., Kopf, M., 2003. Interleukin-6-deficient mice resist development of autoimmune myocarditis associated with impaired upregulation of complement C3. Circulation 107, 320.
Fairweather, D., Rose, N.R., 2002. Type I diabetes: virus infection or autoimmune disease? Nat. Immunol. 3, 338.
Fairweather, D., Kaya, Z., Shellam, G.R., 2001. From infection to autoimmunity. J. Autoimmun. 16, 175.
Fairweather, D., Yusung, S., Frisancho, S., 2003. IL-12Rβ1 and TLR4 increase IL-1β and IL-18-associated myocarditis and Coxsackievirus replication. J. Immunol. 170 4731.
Fearon, D.T., Lockley, R.M., 1996. The instructive role of innate immunity in the acquired immune response. Science 272, 50.
Fong, I.W., 2003. New insights and updates for established entities. In: Fong, I.W (Ed.), Infections and the Cardiovascular System: New Perspectives. Kluwer Academic/Plenum Publishers, New York, p. 20.
Forbes, B.A., 1989. Acquisition of cytomegalovirus infection: an update. Clin. Micro. Rev. 2, 204.
Friman, G., Fohlman, J., 1997. Infectious myocarditis and dilated cardiomyopathy. Cur. Opin. Infect. Dis. 10, 202.
Fujioka, S., Koide, H., Kitaura, Y., 1996. Molecular detection and differentiation of enteroviruses in endomyocardial biopsies and pericardial effusions form dilated cardiomyopathy and myocarditis. Am. Heart J. 131, 760.
Gangaplara, A., Massilamany, C., Brown, D.M., Delhon, G., Pattnaik, A.K. Chapman, N., Rose, N., Steffen, D., Reddy, J., 2012. Coxsackievirus B3 infection leads to the generation of cardiac myosin heavy chain-α-reactive CD4 T cells in A/J mice. Clin. Immunol. 144, 237.
Godeny, E.K., Gauntt, C.J., 1986. Involvement of natural killer cells in Coxsackievirus B3-induced murine myocarditis. J. Immunol. 137, 1695.

Godeny, E.K., Gauntt, C.J., 1987a. Murine natural killer cells limit Coxsackievirus B3 replication. J. Immunol. 139, 913.

Godeny, E.K., Gauntt, C.J., 1987b. In situ immune autoradiographic identification of cells in heart tissues of mice with Coxsackievirus B3-induced myocarditis. Am. J. Pathol. 129, 267.

Gor, D.O., Rose, N.R., Greenspan, N.S., 2003. Th1-Th2: a procrustean paradigm. Nat. Immunol. 4, 503.

Gore, I., Saphir, O., 1947. Myocarditis: a classification of 1402 cases. Am. Heart J. 34, 827.

Gravanis, M.G., Sternby, N.H., 1991. Incidence of myocarditis. Arch. Pathol. Lab. Med. 15, 309.

Grist, N.R., Reid, D., 1993. Epidemiology of viral infections of the heart. In: Banatvala, J.E. (Ed.), Viral Infections of the Heart. Edward Arnold, London, p. 23.

Guthrie, M., Lodge, P.A., Huber, S.A., 1984. Cardiac injury in myocarditis induced by Coxsackievirus group B, type 3 in BALB/c mice is mediated by Lyt2$^+$ cytolytic lymphocytes. Cell. Immunol. 88, 558.

Hashimoto, I., Komatsu, T., 1978. Myocardial changes after infection with Coxsackievirus B3 in nude mice. Br. J. Exp. Pathol. 59, 13.

Henke, A., Huber, S.A., Stelzner, A., 1995. The role of CD8$^+$ T lymphocytes in Coxsackievirus B3-induced myocarditis. J. Virol. 69, 6720.

Hoffmann, J.A., Kafatos, F.C., Janeway Jr., C.A., 1999. Phylogenetic perspectives in innate immunity. Science 284, 1313.

Horwitz, M.S., La Cava, A., Fine, C., 2000. Pancreatic expression of interferon-γ protects mice from lethal Coxsackievirus B3 infection and subsequent myocarditis. Nat. Med. 6, 693.

Hu, Y., Dong, C., Yue, Y., Xiong, S., 2014. In vivo delivery of interleukin-35 relieves coxsackievirus-B3-induced viral myocarditis by inhibiting Th17 cells. Arch. Virol. 159, 2411.

Huber, S.A., 1997. Autoimmunity in myocarditis: relevance of animal models. Clin. Immunol. Immunopathol. 83, 93.

Huber, S.A., Lodge, P.A., 1986. Coxsackievirus B3 myocarditis in mice: evidence for an autoimmune disease. Am. J. Pathol. 122, 284.

Huber, S.A., Job, L.P., Auld, K.R., 1981. Sex-related differences in the rapid production of cytotoxic spleen cells active against infected myofibers during Coxsackievirus B3 infection. J. Immunol. 126, 1336.

Huber, S.A., Polgar, J., Schultheiss, H.-P., 1994. Augmentation of pathogenesis of Coxsackievirus infections in mice by exogenous administration of interleukin-1 and interleukin-2. J. Virol. 68, 195.

Kadowski, N., Antonenko, S., Lau, J.Y.-N., 2000. Natural interferon α/β-producing cells link innate and adaptive immunity. J. Exp. Med. 192, 219.

Kania, G., Siegert, S., Behnke, S., Prados-Rosales, R., Casadevall, A., Lüscher, T.F., Luther, S.A., Kopf, M., Eriksson, U., Blyszczuk, P., 2013. Innate signaling promotes formation of regulatory nitric oxide-producing dendritic cells limiting T-cell expansion in experimental autoimmune myocarditis. Circulation 127, 2285.

Kaplan, M.H., 1988. Coxsackievirus infection in children under 3 months of age. In: Bendinelli, M., Friedman, H. (Eds.), Coxsackievirus: A General Update. Plenum Press, New York, p. 241.

Kaya, Z., Afanasyeva, M., Wang, Y., 2001. Contribution of the innate immune system to autoimmune myocarditis: a role for complement. Nat. Immunol. 2, 739.

Kaya, Z., Dohmen, K.M., Wang, Y., 2002. Cutting edge: a critical role for IL-10 in induction of nasal tolerance in experimental autoimmune myocarditis. J. Immunol. 168, 1552.

Khatib, R., Chason, J.L., Silberberg, B.K., 1980. Age-dependent pathogenecity of group B Coxsackieviruses in Swiss-Webster mice: infectivity for myocardium and pancreas. J. Infect. Dis. 141, 394.

Kong, Q., Wu, W., Yang, F., Liu, Y., Xue, Y., Gao, M., Lai, W., Pan, X., Yan, Y., Pang, Y., Deng, Y., 2012. Increased expressions of IL-22 and Th22 cells in the coxsackievirus B3-induced mice acute viral myocarditis. Virol. J. 9, 232.

Kurrer, M.O., Kopf, M., Penninger, J.M., 2002. Cytokines that regulate autoimmune myocarditis. Swiss Med. Wkly. 132, 408.

Kurt-Jones, E.A., Popova, L., Kwinn, L., 2000. Pattern recognition receptors TLR4 and CD14 mediate response to respiratory syncytial virus. Nat. Immunol. 1, 398.

Lane, J.R., Neumann, D.A., LaFond-Walker, A., 1991. LPS promotes CB3-induced myocarditis in resistant B10.A mice. Cell. Immunol. 136, 219.

Lane, J.R., Neumann, D.A., LaFond-Walker, A., 1992. Interleukin 1 or tumor necrosis factor can promote coxsackievirus B3-induced myocarditis in resistant B10.A mice. J. Exp. Med. 175, 1123.

Lankford, C.S.R., Frucht, D.M., 2003. A unique role for IL-23 in promoting cellular immunity. J. Leukoc. Biol. 73, 49.

Lathbury, L.J., Allan, J.E., Shellam, G.R., 1996. Effect of host genotype in determining the relative roles of natural killer cells and T cells in mediating protection against murine cytomegalovirus infection. J. Gen. Virol. 77, 2605.

Lauer, B., Schannwell, M., Kuhl, U., 2000. Antimyosin autoantibodies are associated with deterioration of systolic and diastolic left ventricular function in patients with chronic myocarditis. J. Am. Coll. Cardiol. 35, 11.

Lawson, C.M., O'Donoghue, H., Reed, W.D., 1989. The role of T cells in mouse cytomegalovirus-induced myocarditis. Immunology 67, 132.

Lawson, C.M., O'Donoghue, H., Bartholomaeus, W.M., 1990. Genetic control of mouse cytomegalovirus-induced myocarditis. Immunology 69, 20.

Lawson, C.M., O'Donoghue, H.L., Reed, W.D., 1992. Mouse cytomegalovirus infection induces antibodies that cross-react with virus and cardiac myosin: a model for the study of molecular mimicry in the pathogenesis of viral myocarditis. Immunology 75, 513.

Lawson, C.M., Yeow, W.-S., Lee, C.M., 1997. In vivo expression of an interferon-α gene by intramuscular injection of naked DNA. J. Int. Cytokine Res. 17, 255.

Lenzo, J.C., Fairweather, D., Shellam, G.R., 2001. Immunomodulation of murine cytomegalovirus-induced myocarditis in mice treated with lipopolysaccharide and tumor necrosis factor. Cell. Immunol. 213, 52.

Lenzo, J.C., Fairweather, D., Cull, V., 2002. Characterisation of murine cytomegalovirus myocarditis: cellular infiltration of the heart and virus persistence. J. Mol. Cell. Cardiol. 34, 629.

Liu, Y., Zhu, H., Su, Z., Sun, C., Yin, J., Yuan, H., Sandoghchian, S., Jiao, Z., Wang, S., Xu, H., 2012. IL-17 contributes to cardiac fibrosis following experimental autoimmune myocarditis by a PKCβ/Erk1/2/NF-κB-dependent signaling pathway. Int. Immunol. 24, 605.

Lodge, P.A., Herzum, M., Olszewski, J., 1987. Coxsackievirus B3 myocarditis: acute and chronic forms of the disease caused by different immunopathogenic mechanisms. Am. J. Pathol. 128, 455.

Lugrin, J., Parapanov, R., Rosenblatt-Velin, N., Rignault-Clerc, S., Feihl, F., Waeber, B., Müller, O., Vergely, C., Zeller, M., Tardivel, A., Schneider, P., Pacher, P., Liaudet, L., January 15, 2015. Cutting edge: IL-1α is a crucial danger signal triggering acute myocardial inflammation during myocardial infarction. J. Immunol. 194 (2), 499–503.

Ma, X., Trinchieri, G., 2001. Regulation of interleukin-12 production by antigen-presenting cells. Adv. Immunol. 79, 55.

Machino-Ohtsuka, T., Tajiri, K., Kimura, T., Sakai, S., Sato, A., Yoshida, T., Hiroe, M., Yasutomi, Y., Aonuma, K., Imanaka-Yoshida, K., 2014. Tenascin-C aggravates autoimmune myocarditis via dendritic cell activation and Th17 cell differentiation. J. Am. Heart Assoc. 3, 001052.

Marboe, C.C., Fenoglio, J.J., 1988. Biopsy diagnosis of myocarditis. In: Waller, B.F. (Ed.), Contemporary Issues in Cardiovascular Pathology. F.A. Davis Co., Philadelphia, p. 137.

Mattner, F., Fischer, S., Guckes, S., 1993. The interleukin-12 subunit p40 specifically inhibits effects of the interleukin-12 heterodimer. Eur. J. Immunol. 23, 2202.

Moser, M., Murphy, K.M., 2000. Dendritic cell regulation of Th1-Th2 development. Nat. Immunol. 1, 199.

Myers, J.M., Cooper, L.T., Kem, D.C., Stavrakis, S., Kosanke, S.D., Shevach, E.M., Fairweather, D., Stoner, J.A., Cox, C.J., Cunningham, M.W., 2016. Cardiac myosin-Th17 responses promote heart failure in human myocarditis. JCI Insight 1.

Nakanishi, K., Yoshimoto, T., Tsutsui, H., 2001. Interleukin-18 regulates both Th1 and Th2 responses. Annu. Rev. Immunol. 19, 423.

Nelms, K., Keegan, A.D., Zamorano, J., 1999. The IL-4 receptor: signaling mechanisms and biologic functions. Annu. Rev. Immunol. 17.

Nepom, B.S., 1993. The role of the major histocompatibility complex in autoimmunity. Clin. Immunol. Immunopathol. 67, S50.

Neu, N., Ploier, B., 1991. Experimentally induced autoimmune myocarditis: production of heart myosin-specific autoantibodies within the inflammatory infiltrate. Autoimmunity 8, 317.

Neu, N., Rose, N.R., Beisel, K.W., 1987. Cardiac myosin induces myocarditis in genetically predisposed mice. J. Immunol. 139, 3630 (.

Neumann, D.A., Lane, J.R., Allen, G.S., 1993. Viral myocarditis leading to cardiomyopathy: do cytokines contribute to pathogenesis? Clin. Immunol. Immunopathol. 68, 181.

O'Garra, A., 1998. Cytokines induce the development of functionally heterogeneous T helper cell subsets. Immunity 8, 275.

O'Neill, L.A.J., Dinarello, C.A., 2000. The IL-1 receptor/toll-like receptor superfamily: crucial receptors for inflammation and host defense. Immunol. Today 21, 206.

Ong, S., Ligons, D.L., Barin, J.G., Wu, L., Talor, M.V., Diny, N., Fontes, J.A., Gebremariam, E., Kass, D.A., Rose, N.R., Čiháková, D., 2015. Natural killer cells limit cardiac inflammation and fibrosis by halting eosinophil infiltration. Am. J. Pathol. 185, 847.

Oppmann, B., Lesley, R., Blom, B., 2000. Novel p19 protein engages IL-12p40 to form a cytokine, IL-23, with biological activities similar as well as distinct from IL-12. Immunity 13, 715.

Parham, C., Chirica, M., Timans, J., 2002. A receptor for the heterodimeric cytokine IL-23 is composed of IL-12Rβ1 and a novel cytokine receptor subunit, IL-23R. J. Immunol. 168, 5699.

Parish, C.R., O'Neill, E.R., 1997. Dependence of the adaptive immune response on innate immunity: some questions answered but new paradoxes emerge. Immunol. Cell Biol. 75, 523.

Penninger, J.M., Neu, N., Timms, E., 1993. The induction of experimental autoimmune myocarditis in mice lacking CD4 or CD8 molecules. J. Exp. Med. 178, 1837.

Penninger, J.M., Pummerer, C., Liu, P., 1997. Cellular and molecular mechanisms of murine autoimmune myocarditis. APMIS 105, 1.

Peters, N.S., Poole-Wilson, P.A., 1991. Myocarditis—a controversial disease. J. R. Soc. Med. 84, 1.

Pirhonen, J., Matikainen, S., Julkunen, I., 2002. Regulation of virus-induced IL-12 and IL-23 expression in human macrophages. J. Immunol. 169, 5673.

Pummerer, C., Berger, P., Fruhwirth, M., 1991. Cellular infiltrate, major histocompatibility antigen expression and immunopathogenic mechanisms in cardiac myosin-induced myocarditis. Lab. Invest. 65, 538.

Pummerer, C., Grassl, G., Neu, N., 1995. Cellular immune mechanisms in myosin-induced myocarditis. Eur. Heart J. 16 (Suppl. O), 71.

Rehren, F., Ritter, B., Dittrich-Breiholz, O., Henke, A., Lam, E., Kati, S., Kracht, M., Heim, A., 2013. Induction of a broad spectrum of inflammation-related genes by Coxsackievirus B3 requires Interleukin-1 signaling. Med. Microbiol. Immunol. 202, 11.

Rose, N.R., 1996. Myocarditis—from infection to autoimmunity. Immunologist 4, 67.

Rose, N.R., 2002. Mechanisms of autoimmunity. Semin. Liver Dis. 22, 387.

Rose, N.R., 2011. Critical cytokine pathways to cardiac inflammation. J. Interferon. Cytokine Res. 31, 705–710.

Rose, N.R., Afanasyeva, M., 2003. From infection to autoimmunity: the adjuvant effect. ASM News 69, 132.

Rose, N.R., Neumann, D.A., Herskowitz, A., 1988. Genetics of susceptibility to viral myocarditis in mice. Pathol. Immunopathol. Res. 7, 266.

Savvatis, K., Müller, I., Fröhlich, M., Pappritz, K., Zietsch, C., Hamdani, N., Grote, K., Schieffer, B., Klingel, K., Van Linthout, S., Linke, W.A., Schultheiss, H.P., Tschöpe, C., 2014. Interleukin-6 receptor inhibition modulates the immune reaction and restores titin phosphorylation in experimental myocarditis. Basic Res. Cardiol. 109, 449.

Scalzo, A.A., Lyons, P.A., Fitzgerald, N.A., 1995. The BALB.B6- Cmv1^r mouse: a strain congenic for Cmv1 and the NK gene complex. Immunogenetics 41, 148.

Schoen, F.J., 1999. The heart. In: Cotran, R.S., Kumar, V., Collins, T. (Eds.), Robbins Pathologic Basis of Disease. W.B. Saunders Co., Philadelphia, p. 544.

Schwimmbeck, P.L., Huber, S.A., Schultheiss, H.-P., 1997. The role of T cells in Coxsackie B-induced disease. In: Tracy, S., Chapman, N.M., Mahy, B.W.J. (Eds.), The Coxsackie B Viruses. Springer, Berlin, p. 283.

Seder, R.A., Gazzinelli, R.T., 1999. Cytokines are critical in linking the innate and adaptive immune responses to bacteria, fungal, and parasitic infection. Adv. Intern. Med. 44, 353.

Smith, S.C., Allen, P.M., 1991. Myosin-induced acute myocarditis is a T cell mediated disease. J. Immunol. 147, 2141.

Smith, S.C., Allen, P.M., 1992a. Expression of myosin-class II major histocompatibility complexes in the normal myocardium occurs before induction of autoimmune myocarditis. Proc. Natl. Acad. Sci. USA 89, 9131.

Smith, S.C., Allen, P.M., 1992b. Neutralization of endogenous tumor necrosis factor ameliorates the severity of myosin-induced myocarditis. Circ. Res. 70, 856.

Smith, S.C., Allen, P.M., 1993. The role of T cells in myosin-induced autoimmune myocarditis. Clin. Immunol. Immunopathol. 68, 100.

Tay, C.H., Szomolanyi-tsuda, E., Welsh, R.M., 1998. Control of infections by NK cells. In: Karre, K., Colonna, M. (Eds.), Current Topics in Microbiology and Immunology: Specificity, Function and Development of NK Cells. Springer, Berlin, p. 193.

Todd, J.A., Acha-Orbea, H., Bell, J.I., 1988. A molecular basis for MHC class II-associated autoimmunity. Science 240, 124.

Valaperti, A., Nishii, M., Liu, Y., Naito, K., Chan, M., Zhang, L., Skurk, C., Schultheiss, H.P., Wells, G.A., Eriksson, U., Liu, P.P., 2013. Innate immune interleukin-1 receptor-associated kinase 4 exacerbates viral myocarditis by reducing CCR5($^+$) CD11b($^+$) monocyte migration and impairing interferon production. Circulation 128, 1542.

Wang, Y., Afanasyeva, M., Hill, S.L., 1999. Characterization of murine autoimmune myocarditis induced by self and foreign cardiac myosin. Autoimmunity 31, 151.

Watford, W.T., O'Shea, J.J., 2003. A case of mistaken identity. Nature 421, 706.

Wiekowski, M.T., Leach, M.W., Evans, E.W., 2001. Ubiquitous transgenic expression of the IL-23 subunit p19 induces multiorgan inflammation, runting, infertility, and premature death. J. Immunol. 166, 7563.

Wolfgram, L.J., Beisel, K.W., Herskowitz, A., Rose, N.R., 1986. Variations in the susceptibility to Coxsactievirus B3-induced myocarditis among different strains of mice. J. Immunol. 136, 1846.

Woodruff, J.F., Woodruff, J.J., 1974. Involvement of T lymphocytes in the pathogenesis of Coxsackievirus B3 heart disease. J. Immunol. 113, 1726.

Yeow, W.-S., Lawson, C.M., Beilharz, M.W., 1998. Antiviral activities of individual murine IFN-α subtypes in vivo: intramuscular injection of IFN expression constructs reduces cytomegalovirus replication. J. Immunol. 160, 2932.

Yoshimoto, T., Takeda, K., Tanaka, T., 1998. IL-12 up-regulates IL-18 receptor expression on T cells, Th1 cells and B cells: synergism with IL-18 for IFN-γ production. J. Immunol. 161, 3400.

Yuan, J., Yu, M., Li, H.H., Long, Q., Liang, W., Wen, S., Wang, M., Guo, H.P., Cheng, X., Liao, Y.H., January 2014. Autophagy contributes to IL-17-induced plasma cell differentiation in experimental autoimmune myocarditis. Int. Immunopharmacol 18 (1), 98–105.

Zempo, H., Sugita, Y., Ogawa, M., Watanabe, R., Suzuki, J., Isobe, M., 2015. A P2X7 receptor antagonist attenuates experimental autoimmune myocarditis via suppressed myocardial $CD4^+$ T and macrophage infiltration and NADPH oxidase 2/4 expression in mice. Heart Vessels 30, 527–533.

Zhang, G.-X., Gran, B., Yu, S., 2003. Induction of experimental autoimmune encephalomyelitis in IL-12 receptor-β2-deficient mice: IL-12 responsiveness is not required in the pathogenesis of inflammatory demyelination in the central nervous system. J. Immunol. 170, 2153.

Zhang, W., Lavine, K.J., Epelman, S., Evans, S.A., Weinheimer, C.J., Barger, P.M., Mann, D.L., 2015. Necrotic myocardial cells release damage-associated molecular patterns that provoke fibroblast activation in vitro and trigger myocardial inflammation and fibrosis in vivo. J. Am. Heart Assoc. 4, e001993.

Zhou, S.F., Yuan, J., Liao, M.Y., Xia, N., Tang, T.T., Li, J.J., Jiao, J., Dong, W.Y., Nie, S.F., Zhu, Z.F., Zhang, W.C., Lv, B.J., Xiao, H., Wang, Q., Tu, X., Liao, Y.H., Shi, G.P., Cheng, X., 2014. IL-17A promotes ventricular remodeling after myocardial infarction. J. Mol. Med. (Berl) 92, 1105.

FURTHER READING

Kos, F.J., Engelman, E.G., 1996. Immune regulation: a critical link between NK cells and CTLs. Immunol. Today 17, 174.

Chapter 2

Organ-Specific Autoimmunity Involvement in Cardiovascular Disease

A.L.P. Caforio,* G. Malipiero,[§] R. Marcolongo[§] and S. Iliceto*
*Division of Cardiology, Department of Cardiological Thoracic and Vascular Sciences, Centro 'V. Gallucci', University of Padova-Policlinico, Padova, Italy; [§]Hematology and Clinical Immunology, University of Padova, Padova, Italy

1. INTRODUCTION

Autoimmune disease occurs as a result of the loss of tolerance to self-antigens, which under physiological conditions is maintained. To be classified as autoimmune in nature a disease must fulfill at least two of the major criteria first proposed by Witebsky and later modified by Rose (Witebsky et al., 1957; Rose and Bona, 1993). There are also minor criteria, some of which are common to all autoimmune conditions, and others that are found in just a few of them. These criteria are summarized in Table 2.1.

Autoimmune disease is characterized by the presence of circulating autoantibodies, which are not always pathogenic but represent markers of ongoing tissue damage. In nonorgan-specific autoimmune disease the autoantibodies are against ubiquitous autoantigens (e.g., nuclear antigens in systemic lupus erythematosus) and tissue damage is generalized. In organ-specific autoimmune disease, immunopathology is restricted to one organ or apparatus within the body, and the autoimmune process, antibody and/or cell-mediated, is directed against autoantigens, which are unique to the affected organ (e.g., thyroid peroxidase in Hashimoto thyroiditis). The histological hallmark of organ-specific autoimmunity is an early mononuclear cell infiltrate in the affected organ, e.g., insulitis in type 1 insulin-dependent diabetes mellitus, with inappropriate expression of human leukocyte antigen (HLA) class II and adhesion molecules. At a later stage, inflammatory cells tend to disappear and the tissue undergoes profound fibrotic changes with ultimate atrophy and organ dysfunction (such as in Hashimoto thyroiditis). However, in other

The Heart in Systemic Autoimmune Diseases.

TABLE 2.1 Criteria of Autoimmune Disease

Major
Mononuclear cell infiltration and abnormal HLA expression in the target organ (organ-specific disease) or in various organs (nonorgan-specific disease)
Circulating autoantibodies and/or autoreactive lymphocytes in patients and unaffected family members
Detection of autoantibody and/or autoreactive lymphocytes in situ within the affected tissue
Identification and isolation of autoantigen(s) involved
Disease induced in animal models following immunization with relevant autoantigen and/or passive transfer of serum, purified autoantibody, and/or lymphocytes
Efficacy of immunosuppressive therapy
Minor
Common to all autoimmune disorders
Middle-aged women most frequently affected
Familial aggregation
HLA association
Hypergammaglobulinemia
Clinical course characterized by exacerbations and remissions
Autoimmune diseases associated in the same patient or family members
Peculiar of organ-specific autoimmune disorders
Presence of autoantigens at low concentration
Autoantibodies directly against organ-specific autoantigens
Immunopathology mediated by type II, IV, V, and VI reactions

instances organ-specific autoimmunity may lead to enhanced target organ function (e.g., Basedow disease).

Organ-specific autoimmune diseases occur as a result of genetic predisposition and environmental influences. The genetic predisposition accounts for the fact that different autoimmune conditions may be associated in patients or their family members, as well as for the well-known feature that single autoimmune diseases often run in families. The inheritance of susceptibility is usually polygenic. Organ-specific autoimmune diseases are commonly associated with specific HLA class II antigens, but the precise mechanisms by which HLA may operate in determining disease predisposition are still undefined. The majority of organ-specific autoimmune diseases are chronic and apparently "idiopathic." Organ- and disease-specific antibodies are found in the affected patients. These antibodies are also detected in family members even years before the development of disease, and thus identify asymptomatic relatives at risk (Bottazzo et al., 1986). Involvement of organ-specific autoimmunity has been suspected in the following cardiovascular diseases: the post-pericardiotomy and post-myocardial infarction (Dressler) syndromes and in idiopathic recurrent acute pericarditis (IRAP), rheumatic carditis, idiopathic forms of inflammatory cardiomyopathy and of brady- or tachyarrhythmias, and systemic arterial hypertension.

2. POST-MYOCARDIAL INFARCTION (DRESSLER) SYNDROME

Post-myocardial infarction (Dressler) pericarditis may occur in 1–4% of patients at 2–4 weeks following an acute myocardial infarction (Dressler, 1956, 1959; Van der Geld, 1964). Clinical features include (1) fever; (2) chest pain, which is often localized to retrosternal and left precordial regions with radiation to the trapezius ridge and neck, or the left arm, sharp or dull in quality, increased by deep inspiration, coughing and recumbence, relieved by sitting up and leaning forward, lasting few days to several weeks; (3) dyspnea of variable extent (mild or severe in the presence of tamponade) and nonproductive cough; (4) pericardial friction rub, of variable intensity in relation to patient posture and pressure of the stethoscope, best heard during inspiration and full expiration with the patient sitting up and leaning forward; and (5) leukocytosis, increased erythrocyte sedimentation rate, and reactive C protein. Pericardial effusion may be present, and is associated with pleural effusion in 70% of the cases of Dressler syndrome. Less than one-third of patients with Dressler syndrome develop pneumonitis, usually at the lung basis. The disease is often self-limiting, but can relapse in the following 28 months.

2.1 Anti-Heart Autoantibodies

Back in 1960, it was demonstrated that in the first 2 weeks following experimentally induced myocardial infarction, rabbits developed circulating anti-heart autoantibodies (Kleinsorge et al., 1960). Subsequently, anti-heart autoantibodies were found using complement fixation test (CFT) or standard indirect immunofluorescence (s-I IFL) in 43–56% of post-myocardial infarction patients with Dressler syndrome and in 10% of those with uncomplicated disease course (Van der Geld, 1964). Antibody titers were reported to reach their highest peak at 4 weeks post-myocardial infarction, with subsequent slow reduction (Itoh et al., 1969). These antibodies were also detected in patients with coronary artery disease without recent myocardial infarction episodes, with variable frequencies, depending upon patient selection criteria and the technique used (Kaplan et al., 1961; Hess et al., 1964; Heine et al., 1966; Bauer et al., 1972; Nicholson et al., 1977; Caforio et al., 1990a). Anti-heart autoantibody frequencies in cardiovascular disease, including ischemic heart disease, are summarized in Tables 2.2 and 2.3.

Two studies emphasized that comparative evaluation of the anti-heart antibody results in various cardiac diseases, particularly in relation to the autoantibody patterns observed by s-I IFL is difficult (Nicholson et al., 1977; Caforio et al., 1990a). In fact, different substrates (e.g., human adult, human neonatal, or rat myocardium) were used and there is no standardized nomenclature for the anti-heart antibody patterns. In addition, some but not all workers tested sera on both skeletal muscle and myocardium; therefore, several studies did not differentiate between organ-specific cardiac and muscle-specific (e.g., cardiac and skeletal muscle reactive) antibody. Taking into account these limitations, the anti-heart antibody patterns seen in ischemic heart disease, with or without Dressler syndrome, were described as

1. more pronounced peripheral sarcoplasmic stain on human or rat heart, with progressive increase of the IFL from the center to the periphery of myofibers, but without clear-cut linear sarcolemmal stain (pattern defined as "sarcolemmal," "subsarcolemmal-sarcoplasmic," "sarcolemmal-subsarcolemmal," or "peripheral");
2. diffuse sarcoplasmic stain, without a tendency to peripheral enhancement (pattern defined as "diffuse-sarcoplasmic" or "diffuse");
3. longitudinal intermyofibrillar sarcoplasmic stain, perpendicular to myofibrillar striations (pattern defined as "intermyofibrillar");
4. patterns defined as combinations of those detailed earlier, or with superimposed striated IFL (pattern defined as "striated" or "antifibrillary");
5. stain of the intercalated disks, isolated or in association with sarcolemmal and/or sarcoplasmic IFL (pattern defined as "antiintercalated disks").

3. POST-PERICARDIOTOMY SYNDROME AND IDIOPATHIC RECURRENT ACUTE PERICARDITIS

Post-pericardiotomy syndrome and pericarditis may occur at 2–4 weeks following heart surgery operations that require opening of the pericardium. In the 1950–70s, it could be observed in up to 40% of the patients, but nowadays it is rare. It is characterized by fever, pericardial or pleuropericardial effusion, chest pain, and pericardial rub; it may relapse (Van der Geld, 1964; Engle et al., 1974). An identical clinical syndrome has been described after cardiac perforation following pacemaker implantation, blunt chest trauma, percutaneous diagnostic left ventricular puncture, and coronary perforation due to balloon angioplasty (Peters et al., 1980; Escaned et al., 1992).

Pericarditis may account for about 5% of presentations to emergency departments for nonischemic chest pain. Recurrences occur in up to 15–32%

TABLE 2.2 Anti-heart Autoantibody Specificities in Miscellaneous Cardiac and Noncardiac Conditions

Autoantibody (Ab)	Disease: Ab Positive (%)	Technique	Autoantigen(s)
Anti-heart antibodies (AHA), skeletal muscle cross-reactive or not tested	Dressler syndrome: 43–56%	s-l IFL, CFT	Sarcolemma, sarcoplasm, myofibrils
	PPS: 73–100%	s-l IFL	Sarcolemma, sarcoplasm, myofibrils
	Rheumatic fever: inactive 12–21%; active 25–87%; carditis 47%	s-l IFL	Sarcolemma, sarcoplasm, myofibrils
Organ-specific AHA	APE: 17%	s-l IFL + absor, s-l IFL, ELISA	Sarcoplasm, α and β MHC
	DCM relatives: 30%		
Anticardiac conducting tissue	Idiopathic CD: 9–34%	s-l IFL on ox heart false tendon	Purkinje fibers
	Nonidiopathic CD: 4–30%		
	RBBB + RA: 76%; RA: 20%		
	Collagenopathy + CD: 14–21%; N: 4–11%		
Anti-β_1 adrenoceptor, stimulating	CD: 28.5%; VA: 47.6%	ELISA	β_1 adrenoceptor
	AA: 13.6%; N: 19%		

Continued

TABLE 2.2 Anti-heart Autoantibody Specificities in Miscellaneous Cardiac and Noncardiac Conditions—cont'd

Autoantibody (Ab)	Disease: Ab Positive (%)	Technique	Autoantigen(s)
Anti-β_2 adrenoceptor, stimulating	CD: 14.3%; VA: 23.8%	ELISA	β_2 adrenoceptor
	AA: 4.5%; N: 14.7%		
Anti-α_1 adrenoceptor, stimulating	I mHTN: 20%; II mHTN: 64%; N: 12%	ELISA	α_1 adrenoceptor
	I HTN: 44%, N:12%	Bioassay	
AT1 receptor, stimulating	I mHTN: 14%; II mHTN: 33%; N: 14%	ELISA	AT1 receptor
	II HTN: 18%	Bioassay	

AA, primary atrial arrhythmias; *absor*, absorption; *APE*, autoimmune polyendocrinopathy; *CD*, conduction disturbances; *CFT*, complement fixation test; *N*, normal subjects; *I HTN*, primary HTN; *I mHTN*, primary malignant hypertension; *II mHTN*, secondary malignant hypertension; *PPS*, post-cardiotomy syndrome; *VA*, ventricular arrhythmias, other abbreviations as in text.

TABLE 2.3 Frequency of Heart Autoantibodies in Acute Myocarditis and DCM

		% Antibody Positive				
Antibody Type	**Method**	**AM**	**DCM**	**OCD**	**Normals**	**References**
Muscle-specific						
ASA	s-I IFL	47[a]	10	NT	25	Maisch et al. (1983a,b)
AMLA	AMC	41[a]	9	NT	12	Maisch et al. (1983a,b)
AFA	s-I IFL	28[a]	24[a]	NT	6	Maisch et al. (1983a,b)
IFA	s-I IFL	32[a]	41[a]	NT	3	Maisch et al. (1983a,b)
Heart-reactive	s-I IFL	59[a]	20[a]	NT	0	Neumann et al. (1990)
	s-I IFL	NT	12–28	21–33	4	Fletcher and Wenger (1968), Camp et al. (1969) and Kirsner et al. (1973)
Anti-s.Na/K-ATPase	ELISA + Western blot	NT	26[a]	NT	2	Baba et al. (2002)
Organ-specific cardiac	s-I IFL + abs	34[a,b]	26[a,b]	1	3	Caforio et al. (1990a, 1997a,b)
Antimitochondrial						
M7	ELISA	13[a]	31[a]	10	0	Klein et al. (1984)
ANT	SPRIA	91[a,b]	57[a,b]	0	0	Schultheiss and Bolte (1985) and Schultheiss et al. (1990)
BCKD-E2	ELISA	100[a,b]	60[a,b]	4	0	Ansari et al. (1994)
Anti-laminin	ELISA	73	78	25–35	6	Wolff et al. (1989)

Continued

TABLE 2.3 Frequency of Heart Autoantibodies in Acute Myocarditis and DCM—cont'd

		% Antibody Positive				
Antibody Type	**Method**	**AM**	**DCM**	**OCD**	**Normals**	**References**
Anti-β1 receptor						
Inhibiting	LBI	NT	30–75[a,b]	37	18	Limas et al. (1989) and Limas and Limas (1991)
	ELISA	NT	31[a,b]	0	12	Magnusson et al. (1990, 1994)
Stimulating	Bioassay	96[a,b]	95[a,b]	8	0	Wallukat et al. (1991)
	ELISA	NT	38[b]	6	19	Chiale et al. (1995)
	ELISA	NT	26[a,b]	10	1	Jahns et al. (1999)
Anti-M2 receptor	ELISA	NT	39[a]	NT	7.5	Fu et al. (1993)
Anti-α and β MHC	Western blot	NT	46[a,b]	8	0	Caforio et al. (1992)
Anti-MLC 1v	Western blot	NT	35	25	15	Caforio et al. (1992)
Non myofibrillar	Western blot	NT	46[a,b]	17	0	Caforio et al. (1992)
Anti-MHC	Western blot	NT	67[b]	42	NT	Latif et al. (1993)
Anti-MLC 1	Western blot	NT	17[b]	0	NT	Latif et al. (1993)
Anti-tropomyosin	Western blot	NT	55[b]	21	NT	Latif et al. (1993)
Anti-actin	Western blot	NT	71[b]	21	NT	Latif et al. (1993)
Anti-HSP-60	Western blot	NT	85[b]	42	NT	Latif et al. (1993)
Anti-HSP-60, 70	Western blot	NT	10–14[b]	1–2	3	Portig et al. (1997)
Anti-β MHC	ELISA	37[a,b]	44[a,b]	16	2.5	Lauer et al. (1994)
Anti-α MHC	ELISA	17[a,b]	20[a,b]	4	2	Goldman et al. (1995) and Caforio (1997a,b)

+*abs*, +absorption; *AFA*, antifibrillary antibody; *AM*, acute myocarditis; *AMC*, antibody-mediated cytotoxicity; *AMLA*, antimyolemmal antibody; *ASA*, antisarcolemmal antibody; *IFA*, antiinterfibrillary; *LBI*, ligand binding inhibition; *NT*, not tested; *OCD*, other cardiac disease; other abbreviations as in Table 2.2 and text.
[a]*P < .05 versus normals.*
[b]*P < .05 versus OCD.*

of patients. Recurrent acute pericarditis is generally idiopathic or post-cardiac injury, and is often a frustrating problem, for both patients and doctors. IRAP is a disease of suspected, yet unproved, immune-mediated pathogenesis.

3.1 Anti-Heart Autoantibodies

Anti-heart autoantibodies, giving staining patterns similar to those described in Dressler syndrome and cross-reacting with skeletal muscle, were found in 73–100% of patients with post-pericardiotomy syndrome (Table 2.2). There was significant correlation between autoantibody titer and severity of symptoms; in addition, the antibodies were undetectable in quiescent intervals between attacks and were again detected during symptomatic recurrent episodes, suggesting a potential pathogenic role (Van der Geld, 1964; Zabriskie et al., 1970; Engle et al., 1974). In a later study, the antibodies were detected in 95% of patients with full clinical criteria, in 72% of those with only some typical clinical features, and in 29% of control subjects who had undergone cardiac surgery without developing symptoms of post-pericardiotomy syndrome (Maisch et al., 1979).

In a recent study (Caforio et al., 2010) anti-heart autoantibodies (organ-specific, cross-reactive 1 and 2 types) and antiintercalated disk autoantibodies were detected in serum samples from patients, at last follow-up, and control subjects by sI-IFL on human myocardium and skeletal muscle. Noncardiac-specific autoantibodies were detected by sI-IFL, and anti-Ro/SSA and anti-La/SSB by enzyme-linked immunosorbent assay (ELISA). The frequencies of cross-reactive 1 anti-heart autoantibodies and of intercalated disk autoantibodies were higher (50%; 25%) in IRAP than in noninflammatory cardiac disease (4%; 4%), ischemic (1%; 2%), or normal subjects (3%; 0%) ($P = .0001$). Anti-heart autoantibodies and/or antiintercalated disk autoantibodies were found in 67.5% patients with IRAP. Of the noncardiac-specific antibodies, only antinuclear autoantibodies at titer $\geq 1/160$ were more common in IRAP (5%) versus normal (0.5%, $P < .04$). Antiintercalated disk autoantibodies in IRAP were associated with a higher number of recurrences ($P = .01$) and hospitalizations ($P = .0001$) and high titer (1/80 or higher) anti-heart autoantibodies with a higher number of recurrences ($P = .02$). These findings support the involvement of autoimmunity in the majority of patients with IRAP.

4. RHEUMATIC CARDITIS

Rheumatic fever is an inflammatory multisystem disease, occurring few weeks to 6 months following group A streptococcal (GAS) infection of the tonsillopharynx. Its diagnosis is based upon Jones criteria (Jones, 1944), which were recently updated (Dajani et al., 1992).

Major criteria include

1. carditis;
2. polyarthritis;
3. chorea;
4. erythema marginatum; and
5. subcutaneous nodules.

Minor criteria are represented by

1. fever;
2. arthralgia;
3. elevated erythrocyte sedimentation rate or C-reactive protein; and
4. prolonged P-R interval on standard 12-lead surface ECG.

If supported by evidence of GAS, e.g., positive throat culture or rapid streptococcal antigen test, elevated or rising streptococcal antibody titer, the presence of two major criteria (or one major and two minor) indicates a high probability of acute rheumatic fever.

The diagnosis of cardiac involvement during acute rheumatic fever is based upon unequivocal fulfillment of any of the following criteria:

1. new onset of nonfunctional cardiac murmurs;
2. cardiac enlargement;
3. signs and symptoms of heart failure; and
4. pericardial friction rubs or accumulation of pericardial fluid.

4.1 Immune Pathogenesis of Rheumatic Carditis

Rheumatic carditis is thought to represent an autoimmune disorder triggered by streptococcal infection via molecular mimicry. Indeed streptococci and heart tissue have several antigenic components for which molecular mimicry has been documented (Robinson and Kehoe, 1992). During rheumatic fever, patients produce both antistreptococcal antibodies and anti-heart autoantibodies, since rheumatogenic streptococci and heart tissue have shared antigens.

4.1.1 Antistreptococcus Antibodies

The external parietal layer of GAS contains distinct M protein types in different strains. More than 80 M protein types are known. M proteins of rheumatogenic streptococci share a long terminal antigen domain (Bessen et al., 1989) and contain epitopes that are shared with human heart tissue, particularly sarcolemmal membrane proteins, cardiac myosin and tropomyosin, as well as with skeletal muscle and smooth muscle and renal glomerular basement membrane (Krisher and Cunningham, 1985; Dale and Beachey, 1986). In addition, shared epitopes have been reported between N-acetylglucosamine of the mid-parietal streptococcus cell layer and glycoproteins of mammalian cardiac valve tissue, and another cross-reaction has been found between streptococcal hyaluronate and protein polysaccharide of mammalian cartilage (Robinson and Kehoe, 1992). In addition, antistreptococcal antibodies, cross-reactive with heart antigens and thalamus and subthalamus components, have been found in some patients with carditis and chorea (reviewed by Kaplan and Frengley, 1969). The heart cross-reactive antistreptococcal antibodies, identified by a combination of immunofluorescent and precipitin-absorption techniques, were present in 55% and 58% of patients with active and inactive rheumatic heart disease, respectively, or with acute glomerulonephritis in 24% of patients with recent streptococcal infection and only rarely (2%) in disease controls without rheumatic heart disease or previous streptococcal infection, but the pathogenetic significance of these antibodies remained to be evaluated (Kaplan and Svec, 1964).

4.1.2 Anti-heart Autoantibodies

Several methods were used, in the earliest studies, for detection of circulating anti-heart autoantibodies in rheumatic fever. These (reviewed by Kaplan and Frengley, 1969) were later abandoned and included agglutination tests with collodion particles coated with saline extracts of the heart and other organs; CFT with saline extracts of the heart, liver, and spleen; tanned red cell hemagglutination test; and antiglobulin consumption with heart homogenate. Subsequently, s-I IFL on cryostat-cut sections became the method of choice; however, tissue substrates were various and included human or rat myocardium (Van der Geld, 1964), normal human myocardium obtained at autopsy or surgery in subjects with congenital heart defects (Zabriskie et al., 1970; Engle et al., 1974), normal human myocardium of blood group O, obtained at surgery in subjects with congenital heart defects (Maisch et al., 1979). Cryostat-cut sections were fixed in acetone (Zabriskie et al., 1970) or unfixed (Engle et al., 1974; Van der Geld, 1964) and then incubated with serum diluted at 1:5 (Zabriskie et al., 1970; Engle et al., 1974) or undiluted (Van der Geld, 1964); sections were washed in PBS and then the autoantibody binding was revealed with fluoresceinated serum antihuman immunoglobulin G (IgG). In a more recent study, patient serum, at 1:10 dilution, was incubated on unfixed cryostat-cut sections and after washing the section was stained with fluoresceinated serum antihuman IgG, IgA, or IgM (Maisch et al., 1979). Clearly, the lack of a standard s-I IFL protocol makes it difficult to compare results from different studies, particularly in terms of anti-heart antibody frequency.

Taking into account such limitations, circulating anti-heart autoantibodies have been found, using s-I IFL, in sera from 25% to 87% of patients with active rheumatic fever, 12–21% of those with inactive rheumatic disease, and 0–4% of normal subjects (Kaplan et al., 1961; Kaplan and Dallenbach,

1961; Hess et al., 1964; Zitnan and Bosmanski, 1966) (Table 2.2). In another study, these have been detected in 81% of patients with streptococcal infection, 80% of those with post-streptococcal nephritis, 87% with acute rheumatic fever, 47% with rheumatic carditis, 100% with post-cardiotomy syndrome, and in none of the control subjects (Zabriskie et al., 1970) (Table 2.2). The autoantibody patterns observed in rheumatic disease were similar to those described in Dressler and post-pericardiotomy syndromes, but the "sarcolemmal-sarcoplasmic" or "peripheral" pattern was found more frequently than the "diffuse" stain (Nicholson et al., 1977). In rheumatic carditis, anticonductive tissue antibodies were also reported (see Section 6.1) (Ledford and Espinoza, 1987). The anti-heart autoantibodies from rheumatic sera could be absorbed out by streptococcal membranes as well as myocardial extracts; conversely, those found in post-pericardiotomy sera reacted exclusively with myocardial extracts, suggesting that the antigenic determinants were different in the two cardiac conditions (Zabriskie et al., 1970). In terms of relations of anti-heart autoantibodies to clinical activity of rheumatic disease, as pointed out by the first investigators in this field (Kaplan and Frengley, 1969), overall the frequency of anti-heart antibodies was higher in clinically active than in clinically inactive disease, in patients with carditis than without and in those with a higher number of previous attacks of rheumatic fever (Hess et al., 1964; Zitnan and Bosmanski, 1966). The titer of autoantibodies in some patients correlated with clinical severity or grade of rheumatic activity and was occasionally reported to be a useful tool in differential diagnosis from other infections or inflammatory conditions (Felsh, 1966). As far as the time course of antibody production is concerned, using s-I IFL or antiglobulin consumption tests, it was shown that anti-heart antibody was detected in some patients before and, in other patients, after the onset of clinical symptoms of rheumatic fever (Hess et al., 1964; Zabriskie, 1967). In the majority of cases, antibody was first detected within the first week of symptom onset, thereafter it rose to maximal titer. Subsequently, antibody titer declined, in some cases rapidly, possibly in relation to steroid treatment; in other cases, a more variable or slower pattern of decay was documented with persistence of low titer antibody up to 2–3 years after an attack of rheumatic fever (Zabriskie, 1967). On the other hand, autoantibodies not detected using s-I IFL or antiglobulin consumption, and directed against aqueous and alcoholic heart tissue extracts, seemed unrelated to clinical findings, suggesting that some but not all antibody specificities produced in rheumatic heart disease may be relevant to pathogenesis (Kaplan and Frengley, 1969). Bound IgG and complement were also identified within the myocardial as well as pericardial and valvular tissues in post-mortem rheumatic hearts and surgical specimens of auricular appendages from patients with rheumatic heart disease (Kaplan and Dallenbach, 1961; Kaplan et al., 1964).

5. DILATED CARDIOMYOPATHY AND MYOCARDITIS

Dilated cardiomyopathy (DCM) is a relevant cause of heart failure and a common indication for heart transplantation. According to the current WHO classification of cardiomyopathies, DCM is characterized by dilatation and impaired contraction of the left or both ventricles; it may be idiopathic, familial/genetic, viral, and/or immune (Richardson et al., 1996). Clinical onset is generally with symptoms/signs of congestive heart failure, brady-/tachyarrhythmia, or thromboembolism. In most cases, the duration of the asymptomatic phase is uncertain. Occasionally, DCM may be diagnosed following the detection of an apical systolic murmur of mitral insufficiency, pathologic ECG, or enlarged cardiac chambers with systolic dysfunction on echocardiography. DCM is familial in 20–30% of cases, has severe prognosis with 40–50% mortality, because of heart failure or sudden death in 2 years following diagnosis. The diagnosis of DCM requires exclusion of known, specific causes of heart failure, including coronary artery disease. Thus in DCM, coronary angiography is normal; on endomyocardial biopsy there is myocyte loss, compensatory hypertrophy, fibrous tissue, and immunohistochemical findings consistent with chronic inflammation (myocarditis) in 30–40% of cases.

Myocarditis is an inflammatory disease of the myocardium and is diagnosed by endomyocardial biopsy using established histological, immunological, and immunohistochemical criteria; it may be idiopathic, infectious, or autoimmune and may heal or lead to DCM (Aretz et al., 1985; Richardson et al., 1996; Caforio et al., 2013, 2015a). The clinical features of myocarditis are quite diverse. Cardiac manifestations may or may not be preceded (1–2 weeks) by a systemic flu-like illness. Myocarditis may be subclinical, causing minor symptoms (palpitation, atypical chest pain), electrocardiographic abnormalities [atrioventricular (AV) conduction disturbance (CD), bundle branch block, ST and T-wave changes] or arrhythmias [paroxysmal atrial fibrillation or ventricular arrhythmias (VAs)] in the absence of demonstrable change in global or regional left or right ventricular function. Pericarditis with or without chest pain, a pericardial effusion, or rub may coexist with myocarditis. Other presentations of myocarditis include syncope, sudden death, acute right or left ventricular failure, cardiogenic shock, or DCM. A syndrome mimicking acute myocardial infarction, but with normal coronary arteries, may also occur.

Prognosis of myocarditis is thought to be good, with complete recovery at least in the majority of patients. However, in neonates and young children, the elderly, and the debilitated, the disease is often severe, causing fulminant and fatal heart failure. Relapses may occur, and a proportion of patients will develop residual mild left ventricular dysfunction or DCM. Thus, in a patient subset, myocarditis and DCM are thought to represent the acute and chronic stages of an inflammatory disease of the myocardium, which can be viral, post-infectious immune, or primarily organ-specific autoimmune (Richardson et al., 1996; Caforio et al., 1994, 2013, 2015a).

5.1 Immune Pathogenesis of Myocarditis and Dilated Cardiomyopathy

Autoimmune features in human myocarditis/DCM include familial aggregation (Baig et al., 1998), HLA association (Meder et al., 2014), lymph mononuclear cell infiltrate, abnormal expression of HLA class II and adhesion molecules on cardiac endothelium, on endomyocardial biopsy, in the affected patients and family members (Caforio et al., 1990b; Mahon et al., 2002), increased levels of circulating cytokines and cardiac autoantibodies in patients and family members (reviewed by Caforio et al., 2002), experimental models of both antibody-mediated and cell-mediated autoimmune myocarditis/DCM following immunization with relevant autoantigen(s), the best characterized of which is cardiac myosin (Rose, 2000; Kuan et al., 2000). Here we mainly focus on the circulating cardiac autoantibodies.

5.2 Anti-Heart Autoantibodies by s-I IFL

Several groups have found antibodies to various cardiac antigens in myocarditis and DCM, but the organ and disease specificity of these antibody types have not been always evaluated (reviewed by Caforio et al., 2002). Using s-I IFL, earlier studies identified antibodies to sarcolemmal and myofibrillar antigens, but these were either cross-reactive or untested on skeletal muscle. In addition, it remained unclear whether these antibodies were disease-specific for myocarditis/DCM because controls with other cardiac disease were not always included.

These autoantibodies were found in 12–75% of DCM/myocarditis patients and 4–34% of normal control subjects (Fletcher and Wenger, 1968; Camp et al., 1969; Kirsner et al., 1973; Maisch et al., 1983a,b) (Table 2.3). The observed antibody patterns were identical to those described in rheumatic heart disease, Dressler and post-pericardiotomy syndromes, the "diffuse" being more frequent than the "sarcolemmal-sarcoplasmic" staining pattern. A more recent study on rat heart tissue sections showed high titer (≥1:20) antibodies of IgG class in 59% of patients with myocarditis, 20% of those with DCM, and in no normal control subjects; interestingly these authors suggested that the three main antibody patterns ("diffuse," "peripheral" or "sarcolemmal," and "fibrillary" or "striated") could coexist (Neumann et al., 1990).

Using indirect s-I IFL on 4-μm thick unfixed fresh frozen cryostat sections of blood group O normal human atrium, ventricle and skeletal muscle, and absorption with human heart and skeletal muscle and rat liver, organ-specific antibodies of IgG class were found in about one-third of myocarditis/DCM patients and their symptom-free family members, 1% of patients with other cardiac disease, 3% of normal subjects, and 17% of patients without cardiac disease, but with autoimmune polyendocrinopathy (Caforio et al., 1990a, 1991, 1994, 1997a) (Tables 2.2 and 2.3). Cardiac antibodies of the cross-reactive 1 type, which exhibited partial organ specificity for heart antigens by absorption, were also more frequently detected in DCM/myocarditis patients or in patients with autoimmune polyendocrinopathy than in controls. Conversely, cardiac antibodies of the cross-reactive 2 type, which were entirely skeletal muscle cross-reactive by absorption, were found in similar proportions among groups. No patients with Dressler or post-pericardiotomy syndromes or active rheumatic heart disease were included in these studies.

Sera were tested at 1/10 dilution; cardiac antibody titers in all sera classified as positive were determined by doubling dilutions of sera in phosphate-buffered saline solution. Immunoglobulin classes of the antibodies in the positive sera were also assessed using fluorescein isothiocyanate–labeled sheep anti-human IgG, IgM, and IgA class-specific antisera (Caforio et al., 1990a, 1991, 1997a). The s-I IFL patterns (figures in Caforio et al., 1990a; Betterle et al., 1997) were as follows:

1. Organ-specific: Sera were observed which gave diffuse cytoplasmic staining of both atrial and ventricular myocytes. The staining was stronger in atrial than in ventricular myocytes. These sera were negative on skeletal muscle. The titer range of these antibodies was 1/10 to 1/80 on atrial tissue and 1/10 to 1/20 on ventricular tissue. All positive sera contained antibodies of IgG class and 10% of IgM class. Organ-specific cardiac antibodies' titers fell after absorption with heart homogenate, but were not affected by incubation with skeletal muscle or rat liver.
2. Cross-reactive 1 or "partially organ-specific": Antibodies that gave a fine striational staining pattern on atrium and to a lesser extent on ventricle, but were negative or only weakly stained skeletal muscle sections were classified as "cross-reactive 1" or "partially organ-specific." Their titers ranged from 1/20 to 1/80 on the atrial substrate and from 1/10 to 1/40 on ventricular tissue. All positive sera contained antibodies of IgG class and a few also contained IgM antibodies. Antibody titers in the sera classified as "cross-reactive 1" or "partially organ-specific" were reduced to the same extent after absorption with heart and skeletal muscle and were not affected by absorption with rat liver.
3. Cross-reactive 2: Antibodies that gave a broad striational pattern on longitudinal sections of heart and skeletal muscle were classified as "cross-reactive 2." This pattern had been previously found in 30–40% of sera from myasthenia gravis patients without thymoma and in all myasthenic patients with thymoma (Zweiman and Arnason, 1987). These striational antibodies have been shown to react with the A band of the myofibrils of

striated muscle and cross-react with thymus myoepithelial cells. Cardiac antibodies in the sera classified as "cross-reactive 2" were absorbed by human skeletal muscle and to a lesser extent by heart tissue and not by rat liver.

5.3 Anti-Heart Autoantibodies by s-I IFL: Technical Considerations and Proposed Nomenclature

1. It is preferable to employ O blood group human heart and skeletal muscle to avoid false positive reactions due to heterophile or anti-ABO antibodies. Testing sera on skeletal muscle is necessary to differentiate heart-specific (organ-specific) from cross-reactive patterns (positive on heart and skeletal muscle), and on rat liver and kidney to detect nonorgan-specific mitochondrial or smooth muscle antibodies, which give false positive "muscle reactive" IFL (Nicholson et al., 1977; Caforio et al., 1990a; Betterle et al., 1997). The pattern defined as "intermyofibrillary" is rather rare and might represent antimitochondrial antibodies (Nicholson et al., 1977). A pseudosarcolemmal or "endomysial" interstitial pattern can be observed on some tissue substrates (heart and muscle). It lacks species and tissue specificity, gives a "brush border" staining on proximal tubules of rat kidney and represents a false-positive reaction (Nicholson et al., 1977; Betterle et al., 1997).
2. More recent studies suggest that there is no pure "sarcolemmal" or "peripheral" pattern; these authors observed that sera giving "striated" patterns seem to react more intensely with the periphery of the myofiber, if the section does not include longitudinally cut fibers (Nicholson et al., 1977; Neumann et al., 1990; Caforio et al., 1990a; Betterle et al., 1997). It is important that the section includes longitudinally cut fibers, in order to identify "striated" patterns, not visible on transverse sections.
3. It is important to use standard positive and negative control sera titrated up to end-dilution in every assay, to minimize inter-assay variability (Caforio et al., 1990a; Betterle et al., 1997).
4. New potentially organ-specific patterns (positive on heart, negative or weak positive on muscle) should be confirmed as heart-specific by absorption (Caforio et al., 1990a; Betterle et al., 1997).
5. If absorption is not performed, patterns of anti-heart autoantibodies by s-I IFL should be classified according to those already described and characterized (Nicholson et al., 1977; Caforio et al., 1990a; Betterle et al., 1997), as follows:
   a. "diffuse" (also defined "diffuse-sarcoplasmic" or "organ-specific");
   b. "striated, nonmyasthenic" (also defined "cross-reactive type 1" or "partially organ-specific" or "antifibrillary");
   c. "striated, myasthenic" (also defined "cross-reactive type 2");

d. "diffuse/striated, nonmyasthenic," if a "striated, nonmyasthenic" pattern is superimposed on a diffuse sarcoplasmic stain resulting in a combination of patterns (a) and (b);
e. "antiintercalated disks," isolated or in combination with diffuse or striated stain.

5.4 Autoantibodies to Myosin Heavy Chain and Other Autoantigens by Immunoblotting Techniques

Two of the autoantigens recognized by the cardiac autoantibodies detected by IFL were identified as α and β myosin heavy chain (MHC) isoforms, as well as ventricular light chain type 1 (MLC-1v), by Western blotting; several bands due to yet unknown antigens were also detected in DCM-positive sera (Caforio et al., 1992). These unknown antigens had apparent molecular weight of 30–35 kDa in 50% of positive sera, 55–60 kDa in 21%, 100 kDa in 14%, and 130–150 kDa in 14% (Caforio et al., 1992). The β MHC is expressed in slow skeletal and ventricular myosin and is therefore only partially cardiac-specific. The α isoform is expressed solely within the atrial myocardium. Antibodies to this molecule represent truly organ-specific cardiac autoantibodies. The identification of α and β MHC as relevant autoantigens in DCM patients parallels what is seen in the experimental model of autoimmune myocarditis/DCM (Neu et al., 1987; Smith and Allen, 1991) and in human myocarditis (Caforio et al., 1997a,b; Neumann et al., 1990; Lauer et al., 2000). The finding of anti-MHC and MLC-1v antibodies of IgG class in DCM patients has been independently confirmed using Western blotting (Latif et al., 1993) or ELISA (Limas et al., 1995; Goldman et al., 1995; Michels et al., 1994); a study has suggested that the disease-specific antimyosin antibodies in DCM sera are mainly of IgG3 subclass (Warraich et al., 1999). By Western blot, antibodies to heat shock protein-60 (HSP-60, tropomyosin, and actin have also been found more frequently in DCM sera than in ischemic heart disease controls, but normal sera were not tested (Latif et al., 1993) (Table 2.3). Portig et al. found antibodies to HSP-60 and -70 at higher frequency in DCM sera than in ischemic or normal control subjects (Table 2.3). Latif et al. (1994) later developed a microcytotoxicity assay and showed complement-mediated cytotoxic activity of DCM sera containing anti-heart antibodies by Western blot. DCM, ischemic, and normal control sera were screened using W1, a transformed human fetal cardiac cell line, and also EA.hy 926, an endothelial and IRB3, a fibroblast cell line. In the presence of complement, sera from 28 (62%) DCM patients showed killing of the W1 cell line as compared to sera from 13 (30%) of ischemic patients ($P < .005$) and 3 (15%) normal subjects. Only one DCM patient showed killing of EA.hy 926 cell line, and one ischemic showed killing of the fibroblast cell line. These in vitro data suggest that a complement-dependent, antibody-mediated mechanism of damage to cardiac myocytes may contribute to the pathogenesis of DCM.

5.5 Autoantibodies to Sarcolemmal Na-K-ATPase

A study, using porcine cerebral cortex Na-K-ATPase as an antigen in ELISA and as a substrate in enzyme activity measurement, tested sera from 100 DCM patients and 100 healthy individuals and found anti-Na-K-ATPase autoantibodies in 26% of DCM and 2% of normal subjects (Baba et al., 2002) (Table 2.3). Western blots showed that the antibodies recognized the α subunit, and 3H-ouabain bindings in the presence of patient IgG showed that dissociation constant was higher in DCM patients with antibodies than in those without, suggesting biologic activity for the antibody. Preliminary unpublished observations of these authors showed that the antibodies reacted with the α-3 and not the α-1 subunit isoform. By multiple regression analysis, the presence of anti-Na-K-ATPase autoantibodies was an independent predictor for the occurrence of ventricular tachycardia. Cardiac sudden death was independently predicted by the presence of antibodies, as well as poor systolic function. The authors speculated that these antibodies may lead to electrical instability, because of abnormal Ca^{2+} handling by reduced Na-K-ATPase activity, and delayed after-depolarizations via reverse-mode operation of the Na^{+}/Ca^{2+} exchanger, resulting from increased intracellular Na^{+} concentrations. Although this represents a tantalizing hypothesis, no definitive conclusions on the functional role of these antibodies can be drawn at present. It remains to be seen whether these antibodies are disease-specific for DCM, since no controls with heart failure from other etiologies were studied. It is worth noting that sarcolemmal Na-K-ATPase does not seem to fulfill strict criteria of organ-specific cardiac autoantigen: the α-1 subunit isoform is expressed in most tissues, the α-2 is predominant in skeletal muscle and can be detected in brain and heart, and the α-3 is found in excitable tissues and the α-4 in testis (Urayama et al., 1989; Muller-Ehmsen et al., 2001). Similarly, the β-1 subunit isoform is fairly ubiquitous, whereas the β-2 and β-3 subunit isoforms are mostly found in skeletal muscle, neural tissues, lung, and liver; in human heart, only α-1β-1, α-2β-1, and α-3β-1 heterodimers are present and are thought to be involved in the actions of cardiac glycosides (Schwinger et al., 1999).

5.6 Autoantibodies to Mitochondrial and to Extracellular Matrix Antigens

Using ELISA, autoantibodies against laminin, a large basement membrane glycoprotein, were found in 73–78% of myocarditis/DCM patients and 6% of normal subjects; the authors did not include ischemic heart disease controls, but they reported unpublished data indicating 25–35% prevalence in coronary artery disease (Wolff et al., 1989) (Table 2.3). Antibodies against distinct mitochondrial antigens, the M7 (Klein et al., 1984; Otto et al., 1998), the adenine nucleotide translocator (ANT) (Schultheiss and Bolte, 1985;

Schultheiss et al., 1990), and the branched chain α-ketoacid dehydrogenase dihydrolipoyl transacylase (BCKD-E2) (Ansari et al., 1994) and other respiratory chain enzymes (Pohlner et al., 1997) have also been detected. The M7 antibodies, detected by ELISA, were of IgG class and were found in 31% of DCM patients, 13% of those with myocarditis, 33% of controls with hypertrophic cardiomyopathy, but not in control subjects with other cardiac disease, other immune-mediated disorders, or in normal subjects (Klein et al., 1984) (Table 2.3). The test antigen was represented by different subcellular and submitochondrial beef heart preparations; sera were also tested on submitochondrial particles from pig kidney and rat liver. Using an indirect micro solid-phase radioimmunoassay and ANT, a protein of the internal mitochondrial membrane, purified from beef heart, liver, and kidney as antigen, anti-ANT antibodies were found in 57–91% of myocarditis/DCM sera, and in no controls with ischemic heart disease, or in normal subjects (Schultheiss and Bolte, 1985; Schultheiss et al., 1990) (Table 2.3). Mitochondrial antigens have generally been classified as nonorgan-specific (Bottazzo et al., 1986; Rose and Bona, 1993). However, the heart specificity of the M7 antibodies was shown by absorption studies, whereas these were not performed with the ANT and the BCKD-E2 antibodies. Experimentally induced affinity-purified anti-ANT antibodies cross-reacted with calcium channel complex proteins of rat cardiac myocytes, induced enhancement of transmembrane calcium current and produced calcium-dependent cell lysis in the absence of complement (Schultheiss et al., 1988, 1990). The authors suggested that such enhancing effect of the antibodies might lead to impaired function of the ANT, imbalance of energy delivery and demand within the myocyte, and subsequent cell death in vivo in patients. The presence of this mechanism of antibody-dependent cell lysis has not been shown using the antibodies present in patients' sera.

5.7 Blocking and Stimulating Autoantibodies to β-Adrenergic Receptors

Several groups have demonstrated antibodies against the β_1-adrenoceptor (Wallukat et al., 1991; Limas et al., 1989; Limas and Limas, 1991; Magnusson et al., 1990, 1994). Using a binding inhibition assay (inhibition of marked [^{3}H] dihydroalprenolol binding to rat cardiac membranes), a significant inhibitory activity, attributed to anti-β_1-adrenoceptor antibodies of IgG class, was found in 30–75% of DCM sera, 37% of ischemic or valvular heart disease controls, and 18% of sera from normal subjects (Limas et al., 1989; Limas and Limas, 1991). Positive DCM sera were also found to immunoprecipitate β-adrenoceptors from solubilized cardiac membranes. Antibody-positive sera induced sequestration and endocytosis of β_1-receptors predominantly dependent on the β-receptor kinase and selectively inhibited isoproterenol-sensitive adenylate cyclase activity (Limas et al., 1989; Limas and Limas, 1991). Magnusson et al. (1990), using as antigens synthetic peptides analogous to the sequences of the second extracellular loop of β_1-and β_2-adrenergic receptors by ELISA, found antibodies in 31% of DCM patients, 12% of normal subjects, and in none of the controls with other cardiac disease. The antibodies from DCM sera exhibited inhibitory activity of isoproterenol binding to the β-adrenergic receptor.

Other studies showed that, when analyzed in a functional test system of spontaneously beating neonatal rat myocytes, antibody-positive DCM sera (Wallukat et al., 1991; Jahns et al., 1999, 2000) or the affinity-purified β_1-receptor antibodies (Magnusson et al., 1994) increased the beating frequency of isolated myocytes in vitro. β_1-blocking drugs (propanolol, bisoprolol, and metoprolol) inhibited the effect of the antibodies. These workers reported that the stimulating anti-β_1-receptor antibodies were present in 96% of myocarditis and 26–95% of DCM sera, 8–10% of controls with ischemic heart disease, and 0–19% of normal subjects (Table 2.3). They also suggested that this antibody-mediated stimulation of the β_1-receptor, observed in vitro, could occur in vivo and account for the accelerated decline in ventricular systolic function in some myocarditis/DCM patients.

5.8 Autoantibodies to M2-Muscarinic Receptors

Fu et al. (1993), using as antigen a synthetic peptide analogous to the 169–193 sequence of the second extracellular loop of human M2-muscarinic receptors and the ELISA method, showed anti-M2 antibodies in 39% of DCM sera and 7% of the normal subjects. The presence of these antibodies correlated with the presence of anti-β-receptor antibodies. A limitation of work involving the antireceptor antibodies is that few disease controls have been studied. These receptors are not organ-specific cardiac autoantigens; in fact, their distribution is not restricted to the heart, and there are no cardiac-specific isoforms (Elalouf et al., 1993; Eglen et al., 1994).

5.9 Cardiac-Specific Antibodies in Myocarditis/DCM: Clinical Correlates and Potential Functional Role

The presence of organ- and disease-specific cardiac antibodies of IgG class against myosin and other unknown antigens in myocarditis/DCM patients supports the involvement of autoimmunity in at least one-third of patients (Caforio et al., 1990a; Neumann et al., 1990; Latif et al., 1993; Michels et al., 1994). These antibodies were associated with shorter duration and minor severity of symptoms at diagnosis, as well as with greater exercise capacity (Caforio et al., 1990a, 1997b, 2001). In many patients who were antibody positive at diagnosis, these markers became undetectable at follow-up (Caforio et al., 1997b). These findings strongly suggest that cardiac-specific autoantibodies are early markers. The absence of antibodies at diagnosis in a proportion of patients could indicate that cell-mediated mechanisms are predominant, and/or that autoimmunity is not involved; since the preclinical stage in DCM may be prolonged, it might also relate to reduction of antibody levels with disease progression (Caforio et al., 1997b). These findings have been obtained using standard autoimmune serology techniques, in particular s-I IFL, ELISA, and immunoblotting, and confirmed by several groups (Neumann et al., 1990; Latif et al., 1993; Michels et al., 1994; Limas et al., 1995). The low frequency of cardiac-specific antibodies in control patients with heart dysfunction not due to myocarditis/DCM (Caforio et al., 1990a; Caforio, 1994; Goldman et al., 1995) and the decrease in antibody titers in advanced DCM (Caforio et al., 1997b, 2001) suggest that these markers are not epiphenomena associated with tissue necrosis of various causes, but represent specific markers of immune pathogenesis. The role of inflammatory cytokines (e.g., the IL-2/sIL-2R system) as markers of T-lymphocyte activation in immune-mediated myocarditis/DCM and its relation to cardiac autoantibodies is a controversial issue (Limas et al., 1995; Caforio et al., 2001). In particular, Limas et al. (1995) found that high titer anti-β_1-receptor antibodies were more common among DCM patients with abnormal sIL-2R serum levels. Others found no association between the cardiac-specific autoantibodies found by IFL and the anti-α-myosin antibodies detected by ELISA and sIL-2R levels (Caforio et al., 2001). sIL-2R may be related with distinct autoantibody specificities, e.g., in Graves disease high sIL-2R was associated with anti-TSH receptor autoantibodies but was unrelated to the autoantibodies to intracellular antigens (antimicrosomal and antithyroglobulin) (Balazs and Farid, 1991). The same may apply to DCM, high sIL-2R being present in association with antibodies to extracellular, e.g., the anti-β_1-receptor, rather than intracellular antigens, e.g., α-myosin and the other cardiac-specific antigens involved in the IFL reaction. The cardiac-specific autoantibodies found by IFL and the anti-α-myosin antibodies detected by ELISA were found in similar proportions of patients with DCM and biopsy-proven myocarditis according to the Dallas criteria, included in the Myocarditis Treatment Trial (Mason et al., 1995), suggesting that conventional histology does not distinguish between patients with and without an ongoing immune-mediated process in myocarditis/DCM (Caforio et al., 1997a, 2013). The Myocarditis Treatment Trial failed to show an improvement in survival in biopsy-proven myocarditis with immunosuppressive therapy; however, no immunohistochemical or serological markers (e.g., increased HLA expression on endomyocardial biopsy and/or detection of cardiac-specific autoantibodies in the serum in the absence of viral genome in myocardial tissue) were used to identify those patients with immune-mediated pathogenesis in whom immunosuppression could have been beneficial (Mason et al., 1995). Interestingly, a subsequent, randomized, placebo control study in DCM patients with HLA upregulation on endomyocardial biopsy showed long-term benefit with immunosuppressive treatment (Wojnicz et al., 2001). In addition, the TIMIC trial showed that immunosuppressive therapy is beneficial in virus-negative myocarditis (Frustaci et al., 2009). Myocarditis/DCM patients with cardiac-specific autoantibodies should be included in future trials of immunosuppressive therapy. A recent European Society of Cardiology expert consensus document recommends immunosuppression in virus-negative myocarditis refractory to standard heart failure and antiarrhythmia treatment (Caforio et al., 2013).

Myosin fulfilled the expected criteria for organ-specific autoimmunity, in that immunization with cardiac but not skeletal myosin reproduced, in susceptible mouse strains, the human disease phenotype of DCM (Neu et al., 1987; Smith and Allen, 1991). In this respect, less experimental data are available with other autoantigens. However, autoimmune diseases are often polyclonal, with production of autoantibodies to different autoantigens. Some of these autoantigens are involved earlier in disease and are more closely related to primary pathogenetic events compared to those, which play a role in secondary immunopathogenesis (Rose and Bona, 1993). Both experimental and clinical evidences, in particular the multiplicity of autoantibody specificities identified so far (Table 2.3), exist that this also applies to myocarditis/DCM. Myosin is an intracellular protein; thus there are two major hypotheses, which may not be mutually exclusive, to explain interruption of tolerance to this autoantigen. These include molecular mimicry, since cross-reactive epitopes between cardiac myosin and infectious agents have been found, and myocyte necrosis due to viral infection or other tissue insults (Horwitz et al., 2000; Galvin et al., 2000; Rose, 2000). Both mechanisms would explain the association of viral infection with autoimmune myocarditis/DCM. Infection with Coxsackie B3 (CB3) virus triggers anti-myosin reactivity and autoimmune myocarditis in many mouse strains, and immunization with cardiac myosin induces disease in the same susceptible strains (Neu et al., 1987; Smith and Allen, 1991). In some strains, such as Balb/c mice, CB3 virus-induced or myosin-induced myocarditis is T cell-mediated (Smith and Allen, 1991), whereas in other strains, such as DBA/2 mice, it is an antibody-mediated disease (Kuan et al., 2000). The same may apply to humans, so that the anti-myosin antibodies may be directly pathogenic in some (Lauer et al., 2000) but not all patients with myocarditis/DCM (Caforio et al., 1997b) according to different immunogenetic backgrounds, isotype (Kuan et al., 2000), and/or subclass specificity of these antibodies (Warraich et al., 1999).

In relation to the proposed functional role of antibodies, e.g., the anti-receptor and some of antimitochondrial antibodies (Table 2.3) in man, passive transfer of the myocarditis/DCM phenotype to genetically susceptible animals by antibody-positive patients' sera would provide conclusive evidence for antibody-mediated pathogenesis. A recent study suggests that serum anti-heart autoantibodies detected by s-I IFL in myocarditis patients passively transfer histologically proven myocarditis to mice (Caforio et al., 2015b). Nonantigen-specific IgG adsorption has recently been used in DCM patients with high titer antibodies to the β_1-receptor, and it has been suggested that it has beneficial clinical effects, accompanied by undetectable antibody titers during follow-up (Muller et al., 2000). This does not imply a direct pathogenic effect of the anti-

β_1-receptor antibodies. The adsorption technique used was nonantigen-specific; in addition, in antibody-mediated disorders the antibody titers rise again at the end of plasmapheresis. However, the authors have recently provided new evidence in favor of the possibility that the beneficial effect of immunoadsorption is related to removal of pathogenic cardiodepressant autoantibodies of IgG3 subclass, although no conclusion is possible on the potential pathogenic role of a specific autoantibody (e.g., β_1-receptor antibody) (Schimke et al., 2001; Felix et al., 2002; Staudt et al., 2002). It may be that this technique has a favorable immunomodulatory/immunosuppressive effect; in addition, IgG substitution performed after immunoadsorption to avoid infective complications of unselective IgG depletion may have contributed to the observed hemodynamic improvement (Mann, 2001; Gullestad et al., 2001); randomized studies are in progress. This does not undermine the possible role of any of the described antibodies (Table 2.3) as predictive markers. Subjects classified as negative for one antibody may be positive for another and combined testing may be advantageous. To this end, standardization of nomenclature and protocols for antibody detection and exchange of sera among laboratories currently assessing the individual antibodies will be useful.

In autoimmune disorders, circulating autoantibodies identify symptom-free subjects at risk years before clinical presentation. So far, the clinical and prognostic significance of cardiac autoantibodies has been prospectively assessed only for serum anti-heart autoantibodies detected by s-I IFL in symptom free relatives of DCM index patients, not for the other published autoantibodies. Healthy relatives of patients with DCM who have echocardiographic changes, including left ventricular enlargement or depressed fractional shortening at baseline, have increased medium-term risk for DCM development (Caforio et al., 2007). Approximately one-third of relatives from both familial and non-familial pedigrees have serum anti-heart autoantibodies detected by s-I IFL at baseline (Caforio et al., 1994). Prospective family studies have shown that anti-heart autoantibodies detected by s-I IFL are independent predictors of DCM development in symptom-free relatives at 5-year follow-up (Caforio et al., 2007).

In conclusion, several groups have shown that a subset of patients with myocarditis/idiopathic DCM and their symptom-free relatives has circulating heart-reactive autoantibodies. These autoantibodies are directed against multiple antigens, some of which are strictly expressed in the myocardium (e.g., organ specific for the heart) and others are expressed in heart and skeletal muscle (e.g., muscle specific). Distinct autoantibodies have also different prevalence in disease and normal controls (e.g., by IFL the organ-specific antibodies are disease specific for DCM, some of the muscle-specific antibodies are not). Different antibody techniques detect one (e.g., ELISA for myosin or for antireceptor antibodies) or more antibody specificities (e.g., indirect IFL), thus they cannot be used interchangeably as screening tools. Antibody frequency in DCM versus controls is expected to be different using distinct techniques; at present it is unknown whether the same subset (30–40%) of patients produces more than one antibody or different patient groups develop autoimmunity to different antigens. Antibodies of IgG class, which are shown to be cardiac and disease specific for myocarditis/DCM, can be used as reliable markers of autoimmune pathogenesis for identifying patients, in whom immunosuppression and/or immunomodulation therapy may be beneficial, and their relatives at risk. Some of these autoantibodies may also have a functional role in patients, as suggested by in vitro data as well as by new clinical observations, but further work is needed to clarify this important issue.

6. IDIOPATHIC TACHY AND BRADYARRHYTHMIAS

Idiopathic AV conduction blocks or other bradyarrhythmias may be seen in association with organ-specific or nonorgan-specific conditions. This led earlier investigators to hypothesize potential immune pathogenetic mechanisms. Cardiac conducting tissue antibodies (CCTA) were first reported by s-I IFI-S in patients with chronic AV block (Fairfax and Doniach, 1976). The antibodies were of IgG class, complement fixing, and with titers between 1/10 and 1/80. More recently, stimulating antibodies against β_1- and β_2-adrenoceptors were found by ELISA in patients with primary electrical cardiac abnormalities, in particular conduction disease or tachyarrhythmia (Chiale et al., 1995). There are nonorgan-specific autoantibodies, which may be associated with cardiac CDs, such as the anti-SSA/Ro anti-nRNP specificities (Scott et al., 1983), but these are covered in another chapter.

6.1 Cardiac Conducting Tissue Antibodies

The s-I IFL substrate for CCTA detection was ox heart false tendon (Fairfax and Doniach, 1976; Villecco et al., 1983; Obiassi et al., 1987). This tissue was used because it is well known that in ox heart, the false tendon contains the right bundle branch block (RBBB) and in ungulates, Purkinje cells are easily distinguishable from ordinary working myocardial cells by light microscopy. The presence of Purkinje cells was also confirmed on tissue sections by histochemical reactions for myosin ATPase and phosphorilase. Cryostat-cut sections were incubated with sera diluted 1/10, and fluorescein-labeled anti-human IgG, A, M, and C3 antisera were used for CCTA detection. In the study by Obiassi et al., CCTA-positive sera stained only Purkinje cells.

Fairfax and Doniach (1976) found CCTA in 8.6% of patients with idiopathic AV block, 4.5% of those with blocks of known cause, and 4.2% of healthy controls (Table 2.2).

CCTA were also found in 76% rheumatoid arthritis (RA) patients with RBBB and 20% of those without RBBB, but were rare in RBBB without RA (Villecco et al., 1983) (Table 2.2).

Obiassi et al. (1987) subsequently reported CCTA reacting only with Purkinje cells in 14–21% of patients with connective tissue disease (systemic lupus erythematosus, AR, Sjogren syndrome, progressive systemic sclerosis) and AV blocks, 30% of patients implanted with permanent pace-makers for nonischemic AV blocks, 34.5% of those with idiopathic block at or below the His bundle, and 11% of normal subjects.

6.2 Stimulating Autoantibodies to β-Adrenergic Receptors

Chiale et al. (1995), using as antigens synthetic peptides analogous to the sequences of the second extracellular loop of β_1- and β_2-adrenergic receptors by ELISA, found stimulating anti-β_1-antibodies at higher frequency in patients with DCM (38%) and in idiopathic VA (47.6%) compared to both normal (19%) and cardiomyopathy controls (6.2%) (Table 2.2). Conversely the antibody frequency in patients with CD (28.5%) or primary atrial arrhythmia (AA) (13.6%) was similar to that seen in normal and cardiomyopathy controls. In addition, they reported a higher frequency of anti-β_2-antibodies in VA (23.8%) compared to cardiopathic (3%) but not the healthy control subjects (14.7%). The authors suggest that the agonist- or catecholamine-like effects mediated by these antibodies may play a role in facilitating the occurrence of VA and the development of chronic myocardial dysfunction and DCM. However, prospective studies are needed to determine whether or not these antibodies are predictive markers of DCM development in patients with idiopathic arrhythmia and normal systolic function.

7. SYSTEMIC ARTERIAL HYPERTENSION

Systemic arterial hypertension is a syndrome of heterogeneous etiology and pathogenesis. An increased frequency of anti-heart autoantibodies to several antigens has recently been reported, suggesting that autoimmune mechanisms might be involved in selected patient subgroups.

7.1 Anti-Heart Autoantibodies by s-I IFL

Caforio et al. (1991) reported organ-specific anti-heart autoantibodies in 17% of sera from patients with autoimmune polyendocrinopathy, in the absence of symptoms and ECG and/or echocardiographic evidence of cardiac dysfunction (Table 2.2). However, a higher frequency of systemic arterial hypertension was found among antibody-positive patients. The authors concluded that the antibodies might represent markers of an autoimmune form of hypertension, although prospective studies were needed to confirm their hypothesis.

7.2 Stimulating Autoantibodies to α_1-Adrenergic Receptors

Fu and Herlitz (1994), using as antigens synthetic peptides analogous to the sequences of the second extracellular loop of α_1-adrenergic receptor by

ELISA, found stimulating anti-α_1-antibodies of mainly IgM isotype in 4 (12%) of 33 normal controls, 3 (20%) of 15 patients with malignant essential hypertension, and 7 (64%) of 11 with secondary malignant hypertension (Table 2.2). The patients' antibodies caused a decrease in tritiated prazosin–binding sites and an increase in heart beating frequency of neonatal cultured rat cardiomyocytes; antibodies purified from the controls had no effect. These workers concluded that these autoantibodies had agonist-like activity, although it remained to be further investigated whether they were merely markers of a subgroup of patients with malignant hypertension or had a pathogenetic role.

Luther et al. (1997) subsequently showed that when analyzed in a functional test system of spontaneously beating neonatal rat myocytes, the Ig fractions of sera from 24 (44%) patients with primary hypertension and 3 (12%) normotensive controls contained antibodies against α_1-adrenergic receptor (Table 2.2). The autoantibodies increased the beating frequency of isolated myocytes in vitro, an effect that was blocked by α_1-adrenergic antagonists. Since the functional characteristics of the autoantibodies showed no desensitization phenomena, the authors suggested that they might play a role in increasing vascular resistance and promoting cardiac hypertrophy in primary hypertension.

7.3 Stimulating Autoantibodies to the Angiotensin Receptor

Fu et al. (2000), using ELISA, studied the presence of autoantibodies against G-protein–coupled cardiovascular receptors in malignant essential hypertension (n = 14), secondary malignant hypertension due to renovascular disease (n = 12), renovascular disease without malignant hypertension (n = 11), and normotensive healthy blood donors (n = 35). They found stimulating anti-angiotensin type 1 receptor (AT1) antibodies in 14%, 33%, 18%, and 14% of patients with malignant essential hypertension, secondary malignant hypertension, renovascular disease, and normotensives, respectively (Table 2.2); no antibodies to bradykinin (B2) or angiotensin II subtype 2 (AT2) receptors.

Wallukat et al. (1999) analyzed in a functional test system of spontaneously beating neonatal rat myocytes, the Ig fractions of sera from 25 preeclamptic patients and compared them with those of 12 normotensive pregnant women and 10 pregnant patients with primary hypertension. Antibodies were detected by the chronotropic response to AT1 receptor–mediated stimulation of the rat myocytes coupled with receptor-specific antagonists. Ig from all preeclamptic patients, but not from controls, stimulated the AT1 receptor; this activity decreased after delivery. Affinity-column purification, peptide inhibition, and Western blot experiments identified this activity as due to agonistic IgG antibodies against the second extracellular AT1 receptor loop. Confocal microscopy of vascular smooth muscle cells showed colocalization of purified patient IgG and AT1 receptor antibody. It was subsequently shown that these antibodies induce vascular cells to express tissue factor and stimulate NADPH oxidase (Dechend et al., 2000, 2003). These data suggest that they may contribute to the pathogenesis of preeclampsia (Roberts, 2000).

REFERENCES

Ansari, A.A., Neckelmann, N., Villinger, F., 1994. Epitope mapping of the branched chain α-ketoacid dehydrogenase dihydrolipoyl transacylase (BCKD-E2) protein that reacts with sera from patients with idiopathic dilated cardiomyopathy. J. Immunol. 153, 4754.

Aretz, H.T., Billingham, M.E., Edwards, W.E., 1985. Myocarditis: a histopathologic definition and classification. Am. J. Cardiol. Pathol. 1, 1.

Baba, A., Yoshikawa, T., Ogawa, S., 2002. Autoantibodies against sarcolemmal Na-K-ATPase: possible upstream targets of arrhythmias and sudden death in patients with dilated cardiomyopathy. J. Am. Coll. Cardiol. 40, 1153.

Baig, M.K., Goldman, J.H., Caforio, A.L.P., 1998. Familial dilated cardiomyopathy: cardiac abnormalities are common in asymptomatic relatives and may represent early disease. J. Am. Coll. Cardiol. 31, 195.

Balazs, C.Z., Farid, N.R., 1991. Soluble IL-2 receptor in sera of patients with Graves' disease. J. Autoimmun. 4, 681.

Bauer, H., Waters, T.J., Talano, J.V., 1972. Antimyocardial antibodies in patients with coronary heart disease. Am. Heart J. 83, 612.

Bessen, D., Jones, K.F., Fischetti, V.A., 1989. Evidence for two distinct classes of streptococcal M protein and their relationship to rheumatic fever. J. Exp. Med. 169, 269.

Betterle, C., Spadaccino, A.C., Pedini, B., 1997. Autoanticorpi nelle malattie autoimmuni del muscolo scheletrico, della giunzione neuro-muscolare e del cuore. In: Betterle, C. (Ed.), Gli autoanticorpi. Manuale-Atlante a colori di diagnostica, p. 313.

Bottazzo, G.F., Todd, I., Mirakian, R., 1986. Organ-specific autoimmunity. A 1986 overview. Immunol. Rev. 94, 137.

Caforio, A.L.P., 1994. Role of autoimmunity in dilated cardiomyopathy. Br. Heart J. 72, S30.

Caforio, A.L., Marcolongo, R., Basso, C., Iliceto, S., 2015. Clinical presentation and diagnosis of myocarditis. Heart 101, 1332.

Caforio, A.L.P., Bonifacio, E., Stewart, J.T., 1990. Novel organ-specific circulating cardiac autoantibodies in dilated cardiomyopathy. J. Am. Coll. Cardiol. 15, 1527.

Caforio, A.L.P., Stewart, J.T., Bonifacio, E., 1990. Inappropriate major histocompatibility complex expression on cardiac tissue in dilated cardiomyopathy. Relevance for autoimmunity? J. Autoimmun. 3, 187.

Caforio, A.L.P., Wagner, R., Jaswinder, S.G., 1991. Organ-specific cardiac antibodies: serological markers for systemic hypertension in autoimmune polyendocrinopathy. Lancet 337, 1111.

Caforio, A.L.P., Grazzini, M., Mann, J.M., 1992. Identification of α and β cardiac myosin heavy chain isoforms as major autoantigens in dilated cardiomyopathy. Circulation 85, 1734.

Caforio, A.L.P., Keeling, P.J., Zachara, E., 1994. Evidence from family studies for autoimmunity in dilated cardiomyopathy. Lancet 344, 773.

Caforio, A.L.P., Goldman, J.H., Haven, A.J., 1997. Circulating cardiac autoantibodies as markers of autoimmunity in clinical and biopsy-proven myocarditis. Eur. Heart J. 18, 270.

Caforio, A.L.P., Goldman, J.H., Baig, K.M., 1997. Cardiac autoantibodies in dilated cardiomyopathy become undetectable with disease progression. Heart 77, 62.

Caforio, A.L.P., Goldman, J.H., Baig, K.M., 2001. Elevated serum levels of soluble interleukin-2 receptor, neopterin and β-2 microglobulin in idiopathic dilated cardiomyopathy: relation to disease severity and autoimmune pathogenesis. Eur. J. Heart Fail. 3, 155.

Caforio, A.L.P., Mahon, N.J., Tona, F., 2002. Circulating cardiac autoantibodies in dilated cardiomyopathy and myocarditis: pathogenetic and clinical significance. Eur. J. Heart Fail. 4, 411.

Caforio, A.L.P., Pankuweit, S., Arbustini, E., 2013. Current state of knowledge on aetiology, diagnosis, management, and therapy of myocarditis: a position statement of the European Society of Cardiology Working Group on Myocardial and Pericardial Diseases. Eur. Heart J. 34, 2636.

Caforio, A.L.P., Mahon, N.G., Baig, M.K., et al., 2007. Prospective familial assessment in dilated cardiomyopathy: cardiac autoantibodies predict disease development in asymptomatic relatives. Circulation 115, 76.

Caforio, A.L.P., Brucato, A., Doria, A., et al., 2010. Anti-heart and anti-intercalated disk autoantibodies: evidence for autoimmunity in idiopathic recurrent acute pericarditis. Heart 96, 779.

Caforio, A.L.P., Angelini, A., Blank, M., et al., 2015. Passive transfer of affinity-purified anti-heart autoantibodies (AHA) from sera of patients with myocarditis induces experimental myocarditis in mice. Int. J. Cardiol. 179, 166.

Camp, F.T., Hess, E.V., Conway, G., 1969. Immunologic findings in idiopathic cardiomyopathy. Am. Heart J. 77, 610.

Chiale, P.A., Rosembaum, M.B., Elizari, M.V., 1995. High prevalence of antibodies against β_1- and β_2-adrenoceptors in patients with primary electrical cardiac abnormalities. J. Am. Coll. Cardiol. 26, 864.

Dajani, A.S., Ayoub, E.M., Bierman, F.Z., 1992. Guidelines for the diagnosis of rheumatic fever: Jones criteria, updated 1992. JAMA 268, 2069.

Dale, J.B., Beachey, E.H., 1986. Sequence of myosin cross-reactive epitopes of streptococcal M protein. J. Exp. Med. 164, 1785.

Dechend, R., Homuth, V., Wallukat, G., 2000. AT1 receptor antibodies from preeclamptic patients cause vascular cells to express tissue factor. Circulation 101, 2382.

Dechend, R., Viedt, C., Muller, D.N., 2003. AT1 receptor agonistic antibodies from preeclamptic patients stimulate NADPH oxidase. Circulation 107, 1632.

Dressler, W.A., 1956. Post-myocardial infarction syndrome: preliminary report of a complication resembling idiopathic recurrent benign pericarditis. JAMA 160, 1379.

Dressler, W., 1959. The Post-myocardial infarction syndrome. A report of forty-four cases. Arch. Intern. Med. 103, 28.

Eglen, R.M., Reddy, H., Watson, N., 1994. Muscarinic acetylcholine receptor subtypes in smooth muscle. Trends Pharmacol. Sci. 15, 114.

Elalouf, J.M., Buhler, J.M., Tessiot, C., 1993. Predominant expression of beta 1-adrenergic receptor in the thick ascending limb of rat kidney: absolute mRNA quantitation by reverse transcription and polymerase chain reaction. J. Clin. Invest. 91, 264.

Engle, M.A., McCabe, J.C., Ebert, P.A., 1974. The postpericardiotomy syndrome and anti-heart antibodies. Circulation 49, 401.

Escaned, J., Ahmad, R.A., Shiu, M.F., 1992. Pleural effusion following coronary perforation during balloon angioplasty: an unusual presentation of the postpericardiotomy syndrome. Eur. Heart J. 13, 716.

Fairfax, J.A., Doniach, D., 1976. Autoantibodies to cardiac conducting tissue and their characterization by immunofluorescence. Clin. Exp. Immunol. 23, 1.

Felix, S.B., Staudt, A., Landsberger, M., 2002. Removal of cardiodepressant antibodies in dilated cardiomyopathy by immunoadsorption. J. Am. Coll. Cardiol. 39, 646.

Felsh, G., 1966. The anti-globulin consumption test in rheumatic carditis. Dtsch. Med. Wochenschr. 91, 2197.

Fletcher, G.F., Wenger, N.K., 1968. Autoimmune studies in patients with primary myocardial disease. Circulation 37, 1032.

Frustaci, A., Russo, M.A., Chimenti, C., 2009. Randomized study on the efficacy of immunosuppressive therapy in patients with virus-negative inflammatory cardiomyopathy: the TIMIC study. Eur. Heart J. 30, 1995.

Fu, L.X., Herlitz, H., 1994. Functional autoimmune epitope on α_1-adrenergic receptors in patients with malignant hypertension. Lancet 344, 1660.

Fu, L.X., Magnusson, Y., Bergh, C.H., 1993. Localization of a functional autoimmune epitope on the muscarinic acetylcholine receptor-2 in patients with idiopathic dilated cardiomyopathy. J. Clin. Invest. 91, 1964.

Fu, L.X., Herlitz, H., Schultze, W., 2000. Autoantibodies against the angiotensin receptor (AT1) in patients with hypertension. J. Hypertens. 18, 945.

Galvin, J.E., Hemric, M.E., Ward, K., 2000. Cytotoxic mAb from rheumatic carditis recognizes heart valves and laminin. J. Clin. Invest. 106, 217.

Goldman, J.H., Keeling, P.J., Warraich, R.S., 1995. Autoimmunity to α-myosin in a subset of patients with idiopathic dilated cardiomyopathy. Br. Heart J. 74, 598.

Gullestad, L., Aass, H., Fjeld, J.G., et al., 2001. Immunomodulating therapy with intravenous immunoglobulin in patients with chronic heart failure. Circulation 103, 220.

Heine, W.I., Friedman, H., Mandell, M.S., 1966. Antibodies to cardiac tissue in acute ischemic heart disease. Am. J. Cardiol. 77, 798.

Hess, E.V., Fink, C.W., Taranta, A., 1964. Heart muscle antibodies in rheumatic fever and other diseases. J. Clin. Invest. 43, 886.

Horwitz, M.S., La Cava, A., Fine, C., 2000. Pancreatic expression of interferon-γ protects mice from lethal coxsackievirus B3 infection and subsequent myocarditis. Nat. Med. 6, 693.

Itoh, K., Ohkumi, H., Kimura, E., 1969. Immuno-serological studies on myocardial infarction and postmyocardial infarction syndrome. Jpn. Heart J. 10, 485.

Jahns, R., Boivin, V., Siegmund, C., 1999. Autoantibodies activating human β1-adrenergic receptors are associated with reduced cardiac function in chronic heart failure. Circulation 99, 649.

Jahns, R., Boivin, V., Krapf, T., 2000. Modulation of β1-adrenoceptor activity by domain-specific antibodies and heart-failure associated autoantibodies. J. Am. Coll. Cardiol. 36, 1280.

Jones, T.D., 1944. The diagnosis of rheumatic fever. JAMA 126, 481.

Kaplan, M.H., Dallenbach, F.D., 1961. Immunologic studies of heart tissue. III. Occurrence of bound gamma globulin in auricular appendages from rheumatic hearts. Relationship to certain histopathologic features of rheumatic heart disease. J. Exp. Med. 113, 1.

Kaplan, M.H., Frengley, D.J., 1969. Autoimmunity to the heart in cardiac disease. Current concepts of the relation of autoimmunity to rheumatic fever, postcardiotomy and postinfarction syndromes and cardiomyopathies. Am. J. Cardiol. 24, 459.

Kaplan, M.H., Svec, K.H., 1964. Immunologic relation of streptococcal and tissue antigens. III. Presence in human sera of streptococcal antibody cross-reactive with heart tissue. Association with streptococcal infection, rheumatic fever, and glomerulonephritis. J. Exp. Med. 119, 651.

Kaplan, M.H., Meyeserian, M., Kushner, I., 1961. Immunologic studies of heart tissue. IV. Serologic reactions with human heart tissue as revealed by immunofluorescent methods: isoimmune, Wassermann, and autoimmune reactions. J. Exp. Med. 113, 17.

Kaplan, M.H., Bolande, R., Rakita, L., 1964. Presence of bound immunoglobulins and complement in the myocardium in acute rheumatic fever. N. Engl. J. Med. 271, 637.

Kirsner, A.B., Hess, E.V., Fowler, N.O., 1973. Immunologic findings in idiopathic cardiomyopathy: a prospective serial study. Am. Heart J. 86, 625.

Klein, R., Maisch, B., Kochsiek, K., 1984. Demonstration of organ specific antibodies against heart mitochondria (anti-M7) in sera from patients with some forms of heart diseases. Clin. Exp. Immunol. 58, 283.

Kleinsorge, H., Dornbusch, S., Romer, R., 1960. Autoimmunization bei entzundlichen und degenerativen Herz krankungen. Int. Arch. Allergy 16, 200.

Krisher, K., Cunningham, M.W., 1985. Myosin: a link between streptococci and heart. Science 227, 413.

Kuan, A.P., Zuckier, L., Liao, L., 2000. Immunoglobulin isotype determines pathogenicity in antibody-mediated myocarditis in naïve mice. Circ. Res. 86, 281.

Latif, N., Baker, C.S., Dunn, M.J., 1993. Frequency and specificity of antiheart antibodies in patients with dilated cardiomyopathy detected using SDS-PAGE and western blotting. J. Am. Coll. Cardiol. 22, 1378.

Latif, N., Smith, J., Dunn, M.J., 1994. Complement-mediated cytotoxic activity of anti-heart antibodies present in the sera of patients with dilated cardiomyopathy. Autoimmunity 19, 99.

Lauer, B., Schannwell, M., Kuhl, U., 2000. Antimyosin autoantibodies are associated with deterioration of systolic and diastolic left ventricular function in patients with chronic myocarditis. J. Am. Coll. Cardiol. 35, 11.

Ledford, D.K., Espinoza, L.R., 1987. Immunologic aspects of cardiovascular disease. JAMA 20, 2974.

Limas, C.J., Limas, C., 1991. β-Receptor antibodies and genetics in dilated cardiomyopathy. Eur. Heart J. 12 (Suppl. D), 175.

Limas, C.J., Goldenberg, I.F., Limas, C., 1989. Autoantibodies against β-adrenoceptors in idiopathic dilated cardiomyopathy. Circ. Res. 64, 97.

Limas, C.J., Goldenberg, I.F., Limas, C., 1995. Soluble interleukin-2 receptor levels in patients with dilated cardiomyopathy. Correlation with disease severity and cardiac autoantibodies. Circulation 91, 631.

Luther, H.P., Homuth, V., Wallukat, G., 1997. α_1-adrenergic receptor antibodies in patients with primary hypertension. Hypertension 29, 678.

Magnusson, Y., Marullo, S., Hoyer, S., 1990. Mapping of a functional autoimmune epitope on the β-adrenergic receptor in patients with idiopathic dilated cardiomyopathy. J. Clin. Invest. 86, 1658.

Magnusson, Y., Wallukat, G., Waagstein, F., 1994. Autoimmunity in idiopathic dilated cardiomyopathy: characterization of antibodies against the β_1-adrenoceptor with positive chronotropic effect. Circulation 89, 2760.

Mahon, N.G., Madden, B., Caforio, A.L.P., 2002. Immunohistochemical evidence of myocardial disease in apparently healthy relatives of patients with dilated cardiomyopathy. J. Am. Coll. Cardiol. 39, 455.

Maisch, B., Berg, P., Kochsiek, K., 1979. Clinical significance of immunopathological findings in patients with post-pericardiotomy syndrome: relevance of antibody pattern. Clin. Exp. Immunol. 38, 189.

Maisch, B., Deeg, P., Liebau, G., 1983. Diagnostic relevance of humoral and cytotoxic immune reactions in primary and secondary dilated cardiomyopathy. Am. J. Cardiol. 52, 1071.

Maisch, B., Deeg, P., Liebau, G., 1983. Diagnostic relevance of humoral and cell-mediated immune reactions in patients with viral myocarditis. Clin. Exp. Immun. 48, 533.

Mann, D.L., 2001. Autoimmunity, immunoglobulin adsorption and dilated cardiomyopathy: has the time come for randomized clinical trials? J. Am. Coll. Cardiol. 38, 184.

Mason, J.W., O'Connell, J.B., Herskowitz, A., 1995. A clinical trial of immunosuppressive therapy for myocarditis. N. Engl. J. Med. 333, 269.

Meder, B., Rühle, F., Weis, T., et al., 2014. A genome-wide association study identifies 6p21 as novel risk locus for dilated cardiomyopathy. Eur. Heart J. 35, 1069.

Michels, V.V., Moll, P.P., Rodeheffer, R.J., 1994. Circulating heart autoantibodies in familial as compared with nonfamilial idiopathic dilated cardiomyopathy. Mayo Clin. Proc. 69, 24.

Muller, J., Wallukat, G., Dandel, M., 2000. Immunoglobulin adsorption in patients with idiopathic dilated cardiomyopathy. Circulation 101, 385.

Muller-Ehmsen, J., Juvvadi, P., Thompson, C.B., 2001. Ouabain and substrate affinities of human Na-K-ATPase α-1β-1, α-2β-1, α-3β-1 when expressed separately in yeast cells. Am. J. Physiol. Cell. Physiol. 281, C1355.

Neu, N., Rose, N.R., Beisel, K.W., 1987. Cardiac myosin induces myocarditis in genetically predisposed mice. J. Immunol. 139, 3630.

Neumann, D.A., Burek, C.L., Baughman, K.L., 1990. Circulating heart-reactive antibodies in patients with myocarditis or cardiomyopathy. J. Am. Coll. Cardiol. 16, 839.

Nicholson, G.C., Dawkins, R.L., McDonald, B.L., 1977. A classification of anti-heart antibodies: differentiation between heart-specific and heterophile antibodies. Clin. Immunol. Immunopathol. 7, 349.

Obiassi, M., Brucato, A., Meroni, P.L., 1987. Antibodies to cardiac Purkinje cell: further characterization in autoimmune diseases and atrioventricular heart block. Clin. Immunol. Immunopathol. 42, 141.

Otto, A., Stahle, I., Klein, R., 1998. Anti-mitochondrial antibodies in patients with dilated cardiomyopathy (anti-M7) are directed against flavoenzymes with covalently bound FAD. Clin. Exp. Immunol. 111, 541.

Peters, R.W., Scheinman, M.M., Raskin, S., 1980. Unusual complications of epicardial pacemakers. Am. J. Cardiol. 45, 1088.

Pohlner, K., Portig, I., Pankuweit, S., 1997. Identification of mitochondrial antigens recognized by antibodies in sera of patients with idiopathic dilated cardiomyopathy by two-dimensional gel electrophoresis and protein sequencing. Am. J. Cardiol. 80, 1040.

Portig, I., Pankuweit, S., Maisch, B., 1997. Antibodies against stress proteins in sera of patients with dilated cardiomyopathy. J. Mol. Cell. Cardiol. 29, 2245.

Richardson, P., McKenna, W.J., Bristow, M., 1996. Report of the 1995 World Health Organization/International Society and Federation of Cardiology Task Force on the definition and classification of cardiomyopathies. Circulation 93, 841.

Roberts, J.M., 2000. Angiotensin-1 receptor autoantibodies. A role in the pathogenesis of preeclampsia? Circulation 101, 2335.

Robinson, J.H., Kehoe, M.A., 1992. Group A streptococcal M proteins: virulence factors and protective antigens. Immunol. Today 13, 362.

Rose, N.R., 2000. Viral damage or 'molecular mimicry'—placing the blame in myocarditis. Nat. Med. 6, 631.

Rose, N.R., Bona, C., 1993. Defining criteria for autoimmune diseases (Witebsky's postulates revisited). Immunol. Today 14, 426.

Schimke, I., Muller, J., Priem, F., 2001. Decreased oxidative stress in patients with idiopathic dilated cardiomyopathy one year after immunoglobulin adsorption. J. Am. Coll. Cardiol. 38, 178.

Schultheiss, H.P., Bolte, H.D., 1985. Immunological analysis of auto-antibodies against the adenine nucleotide translocator in dilated cardiomyopathy. J. Mol. Cell. Cardiol. 17, 603.

Schultheiss, H.P., Ulrich, G., Janda, I., 1988. Antibody mediated enhancement of calcium permeability in cardiac myocytes. J. Exp. Med. 168, 2105.
Schultheiss, H.P., Kuhl, U., Schwimmbeck, P., 1990. Biomolecular changes in dilated cardiomyopathy. In: Baroldi, G., Camerini, F., Goodwin, J.F. (Eds.), Advances in Cardiomyopathies, p. 221.
Schwinger, R.H.G., Wang, J., Frank, K., 1999. Reduced sodium pump α1-, α2-, β1-isoform protein levels and Na,K-ATPase activity but unchanged Na/Ca exchanger protein levels in human heart failure. Circulation 99, 2105.
Scott, J.S., Maddison, P.J., Taylor, P.V., 1983. Connective-tissue disease, antibodies to ribonucleoptrotein, and congenital heart block. N. Engl. J. Med. 309, 209.
Smith, S.C., Allen, P.M., 1991. Myosin-induced myocarditis is a T cell-mediated disease. J. Immunol. 147, 2141.
Staudt, A., Bohm, M., Knebel, F., 2002. Potential role of autoantibodies belonging to the immunoglobulin G-3 subclass in cardiac dysfunction among patients with dilated cardiomyopathy. Circulation 106, 2448.
Urayama, O., Shutt, H., Sweadner, J., 1989. Identification of three isozyme proteins of the catalytic subunit of the Na,K-ATPase in rat brain. J. Biol. Chem. 264, 8271.
Van der Geld, H., 1964. Anti-heart antibodies in the postcardiotomy and postmyocardial infarction syndrome. Lancet II, 617.
Villecco, A.S., De Liberali, E., Bianchi, F.P., 1983. Antibodies to cardiac conduction tissue and abnormalities of cardiac conduction in rheumatoid arthritis. Clin. Exp. Immunol. 53, 536.
Wallukat, G., Morwinski, M., Kowal, K., 1991. Antibodies against the β-adrenergic receptor in human myocarditis and dilated cardiomyopathy: β-adrenergic agonism without desensitization. Eur. Heart J. 12 (Suppl. D), 178.
Wallukat, G., Homuth, V., Fischer, T., 1999. Patients with preeclampsia develop agonist autoantibodies against the angiotensin AT1 receptor. J. Clin. Invest. 103, 945.
Warraich, R.S., Dunn, M.J., Yacoub, M.H., 1999. Subclass specificity of autoantibodies against myosin in patients with idiopathic dilated cardiomyopathy: proinflammatory antibodies in dilated cardiomyopathy patients. Biochem. Biophys. Res. Commun. 259, 255.
Witebsky, E., Rose, N.R., Terplan, K., 1957. Chronic thyroiditis and autoimmunization. JAMA 164, 1439.
Wojnicz, R., Nowalany-Kozielska, E., Wojciechowska, C., 2001. Randomized, placebo controlled study for immunosuppressive treatment of inflammatory dilated cardiomyopathy. Two-year follow-up results. Circulation 104, 39.
Wolff, P.G., Kuhl, U., Schultheiss, H.P., 1989. Laminin distribution and autoantibodies to laminin in dilated cardiomyopathy and myocarditis. Am. Heart J. 117, 1303.
Zabriskie, J.B., 1967. Mimetic relationships between group A streptococci and mammalian tissues. Adv. Immunol. 7, 147.
Zabriskie, J.B., Hs, K.C., Seegal, B.C., 1970. Heart-reactive antibody associated with rheumatic fever: characterization and diagnostic significance. Clin. Exp. Immunol. 7, 147.
Zitnan, D., Bosmanski, K., 1966. Antimyocardial serum factors in rheumatic fever detected by the immunofluorescence method. Acta Rheum. Scand. 12, 267.
Zweiman, B., Arnason, B.G.W., 1987. Immunologic aspects of neurological and neuromuscolar diseases. JAMA 258, 2970.

Chapter 3

Neonatal Lupus Syndromes: Pathogenesis and Clinical Features[a]

A. Brucato,* R. Clancy,§ J.P. Buyon§ and M. Meroni*
*Internal Medicine, Ospedale Papa Giovanni XXIII, Bergamo, Italy; §Hospital for Joint Diseases, New York University School of Medicine, New York, NY, United States

Key Points

- Neonatal lupus is an in vivo model of passively acquired autoimmune disease in which anti-Ro/SSA autoantibodies are transmitted through the placenta from a mother to her fetus.
- The most important clinical feature is congenital heart block, which is usually complete; other conduction abnormalities may be present (sinus bradycardia, PQ prolongation).
- Additional structural cardiac abnormalities may be endocardial fibroelastosis and valve fibrosis; liver and blood elements abnormalities have been also reported, while learning disabilities are probably absent.
- Therapy is based on expert opinion; fluorinated steroids are generally used if the block is incomplete, or recent, or associated with hydrops, myocarditis, and effusions. Intravenous immunoglobulin (IVIG) and also plasmapheresis are sometimes proposed if the block is incomplete or if myocarditis or endocardial fibroelastosis are present.
- Infants are often delivered preterm (on average at 35 weeks gestation); mortality is 15–23%; permanent pacing is required in 51–84%.
- Hydroxychloroquine might have a role in preventing CHB, mediated by interference with TLR, and an open-label prospective trial is currently recruiting to further investigate this association.

a. This chapter is dedicated to the memory of Harriet Buyon.

The Heart in Systemic Autoimmune Diseases.

1. INTRODUCTION

Congenital heart block (CHB) is a characteristic manifestation of the neonatal lupus (NL) syndrome, mainly due to passive transplacental diffusion of maternal antibodies (anti-SSA/Ro and, to a lesser extent, anti-SSB/La) to the fetal circulation. Cardiac NL syndrome typically includes, besides CHB (usually complete), further cardiac abnormalities such as endocardial fibroelastosis (EFE), dilated cardiomyopathy (DCM), and valve fibrosis. Other conduction abnormalities may be present (sinus bradycardia, PR interval prolongation).

The term NL is misleading, since most of the mothers are not affected by systemic lupus erythematosus (SLE), and their infants too are not affected by SLE, but has been used since some of these infants may develop a skin rash resembling that observed in adults with subacute cutaneous lupus erythematosus.

Fluorinated steroids, that do cross the placenta, have been used for some decades, but their efficacy has been recently challenged by several authors, and treatment is currently very controversial (Izmirly et al., 2011; Eliasson et al., 2011; Levesque et al., 2015; Izmirly et al., 2015).

2. EPIDEMIOLOGY AND DEFINITION OF CONGENITAL COMPLETE AVB

CHB is a rare disorder, equally affecting males and females. CHB has an incidence of 1:20,000 live births (Brito-Zéron et al., 2015); these numbers, however, include CHB associated with anatomical malformations, and do not consider in utero deaths. Overall studies of CHB due to all etiologies observe that 14–42% of cases are attributable to anatomical abnormalities; assuming that the remaining geneses are autoimmune, the global incidence of immune-mediated CHB is estimated in 1 in 20,000–30,000 (Kertesz et al., 1997): more precisely, it has recently been established in about 1 in 22,000 live births (Friedman et al., 2003). Recently, the incidence of autoantibody-related atrioventricular block (AVB) of II-III degree was reported as 1/23,300 in Stockholm County.

Confusion exists regarding congenital versus acquired AVB; for these reasons we proposed a new definition: an AVB is defined as congenital if it is diagnosed in utero, at birth, or within the neonatal period (0–27 days after birth). This definition is now generally accepted (Brito-Zéron et al., 2015; Brucato, 2003).

Nonimmune CHB is commonly associated with underlying structural congenital heart disease: among them, left atrial isomerism (often accompanied by atrioventricular septal defect) and levo-transposition of the great arteries. When diagnosed in the postnatal period, approximately one-third of cases of congenital conduction system disease have associated structural disease. In utero, diagnosis of CHB is associated with structural heart disease in approximately one-half of the cases (Kertesz et al., 1997). It can also occur in association with tumors like mesothelioma.

3. ETIOLOGY/PATHOGENESIS

NL clinical manifestations are not only associated, but causally related with the presence of anti-Ro/SSA antibodies (Buyon and Clancy, 2005); their pathogenic role is supported by the fact that, with the only exception of CHB, NL manifestations disappear in temporal relationship with the clearance of antibodies from the baby's circulation. These antibodies, in fact, start crossing the placenta at approximately 12 weeks of gestation, reaching thus the fetal tissues. A study showed that antibodies to native 60-kd and denatured 52-kd Ro/SSA were present only in the heart eluate, and not in the eluates from brain, kidney, and skin of a child who died with congenital complete heart block.

The antibodies-derived pathogenic action may display at least three effects, not mutually exclusive, on cardiac tissues: myocarditis; arrhythmogenesis; and interference with apoptosis.

3.1 Myocarditis

The inflammatory process relevance in NL pathogenesis is supported by the mononuclear cell infiltration in the myocardium, as well as by the deposition of immunoglobulin G (IgG), complement, and fibrin (Nield et al., 2002). The first cardiac lesion may be a pancarditis, resulting in fibrosis of the conducting system. The picture might vary from a clear inflammatory state, to the presence of calcifications only, depending on the time when the pathological evaluation is performed. A generalized myocarditis/cardiomyopathy, possibly associated to EFE, may rarely occur after birth (Alexander et al., 1992).

Llanos described a mononuclear cell (macrophages and giant cells) infiltrated pancarditis (Llanos et al., 2012). Echocardiographic evidence of myocarditis remains extremely rare (Fesslova et al., 2003; Brucato et al., 2011a,b).

3.2 Arrhythmogenesis and Electrophysiological Effects

Boutdjir showed peculiar effects on conduction and heart rate of whole human fetal hearts, obtained after elective termination of normal pregnancy. Perfusion of the heart with purified anti-52-kD SSA/Ro antibody resulted in bradycardia associated with widening of the QRS complex and, after 33 min from perfusion, complete AVB. Reperfusion of the heart with antibody-free solution resulted in recovery. Superfusion of hearts with IgG fractions also induced bradycardia and AV dissociation (Boutjdir et al., 1997).

Several authors showed arrhythmogenic effects of anti-Ro/SSA antibodies in animal or human myocardial tissues (Boutjdir et al., 1998; Mazel et al., 1999), interfering with both L-type and T-type calcium channels. An autoantibody-binding site has been identified on the extracellular loop (domain I, S5-S6) of alpha(1D) L-type Ca channel (the pore-forming subunit of the channel) (Karnabi and Boutjdir, 2010).

Anti-Ro/SSA may also target an extracellular epitope of a1G T-type calcium channels in human fetal cardiomyocytes, but the Buyon's group found this reactivity to be extremely rare and not discriminating in anti-Ro/SSA exposed fetuses with or without CHB (Markham et al., 2015).

A Swedish study showed that pups born to rats immunized with the p200 peptide developed AVB and that p200-specific autoantibodies bound cultured cardiomyocytes, leading to accumulating levels and overload of intracellular Ca^{2+} levels with subsequent loss of contractility and apoptosis. These important findings might be the link between reaction with calcium receptors, arrhythmogenesis, apoptosis, and fibrosis. QT interval may be prolonged in children from anti-Ro/SSA positive mothers (Cimaz et al., 2000), raising the possibility that further ionic channels might be involved. Two different groups observed a prolongation of the corrected QT interval (QTc) in anti-Ro/SSA-positive adults (Lazzerini et al., 2004, 2007; Bourré-Tessier et al., 2011).

More recently, anti-Ro positive sera, purified IgG, and affinity purified anti-52 kDa Ro from patients with autoimmune diseases and QTc prolongation were tested on I_{Kr} using HEK293 cells expressing HERG channel and native cardiac myocytes. Anti-Ro inhibits I_{Kr} to prolong action potential duration by directly binding to the HERG channel protein. 52 kDa Ro antigen immunized guinea-pigs showed QTc prolongation on ECG. The authors concluded that anti-Ro/SSA inhibit I_{Kr} by cross-reacting with the HERG channel likely at the pore region where homology between 52Ro antigen and HERG channel is present. Together, they proposed that adult patients with anti-Ro/SSA with QTc prolongation should receive counseling about drugs that may increase the risk for arrhythmias.

Other interferences of anti-Ro/SSA antibodies have been demonstrated with M1 muscarinic acetylcholine, serotoninergic 5-hydroxytryptamine (5-HT4) receptors (Kamel et al., 2005), and with inner ear antigens, such as Cogan peptide (Lunardi et al., 2002).

3.3 Apoptosis, TGFbeta, TLR, and the Road to Scar

Ro and La antigens are expressed on the surface blebs of apoptotic cells including human fetal myocytes (Miranda et al., 1998). Tran demonstrated the subcellular translocation also of La autoantigen in vivo during apoptosis in the fetal conduction system in mice, and showed that transplacental anti-La autoantibodies bind specifically to apoptotic cells. Impaired clearance of apoptotic cardiocytes is linked to anti-SSA/Ro and -SSB/La antibodies

(Clancy et al., 2006). Accordingly, it has been reported that anti-SSA/Ro autoantibodies, once bound to apoptotic fetal cardiocytes, might promote phagocytosis by macrophages and the secretion of tumor necrosis factor alpha (TNFα) and TGF-beta. TNFα may induce an inflammatory process, but TGF-beta induces a pro-fibrotic activation of myofibroblast. This might be one of the "fetal factors" facilitating fibrosis at the level of the conduction tissue (Clancy et al., 2002). Accordingly, the profibrotic TGF-beta genotype has been detected in a twin with CHB but not in his healthy twin (Cimaz et al., 2006).

To be expressed on the surface of apoptotic fetal cardiomyocytes Ro60 requires binding with its Y3 RNA (Reed et al., 2013). β(2)-glycoprotein I (β_2GPI) interacts with Ro60 on the surface of apoptotic Jurkat cells and inhibits binding of anti-Ro60 IgG, preventing opsonization of apoptotic cardiomyocytes by maternal anti-Ro60 IgG (Reed et al., 2011).

Surface binding of anti-Ro60 to apoptotic cardiocytes activates the urokinase plasminogen activator/urokinase plasminogen activator receptor (uPA/uPAR) system. Subsequent plasmin generation facilitates increased binding of anti-Ro60 by disrupting and cleaving circulating β2GPI, thereby eliminating its protective effect (Briassouli et al., 2013).

Activation of TLR by ssRNA after FcγR-mediated phagocytosis of immune complexes may be relevant. Both macrophage transfection with noncoding ssRNA that bind Ro60 and an immune complex generated by incubation of Ro60-ssRNA with IgG from a CHB mother or affinity purified anti-Ro60 significantly increased TNFα secretion. Dependence on TLR was supported by the significant inhibition of TNFα release by IRS661 and chloroquine. Fibrosis markers were increased in fetal cardiac fibroblasts after incubation with supernatants from macrophages transfected with ssRNA or incubated with the immune complex. Supernatants generated from macrophages with ssRNA in the presence of chloroquine did not cause fibrosis. In a CHB heart, but not a healthy heart, TLR7 immunostaining was localized to a region near the atrioventricular groove. These data support an injury model in CHB, whereby endogenous ligand, Ro60-associated ssRNA, forges a nexus between TLR ligation and fibrosis instigated by binding of anti-Ro Abs to the target protein likely accessible via apoptosis, and explains a possible protective role of chloroquine (Clancy et al., 2010). Recently, transcriptome and epigenetic modifications, which affect transcription factors NF-κB and STAT1, were selected to evaluate the phenotype of macrophages in which TLR7/8 was ligated following treatment with either anti-Ro60/Ro60/hY3 RNA immune complexes or transfection with hY3. Based on microarray, TNF and IL6 were among the most highly upregulated genes in both stimulated conditions, each of which was significantly inhibited by preincubation with hydroxychloroquine (HCQ). In contrast, following stimulation of macrophages with either TNFα or IFN-α, which do not signal through TLR, the resultant gene expression was refractory to HCQ. Ligation of TLR7/8 resulted in increased histone methylation as measured by increased H3K4me2, a requirement for binding of NF-κB at certain promoters, specifically the kB1 region in the TNF promoter (ChIP-qPCR), which was significantly decreased by HCQ. In summary, these results support that the HCQ-sensitive phenotype of hY3-stimulated macrophages reflects the bifurcation of TLR downstream signals involving NF-κB and STAT 1 pathways and for the former dimethylation of H3K4. Accordingly, HCQ may act more as a preventive measure in downregulating the initial production of IFN-α or TNFα and not affect the resultant autacoid stimulation reflected in TNFα and IFN-α responsive genes. The beneficial scope of antimalarials in the prevention of CHB in an anti-Ro offspring or more broadly SLE, may include in part, a mechanism targeting TLR-dependent epigenetic modification (Clancy et al., 2015).

3.4 Genetics

Genetic predisposition may play an important role in disease pathogenesis. Susceptibility genes involve a broad spectrum of candidates ranging from affector pathways, involving antigen presentation (e.g., HLA), to effector pathways, controlling inflammation and fibrosis. Maternal genes HLA DRB1*02 and *03 are strongly associated with the presence of SSA/Ro-SSB/La (Gottenberg et al., 2003). A polymorphism at position -308 on the promoter gene of the TNFα (TNF2) and leucine polymorphism at codon 10 of the TGFβ gene (potentially conferring increased inflammation and scarring development, respectively) occur more frequently in children with CHB than their unaffected siblings (Clancy et al., 2003). Sirén reported an increased frequency of Class I HLA-Cw3 in CHB children. HLA alleles enriched in the mothers were DRB1*03DQB1*02, DQA1*05, and HLACw7 (Colombo et al., 1999). A case of CHB onset in a fetus conceived by in vitro fertilization was described by the authors and demonstrated that the presence of anti-SSA/Ro antibodies is necessary, but not sufficient to provoke autoimmune-associated CHB. HLA-related candidates and single-nucleotide polymorphisms in the promoter region of tumor necrosis factor α and codon 10 in transforming growth factor β1 (TGFβ1) were evaluated in a unique family: the surrogate mother (anti-SSA/Ro positive), the biologic father, and the CHB-affected child (product of ovodonation). There was an HLA mismatch between the affected child and the surrogate mother. However, both the biologic and the surrogate mothers shared DQ2 and the profibrosing leucine polymorphism at codon 10 of TGFβ. CHB can therefore develop in a genetically unrelated child exposed in utero to anti-SSA/Ro antibodies (Brucato et al., 2010).

A Swedish group recently performed a genotype analysis in 86 families. HLA-DRB1*04 and HLA-Cw*05 variants were significantly more frequently transmitted to CHB cases, whilst HLA-DRB1*13 and HLA-Cw*06 were significantly less often transmitted. Furthermore a marked association of increased paternal (but not maternal) HLA-DRB1*04 transmission to affected offspring was observed. The authors concluded that HLA-DRB1*04 and HLA-Cw*05 were identified as novel fetal HLA allele variants that confer susceptibility to CHB, whilst DRB1*13 and Cw*06 emerged as protective alleles. Additionally, a paternal contribution to fetal susceptibility to CHB was demonstrated (Meisgen et al., 2014).

3.5 Evaluation of the Fine Specificities of the Maternal Autoantibody Profile

SSA/Ro is a complex system, associated with RNA, the function of which is not completely known, that comprises at least two polypeptides of molecular weight of 52 and 60 kD, respectively.

Novel interest was raised by a small central portion of 52 kD Ro, from 200 to 239 amino acids, named p200 that could represent the fine specificity of anti-Ro Ab associated to CHB. Salomonsson described the presence of anti-p200 in nine out of nine mothers who delivered babies with CHB, and demonstrated that anti-p200 inoculation in rat pups was associated to cardiocytes Ca^{2+}-homeostasis dysregulation, leading to an increase in heart cell death, atrium-ventricular conduction prolongation, and to CHB; Clancy (Clancy et al., 2005) did not confirm these findings as being specific to only pregnancies resulting in CHB. Strandberg showed an association between high titers of maternal anti-p200 Ab and CHB in a wide multicenter study. An animal model demonstrated that the inoculation of anti-p200, but not of anti-52 kD Ro Ab without p200 peptide specificity, was able to cause heart block in rat pups (Ambrosi et al., 2012a).

In a study of 115 anti-Ro positive mothers, both maternal anti-Ro52 and p200 autoantibodies were less than 50% specific for cardiac NL, but anti-p200 was the least likely of the Ro autoantibodies to be false-positive in mothers who have never had an affected child (Reed et al., 2012).

We retrospectively evaluated 207 Italian women carrying anti-Ro/SSA Ab. CHB occurred in 42 children, whereas 165 were not affected. Anti-p200 was more frequently positive (81.0% vs. 59.1%, $p = .013$) and at a higher titer in CHB mothers [Odds Ratio (OR) for CHB: 2.98]. CHB risk significantly decreased in the absence of this specificity (OR: 0.34). However, while the negative predictive value related to anti-Ro/SSA 60 kD Ab ELISA was 100%, almost 20% of mothers negative for anti-p200 Ab delivered babies with CHB. An ELISA screening for anti-Ro/SSA 60 kD Ab is mandatory, given the probability of developing CHB also in the absence of anti-p200 Ab.

3.6 Other Pathogenetic Mechanisms

Moving from the observation that only a minority (1–2%) of mothers with anti-Ro and anti-La antibodies deliver an affected child, others pathogenetic mechanisms appear to be relevant. In particular, an intriguing discordance on the occurrence of complete CHB was reported in monozygotic twins. The persistent presence of maternal cells in the fetal heart (microchimerism) is a hypothesis to explain a local immune-mediated response.

CHB was associated with higher maternal age and displayed a seasonal birth pattern in a Swedish study, eventually due to lower levels of vitamin D due to decreased sunlight exposure during winter months (Jaeggi et al., 2011). Recently cord blood and maternal vitamin D levels were not significantly associated with cardiac NL, but average maternal vitamin D level during pregnancy was positively associated with longer time to postnatal pacemaker placement, so maternal levels should be optimized.

4. RISK OF DELIVERING A CHILD WITH COMPLETE CHB

In a prospective study we found that the prevalence of complete CHB in newborns of 100 women already known to be anti-Ro/SSA positive and with known connective tissue disease was 2% (95% confidence interval 0.2–7%) (Brucato et al., 2001). We only studied mothers who had been found to be anti-Ro/SSA positive by counterimmunoelectrophoresis, a method with high specificity and low sensitivity, to exclude women with low or dubious titers of anti-Ro/SSA. This finding has been now confirmed by other groups: Gladman reported no cases of CHB in 100 live births in 96 women (Gladman et al., 2002); Cimaz observed two cases of CCHB out of 128 infants (1.6%), and Costedoat-Chalumeau one case out of 99 infants (1%) (Costedoat-Chalumeau et al., 2004). Motta observed a prevalence of 1/50 (2%) (Motta et al., 2007), Gerosa 1/60 (1.7%) (Gerosa et al., 2007), Friedman 2/74 (2.7%) (Friedman et al., 2008), Rein 0/70 (0%), and Jaeggi 1/165 (0.6%) (Jaeggi et al., 2011). Overall a meta-analysis including all the studies available would give a prevalence of 10 out of 746 cases (1.3%) in women with anti-SSA/Ro and no history of a previous child with NL.

If the mother is anti-La/SSB positive the risk might increase to 3%, while if negative might decrease to 0.9% (Gordon et al., 2004).

If the mother has antithyroid Ab or is hypothyroid the risk should increase, with an estimated OR of 8.6. In a separate study, Askanase reported that mothers of children with NL in the Research Registry for Neonatal Lupus were more likely to have anti-TG antibodies than women with primary Sjögren's syndrome and historical healthy controls, anti-TG antibodies being present in one-third of the mothers tested. However, whether these antibodies specifically segregate between affected and unaffected pregnancies was not evaluated (Askanase et al., 2006).

We observed that the risk for CHB was <1% in women who were anti-p200 negative.

The Canadian group tested in ELISA 186 anti-Ro/SSA positive women and found that all cardiac complications of NL were associated with at least moderate titer of anti-SSA (>50 U/mL): no case of cardiac NL was observed in mothers low positive for anti-Ro (<50 U/mL) (Jaeggi et al., 2010).

In practice, positivity for anti-Ro/SSA must be reliable, and ELISA low titers probably are not relevant. These findings might be relevant in deciding which woman to monitor during pregnancy.

The risk of recurrence of CHB is 15–20% (Buyon et al., 1998; Julkunen and Eronen, 2001). This probability seems lower in Sweden: 12% (Ambrosi et al., 2012b). The risk of CHB seems similar even after a case of skin rash only (Brito-Zéron et al., 2015); however, Izmirly reported the recurrence to be slightly lower following skin rash (13%) compared to 17% following CHB.

5. CLINICAL MANIFESTATIONS

5.1 Cardiac Manifestations

Cardiac manifestations are a hallmark of NL. CHB is the most severe consequence, since it is irreversible and carries a high morbidity and mortality rate, mainly related to the ventricular rate, which usually ranges between 30 and 80 beats/min; the lower the rate, the higher the possibility of fetal hydrops, neonatal cardiac failure, and death (Izmirly et al., 2011; Eliasson et al., 2011; Lopes et al., 2008).

In 2011 two large series of cardiac NL were published, one from Europe (report form the Fetal Working Group of the European Association of Pediatric Cardiology) and one from USA. Recently, the French group also published a large series of 214 CHB (Levesque et al., 2015).

The main findings from these studies are summarized in Table 3.1, together with those from a large Brazilian study (Lopes et al., 2008).

CHB is most frequently detected in utero by prenatal ultrasound, between 16–18 and 24 weeks of gestational age. This "window" is related to the timing of transplacental passage of autoantibodies (that does not start before the third month of gestation) and to the ontogenic development of the cardiac conduction system that is not fully developed until the 22nd week (Lopes et al., 2008).

The rapidity of clinically detectable injury is supported by the report of fetuses experiencing normal sinus rhythm, then progressing to irreversible third-degree block within 1 week, observed in USA, Sweden, and Italy (Friedman et al., 2008). Most of these infants are delivered preterm (35 weeks gestation) (Izmirly et al., 2011; Eliasson et al., 2011; Brucato et al., 2000; Eronen et al., 2000).

In utero death is usually related to intractable heart failure, but may occur suddenly (Fesslova et al., 2009).

Other electrocardiographic abnormalities entail incomplete AVBs (first- and second-degree) and sinus bradycardia (Brucato et al., 2000; Cimaz et al., 1997). This last finding is of importance, since it suggests that also the sinus

TABLE 3.1 Outcome of Infants With Cardiac NL in Four Large International Series

	Lopes et al. (2008)	Eliasson et al. (2011)	Izmirly et al. (2011)	Levesque et al. (2015)
No. of fetuses	57 with normal cardiac anatomy	175	325	214
Total mortality	13 (23%)	27 (15%)	57 (17.5%)	49 (23%)
Mortality in utero	6 (10%)	16 (9%)	19 (6%)	27 (with 14 for elective termination of pregnancy) (13%)
Perinatal mortality	7 (12%)	11 (7%)	38 (12%)	8 (4%)
Pacemaker implantation	51%	66%	70%	79%
Late-onset cardiomiopathy	3%	4.6%	4 cases of heart transplantation	18% (but diagnosed at a mean age of 5 months)
Treated with fluorinated corticosteroids	10%	38%	90%	79 (39%)
Effects of corticosteroids	None	None on mortality; possibly reversal on incomplete AVB	Possibly reversal on incomplete AVB	None
Reversal of second-degree AV after fluorinated corticosteroids	None	In 3/7 fetuses treated versus 0/8 untreated	In 4/13 fetuses treated versus 1/8 untreated	In 1/13 treated versus 1/11 untreated
Variables associated with death	Atrial rate <120 bpm, ventricular rate <55 bpm, hydrops	Gestational age <20 weeks, ventricular rate <50 bpm, hydrops, impaired left ventricular function	Earlier gestational age, lower ventricular rate, hydrops, EFE	Hydrops, prematurity (less than 37 weeks gestation)
Survival at 10 years for a child born alive			86%	88%
Maternal anti-Ro/SSA antibodies	72%	80% of 162 pregnancies with documented antibody status	100%	99.5%

node can be transiently affected. Cimaz described QT prolongation in infants from mothers with anti-SSA/Ro antibodies (Cimaz et al., 2000). The French group has not confirmed this finding in 152 pregnancies in 96 anti-SSA positive women (Costedoat-Chalumeau et al., 2004). On the other hand a QT interval prolongation has been reported also in adults positive for anti-SSA/Ro (Lazzerini et al., 2004, 2007; Bourré-Tessier et al., 2011), and recently it has been shown that anti-Ro positive sera inhibit I_{Kr} to prolong action potential duration by directly binding to the HERG channel protein inducing QTc prolongation. This topic, therefore, is still a matter of debate.

Two relevant papers, prospective controlled observational Italian studies, described ECGs abnormalities in infants born from anti-Ro/SSA positive mothers.

Gerosa prospectively followed 60 anti-Ro-positive and 36 anti-Ro-negative women before/during pregnancy and underwent weekly fetal echocardiography from the 18th to 26th weeks of gestational age. Infants' ECG and/or ECG-Holter were performed at 1, 3, 6, and 12 months. ECGs of 200 consecutive neonates were used as a healthy control group. One of 61 fetuses of anti-Ro-positive mothers developed CHB; another anti-Ro-positive baby developed second-degree AVB (30th week). The prevalence of transient first-degree AVB detected postnatally was significantly higher in the anti-Ro-positive group ($p = .002$). No differences in QTc interval prolongation prevalence (≥ 440 ms) was observed between the anti-Ro-positive and -negative groups, but both were significantly higher than that of the control normal population ($p < .001$). ECG-Holter showed QTc prolongation in 59% of infants of anti-Ro-positive and in 60% of infants of anti-Ro-negative mothers. Holter QTc was ≥ 470 ms in four infants of anti-Ro-positive group and two of anti-Ro-negative group. This prospective study confirmed that ECG abnormalities (first-degree AVB and QTc interval prolongation) are frequent in infants of mothers with autoimmune diseases, independently of maternal disease, autoantibody profile, and treatment during pregnancy (Gerosa et al., 2007).

Motta evaluated neonates born from mothers with connective tissue disease and positive (51 infants) or negative (50 control infants) for anti-SSA/Ro antibodies. No infant showed sinus bradycardia. A first-degree AVB at birth was observed in five study group and no control group infants ($p = .023$). AVBs spontaneously reverted or remained stable during the first year of life. Mean QTc of infants born from anti-SSA/Ro-positive mothers was slightly prolonged as compared with the control group (0.404 ± 0.03 s vs. 0.395 ± 0.02 s; $p = .060$) (Motta et al., 2007).

These two studies overall concluded that several minor ECG abnormalities may be present in infants born form anti-SSA positive mothers, but also born from women with autoimmune diseases who are anti-SSA negative, and that their clinical relevance is modest.

Immunomediated valvular disease caused by the dysfunction of the atrioventricular valve tensor apparatus may be a severe complication of NL

(Llanos et al., 2012), reported in 14/255 (5.5%) babies (Izmirly et al., 2011). A single study has detailed the clinical approach of six affected babies (Cuneo et al., 2011).

Fetal EFE has been associated with maternal anti-Ro/SSA antibodies, both with and without conduction disorders (Nield et al., 2002; Llanos et al., 2012; Guettrot-Imbert et al., 2011); prenatal echocardiographic signs of EFE are manifest as areas of patchy echogenicity (fibrosis) on the endocardial surfaces. The long-term implication of this finding is not clear, but EFE may be linked to the development of severe cardiomiopathy.

A subset of patients with CHB may in fact develop late-onset DCM (approximately 4–8%) (Izmirly et al., 2011; Eliasson et al., 2011, 2015; Eronen et al., 2000; Moak, 2001). Biopsy revealed hypertrophy, interstitial fibrosis, and rarely myocyte degeneration. A majority of affected children die from congestive heart failure or require cardiac transplantation, while a recovery was reported in few cases (Moak et al., 2001).

5.2 Non-Cardiac Manifestations

A skin rash can be present in the neonatal period, but more frequently it appears between the second and third month of life (Neiman et al., 2000). Unlike CHB, it disappears with the clearance of maternal autoantibodies from the baby's circulation, usually without any residuals. The rash is erythematous and scaly, similar to subacute cutaneous lupus erythematosus (and this is the origin of the name "Neonatal Lupus"). It is frequently annular in shape, and mostly located in sun-exposed area with a characteristic predilection for the periorbital area. Ultraviolet exposure may be an exacerbating factor. Data regarding skin pathology are scanty. Peñate described five cases and reviewed the literature, observing vacuolar alteration at the dermoepidermal interface and adnexal structures. Some cases exhibit a superficial and deep perivascular and periadnexal lymphocytic infiltrate without epidermal alteration (Peñate et al., 2009). Since these lesions are self-limiting, usually no treatment is required.

Regarding laboratory abnormalities, anemia, thrombocytopenia, and neutropenia have been described (Kanagasegar et al., 2002). Hepatic involvement has also been described (Laxer et al., 1990; Lee et al., 1993): it can vary from asymptomatic increase in transaminases to severe cholestasis. This has been noted to be present at birth in some cases but has not been clinically evident until several weeks in others. We observed hematologic abnormalities in 27% of the babies and elevation of liver enzymes in 26%. As for skin rash, these manifestations are transient and usually do not need medical treatment.

At variance with previous studies, Motta observed a low frequency of hematologic abnormalities and no cases of hepatobiliary disease in 50 infants (Motta et al., 2007).

Neurological manifestations have been reported in NL syndrome: hydrocephalus and macrocephaly have been occasionally suggested; furthermore the presence of maternal anti-Ro/SSA antibodies per se might be associated with learning disabilities in the offspring.

Animal (Huang et al., 2001; Matthews, 2000) and human (Abbasi et al., 2000) observations suggest that repeated antenatal steroid doses can interfere with the development of the immature brain, suggesting that dexamethasone may negatively affect the child's neuropsychological development. In light of these findings CHB babies who are both treated in utero with high-dose dexamethasone and exposed to maternal anti-Ro/SSA antibodies could be at risk for neurodevelopmental defects. We have therefore tested 16 CCHB patients for neuropsychological development, IQ, and learning disabilities. The children had been exposed in utero to a mean dose of 186.6 mg of dexamethasone. IQ levels were always normal; only one child had a learning disability, of borderline clinical significance, but this child had never been exposed to dexamethasone (Brucato et al., 2006).

The issue has been further studied. Questionnaires related to neuropsychiatric development were sent to all mothers enrolled in the Research Registry for NL. Controls consisted of healthy friends; 121 anti-Ro exposed children and 22 friend controls were studied. Forty percent of the anti-Ro exposed children were reported to have a neuropsychiatric disorder, compared with 27% of the friend controls ($p = .34$). The prevalence of depression, anxiety, developmental delays, learning, hearing, and speech problems were not significantly different between groups. Parental reporting of neuropsychiatric abnormalities was high in anti-Ro exposed children, regardless of the NL manifestation. However, it did not reach significance (Askanase et al., 2010).

Medical records of a Swedish cohort of siblings with (n = 60) and without (n = 54) CHB born to anti-Ro/SSA-positive mothers were retrieved from primary healthcare centers. Impaired neurodevelopment was reported in 16% (18/114) during the follow-up of 13 years. Reported problems included speech (9%), motor (8%) and learning (8%) impairment, attention deficit (5%), and behavioral impairment (4%). Learning impairment was significantly influenced by maternal SLE ($p < .005$), while attention deficits was influenced by both maternal SLE ($p < .05$) and CHB in the child ($p < .05$). The authors concluded that, in addition to well-established factors, such as male sex and being born preterm, both maternal SLE and CHB may influence neurodevelopment.

The Canadian group confirmed these reassuring findings by performing a prospective, blinded assessment of the cognitive functioning of children aged 6–16 years, exposed in utero to maternal anti-Ro antibodies. The population consisted in the following three groups: subjects free from CHB and from prenatal dexamethasone treatment (n = 14); CHB affected, without having received prenatal treatment (n = 10); and CHB subjects, despite with prenatal dexamethasone treatment (n = 16). Parameters evaluation included abstract intelligence, visual perceptual and motor skills, auditory and visual attention, verbal learning and memory, visual memory, executive function, and behavior. All cohorts scored within the normal range and were not significantly different in any domains. There were no relevant associations between the neurocognitive function scores, the minimal fetal heart rate, and either the duration or dosage of dexamethasone therapy (Kelly et al., 2014).

Despite the possibility that repeated courses of dexamethasone may be detrimental to the newborn's neurodevelopment, a child's final intellectual maturation remains a complex process, involving the interplay of biological, social, and cultural factors. The Canadian group and the writing authors did not notice negative effects on the neurodevelopment patients, sometimes exposed to very high doses of dexamethasone (much higher than those used to enhance fetal lung maturity). CHB is a rare disease, but these reassuring findings might be clinically relevant, even more for the reason that a large number of newborns are often treated with repeated courses of antenatal fluorinated steroids to induce fetal lung maturity.

6. TREATMENT

There is no known effective therapy for CHB. Prenatal interventions try to diminish the autoimmune response and/or the cardiac inflammatory injury and increase fetal heart rate.

6.1 Fluorinated Corticosteroids

Fluorinated corticosteroids (FS) (dexamethasone and betametasone) are frequently used, since they are not metabolized by the placenta and are available to the fetus in an active form. Steroid therapy has been reported as potentially effective in the resolution of inflammatory signs (pleural effusions, ascites, and hydrops) in some case reports (Raboisson et al., 2005) and in a recently published paper (Ho et al., 2015). Two systematic retrospective analyses of major NL registries (the American and the French one, respectively), however, showed that this kind of treatment is not able to revert third-degree heart block, presumably due to the fibrosis of conducting system (Levesque et al., 2015; Izmirly et al., 2015). These data are aligned with previous publications. A European task force reported 175 fetuses outcome; among them, 67 cases (38%) were treated with fluorinated CS. In the steroid-treated arm, intrauterine survival was 91%: a percentage superposable to those of nontreated subjects (Eliasson et al., 2011). The Canadian group came to an opposite conclusion. They observed 37 cases of fetal CHB. Twenty-one fetuses were treated with dexamethasone and had a 1-year survival rate of 90%, compared with a 46% rate of patients free from FS treatment ($p < .02$). Immune-mediated conditions (myocarditis, hepatitis, cardiomyopathy), resulting in postnatal death or heart transplantation, were significantly more common in untreated subjects, compared with FS-treated patients (0/18 vs. 4/9 live births; $p < .007$) (Jaeggi et al., 2004). The American group recently published a large retrospective study to evaluate whether fluorinated steroids given to manage isolated advanced block prevented development of disease beyond the AV node and found that fluorinated steroids did not confer a survival benefit. They studied fetuses with isolated advanced heart block in utero who either received fluorinated steroids within 1 week of detection (n = 71) or no treatment (n = 85). Outcomes evaluated were development of EFE, DCM, and/or hydrops fetalis; mortality; and pacemaker implantation. In Cox proportional hazards regression analyses, fluorinated steroids did not significantly prevent development of disease beyond the AV node (adjusted HR = 0.90; 95% CI 0.43−1.85; $p = .77$), reduce mortality (HR = 1.63; 95% CI 0.43−6.14; $p = .47$), or forestall/prevent pacemaker implantation (HR = 0.87; 95% CI 0.57−1.33; $p = .53$). No risk factors for development of disease beyond the AV node were identified. The authors concluded that their data do not provide evidence to support the use of fluorinated steroids to prevent disease progression or death in cases presenting with isolated heart block (Izmirly et al., 2015).

A particular case is the possible role of fluorinated steroids in the regression of second-degree AVB. Permanent reversal of fetal second-degree AVB is rare, and only two cases of spontaneous resolution of second-degree AVB in fetuses of anti-Ro/SSA positive mothers have been reported (Izmirly et al., 2011; Levesque et al., 2015), whereas cases of reversal after steroid treatment have been described (Raboisson et al., 2005; Izmirly et al., 2011; Eliasson et al., 2011) (see Table 3.1).

However, to differentiate incomplete from complete AVB is very difficult in utero, requiring a particular expertise.

Overall also fetal cardiologists have no reached a consensus on treatment: some authors suggest FS use (Jaeggi et al., 2004), whereas others discourage it (Lopes et al., 2008), even in the most severe cases (Eliasson et al., 2011).

As previously reported, repeated courses of steroids are known to potentially induce harmful side effects in both mother and child. The negative effects seem to be more linked to dexamethasone use: since that, betamethasone use, when available, is preferred. A past Cochrane review showed that only betamethasone, and not dexamethasone, significantly reduces neonatal mortality (Crowley, 2000). On the other hand, a more recent Cochrane review observed that dexamethasone may have some benefits, compared with betamethasone: namely, less intraventricular hemorrhage and a shorter length of stay in the neonatal intensive care unit for the newborns (Brownfoot et al., 2013). Generally speaking, the need of trials comparing the more commonly used corticosteroids is absolutely urgent.

Therapy choice, at the end, remains based on expert opinion. In the case of an incomplete block (e.g., second-degree), fluorinated corticosteroids 4 mg (once or twice daily) to the mother are often started, with a note of caution:

differentiating incomplete from complete AVB may be difficult in utero. In particular a differential diagnosis is blocked atrial premature contractions versus second-degree AVB, and the former is a normal variant probably and resolves spontaneously. If the block is recent (the more common clinical situation), some clinicians start FS as well; the dose is tapered and FS are discontinued if no change occurs after some weeks. If the block is associated with signs of myocarditis, heart failure, or hydropic changes, FS is once more recommended. If the block is complete and established from more than 2–4 weeks, with no effusions and no signs of hydrops, only serial echograms might be performed, since no evidence of effective therapy is available.

6.2 Other Possible Therapies

Some positive neonatal outcomes were reached by intravenous immunoglobulin (IVIG) administration. Ruffatti treated two consecutive cases of anti-Ro/La-related second-degree block with betamethasone (4 mg/day), weekly plasmapheresis, and IVIG (1 g/kg), administered every 15 days. This regimen was started shortly after CHB was detected and then continued until delivery. The newborns, too, were treated with IVIG (1 g/kg) fortnightly until anti-Ro/La antibody levels became undetectable. In both cases, second-degree AVB reverted to a stable sinus rhythm with a first-degree AVB. The tricky and very important point, however, is that other authors reported similar outcomes even without any therapy (Lopes et al., 2008).

The group of David, similarly, administered IVIG to prevent progression of incomplete early AVB, at the dose of 400 mg/kg/d for 5 days; after two maternal infusions, fetal heart rate reverted to sinus rhythm (David et al., 2010). Brucato treated two fetuses with incomplete AVB with IVIG, without any benefit (Brucato, 2011a,b).

Probably, IVIG might be useful in treating fetal myocarditis. Brucato treated with IVIG (400 mg/kg/d for 5 days) a mother whose fetus had CCHB and clear echocardiographic evidence of myocarditis: the myocarditis quickly resolved, but the complete AVB persisted (Brucato, 2011a,b). The therapeutic efficacy of IVIG use in the early treatment of complete or incomplete AVB is still under debate (David et al., 2010; Kaaja and Julkunen, 2003).

On the other hand, IVIG were found ineffective in preventing the recurrence of CHB in women who previously had a fetus with NL; in examined papers, IVIG were administered at a replacement dose, not a true antiinflammatory dose: 400 mg/kg at weeks 12, 15, 18, 21, and 24 of pregnancy (Pisoni et al., 2010; Friedman et al., 2010).

In another study IVIG was also effective in treating fetuses with EFE.

Terbutaline or salbutamol, selective beta 2 adrenergic agonists, may increase the fetal heart rate, improving ventricular function. In particular, they may have an importance role as "bridge therapy," in order to reach a more advanced gestational age and a safer baby weight (Fesslova et al., 2003). Salbutamol can be given orally to the mother, at a dosage of 2 mg 6 to 10 times daily, according to maternal compliance.

HCQ is an inhibitor of toll-like receptor (TLR) ligation. TLR signaling involvement has been frequently suggested (Brucato et al., 2003) and recently confirmed as fundamental in the pathogenesis of cardiac NL, thus representing a potential target for prevention of the disease (Clancy et al., 2015).

Two retrospective case-control studies showed a benefit of HCQ in lowering the risk of CHB (Izmirly et al., 2010a,b, 2015). The first study was limited to children born to Ro/SSA positive SLE mothers, including 50 cardiac NL cases and 151 noncardiac NL controls (Izmirly et al., 2010a,b). Seven (14%) cardiac NL children were exposed to HCQ, compared with 56 (37%) controls ($p = .002$; OR = 0.28). A successive study was performed to evaluate HCQ independent of maternal disease (Izmirly et al., 2015): 257 pregnancies were evaluated, collected among women who previously gave birth to children with cardiac NL (40 exposed, 217 unexposed to HCQ). The recurrence rate of CHB in fetuses exposed to HCQ was 7.5% (3/40), compared with 21.2% (46/217) in the unexposed group ($p = .05$). There were no deaths in the HCQ exposed group, compared with a case fatality rate of 22% in the unexposed group. These data suggest that HCQ may exert a protective action to fetus. HCQ has been used safely and regularly during pregnancy and has been associated with prevention of SLE flares (Levy et al., 2001; Clowse et al., 2006).

The Preventive Approach to Congenital Heart Block with Hydroxychloroquine (PATCH) is an open-label prospective trial, currently recruiting, in order to assess the utility of HCQ to prevent the recurrence of CHB in high-risk women with a previously affected child (ClinicalTrials.gov).

6.3 Postnatal Treatment

Postnatal treatment of CCHB is based on pace-maker implantation, frequently in the neonatal period; the device is implanted by thoracotomy route, with an electrode on the epicardial surface connected to an impulse generator placed in an abdominal subfascial pouch. In the presence of extreme bradycardia, isoproterenol (0.1−0.3 mcg/kg/min) may be administered as well. Pacemaker implantation in these preterm infants should not be considered a routine, but a surgical procedure to be used in presence of clinical conditions requiring pacing (heart failure, failure to thrive) (Fesslova et al., 2009). The percentage of paced children is reported in Table 3.1, and ranges from 50% to 80%.

Non cardiac NL manifestations, such as skin rash or hematology abnormalities, do not require any specific treatment: in fact, they spontaneously disappear, usually during the second semester of life.

7. OBSTETRIC MANAGEMENT OF PREGNANCIES AT RISK OF DEVELOPING CCHB

A woman is at risk if she is definitely anti-Ro/SSA positive. If the positivity is uncertain, or the titer is very low, we advise to confirm it with standard methods or in reference laboratories.

The management of anti-Ro/SSA positive women is based on expert opinion. Routine management might differ from management in research centers. Protocols vary from weekly serial sonograms to no particular screening (Brucato et al., 2011a,b).

Most centers perform serial echocardiograms and obstetric sonograms at least every 1 weeks starting from the 16 weeks gestation. The goal is to detect early fetal abnormalities, such as mechanical PR prolongation (first-degree AVB), echodensities, pericardial or pleural effusions, decreased contractility, valvular regurgitations, that might precede complete AVB and that might be a target of preventive therapy.

Prophylactic therapy with dexamethasone or betamethasone is not recommended, because of the low risk of CCHB and the potential side effects (Costedoat-Chalumeau et al., 2003). Other steroids are not useful since they do not cross the placenta in active form.

8. PROGNOSIS

8.1 Infants

CCHB is a severe disease (Table 3.1). Mortality, usually in utero or in the first three months of life, can reach 30%. In perinatal life pacemaker implantation is considered only if clinically indicated, while in the following years prophylactic pacemaker treatment might be considered even in asymptomatic patients because of unpredictable Stokes-Adams attacks; overall 60–70% of these children are paced (Brito-Zéron et al., 2015; Eliasson et al., 2011).

Median age at pacemaker implantation was 3.2 years in 127 Swedish children (Eliasson et al., 2015).

The probability to develop left ventricular disfunction or cardiomyopathy over time is 4–18% (Izmirly et al., 2011; Eliasson et al., 2011; Eronen et al., 2000; Moak et al., 2001; Eliasson et al., 2015; Levesque et al. 2015).

After pacemaker implantation, most of these children can live an almost normal life. The possibility for these children to develop SLE or another connective tissue disease in later life seems to be rare (Brucato et al., 1995; Martin et al., 2002), not higher than in asymptomatic children of mothers with autoimmune diseases (Martin et al., 2002; Cimaz, 2004).

8.2 Maternal

Most mothers are asymptomatic at the time of NL detection. In a review of 856 mothers more than half were classified as asymptomatic, and in the remaining cases SLE or primary Sjogren's syndrome were diagnosed in the majority of cases (Brito-Zerón et al., 2015).

The long-term prognosis of these mothers is good, since only half of them eventually develop a connective tissue disease, mild and non-life-threatening in most cases (Brucato et al., 1995; Julkunen et al., 1993; Press et al., 1996).

Rivera showed that the probability of an asymptomatic mother developing SLE by 10 years was 18.6%, and developing probable/definite Sjogren was 27.9%.

9. OTHER PREGNANCY OUTCOMES IN WOMEN WITH ANTI-RO/SSA ANTIBODIES

It is not clear if anti-Ro/SSA antibodies are linked to other adverse pregnancy outcomes, both in (SLE) and in non-SLE women. Most of the available data come from retrospective studies. In a large multicenter study we have prospectively followed 100 anti-Ro/SSA positive women (53 SLE) and 107 anti-Ro/SSA negative women (58 SLE) (Brucato et al., 2002). Mean gestational age at delivery (38 vs. 37.9 weeks), pregnancy loss (9.9% vs. 18.6%), preterm birth (21.3% vs. 13.9%), cesarean sections (49.2% vs. 53.4%), preeclampsia (6.6% vs. 8%), and intrauterine growth retardation (0% vs. 2.3%) were similar in anti-Ro/SSA positive and negative mothers: we concluded that anti-Ro/SSA antibodies cause CHB but do not affect other pregnancy outcomes, both in SLE and in non-SLE women.

10. ANTI-RO/SSA NEGATIVE CHB

Anti-Ro/SSA negative cases of fetal AVB have been reported. Of course the possible explanation is incomplete testing, mainly in cardiological series (Brito-Zerón et al., 2015). Still we studied 45 consecutive unselected cases with a wide battery of tests in a multilab workup, and 9 (20%) were definitely anti-Ro/SSA negative. These blocks are more often incomplete, and infant deaths more often occurred from noncardiac causes (Brucato et al., 2009).

ACKNOWLEDGMENT

We acknowledge grant support by a National Institutes of Health Merit Award [R37 AR042455, 3R37AR042455-21S1, 3R37AR042455-21S2 (J.P.B.)], the Research Registry for Neonatal Lupus [N01-AR-4-2220 (J.P.B.)], a Lupus Foundation of America Lifeline grant (J.P.B.), the National Institutes of Health [R03 HD069986 and R01 HD079951-01A1 (J.P.B.)], and the Italian Society of Rheumatology (M.M.)

REFERENCES

Abbasi, S., Hirsch, D., Davis, J., Tolosa, J., Stouffer, N., Debbs, R., et al., 2000. Effect of single versus multiple courses of antenatal corticosteroids on maternal and neonatal outcome. Am. J. Obstet. Gynecol. 182, 1243.

Alexander, E., Buyon, J.P., Provost, T.T., Guarnieri, T., 1992. Anti-Ro/SS-A antibodies in the pathophysiology of congenital heart block in neonatal lupus syndrome, an experimental model. Arthritis Rheum. 35, 176.

Ambrosi, A., Dzikaite, V., Park, J., Strandberg, L., Kuchroo, V.K., Herlenius, E., et al., 2012. Anti-Ro52 monoclonal antibodies specific for amino acid 200-239, but not other Ro52 epitopes, induce congenital heart block in a rat model. Ann. Rheum. Dis. 71, 448.

Ambrosi, A., Salomonsson, S., Eliasson, H., Zeffer, E., Skog, A., Dzikaite, V., et al., 2012. Development of heart block in children of SSA/SSB-autoantibody-positive women is associated with maternal age and displays a season-of-birth pattern. Ann. Rheum. Dis. 71, 334.

Askanase, A., Iloh, I., Buyon, J.P., 2006. Hypothyroidism and antithyroglobulin and antithyroperoxidase antibodies in the pathogenesis of autoimmune associated congenital heart block. J. Rheumatol. 33, 2099.

Askanase, A.D., Izmirly, P.M., Katholi, M., Mumtaz, J., Buyon, J.P., 2010. Frequency of neuropsychiatric dysfunction in anti-SSA/SSB exposed children with and without neonatal lupus. Lupus 19, 300.

Bourré-Tessier, J., Clarke, A.E., Huynh, T., Bernatsky, S., Joseph, L., Belisle, P., et al., 2011. Prolonged corrected QT interval in anti-Ro/SSA-positive adults with systemic lupus erythematosus. Arthritis Care Res. 63, 1031.

Boutjdir, M., Chen, L., Zhang, Z.H., Tseng, C.E., Di Donato, F., Rashbaum, W., et al., 1997. Arrhythmogenicity of IgG and anti-52-kD SSA/Ro affinity-purified antibodies from mothers of children with congenital heart block. Circ. Res. 8, 354.

Boutjdir, M., Chen, L., Zhang, Z.H., Tseng, C.E., El-Sherif, N., Buyon, J.P., 1998. Serum and immunoglobulin G from the mother of a child with congenital heart block induce conduction abnormalities and inhibit L-type calcium channels in a rat heart model. Pediatr. Res. 44, 11.

Briassouli, P., Halushka, M.K., Reed, J.H., Molad, Y., Fox-Talbot, K., Buyon, L., et al., 2013. A central role of plasmin in cardiac injury initiated by fetal exposure to maternal anti-Ro autoantibodies. Rheumatology 52, 1448.

Brito-Zéron, P., Izmirly, P.M., Ramos-Casals, M., et al., 2015. The clinical spectrum of autoimmune congenital heart block. Nat. Rev. Rheumatol. 11, 301.

Brownfoot, F., Gagliardi, D., Bain, E., Middleton, P., Crowther, C., 2013. Different corticosteroids and regimens for accelerating fetal lung maturation for women at risk of preterm birth. Cochrane Database Syst. Rev. 8, CD006764.

Brucato, A., Gasparini, M., Vignati, G., Riccobono, S., De Juli, E., Quinzanini, M., et al., 1995. Isolated congenital complete heart block: longterm outcome of children and immunogenetic study. J. Rheumatol. 22, 541.

Brucato, A., Cimaz, R., Catelli, L., Meroni, P., 2000. Anti-Ro-associated sinus bradycardia in newborns. Circulation 102, E88.

Brucato, A., Frassi, M., Franceschini, F., Cimaz, R., Faden, D., Pisoni, M.P., et al., 2001. Risk of congenital complete heart block in newborns of mothers with anti-Ro/SSA antibodies detected by counterimmunoelectrophoresis: a prospective study of 100 women. Arthritis Rheum. 44, 1832.

Brucato, A., Doria, A., Frassi, M., Castellino, G., Franceschini, F., Faden, D., et al., 2002. Pregnancy outcome in 100 women with autoimmune diseases and anti-Ro/SSA antibodies: a prospective controlled study. Lupus 11, 716.

Brucato, A., Jonzon, A., Friedman, D., 2003. Proposal for a new definition of congenital complete atrioventricular block. Lupus 12, 427.

Brucato, A., Astori, M.G., Cimaz, R., Villa, P., Li Destri, M., Chimini, L., et al., 2006. Normal neuropsychological development in children with congenital complete heart block who may or may not be exposed to high-dose dexamethasone in utero. Ann. Rheum. Dis. 65, 1422.

Brucato, A., Grava, C., Bortolati, M., Ikeda, K., Milanesi, O., Cimaz, R., et al., 2009. Congenital heart block not associated with anti-Ro/La antibodies: comparison with anti-Ro/La-positive cases. J. Rheumatol. 36, 1744.

Brucato, A., Ramoni, V., Penco, S., Sala, E., Buyon, J., Clancy, R., 2010. Passively acquired anti-SSA/Ro antibodies are required for congenital heart block following ovodonation but maternal genes are not. Arthritis Rheum. 62, 3119.

Brucato, A., Cimaz, R., Caporali, R., Ramoni, V., Buyon, J., 2011. Pregnancy outcomes in patients with autoimmune diseases and anti-Ro/SSA antibodies. Clin. Rev. Allergy Immunol. 40, 27.

Brucato, A., Ramoni, V., Gerosa, M., Pisoni, M.P., 2011. Congenital fetal heart block: a potential therapeutic role for intravenous immunoglobulin. Obstet. Gynecol. 117, 177.

Buyon, J.P., Heibert, R., Copel, J., et al., 1998. Autoimmune-associated congenital heart block: demographics, mortality, morbidity, and recurrence rates obtained from a national neonatal lupus registry. J. Am. Coll. Cardiol. 31, 1658.

Buyon, J.P., Clancy, R.M., 2005. Autoantibody-associated congenital heart block: TGF beta and the road to scar. Autoimmun. Rev. 4, 1.

Cimaz, R., Airoldi, M., Careddu, P., Centinaio, G., Catelli, L., Franceschini, F., et al., 1997. Transient neonatal bradycardia without heart block associated with anti-Ro antibodies. Lupus 6, 487.

Cimaz, R., Stramba-Badiale, M., Brucato, A., Catelli, L., Panzeri, P., Meroni, P.L., 2000. QT interval prolongation in asymptomatic anti-SSA/Ro-positive infants without congenital heart block. Arthritis Rheum. 43, 1049.

Cimaz, R., 2004. Any increased risk of autoimmune disease? Lupus 13, 736.

Cimaz, R., Borghi, M.O., Gerosa, M., Biggioggero, M., Raschi, E., Meroni, P.L., 2006. Transforming growth factor beta1 in the pathogenesis of autoimmune congenital complete heart block: lesson from twins and triplets discordant for the disease. Arthritis Rheum. 54, 356.

Clancy, R.M., Askanase, A.D., Kapur, R.P., Chiopelas, E., Azar, N., Miranda-Carus, M.E., et al., 2002. Transdifferentiation of cardiac fibroblasts, a fetal factor in anti-SSA/Ro-SSB/La antibody-mediated congenital heart block. J. Immunol. 169, 2156.

Clancy, R.M., Backer, C.B., Yin, X., Kapur, R.P., Molad, Y., Buyon, J.P., 2003. Cytokine polymorphisms and histologic expression in autopsy studies: contribution of TNF-alpha and TGF-beta 1 to the pathogenesis of autoimmune-associated congenital heart block. J. Immunol. 171, 3253.

Clancy, R.M., Buyon, J.P., Ikeda, K., Nozawa, K., Argyle, D.A., Friedman, D.M., et al., 2005. Maternal antibody responses to the 52-kd SSA/Ro p200 peptide and the development of fetal conduction defects. Arthritis Rheum. 52, 3079.

Clancy, R.M., Neufing, P.J., Zheng, P., O'Mahony, M., Nimmerjahn, F., Gordon, T.P., et al., 2006. Impaired clearance of apoptotic cardiocytes is linked to anti-SSA/Ro and -SSB/La antibodies in the pathogenesis of congenital heart block. J. Clin. Invest. 116, 2413.

Clancy, R.M., Alvarez, D., Komissarova, E., Barrat, F.J., Swartz, J., Buyon, J.P., 2010. Ro60--associated single-stranded RNA links inflammation with fetal cardiac fibrosis via ligation of TLRs: a novel pathway to autoimmune-associated heart block. J. Immunol. 184, 2148.

Clancy, R.M., Markham, A.J., Reed, J.H., Blumenberg, M., Halushka, M.K., Buyon, J.P., 2015. Targeting downstream transcription factors and epigenetic modifications following toll-like receptor 7/8 ligation to forestall tissue injury in anti-Ro60 associated heart block. J. Autoimmun. http://dx.doi.org/10.1016/j.jaut.2015.09.003 pii:S0896−8411(15)30042-1.

Clowse, M.E.B., Magder, L., Witter, F., Petri, M., 2006. Hydroxychloroquine in lupus pregnancy. Arthritis Rheum. 54, 3640.

Colombo, G., Brucato, A., Coluccio, E., Compasso, S., Luzzana, C., Franceschini, F., et al., 1999. DNA typing of maternal HLA in congenital complete heart block: comparison with systemic lupus erythematosus and primary Sjogren's syndrome. Arthritis Rheum. 42, 1757.

Costedoat-Chalumeau, N., Amoura, Z., Le Thi Hong, D., Wechsler, B., Vauthier, D., Ghillani, P., et al., 2003. Questions about dexamethasone use for the prevention of anti-SSA related congenital heart block. Ann. Rheum. Dis. 62, 1010.

Costedoat-Chalumeau, N., Amoura, Z., Lupoglazoff, J.M., Huong, D.L., Denjoy, I., Vauthier, D., et al., 2004. Outcome of pregnancies in patients with anti-SSA/Ro antibodies: a study of 165 pregnancies, with special focus on electrocardiographic variations in the children and comparison with a control group. Arthritis Rheum. 50, 3187.

Crowley, P., 2000. Prophylactic corticosteroids for preterm birth. Cochrane Database Syst. Rev. 2, CD000065.

Cuneo, B.F., Fruitman, D., Benson, D.W., Ngan, B.Y., Liske, M.R., Wahren-Herlineus, M., et al., 2011. Spontaneous rupture of atrioventricular valve tensor apparatus as late manifestation of anti-Ro/SSA antibody-mediated cardiac disease. Am. J. Cardiol. 107, 761.

David, A.L., Ataullah, I., Yates, R., Sullivan, I., Charles, P., Williams, D., 2010. Congenital fetal heart block: a potential therapeutic role for intravenous immunoglobulin. Obstet. Gynecol. 116 (Suppl. 3), 43.

Eliasson, H., Sonesson, S.E., Sharland, G., et al., 2011. Isolated atrioventricular block in the fetus: a retrospective, multinational, multicenter study of 175 patients. Circulation 124, 1919.

Eliasson, H., Sonesson, S., Salomonsson, S., Skog, A., Wahren-Herlenius, M., Gadler, F., 2015. Outcome in young patients with isolated complete atrioventricular block and permanent pacemaker treatment — a nationwide study of 127 patients. Hear Rhythm 12, 2278.

Eronen, M., Sirén, M.K., Ekblad, H., Tikanoja, T., Julkunen, H., Paavilainen, T., 2000. Short- and long-term outcome of children with congenital complete heart block diagnosed in utero or as a newborn. Pediatrics 106, 86.

Fesslova, V., Mannarino, S., Salice, P., Boschetto, C., Trespidi, L., Acaia, B., et al., 2003. Neonatal lupus: fetal myocarditis progressing to atrioventricular block in triplets. Lupus 12, 775.

Fesslova, V., Vignati, G., Brucato, A., De Sanctis, M., Butera, G., Pisoni, M.P., et al., 2009. The impact of treatment of the fetus by maternal therapy on the fetal and postnatal outcomes for fetuses diagnosed with isolated complete atrioventricular block. Cardiol. Young 19, 282.

Friedman, D.M., Duncanson, L.I., Glickstein, J., Buyon, J.P., 2003. A review of congenital heart block. Images Paediatr. Cardiol. 5, 36.

Friedman, D.M., Kim, M.Y., Copel, J.A., Davis, C., Phoon, C.K.L., Glickstein, J.S., et al., 2008. Utility of cardiac monitoring in fetuses at risk for congenital heart block : the PR interval and dexamethasone evaluation (PRIDE) prospective study. Circulation 117, 485.

Friedman, D.M., Llanos, C., Izmirly, P.M., Brock, B., Byron, J., Copel, J., et al., 2010. Evaluation of fetuses in a study of intravenous immunoglobulin as preventive therapy for congenital heart block: results of a multicenter, prospective, open-label clinical trial. Arthritis Rheum. 62, 1138.

Gerosa, M., Cimaz, R., Stramba-Badiale, M., Goulene, K., Meregalli, E., Trespidi, L., et al., 2007. Electrocardiographic abnormalities in infants born from mothers with autoimmune diseases—a multicentre prospective study. Rheumatology 46, 1285.

Gladman, G., Silverman, E.D., Yuk-Law, Luy, L., Boutin, C., Laskin, C., et al., 2002. Fetal echocardiographic screening of pregnancies of mothers with anti-Ro and/or anti-La antibodies. Am. J. Perinatol. 73.

Gordon, P., Khamashta, M.A., Rosenthal, E., Simpson, J.M., Sharland, G., Brucato, A., et al., 2004. Anti-52 kDa Ro, anti-60 kDa Ro, and anti-La antibody profiles in neonatal lupus. J. Rheumatol. 31, 2480.

Gottenberg, J.E., Busson, M., Loiseau, P., Cohen-Solal, J., Lepage, V., Charron, D., et al., 2003. In primary Sjogren's syndrome, HLA class II is associated exclusively with autoantibody production and spreading of the autoimmune response. Arthritis Rheum. 48, 2240.

Guettrot-Imbert, G., Cohen, L., Fermont, L., Villain, E., Francès, C., Thiebaugeorges, O., et al., 2011. A new presentation of neonatal lupus: 5 cases of isolated mild endocardial fibroelastosis associated with maternal anti-SSA/Ro and anti-SSB/La antibodies. J. Rheumatol. 38, 378.

Ho, A., Gordon, P., Rosenthal, E., Simpson, J., Miller, O., Sharland, G., 2015. Isolated complete heart block in the fetus. Am. J. Cardiol. 116, 142.

Huang, W.L., Harper, C.G., Evans, S.F., Newnham, J.P., Dunlop, S.A., 2001. Repeated prenatal corticosteroid administration delays astrocyte and capillary tight junction maturation in fetal sheep. Int. J. Dev. Neurosci. 19, 487.

Izmirly, P.M., Kim, M.Y., Llanos, C., Le, P.U., Guerra, M.M., Askanase, A.D., et al., 2010. Evaluation of the risk of anti-SSA/Ro-SSB/La antibody-associated cardiac manifestations of neonatal lupus in fetuses of mothers with systemic lupus erythematosus exposed to hydroxychloroquine. Ann. Rheum. Dis. 69, 1827.

Izmirly, P.M., Llanos, C., Lee, L.A., Askanase, A., Kim, M.Y., Buyon, J.P., 2010. Cutaneous manifestations of neonatal lupus and risk of subsequent congenital heart block. Arthritis Rheum. 62, 1153.

Izmirly, P.M., Saxena, A., Kim, M.Y., et al., 2011. Maternal and fetal factors associated with mortality and morbidity in a multi-racial/ethnic registry of anti-SSA/Ro-associated cardiac neonatal lupus. Circulation 124, 1927.

Izmirly, P.M., Saxena, A., Sahl, S.K., Shah, U., Friedman, D.M., Kim, M.Y., Buyon, J.P., 2015. Assessment of fluorinated steroids to avert progression and mortality in anti-SSA/Ro-associated cardiac injury limited to the fetal conduction system. Ann. Rheum. Dis.. http://dx.doi.org/10.1136/annrheumdis-2015−208311.

Jaeggi, E.T., Fouron, J.C., Silverman, E.D., Ryan, G., Smallhorn, J., Hornberger, L.K., 2004. Transplacental fetal treatment improves the outcome of prenatally diagnosed complete atrioventricular block without structural heart disease. Circulation 110, 1542.

Jaeggi, E., Laskin, C., Hamilton, R., Kingdom, J., Silverman, E., 2010. The importance of the level of maternal anti-Ro/SSA antibodies as a prognostic marker of the development of cardiac neonatal lupus erythematosus a prospective study of 186 antibody-exposed fetuses and infants. J. Am. Coll. Cardiol. 55, 2778.

Jaeggi, E.T., Silverman, E.D., Laskin, C., Kingdom, J., Golding, F., Weber, R., 2011. Prolongation of the atrioventricular conduction in fetuses exposed to maternal anti-Ro/SSA and anti-La/SSB antibodies did not predict progressive heart block. A prospective observational study on the effects of maternal antibodies on 165 fetuses. J. Am. Coll. Cardiol. 57, 1487.

Julkunen, H., Kurki, P., Kaaja, R., Heikkilä, R., Immonen, I., Chan, E.K., et al., 1993. Isolated congenital heart block. Long-term outcome of mothers and characterization of the immune response to SS-A/Ro and to SS-B/La. Arthritis Rheum. 36, 1588.

Julkunen, H., Eronen, M., 2001. The rate of recurrence of isolated congenital heart block: a population-based study. Arthritis Rheum. 44, 487.

Kaaja, R., Julkunen, H., 2003. Prevention of recurrence of congenital heart block with intravenous immunoglobulin and corticosteroid therapy: comment on the editorial by Buyon et al [letter]. Arthritis Rheum. 48, 280.

Kamel, R., Eftekhari, P., Garcia, S., Berthouze, M., Berque-Bestel, I., Peter, J.C., et al., 2005. A high-affinity monoclonal antibody with functional activity against the 5-hydroxytryptaminergic (5-HT4) receptor. Biochem. Pharmacol. 70, 1009.

Kanagasegar, S., Cimaz, R., Kurien, B.T., Brucato, A., Scofield, R.H., 2002. Neonatal lupus manifests as isolated neutropenia and mildly abnormal liver functions. J. Rheumatol. 29, 187.

Karnabi, E., Boutjdir, M., 2010. Role of calcium channels in congenital heart block. Scand. J. Immunol. 72, 226.

Kelly, E., Sananes, R., Chiu-Man, C., Silverman, E., Jaeggi, E., 2014. Prenatal anti-Ro antibody exposure, congenital complete atrioventricular heart block, and high-dose steroid therapy: impact on neurocognitive outcome in school-age children. Arthritis Rheumatol. 66, 2290.

Kertesz, N.J., Fenrich, A.L., Friedman, R.A., 1997. Congenital complete atrioventricular block. Tex. Heart Inst. J. 24, 301.

Laxer, R.M., Roberts, E.A., Gross, K.R., Britton, J.R., Cutz, E., Dimmick, J., et al., 1990. Liver disease in neonatal lupus erythematosus. J. Pediatr. 116, 238.

Lazzerini, P.E., Acampa, M., Guideri, F., Capecchi, P.L., Campanella, V., Morozzi, G., et al., 2004. Prolongation of the corrected QT interval in adult patients with anti-Ro/SSA-positive connective tissue diseases. Arthritis Rheum. 50, 1248.

Lazzerini, P.E., Capecchi, P.L., Guideri, F., Bellisai, F., Selvi, E., Acampa, M., et al., 2007. Comparison of frequency of complex ventricular arrhythmias in patients with positive versus negative anti-Ro/SSA and connective tissue disease. Am. J. Cardiol. 100, 1029.

Lee, L.A., Reichlin, M., Ruyle, S.Z., Weston, W.L., 1993. Neonatal lupus liver disease. Lupus 2, 333.

Levesque, K., Morel, N., Maltret, A., Baron, G., Masseau, A., Orquevaux, P., Piette, J.C., Barriere, F., Le Bidois, J., Fermont, L., Fain, O., Theulin, A., Sassolas, F., Pezard, P., Amoura, Z., Guettrot-Imbert, G., Le Mercier, D., Georgin-Lavialle, S., Deligny, C., Hachulla, E., Mouthon, L., Ravaud, P., Villain, E., Bonnet, D., Costedoat-Chalumeau, N., 2015. Description of 214 cases of autoimmune congenital heart block: results of the French neonatal lupus syndrome. Autoimmun. Rev. 14, 1154.

Levy, R.A., Vilela, V.S., Cataldo, M.J., Ramos, R.C., Duarte, J.L., Tura, B.R., et al., 2001. Hydroxychloroquine (HCQ) in lupus pregnancy: double-blind and placebo-controlled study. Lupus 10, 401.

Llanos, C., Friedman, D.M., Saxena, A., Izmirly, P.M., Tseng, C.E., Dische, R., et al., 2012. Anatomical and pathological findings in hearts from fetuses and infants with cardiac manifestations of neonatal lupus. Rheumatology 51, 1086.

Lopes, L.M., Tavares, G.M., Damiano, A.P., Lopes, M.A., Aiello, V.D., Schultz, R., et al., 2008. Perinatal outcome of fetal atrioventricular block: one-hundred-sixteen cases from a single institution. Circulation 118, 1268.

Lunardi, C., Bason, C., Leandri, M., Navone, R., Lestani, M., Millo, E., et al., 2002. Autoantibodies to inner ear and endothelial antigens in Cogan's syndrome. Lancet 360, 915.

Markham, A.J., Rasmussen, S.E., Salmon, J.E., Martinez-Ortiz, W., Cardozo, T.J., Clancy, R.M., et al., 2015. Reactivity to the p305 epitope of the α1G T-type calcium channel and autoimmune-associated congenital heart block. J. Am. Heart Assoc. 4, e001836.

Martin, V., Lee, L.A., Askanase, A.D., Katholi, M., Buyon, J.P., 2002. Long-term followup of children with neonatal lupus and their unaffected siblings. Arthritis Rheum. 46, 2377.

Matthews, S.G., 2000. Antenatal glucocorticoids and programming of the developing CNS. Pediatr. Res. 47, 291.

Mazel, J.A., El-Sherif, N., Buyon, J., Boutjdir, M., 1999. Electrocardiographic abnormalities in a murine model injected with IgG from mothers of children with congenital heart block. Circulation 99, 1914.

Meisgen, S., Östberg, T., Salomonsson, S., Ding, B., Eliasson, H., Mälarstig, A., et al., 2014. The HLA locus contains novel foetal susceptibility alleles for congenital heart block with significant paternal influence. J. Intern. Med. 275, 640.

Miranda, M.E., Tseng, C.E., Rashbaum, W., Ochs, R.L., Casiano, C.A., Di Donato, F., et al., 1998. Accessibility of SSA/Ro and SSB/La antigens to maternal autoantibodies in apoptotic human fetal cardiac myocytes. J. Immunol. 161, 5061.

Moak, J.P., Barron, K.S., Hougen, T.J., Wiles, H.B., Balaji, S., Sreeram, N., et al., 2001. Congenital heart block: development of late-onset cardiomyopathy, a previously underappreciated sequela. J. Am. Coll. Cardiol. 37, 238.

Motta, M., Rodriguez-Perez, C., Tincani, A., Lojacono, A., Chirico, G., 2007. Outcome of infants from mothers with anti-SSA/Ro antibodies. J. Perinatol. 27, 278.

Neiman, A.R., Lee, L.A., Weston, W.L., Buyon, J.P., 2000. Cutaneous manifestations of neonatal lupus without heart block: characteristics of mothers and children enrolled in a national registry. J. Pediatr. 137, 674.

Nield, L.E., Silverman, E.D., Smallhorn, J.F., Taylor, G.P., Brendan, J., Mullen, M., et al., 2002. Endocardial fibroelastosis associated with maternal anti-Ro and anti-La antibodies in the absence of atrioventricular block. J. Am. Coll. Cardiol. 40, 796.

Peñate, Y., Guillermo, N., Rodríguez, J., Hernández-Machín, B., Montenegro, T., Afonso, J.L., et al., 2009. Histopathologic characteristics of neonatal cutaneous lupus erythematosus: description of five cases and literature review. J. Cutan. Pathol. 36, 660.

Pisoni, C.N., Brucato, A., Ruffatti, A., Espinosa, G., Cervera, R., Belmonte-Serrano, M., et al., 2010. Failure of intravenous immunoglobulin to prevent congenital heart block: findings of a multicenter, prospective, observational study. Arthritis Rheum. 62, 1147.

Press, J., Uziel, Y., Laxer, R.M., Luy, L., Hamilton, R.M., Silverman, E.D., 1996. Long-term outcome of mothers of children with complete congenital heart block. Am. J. Med. 100, 328.

Raboisson, M.J., Fouron, J.C., Sonesson, S.E., Nyman, M., Proulx, F., Gamache, S., 2005. Fetal Doppler echocardiographic diagnosis and successful steroid therapy of Luciani-Wenckebach phenomenon and endocardial fibroelastosis related to maternal anti-Ro and anti-La antibodies. J. Am. Soc. Echocardiogr. 18, 375.

Reed, J.H., Clancy, R.M., Purcell, A.W., Kim, M.Y., Gordon, T.P., Buyon, J.P., 2011. β_2-glycoprotein I and protection from anti-SSA/Ro60-associated cardiac manifestations of neonatal lupus. J. Immunol. 187, 520.

Reed, J.H., Clancy, R.M., Lee, K.H., Saxena, A., Izmirly, P.M., Buyon, J.P., 2012. Umbilical cord blood levels of maternal antibodies reactive with p200 and full-length Ro 52 in the assessment of risk for cardiac manifestations of neonatal lupus. Arthritis Care Res. 64, 1373.

Reed, J.H., Sim, S., Wolin, S.L., Clancy, R.M., Buyon, J.P., 2013. Ro60 requires y3 RNA for cell surface exposure and inflammation associated with cardiac manifestations of neonatal lupus. J. Immunol. 191, 110.

Chapter 4

Subclinical Cardiovascular Damage in Systemic Rheumatic Diseases

C. Nardin, M. Rattazzi and P. Pauletto
Department of Medicine – DIMED, University of Padova Medical School and Medicina Interna 1, University Hospital Cà Foncello, Treviso, Italy

1. INTRODUCTION

Key points

- Compared to the general population, patients affected by systemic autoimmune rheumatic diseases carry an increased risk of developing cardiovascular comorbidities, which occur earlier than in the general population.
- This could be explained by the interrelation between traditional and specific disease-related cardiovascular risk factors that accelerate the progression of atherosclerosis.
- The spectrum of cardiovascular manifestations includes myocardial infarction, congestive heart failure, and cerebrovascular accidents.

Evidence collected in the last 2 decades suggests that, compared to the general population, patients affected by systemic autoimmune rheumatic diseases (SADs) carry an increased risk of developing cardiovascular (CV) comorbidities in a context of accelerated atherosclerosis. Moreover, CV manifestations occur earlier than in the general population, thus having a relevant effect on mortality of patients with SADs (Nurmohamed et al., 2015; Avina-Zubieta et al., 2012). This is explained by the coexistence in this group of patients of a high prevalence of traditional (such as hypertension, dyslipidemia, diabetes) and specific disease-related risk factors that accelerate the progression of vascular damage. In this context, not only inflammatory mechanisms and immunologic abnormalities, but also genetic factors and treatment effects may contribute to CV comorbidities (Hollan et al., 2013).

However, the processes that are responsible for accelerated atherosclerosis in SADs remain incompletely understood.

In the present chapter we will summarize the spectrum of CV manifestations affecting patients with SADs, with a specific focus on early vascular damage and the effects of therapeutic interventions.

2. EPIDEMIOLOGY AND ROLE OF TRADITIONAL RISK FACTORS

2.1 Rheumatoid Arthritis

Several clinical studies showed that rheumatoid arthritis (RA) is associated with a significant increase in the risk of CV mortality (up to 50%) (Avina-Zubieta et al., 2008), reaching a level similar to what is predicted in patients with type 2 diabetes (Prasad et al., 2015; Peters et al., 2009).

Unlike than expected, the highest relative CV risk is observed in younger people (less than 55 years old) and women, independently from the presence of traditional risk factors (Symmons and Gabriel, 2011; Bartoloni et al., 2010). This is especially the case for RA patients with extraarticular manifestations and high level of disease activity. A clear association between CV comorbidity and time-average disease activity has been demonstrated (Solomon et al., 2015).

Of note, CV risk mortality in patients with RA is increased not only in long-lasting disease, but also within the first 5 years after the diagnosis and, according to the most recent evidence, even before the onset of RA symptoms (Bartoloni et al., 2010). Some studies showed that atherosclerosis may quicken in the preclinical phase of RA, and CV events can occur even within the first year after RA diagnosis (Kerola et al., 2012; Kremers et al., 2008).

CV events include myocardial infarction (MI), congestive heart failure (CHF), and cerebrovascular accidents (CVA). In order to analyze the occurrence of MI, CHF, and CVA in RA, Avina-Zubieta et al. have screened several observational studies and databases. They described in both women and men an overall 48% increase in the incidence of CV events, with an estimated relative risk (RR) for MI and CHF of 1.68 and 1.87, respectively. These studies also showed a relative lower incidence of CVA (RR 1.41), thus suggesting a differential involvement of the brain and the heart during the RA progression (Avina-Zubieta et al., 2012).

Ischemic heart disease is the most frequent cause of CV death in patients with RA. As mentioned earlier, the incidence of MI in these subjects is more than two-fold compared with age- and sex-matched individuals without RA (Hollan et al., 2013; Prasad et al., 2015). In particular, RA is associated with a higher risk of death at 30 days (Van Doornum et al., 2006), together with an increased risk of sudden cardiac death (two-fold excess) and unrecognized MI (Symmons and Gabriel, 2011). Ischemic heart disease in RA patients is often clinically silent, with a low frequency of the typical symptoms of angina and can precede the clinical onset of the rheumatic disease (Maradit-Kremers et al., 2005). This is in agreement with the demonstration that systemic inflammation and immunologic abnormalities can precede many years of the clinical diagnosis of RA. The cardiac vascular damage is mainly characterized for the presence of microvascular dysfunction, with a relatively low prevalence of advanced atherosclerotic lesions and obstructive coronary artery disease (Toutouzas et al., 2013). Consequently, there is a less frequent use of coronary artery by-pass grafting in RA patients as compared to other populations (Maradit-Kremers et al., 2005).

Patients with RA have also increased risk of CHF, which arises independently from the presence of traditional CV risk factors (Prasad et al., 2015; Symmons and Gabriel, 2011). When compared with CHF observed in the general population, the disease occurring in RA patients is characterized by low prevalence of the typical signs/symptoms, presence of preserved ejection fraction and worse clinical outcome (in particular a two-fold excess of sudden death) (Davis et al., 2008).

Other cardiac manifestations commonly seen in RA patients are valvular and pericardial disorders, in particular mitral regurgitation, which affects up to 80% of the patients, and pericarditis, which are generally clinically silent (Van Doornum et al., 2010). Patients with cardiac rheumatoid nodules can also have ECG abnormalities such as ST segment depression (Kremers et al., 2008) or QT dispersion (Peters et al., 2009) that have been both associated with a high risk of ventricular arrhythmias and sudden cardiac death.

The role played by traditional risk factors in determining the CV risk profile of RA patients is still a matter of debate. Although their prevalence is higher in patients with RA the actual association with CV disease progression is weaker than expected (Skeoch and Bruce, 2015). Dyslipidemia is commonly observed in RA patients and it is characterized by a particular lipid profile with reduced levels of both LDL and HDL cholesterol. Of note, HDL usually presents a greater decline than LDL levels, thus generating a more atherogenic profile (Nurmohamed et al., 2015; Skeoch and Bruce, 2015). This phenomenon is known as the "lipid paradox," according to which the reduction of LDL levels is associated with a higher risk of CV events. In particular, it has been postulated that inflammation could modify lipid function and structure, altering the cholesterol efflux capacity of HDL and leading to an impairment of their antiatherogenic function (Charles-Schoeman et al., 2012). Therefore, this phenomenon is particularly evident among RA patients with high disease activity, where elevated systemic inflammation might negatively impact lipid metabolism. Of interest, several studies described the existence of a "pro-inflammatory" phenotype of HDL, the so-called "piHDL." These particles seem to be associated with the circulating levels of several inflammatory molecules such as fibrinogen, haptoglobin, and complement factors, and might actively contribute to the accelerated atherosclerosis. In addition, a high inflammatory activity of the disease has been associated with the loss of antioxidant functions of HDL (Charles-Schoeman et al., 2012). Hypertension is one of the most important risk factors for CV disease and the development of subclinical atherosclerosis and cardiac organ damage. There are conflicting data regarding the prevalence of hypertension in RA. Some studies indicate that hypertension is increased in RA patients compared with the general population (Panoulas et al., 2008), whereas other investigations showed a similar prevalence of hypertension in subjects with or without RA (Boyer et al., 2011). Moreover, according to other evidences hypertension seems to be underdiagnosed and undertreated in patients with RA (Boyer et al., 2011). In particular, Protogerou et al. found a global 54% prevalence of hypertension among RA patients, with 10% of the subjects unaware of being hypertensive and 29% with uncontrolled hypertension. The same authors also found that the "white coat" phenomenon was very common in this population (one of every five patients) and that was associated with the presence of subclinical vascular damage (Protogerou et al., 2013). Several clinical data also suggest that there is no correlation between the presence of hypertension and the disease activity (Panoulas et al., 2008). Nevertheless, some mechanisms have been proposed to explain the increase in blood pressure observed in RA patients, including the corticosteroid use and the vascular effects of circulating inflammatory mediators (Panoulas et al., 2008).

Several studies also found an increased prevalence of diabetes in RA patients, compared with the general population (Boyer et al., 2011). In particular, a strong correlation between high disease activity, seropositivity to rheumatoid factor (RF), and insulin resistance has been described, suggesting a central role for inflammation in the pathogenesis of insulin resistance (Chung et al., 2008). In agreement with this possibility, it has been shown that antiinflammatory treatments [in particular TNF inhibitors and hydroxychloroquine (HCQ)] can reduce insulin resistance and that this positive effect was more evident among patients with normal body mass index (BMI) (Stavropoulos-Kalinoglou et al., 2012). Although the prevalence of central obesity is higher in patients with RA, there are evidence showing that subjects with low BMI (<20 kg/m^2) have increased risk of CV disease and death when compared to individuals without RA and normal BMI. This is probably due to a correlation between high disease activity and the catabolic state, in which muscle mass is destroyed more rapidly than fat (rheumatoid cachexia) (Kremers et al., 2004).

2.2 Systemic Lupus Erythematosus

As described for RA, patients affected by systemic lupus erythematosus (SLE) display an increased risk of CV disease. The latter is correlated with the disease duration, average disease activity, the titer of anti-dsDNA, and corticosteroid therapy. CV events are more frequent in young people (less than 40 years old) although a bimodal mortality pattern has been described. In particular, the first peak occurs within 3 years after the diagnosis and it is mainly associated with the disease activity; the second peak instead occurs later and mainly reflects the impact of the CV diseases. While the first peak has been reduced by the improvement in the management of SLE complications, the second peak remains the main cause of death in these patients (Schoenfeld et al., 2013).

Although traditional CV risk factors are present in SLE patients, some SLE-specific risk factors have been associated with CV mortality. These include C-reactive protein (CRP), cytokines, antiphospholipid antibodies, and other autoantibodies (Doria et al., 2005).

Similar to RA, several clinical studies observed an increased risk of MI in SLE patients (2- to 10-fold increase) especially among younger people, who in fact carry the higher relative risk. Interestingly, unlike than expected, CV risk is particularly elevated among young women, especially among those in the premenopausal age, who have the higher relative risk of MI (8.7-fold increase). No differences in CV risk have been described between older SLE patients and controls (Schoenfeld et al., 2013).

SLE is often associated also with ventricular hypertrophy and cardiomyopathy. The negative cardiac remodeling can be due to traditional risk factors such as hypertension, but also can be in some cases attributed to pharmacological treatment (such as hydroxychloroquine). As for the ischemic disease, the risk of CHF is particularly elevated among younger SLE patients (18–44 years old) (Roman and Salmon, 2007).

Valvular manifestations, such as valvular regurgitation and other abnormalities are very frequent during SLE (>50%). In particular, valvular nodules and endocarditis are the most common valve diseases but they are often clinically silent and underdiagnosed (Roman and Salmon, 2007). Libman-Sacks endocarditis, which is characterized by nonbacterial vegetations, occurs in mitral (15%) or aortic (19%) valve and it is often correlated with positivity for antiphospholipid antibodies. Pericarditis is commonly seen in SLE patients (20–50%) but they are usually mild without significant cardiac tamponade (Owlia et al., 2012). Sinus tachycardia, atrial fibrillation, and ectopic atrial beats are frequently seen in patients with SLE and are often correlated with the disease activity. Moreover, the presence of antibodies for small cytoplasmic ribonucleoproteins has been associated with development of sinus bradycardia and prolonged QT interval (Lazzerini et al., 2011).

The prevalence of stroke, both ischemic and hemorrhagic, is increased in SLE patients compared to healthy individuals (10–15% of deaths) and it is accompanied by a worse clinical outcome. The higher relative risk was observed, once again, in younger people and the presence of traditional risk factors, such as hypertension, is not sufficient to explain this clinical outcome. Other SLE-specific risk factors such as intracranial vasculitis, antiphospholipid syndrome, valvular immune deposits, and others, might play an important pathogenic role (Holmqvist et al., 2015).

SLE patients with CV manifestations present less frequently traditional risk factors as compared to the general population. In line with findings in RA patients, also in SLE the relative contribution of classic risk factors to CV disease is weaker. According to several studies, the presence of dyslipidemia in SLE and in the general population is similar. Data derived from Urowitz et al. (2007, 2008) reported a prevalence of lipid disorders in SLE patients ranging from 36.3% at diagnosis and 60% after the first 3 years with the more severe dyslipidemia occurring in patients with chronic kidney disease (lupus nephritis) (Chong et al., 2011). Nevertheless, the interaction between SLE and lipid abnormalities can produce a synergistic pathogenic effect that explains the higher risk of MI observed in these patients. SLE patients display a peculiar lipid phenotype called "*lupus pattern of dyslipidemia*," which is characterized by elevated VLDL and triglycerides (TG) as well as reduced HDL. Of note, this atherogenic pattern is already evident at the moment of disease diagnosis and the levels of piHDL (proinflammatory phenotype of HDL) are more elevated in SLE than in RA patients (45% vs. 20%) (Symmons and Gabriel, 2011). Several pathogenetic mechanisms have been proposed to explain these modifications, including impaired lipid metabolism induced by autoantibodies and cytokines [tumor necrosis factor alpha (TNFα)] as well as the negative impact of some drugs (in particular prednisone therapy) (Wijaya et al., 2005). Clinical studies also indicate that the prevalence of hypertension is increased in SLE patients, in particular among women younger than 40 years old (74% during SLE vs. 2.7–14% in the general population). Pathogenesis of hypertension in SLE is mainly supported by the presence of hyperrenin state (due to the renal damage) and by the development of autonomic dysfunction (reduction of parasympathetic activity and relative increase of the sympathetic tone) (Mathis, 2015). Even diabetes and insulin resistance are more frequent in SLE women than in the healthy controls and are considered independent risk factors for CV events in these patients (Schoenfeld et al., 2013).

2.3 Psoriatic Arthritis

Psoriatic arthritis (PsA) is a rheumatic disorder that occurs in 14–30% of patients with psoriasis (Eder and Gladman, 2015). Although epidemiologic data are still limited, similarly to psoriasis (PsO), PsA is also associated with a 40% increase in the risk of CV events, in particular MI and stroke (Eder et al., 2014). Recent studies reported an overall CV risk in PsA patients higher than those with PsO alone. Despite the significant contribution to CV morbidity and mortality of traditional risk factors, such as metabolic and lipid alterations, PsA per se should be considered as an independent CV risk factor (Zhu et al., 2012). In this context an important role could be attributed to PsA-related risk factors such as the disease activity and the extent of systemic inflammation. As a matter of fact, indicators of disease severity and markers of inflammation [such as number of joints involved, erythrocyte sedimentation rate (ESR), number of dactylitic digits, and leukocyte count] have been associated with accelerated atherosclerosis and clinical CV manifestations (Eder et al., 2016).

In a population-based study Husted et al. have found that, compared to patients with PsO alone, PsA subjects showed higher prevalence of the majority of the CV traditional risk factors, including hypertension (37.1% vs. 26.5%), dyslipidemia (20.7% vs. 14.5%), and diabetes (12% vs. 6.7%). Other studies confirmed that hypertension is the most common CV risk factor observed in PsA and that its prevalence is increased in these patients compared to the general population (Eder et al., 2016; Husted et al., 2011). The risk of developing diabetes is elevated in PsA subjects (up to 70%, according to data derived from Dubreuil et al., 2014) and it is often associated with obesity, smoking, and alcohol consumption (Zhu et al., 2012). Moreover, patients with PsA have higher BMI as compared to healthy controls, PsO alone, or RA patients. The overall prevalence of metabolic syndrome is also increased in PsA patients and its presence has been shown to correlate with the disease activity and the levels of serum adipokines (Eder et al., 2012). According to data derived from Mok et al. (2011b), the risk of developing metabolic syndrome is 2.44-fold increased in PsA patients with respect to those with RA or ankylosing spondylitis (AS). Data on lipid pattern in PsA are controversial. For instance, some authors described a lipid profile characterized by a reduction in HDL_3 cholesterol with an increase in LDL_3 cholesterol, whereas others reported opposite modification with increase in HDL and reduction in total and LDL cholesterol (Zhu et al., 2012).

2.4 Ankylosing Spondylitis

It is well established that AS represents an independent CV risk factor. AS patients carry a significant increased risk of CV, in particular for ischemic heart disease and MI (Szabo et al., 2011). Data derived from a recent population-based study on a Canadian cohort reported a risk up to 25–60% of CV disease among AS patients (Szabo et al., 2011). However, in their meta-analysis, Mathieu et al. observed that nowadays the incidence of MI in AS is reduced as compared to previous clinical investigations. An opposite trend was instead observed for the incidence of stroke that is now more elevated than in the past. These changes are probably due to concomitant improvement in the recent years in both the clinical management of ischemic heart disease and stroke diagnosis (Mathieu et al., 2010b). As already previously described in other rheumatic diseases such as AR and SLE, also younger patients with AS carry the highest RR for CV events (Szabo et al., 2011). Interestingly, Huang et al. (2013) found an increased CV risk among patients with recent diagnosis of the disease, suggesting that atherosclerosis may be accelerated in the preclinical phase of AS.

Indeed, the risk of developing CV events in AS patients remains high even after correction for traditional risk factors, suggesting the existence of an independent pathogenic role for systemic inflammation. This is supported by data derived from the literature describing an association between the risk of premature CV death and the disease activity as measured by CRP levels. Interestingly, it was also shown that women with AS had a lower degree of inflammation and only men had an increased CV mortality compared to healthy controls (Berg et al., 2015).

Some authors reported an increased prevalence of heart failure with preserved ejection fraction (HFpEF) in AS patients, compared to healthy controls. It has been hypothesized that inflammatory mechanisms can lead to cardiac hypertrophy and diastolic dysfunction of the left ventricle, by reducing cardiac elasticity and compliance. Moreover, inflammatory processes could also lead to fibrosis of intraventricular septum, causing electrical disturbances such as ventricular extrasystoles (Nurmohamed et al., 2012).

Aortic insufficiency occurs in the 5–26% of AS patients and it is associated with early hospitalization. This aortic regurgitation is derived from an inflammatory process characterized by destruction of elastic tissue and fibrosis, which involve the aortic root, the ascending aorta, and the valve. The resulting aortic insufficiency can remain asymptomatic for several years (Palazzi et al., 2010).

In patients with AS the prevalence of traditional CV risk factors is increased, but even in this case they can only partially explain the elevated vascular risk profile of these subjects (Haroon et al., 2015). A "proatherogenic" lipid pattern has been described in AS patients, which is characterized by low HDL cholesterol levels and a high total/HDL cholesterol ratio. Moreover, in their systematic review of the literature, Mathieu et al. (2011) described the existence of an inverse correlation between HDL cholesterol levels and the intensity of inflammation.

The prevalence of hypertension among AS patients is increased compared to healthy subjects. The chronic treatment with nonsteroidal antiinflammatory drugs (NSAIDs) could lead to organ damage and contribute to increase of blood pressure in these patients. AS patients also present an elevated prevalence of diabetes and metabolic syndrome. Data derived from the literature about the role of BMI are contrasting. Indeed, while most recent population-based studies reported a higher BMI in AS subjects (Haroon et al., 2015), other researches showed reduction in BMI in AS compared to the general population (Papagoras et al., 2013).

2.5 Systemic Sclerosis

Recent evidences showed that systemic sclerosis (SSc) carries an increased risk of premature CV death (up to 30%), so that SSc per se and can be considered an independent CV risk factor. SSc patients have a higher risk of hospitalization for CV events and a worse outcome compared to unaffected controls (Ali et al., 2015). Similar data have been reported by Avina-Zubieta et al. who highlighted that CV events usually occur in the early phase of the disease, especially in the first year after the diagnosis. Several mechanisms have been proposed to explain the increase of CV events in SSc patients. Besides the well-known macrovascular damage induced by systemic inflammation, microvascular abnormalities per se seem to have an important independent role in the pathogenesis of accelerated atherosclerosis (Avina-Zubieta et al., 2015).

A peculiar characteristic of the CV manifestations in SSc is the frequent involvement of the right ventricle. According to Meune et al., the right ventricle is affected early after the diagnosis showing features of diastolic dysfunction (25% vs. 5% of systolic dysfunction). This occurs regardless of the presence of pulmonary arterial hypertension and is probably due to a vascular damage of both heart and lung in the context of the so-called "myocardial Raynaud's phenomenon," a process leading to myocardial fibrosis (Meune et al., 2015). Patients with diffuse SSc also show a higher prevalence of atrial arrhythmias (20–30%), especially atrial fibrillation (Giallafos et al., 2014). The latter is often correlated with left ventricle dysfunction, left atrial dilatation, and high BNP levels. Unlike the other rheumatic diseases, the prevalence of traditional CV risk factors among SSc patients is similar or even lower compared with the general population. However, some studies showed that even in SSc can be found an increase in piHDL levels or the presence of a proatherogenic lipid profile (Tsifetaki et al., 2010).

3. SUBCLINICAL ATHEROSCLEROSIS

Key points

- The presence of early vascular damage can be detected through the measurement of carotid intima-media thickness (CIMT), the analysis of pulse wave velocity (PWV), and flow-mediated dilatation (FMD).
- The majority of evidence derived from literature reported an increase of CIMT and PWV and a decrease of FMD in the rheumatic diseases, suggesting the presence of an early vascular damage that precedes the onset of clinical events.

As mentioned earlier the clinical history of SADs can be characterized by the development of early vascular damage that precedes the onset of clinical events. For this reason a precocious detection of subclinical atherosclerosis can be of importance for the clinical management of these groups of patients. The presence of early vascular damage can be detected through noninvasive, simple, and inexpensive methods such as the measurement of carotid IMT (CIMT), the analysis of pulse wave velocity

TABLE 4.1 Markers of Subclinical Atherosclerosis in Rheumatic Diseases

	Carotid Intima-Media Thickness (CIMT)	Pulse Wave Velocity (PWV)	Flow-Mediated Dilatation
Rheumatoid arthritis	↑ (Kurt et al., 2015; Chatterjee Adhikari et al., 2012)	↑ (Maki-Petaja et al., 2006; Kocabay et al., 2012)	↓ (Chatterjee Adhikari et al., 2012; Watanabe et al., 2014; Gonzalez-Juanatey et al., 2003)
Systemic lupus erythematosus	↑ (Doria et al., 2003; Przywara-Chowaniec et al., 2014)	↑ (Djokovic et al., 2014; Liu et al., 2014)	↓ (Wang et al., 2014)
Psoriatic arthritis	↑ (Di Minno et al., 2011; Contess et al., 2009; Mazlan et al., 2009)	Limited data	↓ (Puato et al., 2014; Sharma et al., 2016)
Ankylosing spondylitis	↓ (Choe et al., 2008), ↑ (Mathieu et al., 2008)	↑ (Mathieu et al., 2008)	↓ (Choe et al., 2008)
Systemic sclerosis	↑ (Turiel et al., 2013; Au et al., 2011)	↑ (Timar et al., 2008; Liu et al., 2011)	↓ (Au et al., 2011; Szucs et al., 2007), ↑ (Andersen et al., 2002)

(PWV), and of FMD (Table 4.1). In the following paragraphs we will review the evidence about the impact of SADs on arterial disease as established through the use of these noninvasive procedures.

3.1 Rheumatoid Arthritis

A number of longitudinal investigations, performed in different clinical settings, clearly demonstrated that CIMT is a reliable marker of preclinical atherosclerosis and an independent predictor of CV events (Qu and Qu, 2015). Several studies reported a significant increase of CIMT in RA patients compared with the general population, even after adjustment for traditional risk factors. Moreover, this association was evident even among patients without conventional risk factors or CV symptoms, thus suggesting an independent effect of RA in generating the vascular injury (Kurt et al., 2015). Clinical features of RA correlated with CIMT are the African race, age less than 45 years old, a disease duration $\geq$5 years and BMI $\geq$25 (Wang et al., 2015). As for the association between CIMT and disease duration, other authors observed an increased CIMT also among RA subjects at early stage of the disease (Chatterjee Adhikari et al., 2012). Conversely, other investigators have questioned these previous findings and found similar values of CIMT between RA patients and control subjects. Probably, this discrepancy can be explained by the difference in disease activity observed among RA patients enrolled in the different studies. Several researches also evaluated the relationship between the presence of subclinical atherosclerosis, detected through CIMT, and the levels of different circulating markers of systemic inflammation, which reflect the disease activity. However, the data derived from literature are conflicting. Infact, the strong association described by some authors between CIMT and serum levels of CRP, erythrocyte sedimentation rate (ESR), interleukin-6 (IL-6), osteoprotegerin (OPG), and TNFα (Vazquez-Del Mercado et al., 2015) was not confirmed by others (van Breukelen-van der Stoep et al., 2015). This suggests that, in addition to systemic inflammation, concomitant immunologic abnormalities might actively contribute in generating the vascular damage. In line with this possibility, it has been recently shown that increased levels of RF, anticyclic citrullinated peptide antibodies and thyroid peroxidase antibodies are directly associated with CIMT (Raterman et al., 2013). These data also indicate that autoantibodies may play a role in the pathogenesis of the early vascular damage observed in RA.

PWV is a noninvasive and inexpensive method to detect arterial stiffness, an early marker of arterial dysfunction that is strongly correlated with the presence of endothelial impairment, atherogenesis and arterial fibrosis/calcification. PWV is inversely correlated to arterial compliance and represents an independent predictor of future CV events. Data collected in RA patients have shown that subjects affected by the rheumatic disease had a significant increase in aortic PWV, compared to healthy controls (Maki-Petaja et al., 2006). Of note, this alteration was also evident among patients with early RA, suggesting, once again, that arterial degenerative processes occur at early stages of the disease (Kocabay et al., 2012). The relationship between PWV and systemic inflammation remains unclear. According to some studies, arterial stiffness is directly correlated to circulating levels of markers of inflammation and disease duration. However, other authors did not confirm these data and described instead the presence of a current but nonpersistent association (Maki-Petaja et al., 2006). Interestingly, Turkyilmaz et al. reported in early RA an association between PWV and increased serum levels of YKL-40. The latter is a glycoprotein that can be considered as a potential biomarker of endothelial dysfunction and local inflammation (Turkyilmaz et al., 2013).

FMD is a noninvasive approach to detect the endothelial impairment occurring at the early phases of atherogenesis. Several studies showed that FMD is significantly lower in RA patients than healthy controls. These differences remained significant even after correction for traditional risk factors, thus suggesting that the impaired vascular function is independently correlated with the presence of RA (Chatterjee Adhikari et al., 2012). Reduction in FMD is also evident in early RA and it is directly associated with the activity and the duration of the disease (Watanabe et al., 2014), although some studies indicated that FMD is impaired in patients with both high and low disease activity (Gonzalez-Juanatey et al., 2003). The studies that have correlated in RA the presence of both structural (CIMT) and functional (FMD) damage returned conflicting evidence. In fact, while previous works did not find statistically significant relationships between CIMT and FMD (Gonzalez-Juanatey et al., 2011), other studies described a positive correlation between the presence of carotid lesions and endothelial dysfunction, an association that was mainly dependent on disease duration (more evident after 7 years from diagnosis) (Mohan et al., 2014). Interestingly, Temiz et al. recently reported in RA patients an association between FMD, CIMT, and the thickness of the epicardial adipose tissue. The latter is a surrogate of visceral adiposity, which is also increased in RA and it is correlated to the risk of CV events (Temiz et al., 2015).

3.2 Systemic Lupus Erythematosus

Studies performed in SLE subjects showed that CIMT can be considered a predictor of future CV events, in analogy with observations in RA patients (Kao et al., 2013). Clinical investigations also showed that SLE patients have a significantly higher CIMT and increased incidence of atherosclerotic plaques as compared to healthy controls (Doria et al., 2003). Some authors reported a difference of 0.2−0.3 mm between CIMT of patients with SLE and control individuals (Przywara-Chowaniec et al., 2014), an increment that can translate in more than 10−15% increase in the risk of MI (Lorenz et al., 2007). Of note, SLE women not only develop carotid plaques earlier, but also display a faster disease progression. A population-based study performed by Leonard et al. evaluated the role of conventional CIMT to detect the presence of atherosclerotic plaques in SLE premenopausal women. They found that SLE patients have a decrease in the thickness of the carotid media layer and an increase in the intima layer, resulting in a higher intima/media ratio (Leonard et al., 2011). Although the correlation between CIMT, classical risk factors and systemic inflammatory markers remains nowadays unclear, SLE per se can probably be considered an independent risk factor for early carotid vascular damage. While several population-based studies reported a significant association between CIMT and both classical (such as increased BMI, dyslipidemia, and hypertension) (Gheita et al., 2013) and SLE-related risk factors (such as disease duration/activity and age at onset) (Hassan et al., 2013), others investigators did not confirm these findings (Belibou et al., 2012). For instance Kisiel et al. (2015b) and Kiani et al. (2011a) showed a direct, positive association between CIMT and disease duration, but not with disease activity. In addition, Ammirati et al. (2014) found that SLE patients with higher CIMT had an increase in BMI and systolic blood pressure (SBP), without showing associations with disease duration, age at the onset, or levels of systemic inflammatory markers, such as CRP. Djokovic et al. (2014) demonstrated that the presence of antiphospholipid antibodies represents an independent predictor for higher CIMT regardless of the prevalence of traditional risk factors. A study performed by our group in 78 SLE patients showed a 17% and a 28% prevalence of carotid plaques and CIMT, respectively. We also observed that prednisone cumulative dose, chronic kidney disease, and SLE disease activity were the most important SLE-related risk factors for subclinical atherosclerosis (Doria et al., 2003). The conflicting data derived from the literature could be explained by the presence of a complex interplay between conventional CV risk factors, inflammation, and immunologic alterations, that can have independent or synergistic effects during the atherogenic process.

Compared to healthy subjects, SLE patients also showed increased aortic PWV. In particular, Liu et al. (2014) demonstrated that, regardless of disease duration, instantaneous wave intensity, used to measure carotid elasticity, was higher in SLE premenopausal women without cardiovascular risk factors. In SLE, small artery elasticity (SAE) is also impaired and significantly associated with SLE-related risk factors. Of interest, these modifications have been described in patients without increase in CIMT, suggesting that SAE might occur at very early stage of atherosclerosis (Nienhuis et al., 2010). Data about the contribution of traditional and SLE-specific risk factors to the arterial stiffness are conflicting. Some studies described the presence of a correlation between metabolic syndrome and PWV (Sabio et al., 2009), whereas other investigators reported a positive association with SBP but not with the disease activity or duration (Sacre et al., 2014). A positive correlation between plasma homocysteine levels and brachial ankle PWV was also observed (Tso et al., 2006), but these findings were not confirmed by other researches (Sacre et al., 2014).

Several population-based studies also compared FMD values between SLE patients and healthy controls. However, these researches provided inconsistent findings, probably because of a significant heterogeneity among the groups under investigation. Nevertheless, a recent meta-analysis performed by Wang et al. reported a significant decrease in FMD among SLE patients as compared to the general population. Additional investigations are needed to evaluate the correlation between FMD and traditional CV or SLE-related risk factors (Wang et al., 2014).

3.3 Psoriatic Arthritis

A number of ultrasonographic studies showed the presence of increased CIMT in PsA patients compared to the general population (Di Minno et al., 2011; Contessa et al., 2009). In particular Mazlan et al. (2009) reported a prevalence of increased CIMT in 15.9% of PsA subjects. Data dissecting the correlation between CIMT and traditional and PsA-specific risk factors are modest. Some authors showed that PsA patients have a positive correlation between the extent of CIMT and BMI, diabetes, SBP, total cholesterol, and LDL cholesterol (Contessa et al., 2009; Gonzalez-Juanatey et al., 2007). However, Di Minno et al. reported the presence of a lower CIMT in PsA patients compared to controls, when taking into account the presence of traditional risk factors. These data suggested a minor role for PsA per se in promoting carotid vascular damage (Di Minno et al., 2011). Our group recently investigated the role of hypertension in the progression of subclinical atherosclerosis in this rheumatic population. We demonstrated that PsA hypertensive patients had higher increase in CIMT as compared to normotensive subjects. These data indicate that mechanisms involved in hypertension may play an important amplificatory role in the generation of vascular damage. On the contrary, we could not find any differences in FMD values, which was in fact equally impaired in both groups regardless of blood pressure values. Moreover, a significant correlation was found between OPG levels, an independent predictor of CV events, and the extent of CIMT, particularly among the hypertensive patients (Puato et al., 2014a). As for PsA-related risk factors, such as disease activity/duration, CRP, and fibrinogen levels, a positive association with CIMT has been described by Kimhi et al. (2007), but not by Mazlan et al. (2009). Similar to our findings, other investigators found a significant decrease in FMD among PsA patients, which seems to occur earlier than CIMT (Sharma et al., 2016).

3.4 Ankylosing Spondylitis

A number of clinical studies reported an increased CIMT in AS patients compared with matched controls, regardless of the prevalence of classical CV risk factors (Mathieu et al., 2008). However, these findings were not confirmed by others (Choe et al., 2008). Perrotta et al. observed that increase in CIMT was confined at the carotid bulb segment. These authors also found an association between carotid bulb CIMT and ESR values (Perrotta et al., 2013). This observation was not entirely confirmed by Gonzalez et al. who reported a positive correlation between ESR and the presence of carotid plaques, but not with the extent of CIMT (Gonzalez-Juanatey et al., 2009).

Data about the role of traditional and AS-related risk factors are ambiguous. A positive correlation between CIMT and disease duration was described by the majority of the studies so far performed, revealing that a prolonged systemic inflammation plays an important role in accelerated atherogenesis. Conversely, no association was found with disease activity and markers of systemic inflammation such as CRP (Gonzalez-Juanatey et al., 2009). In addition, Mathieu et al. (2008), in their investigations, reported a correlation between CIMT, smoking, and SBP.

Modifications in PWV and FMD in AS patients have been investigated in a limited number of studies. Some reports showed that PWV values are higher among AS cases than controls (Mathieu et al., 2008), although additional studies are needed to confirm these data and to evaluate the contribution of traditional and AS-related risk factors to arterial stiffness. Some authors also reported a reduction in FMD in AS patients as compared to the general population, suggesting the presence of early endothelial dysfunction in this group of patients (Choe et al., 2008). However, these findings were not confirmed by Perrotta et al. (2013) who did not find any differences in FMD values between cases and controls.

3.5 Systemic Sclerosis

Differently from previous investigations (Hettema et al., 2008), recent studies described a significant increment of CIMT in SSc patients as compared to the general population and nonsystemic sclerosis (noScc) subjects, although no differences were seen in the prevalence of carotid plaques. Similar findings have been reported in some meta-analysis (Turiel et al., 2013). Other investigators, such as for instance Au et al. (2011) observed a 0.11 mm difference in CIMT between cases and controls. Interestingly, Schiopu et al. (2014) demonstrated that CIMT was directly correlated to the serum levels of proteins and cytokines involved in fibrosis and vasculopathy, whereas Bartoli et al. (2007a) found an association between CIMT and the deletion polymorphism of the angiotensin-converting enzyme gene. Nevertheless, additional studies are needed to elucidate the role of traditional and disease-related risk factors in the pathogenesis of vascular damage. So far, only age seems to be associated with accelerated atherosclerosis in SSc (Sherer et al., 2007). The presence of an early vascular damage in SSc patients was also confirmed by studies evaluating the presence of arterial stiffness and endothelial dysfunction. An increase in PWV was observed in SSc subjects, and this increase of markers of vascular damage was independent from the presence of conventional risk factors (Timar et al., 2008). Interestingly, Liu et al. (2011) showed that regional, but not aortic, PWV was increased prior to the increment of CIMT; this could be explained by the fact that the reduction of arterial elasticity affects the muscular arteries prior than the large vessels (such as the aorta and its branches). According to a population-based studies performed by Timar et al., PWV seems to be higher in patients with limited than diffuse cutaneous scleroderma, suggesting the existence of different vascular pathogenetic mechanisms between these two clinical forms. In addition, presence of arterial stiffness has been associated with disease duration, positivity of anticentromere antibodies (Timar et al., 2008) as well as circulating levels of soluble endothelial adhesion molecules (Andersen et al., 2002). The development of endothelial dysfunction is another early event in the course of SSc; indeed many authors described a lower FMD in SSc patients when compared to healthy subjects (Szucs et al., 2007), although some researches did not confirm these findings (Andersen et al., 2002). A meta-analysis performed by Au et al. (2011) reported a difference in FMD of 3.07% between patients with SSc and controls with similar evidences for nitroglycerin-mediated dilatation, an endothelium-independent vasodilatation (Andersen et al., 2002).

Limited data exist about the contribution of traditional and SSc-related risk factors on endothelial dysfunction. The studies available so far revealed no correlation between impairment of FMD and SSc disease duration or presence of CV risk factors (such as hypertension, smoke and dyslipidemia) (Bartoli et al., 2007b).

4. CARDIOVASCULAR EFFECTS OF PHARMACOLOGICAL TREATMENTS

Key points

- Several clinical studies suggested a beneficial cardiovascular effect of disease-modifying antirheumatic drugs, which may slow the progression of subclinical atherosclerosis and improve the clinical outcome.

4.1 Rheumatoid Arthritis

As described earlier, increased CV risk in RA has been well established, although the specific contribution and interrelation between traditional and RA-related risk factors remain nowadays unclear. As systemic inflammation represents a major contributor to CV disease, antiinflammatory therapeutic approaches could furnish at least ancillary effects and improve the CV risk in RA as well as in other rheumatic diseases. We will now focus on the impact on CV risk of the main pharmacological therapies currently available for RA patients.

4.1.1 Nonsteroidal Antiinflammatory Drugs

Data about the CV risk associated with the use of NSAIDs in RA are conflicting. NSAIDs should be prescribed at the lowest possible dose and with the lowest frequency (Dhillon and Liang, 2015; Pieringer et al., 2014). While some population-based studies showed that the use of NSAIDs is correlated with increased CV morbidity in RA (Garner et al., 2005), others researches observed a decrease of CV events in RA patients treated with NSAIDs compared to control subjects undergoing similar therapy. However, this protective effect was not reported for diclofenac and rofecoxib (Hollan et al., 2015). As for Aspirin, despite its well-established use for CV prevention in the general population, further studies are needed to clarify its potential role in primary prevention in RA.

4.1.2 Glucocorticoids

Glucocorticoids (GC) are commonly used in RA and many studies have been performed in order to establish their impact on CV events. It is well known that GC therapy has beneficial, fast effects on the control of the disease activity but also carries multiple adverse metabolic effects in term of glycemic control, increase of body fat, development of hypertension, and so on. Taking into account the difficulty of distinguishing the contribution of the underlying disease activity from the effects of GC therapy itself, it should be also noted that several authors observed an increase in CV risk among RA patients (by up to 68% for MI, by 14% per 5 mg/day) treated with GC (Pieringer et al., 2014; Barbhaiya and Solomon, 2013; Avina-Zubieta et al., 2013). In particular, Avina-Zubieta et al. (2011) found that, while the risk of MI and CHF is increased during GC therapy, no differences were found in the rate of cerebrovascular accidents. This phenomenon was observed not only in case of cumulative supraphysiologic doses and long exposure, but also for prednisone daily dosage less than 10 mg (Barbhaiya and Solomon, 2013). In line with these findings, Del Rincòn et al. demonstrated that 8 mg was the prednisone daily threshold dose correlated with an increased risk of CV death. Thus, according to these data, RA patients should be preferentially treated by using a daily prednisone dose of less than 7.5 mg and a cumulative dose of less than 40 mg (del Rincon et al., 2014). Notably, the RF positivity was reported to be associated with a greater CV morbidity during GC treatment compared to FR negativity, thus suggesting a potential interaction between GC and autoantibodies in the pathogenesis of the vascular damage (van Sijl et al., 2014); these findings add to other pathogenic mechanisms independently induced by GC such as the destabilization of atherosclerotic plaques or the development of vascular calcification (Preusch et al., 2008).

Some authors also investigated the impact of GC on lipid profile. In particular, Schroeder et al. demonstrated that a daily prednisone dose of $\geq$7.5 mg led to an increase in HDL cholesterol levels, whereas no effects were seen in LDL and total cholesterol levels These data were confirmed by other studies of pharmacological association, which highlighted that this improvement in lipid profile was specific for GC activity and was not observed when using other drugs. However, the impact of this modification of lipid profile on vascular disease progression is currently unknown (Schroeder et al., 2015).

4.1.3 Nonbiologic Disease-Modifying Antirheumatic Drugs

Methotrexate (MTX) is one of the most commonly used nonbiologic disease-modifying drugs (DMARDs). Data derived from the literature reported a favorable impact of MTX on CV disease, with a decrease in mortality that ranges from 15% to 80% depending on the studies (Barbhaiya and Solomon, 2013). These positive effects were also seen in early RA and when the drug was administered as monotherapy or in combination with sulfasalazine (SSZ), HCQ as well as other biologic therapies (Zha et al., 2015). Interestingly, MTX treatment was also associated with a reduction in cerebrovascular accidents, with an 11% decrease in the risk of stroke (Naranjo et al., 2008).

Several studies also highlighted a positive impact of MTX in preventing the onset of subclinical atherosclerosis in RA patients. In particular, Je Kim et al. demonstrated a decrease in CIMT among RA patients who were treated with MTX, an effect that remained significant even after correction for age, disease activity, and level of inflammation. These data were confirmed by Kisiel et al. who reported an improvement in CIMT and femoral intima-media thickness (FIMT) in RA patients treated with MTX $\geq$20 mg/week, regardless of the disease activity. Moreover, they did not observe a significant difference in CIMT and FIMT between MTX and other biologic therapies (Kisiel et al., 2015a). Hannawi et al. (2009) deepened these findings showing that patients treated with MTX, HCQ, and SSZ also had significant improvement in endothelial function as established through FMD. Overall, these clinical data strongly suggest the existence of an independent atheroprotective effect of the therapy with MTX.

Several studies have been performed also to dissect the impact of MTX on traditional CV risk factors. However, the data collected so far are inconclusive. In particular, Dessein et al. (2002) did not find significant modifications in the lipid profile of patients treated with MTX. Instead, the COBRA (combination therapy in rheumatoid arthritis) study revealed that SSZ therapy was associated with a significant increase in total/HDL cholesterol ratio and a decrease in the atherogenic index compared to a combination therapy with SSZ, MTX, and prednisone (Boers et al., 2003). Of note, MTX treatment has been associated with an increase in the levels of homocysteine, which might have a negative impact on CV risk (Landewe et al., 2000). Toms et al. also found a negative association between MTX therapy and the presence of metabolic syndrome, in particular, among patients >60 years. These data suggest that MTX treatment per se can have protective metabolic effects, thus partly explaining the favorable CV outcomes described earlier (Toms et al., 2009).

4.1.4 Biologic Disease-Modifying Antirheumatic Drugs

TNFα inhibitors. A number of basic science studies clearly demonstrated that TNFα can exert significant pathogenic effects during all the phases of atherogenesis. TNFα has been implicated in the initiation of endothelial dysfunction, in the amplification of intimal inflammatory processes as well as in the events associated with plaque rupture. Thus, overproduction of TNFα has been considered as major contributor to the cardiovascular damage observed in RA patients, and its pharmacological inhibition is expected to exert ancillary cardioprotective effects. In line with this possibility, a long-term therapy with TNFα inhibitors, both as monotherapy or in combination with MTX, has been associated in RA patients with a significant reduction in all causes of CV death (mainly MI and stroke) (Dhillon and Liang, 2015), whereas data about the effects on the risk of CHF are conflicting. In particular, Solomon et al. showed that the decrease in CV risk was greater in the first 6 months of treatment with TNFα inhibitors. This was especially true for patients >65 years old (Solomon et al., 2013). In the CORRONA registry, Greenberg at al. reported a major reduction of CV events in patients treated with TNFα inhibitors, compared to those treated with other DMARDs (Greenberg et al., 2011), although others did not confirm these findings (Kisiel et al., 2015a). Several mechanisms have been proposed to explain the CV risk reduction observed during anti-TNFα therapy, including systemic antiinflammatory effects, improvement of lipid profile, plaque stabilization, and others (Popa et al., 2005).

Anti-TNFα therapy might also have a significant impact on subclinical atherosclerosis, which is accelerated in RA patients. In their review of the literature Tam et al. (2014), reported a significant improvement in CIMT and aortic PWV among subjects treated with long-term anti-TNFα and who responded to the therapy. Interestingly, Vassilopoulos et al. (2014) demonstrated that adalimumab decreased aortic stiffness regardless of its effects on disease activity. However, Komai et al. (2007) did not find differences in PWV during anti-TNFα therapy. Other investigators reported an improvement in FMD following anti-TNFα therapy, although this effect was reduced in the long-term (Mazzoccoli et al., 2010).

Data about modifications in the lipid profile during anti-TNFα therapy are conflicting. Some studies showed that TNFα inhibitors can induce a rapid and transient increase in both total and HDL cholesterol and lead to an improvement of the atherogenic index in the long-term (Popa et al., 2005). However, additional studies are needed to understand whether these changes are attributable to the control of systemic inflammation or instead can be considered specific pharmacological effects. In addition, Stagakis et al. (2012) described an improvement in insulin sensitivity and in beta cell function, among RA patients with high insulin resistance treated for 12 weeks with TNFα blockers. Moreover, anti-TNAα therapy, infliximab in particular, have been associated with a significant improvement of blood pressure control as compared to other treatments (Klarenbeek et al., 2010).

IL-6 receptor inhibitors. In analogy with anti-TNFα therapy treatment with tocilizumab, an IL-6 receptor inhibitor has also been shown to exert beneficial effects on CV risk. In particular, a 3-month therapy with tocilizumab was followed by a significant reduction in PWV and improvement in FMD, along with an improvement of systemic inflammation (Protogerou et al., 2011). However, as therapy with tocilizumab has been associated with a worsening of the lipid profile (increase of total and LDL cholesterol), further studies are needed to clarify whether these changes might have detrimental effects on CV risk in the long-term.

Rituximab. Although data derived from literature are limited, patients treated with rituximab (RTX), an anti-CD20 monoclonal antibody, showed an improvement in FMD (Pieringer et al., 2014). The data about the effects of RTX on lipid levels are conflicting with some studies showing a beneficial impact (Pieringer et al., 2014), and others demonstrating no effects (Mathieu et al., 2012).

Abatacept. Studies performed in patients treated with abatacept showed that a 6-month treatment was followed by an increase in aortic stiffness (Mathieu et al., 2013a). Further studies are needed to establish whether this new drug exert negative impact on CV risk.

4.1.5 Statins

Statin therapy is known to have protective effects on CV events in both primary and secondary prevention. These drugs have been shown to promote atherosclerotic plaque stabilization mainly through the reduction of inflammatory mechanisms (Puato et al., 2010; Puato et al., 2014b). However, data about the effects of statin therapy in RA patients are limited. In the TARA trial (Trial of Atorvastatin in Rheumatoid Arthritis), Mc Carey et al. reported beneficial effects on both inflammation and lipid profile in the patients with RA treated with 40 mg of atorvastatin for 6 months (McCarey et al., 2004). In the RORA-AS trial (Rosuvastatin in Rheumatoid Arthritis, Ankylosing Spondylitis and Other Inflammatory Joint Diseases), Ikdahl et al. (2015), demonstrated a significant reduction of atherosclerotic plaques, LDL cholesterol, and systemic markers of inflammation during the statin treatment. Akiyama et al. (2015) in a recent work based on RA Japanese population, found that a low dose of atorvastatin (5–10 mg) led to an improvement of the lipid profile without any effects on disease activity. Interestingly, Tam et al. (2011a) showed a possible improvement of subendocardial perfusion in patients treated with rosuvastatin. According to these observations, further prospective studies should be conducted to evaluate whether statin therapy should be recommended for primary prevention in RA patients.

4.2 Systemic Lupus Erythematosus

Despite the increased prevalence of CV events in SLE patients described earlier it is still unclear whether specific lupus treatments could have some impact on the CV risk of these patients.

4.2.1 Glucocorticoids

GC are commonly used in SLE for their efficacy in the control of disease activity. However, as already mentioned, their negative impact on traditional risk factors such as glycemic control, lipid profile, and hypertension, might have detrimental consequences on the CV risk profile of SLE patients. In line with this possibility, some cohort studies described the existence of an association between GC use and the increase in CV risk. For instance, Moya et al. (2016) showed the presence of a linear relationship between the cumulative GC dose and future CV events, while Al Sawah et al. (2015) in the Hopkins Lupus Cohort, reported a higher risk of organ damage in patients treated with a prednisone dose of $\geq$7.5 mg/d. These data are in agreement with other investigations (Tanay et al., 2007). In a recent study Croca et al. (2015) found that high GC dose was correlated with the levels of anti-ApoA1 antibodies, which are present in SLE and represent a surrogate of high degree of disease activity.

4.2.2 Hydroxychloroquine

HCQ is an antimalarial agent widely used to treat SLE patients and to obtain a rapid control of disease activity. Although an HCQ-induced cardiomyopathy has been described (Yogasundaram et al., 2014), several cohort studies reported a cardioprotective effect of this drug during long-term therapy. This protective effect is probably due to interference of the drug with the TLR7 and TLR9 pathways (Sun et al., 2007). Tanay et al. (2007) demonstrated that, compared to steroids, HCQ led to a lower vascular damage, while Virdis et al. (2015) observed that HCQ improved the endothelial dysfunction in a murine model of SLE, probably through antioxidant-mediated effects.

Clinical studies also showed that treatment with HCQ could have significant impact on traditional CV risk factors. In particular HCQ has been shown to reduce total cholesterol levels and to increase insulin sensitivity, leading to improvement in glycemic control (Rahman et al., 1999).

4.2.3 Immunosuppressive Treatment

Some studies indicated that immunosuppressive agents, namely Mycophenolate mofetil (MMF) and cyclosporine A (CyA), can have beneficial impact on atherogenesis in SLE, mainly in term of reduction in CIMT progression (Kisiel et al., 2015b).

Despite its well-recognized antiinflammatory role, there are conflicting data about the effects of MMF on atherosclerosis in SLE. While Richez et al. (2013) observed a decrease in molecules involved in atherogenesis in a murine model of SLE (*gld.apoE−/−*) treated with MMF, a longitudinal cohort study performed by Kiani et al. (2011b) did not report changes in CIMT of SLE patients treated for 2 years with MMF. On the other side, some studies suggested the existence of an atheroprotective role of CyA, which in fact has been associated with a reduction of CIMT in SLE patients (Oryoji et al., 2014). However, further longitudinal investigations are needed in order to elucidate the real impact of immunosuppressive treatment on traditional CV risk factors and CV events.

4.2.4 Statins

Similar to RA, some investigations indicate the existence of a beneficial impact of statin therapy in preventing atherogenesis in SLE patients. However, mechanisms driving these protective effects are still unclear and might be partly explained by existence of pleiotropic activities of statins, which are independent from the lipid-lowering action. The net result is an improvement in CV outcomes in SLE patients, with an overall reduction in CV morbidity and mortality (Yu et al., 2015). The potential antiinflammatory effects of statins are supported by studies showing a relevant decrease of CRP levels in SLE patients treated with these drugs (Sahebkar et al., 2015). These results are in agreement with previous studies performed by Mok et al. (2011a) and Ruiz-Limon et al. (2014) that also underscored the importance of antioxidant effects associated with the use of these compounds.

Nevertheless, data about the effects of the statins on subclinical atherosclerosis in SLE are discordant. For instance, Mok et al. (2011a) reported a relevant decrease of CIMT, LDL cholesterol, and hs-CRP in SLE patients treated with rosuvastatin, 10 mg/day, up to 24 months. Moreover, an 8-week treatment with atorvastatin, 20 mg, was found to improve FMD (Ferreira et al., 2007). However, in the Lupus Atherosclerosis Prevention Study (LAPS), Petri et al. (2011) did not find differences in CIMT progression among patients treated with atorvastatin 40 mg/day for 2 years. Similar results have been observed in the APPLE (Atherosclerosis Prevention in Pediatric Lupus Erythematosus) study after 36 months of treatment with atorvastatin (Schanberg et al., 2012). In particular, in this latter study, the treatment was not associated with reduction in CIMT progression.

4.3 Psoriatic Arthritis

Data about the impact of antipsoriatic drugs on CV morbidity and mortality in PsA patients are limited and less conclusive when compared with those obtained in RA patients. We will focus especially on biologic DMARDs (TNFα inhibitors), which have been the target of many studies in the recent years.

4.3.1 Biologic Disease-Modifying Antirheumatic Drugs

Several clinical studies suggested the existence of beneficial CV effects of anti-TNFα agents in PsA patients. In particular these drugs may slow the progression of subclinical atherosclerosis and seem to improve the CV risk of PsA patients. Indeed, a higher decrease in CIMT among PsA patients treated with etanercept compared with patients treated with conventional DMARDs, has been recently described (Di Minno et al., 2015). These data are in agreement with previous cohort studies performed by Tam at al. and Di Minno et al. The latter authors also highlighted a relationship with the treatment duration (Di Minno et al., 2015; Tam et al., 2011). In addition, TNFα inhibitors have been shown to produce an improvement in endothelial function, which is known to be impaired in PsA. In particular, Mazzoccoli et al. evaluated the impact of infliximab and etanercept on brachial FMD after 8−12 weeks of treatment. Surprisingly, they found a transitory effect on FMD, which is initially increased and then decreased in the following few weeks of treatment (Mazzoccoli et al., 2010). As for the effect on PWV, there are evidence showing that the long-term anti-TNFα therapy seems to increment aortic elasticity in patients with inflammatory arthropathies. Our group investigated the impact of 2 years of anti-TNFα therapy on subclinical atherosclerosis in a cohort of 32 PsA patients. We reported that, despite clinical improvement, the treatment was not able to slow down the progression of arterial remodeling. While there were no changes in FMD, CIMT showed a higher increase (four-fold excess) compared to age-matched healthy controls (Ramonda et al., 2014).

Besides their well-established antiinflammatory effects, biologic DMARDs have an impact also on conventional CV risk factors. Anti-TNFα therapy has been associated in PsA patients with lower prevalence of metabolic syndrome compared to other treatments. However, data about the effects on lipid profile are conflicting. While Spanakis et al. (2006) reported an increase in HDL cholesterol levels during treatment with infliximab, Cauza et al. (2002) observed a worsening in lipid profile mainly through an increment of TG levels. Costa et al. performed a prospective study with the aim to evaluate the prevalence of metabolic syndrome in patients treated with etanercept, infliximab, and MTX. After 24 months of therapy they found a lower prevalence of metabolic syndrome in patients treated with TNFα inhibitors, as compared to those treated with MTX (Costa et al., 2014).

4.4 Ankylosing Spondylitis

The impact of antirheumatic therapy on CV risk in AS patients remains, nowadays, unclear, although many evidences suggest a potential cardioprotective effect of TNFα inhibitors.

4.4.1 Biologic Disease-Modifying Antirheumatic Drugs

Researches performed in recent years about the impact of DMARDs on CV risk in AS patients were mainly focused on subclinical atherosclerosis and its surrogates. TNFα blocking therapy could exert its beneficial cardioprotective effects through its impact on both AS-related and conventional CV risk factors. van Sijl et al. (2015) found a slower progression of CIMT in patients undergoing continuous treatment with anti-TNFα as compared to those treated discontinuously. These results are in agreement with evidences derived from previous studies (Angel et al., 2012).However, despite a persistent reduction of disease activity, no changes in PWV were found in AS patients during anti-TNFα treatment (Mathieu et al., 2013b). On the contrary, some authors observed a significant improvement of FMD after prescription of infliximab (Syngle et al., 2010) or etanercept (van Eijk et al., 2009). In addition, an inverse correlation between increase of FMD and decrease of CRP levels was found in AS patients treated with infliximab (Syngle et al., 2010). Interestingly, Genre et al. (2015) reported a significant and rapid reduction of circulating markers of endothelial cell activation such as sVCAM-1 and sE-selectin, after administration of a single dose of infliximab. Notably, an antiarrhythmic effect of infliximab has also been described, in term of shortening of QT interval which is usually prolonged in AS patients (Senel et al., 2011).

Some authors also showed that anti-TNFα therapy is followed by an improvement of lipid profile which is characterized by an increment of both total and HDL cholesterol in the absence of changes of atherogenic index (Mathieu et al., 2010a).

4.4.2 Statins

In a recent work, Garg et al. evaluated the impact of rosuvastatin (10 mg/day) treatment on endothelial dysfunction in AS patients. Of note, they found a significant improvement in FMD after statin therapy, which was paralleled by a decrease of the disease activity. These data confirmed, once again, the coexistence of antiinflammatory and immunomodulatory effects associated with statin therapy (Garg et al., 2015). Given these encouraging evidences, further studies are needed in order to clarify the role of statin treatment in the management of CV risk in AS patients.

4.5 Systemic Sclerosis

Although the increased CV risk and the accelerated atherosclerosis in SSc are both well established, only in recent years the effects of antirheumatic drugs on CV mortality have been investigated. However, data derived from the literature are limited, inconclusive, and focus mainly on statin treatment. Timar et al. investigated the impact of rosuvastatin (20 mg/day) on subclinical atherosclerosis in SSc patients. They found that the statin therapy was accompanied by a significant increase of FMD without changes in PWV and CIMT (Timar et al., 2013). However, these results are in disagreement with previous data by Sadik et al. (2010) who did not find modifications in endothelial function after 8 weeks of treatment with atorvastatin 20 mg/day. Further prospective studies are mandatory to improve the management of CV risk in SSc patients.

REFERENCES

Akiyama, M., et al., 2015. Prevalence of dyslipidemia in Japanese patients with rheumatoid arthritis and effects of atorvastatin treatment. Clin. Rheumatol. 34 (11), 1867–1875.

Al Sawah, S., et al., 2015. Effect of corticosteroid use by dose on the risk of developing organ damage over time in systemic lupus erythematosus-the Hopkins Lupus Cohort. Lupus Sci. Med. 2 (1), e000066.

Ali, H., Ng, K.R., Low, A.H., 2015. A qualitative systematic review of the prevalence of coronary artery disease in systemic sclerosis. Int. J. Rheum. Dis. 18 (3), 276–286.

Ammirati, E., et al., 2014. Cardiometabolic and immune factors associated with increased common carotid artery intima-media thickness and cardiovascular disease in patients with systemic lupus erythematosus. Nutr. Metab. Cardiovasc. Dis. 24 (7), 751–759.

Andersen, G.N., et al., 2002. Assessment of vascular function in systemic sclerosis: indications of the development of nitrate tolerance as a result of enhanced endothelial nitric oxide production. Arthritis Rheum. 46 (5), 1324–1332.

Angel, K., et al., 2012. Effect of 1-year anti-TNF-alpha therapy on aortic stiffness, carotid atherosclerosis, and calprotectin in inflammatory arthropathies: a controlled study. Am. J. Hypertens. 25 (6), 644–650.

Au, K., et al., 2011. Atherosclerosis in systemic sclerosis: a systematic review and meta-analysis. Arthritis Rheum. 63 (7), 2078–2090.

Avina-Zubieta, J.A., et al., 2008. Risk of cardiovascular mortality in patients with rheumatoid arthritis: a meta-analysis of observational studies. Arthritis Rheum. 59 (12), 1690–1697.

Avina-Zubieta, J.A., et al., 2011. Risk of cerebrovascular disease associated with the use of glucocorticoids in patients with incident rheumatoid arthritis: a population-based study. Ann. Rheum. Dis. 70 (6), 990–995.

Avina-Zubieta, J.A., et al., 2012. Risk of incident cardiovascular events in patients with rheumatoid arthritis: a meta-analysis of observational studies. Ann. Rheum. Dis. 71 (9), 1524–1529.

Avina-Zubieta, J.A., et al., 2013. Immediate and past cumulative effects of oral glucocorticoids on the risk of acute myocardial infarction in rheumatoid arthritis: a population-based study. Rheumatology 52 (1), 68–75.

Avina-Zubieta, J.A., et al., 2015. Early cardiovascular disease after the diagnosis of systemic sclerosis. Am. J. Med. 129 (3), 324–331.

Barbhaiya, M., Solomon, D.H., 2013. Rheumatoid arthritis and cardiovascular disease: an update on treatment issues. Curr. Opin. Rheumatol. 25 (3), 317–324.

Bartoli, F., et al., 2007a. Angiotensin-converting enzyme I/D polymorphism and macrovascular disease in systemic sclerosis. Rheumatology 46 (5), 772–775.

Bartoli, F., et al., 2007b. Flow-mediated vasodilation and carotid intima-media thickness in systemic sclerosis. Ann. N.Y. Acad. Sci. 1108, 283–290.

Bartoloni, E., et al., 2010. How early is the atherosclerotic risk in rheumatoid arthritis? Autoimmun. Rev. 9 (10), 701–707.

Belibou, C., et al., 2012. Carotid intima-media thickness and plaque as surrogate biomarkers of atherosclerosis among consecutive women with systemic lupus erythematosus. Rom. J. Morphol. Embryol. 53 (1), 29–34.

Berg, I.J., et al., 2015. CRP and ASDAS are associated with future elevated arterial stiffness, a risk marker of cardiovascular disease, in patients with ankylosing spondylitis: results after 5-year follow-up. Ann. Rheum. Dis. 74 (8), 1562–1566.

Boers, M., et al., 2003. Influence of glucocorticoids and disease activity on total and high density lipoprotein cholesterol in patients with rheumatoid arthritis. Ann. Rheum. Dis. 62 (9), 842–845.

Boyer, J.F., et al., 2011. Traditional cardiovascular risk factors in rheumatoid arthritis: a meta-analysis. Jt. Bone Spine 78 (2), 179–183.

Cauza, E., et al., 2002. Treatment of psoriatic arthritis and psoriasis vulgaris with the tumor necrosis factor inhibitor infliximab. Rheumatol. Int. 22 (6), 227–232.

Charles-Schoeman, C., et al., 2012. Cholesterol efflux by high density lipoproteins is impaired in patients with active rheumatoid arthritis. Ann. Rheum. Dis. 71 (7), 1157–1162.

Chatterjee Adhikari, M., et al., 2012. Subclinical atherosclerosis and endothelial dysfunction in patients with early rheumatoid arthritis as evidenced by measurement of carotid intima-media thickness and flow-mediated vasodilatation: an observational study. Semin. Arthritis Rheum. 41 (5), 669–675.

Choe, J.Y., et al., 2008. No differences of carotid intima-media thickness between young patients with ankylosing spondylitis and healthy controls. Jt. Bone Spine 75 (5), 548–553.

Chong, Y.B., et al., 2011. Dyslipidaemia in patients with lupus nephritis. Nephrology 16 (5), 511–517.

Chung, C.P., et al., 2008. Inflammation-associated insulin resistance: differential effects in rheumatoid arthritis and systemic lupus erythematosus define potential mechanisms. Arthritis Rheum. 58 (7), 2105–2112.

Contessa, C., et al., 2009. Subclinical atherosclerosis in patients with psoriatic arthritis: a case-control study. Preliminary data. Reumatismo 61 (4), 298–305.

Costa, L., et al., 2014. Impact of 24-month treatment with etanercept, adalimumab, or methotrexate on metabolic syndrome components in a cohort of 210 psoriatic arthritis patients. Clin. Rheumatol. 33 (6), 833–839.

Croca, S., et al., 2015. IgG anti-apolipoprotein A-1 antibodies in patients with systemic lupus erythematosus are associated with disease activity and corticosteroid therapy: an observational study. Arthritis Res. Ther. 17, 26.

Davis 3rd, J.M., et al., 2008. The presentation and outcome of heart failure in patients with rheumatoid arthritis differs from that in the general population. Arthritis Rheum. 58 (9), 2603–2611.

del Rincon, I., et al., 2014. Glucocorticoid dose thresholds associated with all-cause and cardiovascular mortality in rheumatoid arthritis. Arthritis Rheumatol. 66 (2), 264–272.

Dessein, P.H., Joffe, B.I., Stanwix, A.E., 2002. Effects of disease modifying agents and dietary intervention on insulin resistance and dyslipidemia in inflammatory arthritis: a pilot study. Arthritis Res. 4 (6), R12.

Dhillon, N., Liang, K., 2015. Prevention of stroke in rheumatoid arthritis. Curr. Treat Options Neurol. 17 (7), 356.

Di Minno, M.N., et al., 2011. Carotid intima-media thickness in psoriatic arthritis: differences between tumor necrosis factor-alpha blockers and traditional disease-modifying antirheumatic drugs. Arterioscler. Thromb. Vasc. Biol. 31 (3), 705–712.

Di Minno, M.N., et al., 2015. Cardiovascular effects of etanercept in patients with psoriatic arthritis: evidence from the cardiovascular risk in rheumatic diseases database. Expert Opin. Drug Saf. 14 (12), 1905–1913.

Djokovic, A., et al., 2014. Does the presence of secondary antiphospholipid syndrome in patients with systemic lupus erythematodes accelerate carotid arteries intima-media thickness changes? Rheumatol. Int. 34 (3), 321–327.

Doria, A., et al., 2003. Risk factors for subclinical atherosclerosis in a prospective cohort of patients with systemic lupus erythematosus. Ann. Rheum. Dis. 62 (11), 1071–1077.

Doria, A., et al., 2005. Inflammation and accelerated atherosclerosis: basic mechanisms. Rheum. Dis. Clin. N. Am. 31 (2), 355–362 viii.

Dubreuil, M., et al., 2014. Diabetes incidence in psoriatic arthritis, psoriasis and rheumatoid arthritis: a UK population-based cohort study. Rheumatology 53 (2), 346–352.

Eder, L., Gladman, D.D., 2015. Atherosclerosis in psoriatic disease: latest evidence and clinical implications. Ther. Adv. Musculoskelet. Dis. 7 (5), 187–195.

Eder, L., et al., 2012. Serum adipokines in patients with psoriatic arthritis and psoriasis alone and their correlation with disease activity. Ann. Rheum. Dis. 72 (12), 1956–1961.

Eder, L., et al., 2014. Increased burden of inflammation over time is associated with the extent of atherosclerotic plaques in patients with psoriatic arthritis. Ann. Rheum. Dis. 74 (10), 1830–1835.

Eder, L., et al., 2016. Incidence and predictors for cardiovascular events in patients with psoriatic arthritis. Ann. Rheum. Dis. 75 (9), 1680–1686.

Ferreira, G.A., et al., 2007. Atorvastatin therapy improves endothelial-dependent vasodilation in patients with systemic lupus erythematosus: an 8 weeks controlled trial. Rheumatology 46 (10), 1560–1565.

Garg, N., Krishan, P., Syngle, A., 2015. Rosuvastatin improves endothelial dysfunction in ankylosing spondylitis. Clin. Rheumatol. 34 (6), 1065–1071.

Garner, S.E., et al., 2005. Rofecoxib for rheumatoid arthritis. Cochrane Database Syst. Rev. 1, CD003685.

Genre, F., et al., 2015. Anti-TNF-alpha therapy reduces endothelial cell activation in non-diabetic ankylosing spondylitis patients. Rheumatol. Int. 35 (12), 2069–2078.

Gheita, T.A., et al., 2013. Metabolic syndrome and insulin resistance comorbidity in systemic lupus erythematosus. Effect on carotid intima-media thickness. Z. Rheumatol. 72 (2), 172–177.

Giallafos, I., et al., 2014. Incident atrial fibrillation in systemic sclerosis: the predictive role of B-type natriuretic peptide. Hell. J. Cardiol. 55 (4), 313–321.

Gonzalez-Juanatey, C., et al., 2003. HLA-DRB1 status affects endothelial function in treated patients with rheumatoid arthritis. Am. J. Med. 114 (8), 647–652.

Gonzalez-Juanatey, C., et al., 2007. High prevalence of subclinical atherosclerosis in psoriatic arthritis patients without clinically evident cardiovascular disease or classic atherosclerosis risk factors. Arthritis Rheum. 57 (6), 1074–1080.

Gonzalez-Juanatey, C., et al., 2009. The high prevalence of subclinical atherosclerosis in patients with ankylosing spondylitis without clinically evident cardiovascular disease. Medicine 88 (6), 358–365.

Gonzalez-Juanatey, C., Llorca, J., Gonzalez-Gay, M.A., 2011. Correlation between endothelial function and carotid atherosclerosis in rheumatoid arthritis patients with long-standing disease. Arthritis Res. Ther. 13 (3), R101.

Greenberg, J.D., et al., 2011. Tumour necrosis factor antagonist use and associated risk reduction of cardiovascular events among patients with rheumatoid arthritis. Ann. Rheum. Dis. 70 (4), 576–582.

Hannawi, S., Marwick, T.H., Thomas, R., 2009. Inflammation predicts accelerated brachial arterial wall changes in patients with recent-onset rheumatoid arthritis. Arthritis Res. Ther. 11 (2), R51.

Haroon, N.N., et al., 2015. Patients with ankylosing spondylitis have increased cardiovascular and cerebrovascular mortality: a population-based study. Ann. Intern. Med. 163 (6), 409–416.

Hassan, A.A., Habib, H.M., Eissa, A.A., 2013. Peripheral arterial disease in patients with systemic lupus erythematosus: a prospective controlled study. Int. J. Rheum. Dis. 16 (3), 319–324.

Hettema, M.E., et al., 2008. Early atherosclerosis in systemic sclerosis and its relation to disease or traditional risk factors. Arthritis Res. Ther. 10 (2), R49.

Hollan, I., et al., 2013. Cardiovascular disease in autoimmune rheumatic diseases. Autoimmun. Rev. 12 (10), 1004–1015.

Hollan, I., et al., 2015. Prevention of cardiovascular disease in rheumatoid arthritis. Autoimmun. Rev. 14 (10), 952–969.

Holmqvist, M., et al., 2015. Stroke in systemic lupus erythematosus: a meta-analysis of population-based cohort studies. RMD Open 1 (1), e000168.

Huang, Y.P., Wang, Y.H., Pan, S.L., 2013. Increased risk of ischemic heart disease in young patients with newly diagnosed ankylosing spondylitis—a population-based longitudinal follow-up study. PLoS One 8 (5), e64155.

Husted, J.A., et al., 2011. Cardiovascular and other comorbidities in patients with psoriatic arthritis: a comparison with patients with psoriasis. Arthritis Care Res. 63 (12), 1729—1735.

Ikdahl, E., et al., 2015. Rosuvastatin improves endothelial function in patients with inflammatory joint diseases, longitudinal associations with atherosclerosis and arteriosclerosis: results from the RORA-AS statin intervention study. Arthritis Res. Ther. 17, 279.

Kao, A.H., et al., 2013. Relation of carotid intima-media thickness and plaque with incident cardiovascular events in women with systemic lupus erythematosus. Am. J. Cardiol. 112 (7), 1025—1032.

Kerola, A.M., et al., 2012. How early in the course of rheumatoid arthritis does the excess cardiovascular risk appear? Ann. Rheum. Dis. 71 (10), 1606—1615.

Kiani, A.N., et al., 2011a. Predictors of progression in atherosclerosis over 2 years in systemic lupus erythematosus. Rheumatology 50 (11), 2071—2079.

Kiani, A.N., Magder, L.S., Petri, M., 2011b. Mycophenolate mofetil (MMF) does not slow the progression of subclinical atherosclerosis in SLE over 2 years. Rheumatol. Int. 32 (9), 2701—2705.

Kimhi, O., et al., 2007. Prevalence and risk factors of atherosclerosis in patients with psoriatic arthritis. Semin. Arthritis Rheum. 36 (4), 203—209.

Kisiel, B., et al., 2015a. Methotrexate, cyclosporine a, and biologics protect against atherosclerosis in rheumatoid arthritis. J. Immunol. Res. 2015, 759610.

Kisiel, B., et al., 2015b. Systemic lupus erythematosus: the influence of disease-related and classical risk factors on intima media thickness and prevalence of atherosclerotic plaques—a preliminary report. Beneficial effect of immunosuppressive treatment on carotid intima media thickness. Acta Cardiol. 70 (2), 169—175.

Klarenbeek, N.B., et al., 2010. Blood pressure changes in patients with recent-onset rheumatoid arthritis treated with four different treatment strategies: a post hoc analysis from the BeSt trial. Ann. Rheum. Dis. 69 (7), 1342—1345.

Kocabay, G., Hasdemir, H., Yildiz, M., 2012. Evaluation of pulse wave velocity in systemic lupus erythematosus, rheumatoid arthritis and Behcet's disease. J. Cardiol. 59 (1), 72—77.

Komai, N., et al., 2007. Anti-tumor necrosis factor therapy increases serum adiponectin levels with the improvement of endothelial dysfunction in patients with rheumatoid arthritis. Mod. Rheumatol. 17 (5), 385—390.

Kremers, H.M., et al., 2004. Prognostic importance of low body mass index in relation to cardiovascular mortality in rheumatoid arthritis. Arthritis Rheum. 50 (11), 3450—3457.

Kremers, H.M., et al., 2008. High ten-year risk of cardiovascular disease in newly diagnosed rheumatoid arthritis patients: a population-based cohort study. Arthritis Rheum. 58 (8), 2268—2274.

Kurt, T., et al., 2015. Can the ankle brachial pressure index (ABPI) and carotis intima media thickness (CIMT) be new early stage markers of subclinical atherosclerosis in patients with rheumatoid arthritis? Wien. Klin. Wochenschr. 127 (13—14), 529—534.

Landewe, R.B., et al., 2000. Methotrexate effects in patients with rheumatoid arthritis with cardiovascular comorbidity. Lancet 355 (9215), 1616—1617.

Lazzerini, P.E., et al., 2011. Anti-Ro/SSA-associated corrected QT interval prolongation in adults: the role of antibody level and specificity. Arthritis Care Res. 63 (10), 1463—1470.

Leonard, D., et al., 2011. Increased carotid intima thickness and decreased media thickness in premenopausal women with systemic lupus erythematosus: an investigation by non-invasive high-frequency ultrasound. Scand. J. Rheumatol. 40 (4), 279–282.

Liu, J., et al., 2011. Preferential macrovasculopathy in systemic sclerosis detected by regional pulse wave velocity from wave intensity analysis: comparisons of local and regional arterial stiffness parameters in cases and controls. Arthritis Care Res. 63 (4), 579–587.

Liu, C.L., et al., 2014. Early evaluation of carotid elasticity by an instantaneous wave intensity technique in patients with systemic lupus erythematosus. J. Ultrasound Med. 33 (12), 2125–2129.

Lorenz, M.W., et al., 2007. Prediction of clinical cardiovascular events with carotid intima-media thickness: a systematic review and meta-analysis. Circulation 115 (4), 459–467.

Maki-Petaja, K.M., et al., 2006. Rheumatoid arthritis is associated with increased aortic pulse-wave velocity, which is reduced by anti-tumor necrosis factor-alpha therapy. Circulation 114 (11), 1185–1192.

Maradit-Kremers, H., et al., 2005. Increased unrecognized coronary heart disease and sudden deaths in rheumatoid arthritis: a population-based cohort study. Arthritis Rheum. 52 (2), 402–411.

Mathieu, S., et al., 2008. Trend towards increased arterial stiffness or intima-media thickness in ankylosing spondylitis patients without clinically evident cardiovascular disease. Rheumatology 47 (8), 1203–1207.

Mathieu, S., et al., 2010a. Effects of 14 weeks of TNF alpha blockade treatment on lipid profile in ankylosing spondylitis. Jt. Bone Spine 77 (1), 50–52.

Mathieu, S., et al., 2011. Cardiovascular profile in ankylosing spondylitis: a systematic review and meta-analysis. Arthritis Care Res. 63 (4), 557–563.

Mathieu, S., et al., 2012. No significant change in arterial stiffness in RA after 6 months and 1 year of rituximab treatment. Rheumatology 51 (6), 1107–1111.

Mathieu, S., et al., 2013a. Effects of 6 months of abatacept treatment on aortic stiffness in patients with rheumatoid arthritis. Biologics 7, 259–264.

Mathieu, S., et al., 2013b. No significant changes in arterial stiffness in patients with ankylosing spondylitis after tumour necrosis factor alpha blockade treatment for 6 and 12 months. Rheumatology 52 (1), 204–209.

Mathieu, S., Motreff, P., Soubrier, M., 2010b. Spondyloarthropathies: an independent cardiovascular risk factor? Jt. Bone Spine 77 (6), 542–545.

Mathis, K.W., 2015. An impaired neuroimmune pathway promotes the development of hypertension in systemic lupus erythematosus. Am. J. Physiol. Regul. Integr. Comp. Physiol. 309 (9), R1074–R1077.

Mazlan, S.A., et al., 2009. A study of intima media thickness and their cardiovascular risk factors in patients with psoriatic arthritis. Acta Med. 52 (3), 107–116.

Mazzoccoli, G., et al., 2010. Anti-tumor necrosis factor-alpha therapy and changes of flow-mediated vasodilatation in psoriatic and rheumatoid arthritis patients. Intern. Emerg. Med. 5 (6), 495–500.

McCarey, D.W., et al., 2004. Trial of atorvastatin in rheumatoid arthritis (TARA): double-blind, randomised placebo-controlled trial. Lancet 363 (9426), 2015–2021.

Meune, C., et al., 2015. A right ventricular diastolic impairment is common in systemic sclerosis and is associated with other target-organ damage. Semin. Arthritis Rheum. 45 (4), 439–445.

Mohan, A., et al., 2014. Subclinical atherosclerosis in patients with rheumatoid arthritis by utilizing carotid intima-media thickness as a surrogate marker. Indian J. Med. Res. 140 (3), 379–386.

Mok, C.C., et al., 2011a. Effects of rosuvastatin on vascular biomarkers and carotid atherosclerosis in lupus: a randomized, double-blind, placebo-controlled trial. Arthritis Care Res. 63 (6), 875–883.
Mok, C.C., et al., 2011b. Prevalence of atherosclerotic risk factors and the metabolic syndrome in patients with chronic inflammatory arthritis. Arthritis Care Res. 63 (2), 195–202.
Moya, F.B., Pineda Galindo, L.F., Garcia de la Pena, M., 2016. Impact of chronic glucocorticoid treatment on cardiovascular risk profile in patients with systemic lupus erythematosus. J. Clin. Rheumatol. 22 (1), 8–12.
Naranjo, A., et al., 2008. Cardiovascular disease in patients with rheumatoid arthritis: results from the QUEST-RA study. Arthritis Res. Ther. 10 (2), R30.
Nienhuis, H.L., et al., 2010. Small artery elasticity is decreased in patients with systemic lupus erythematosus without increased intima media thickness. Arthritis Res. Ther. 12 (5), R181.
Nurmohamed, M.T., van der Horst-Bruinsma, I., Maksymowych, W.P., 2012. Cardiovascular and cerebrovascular diseases in ankylosing spondylitis: current insights. Curr. Rheumatol. Rep. 14 (5), 415–421.
Nurmohamed, M.T., Heslinga, M., Kitas, G.D., 2015. Cardiovascular comorbidity in rheumatic diseases. Nat. Rev. Rheumatol. 11 (12), 693–704.
Oryoji, K., et al., 2014. Reduced carotid intima-media thickness in systemic lupus erythematosus patients treated with cyclosporine A. Mod. Rheumatol. 24 (1), 86–92.
Owlia, M.B., Mostafavi Pour Manshadi, S.M., Naderi, N., 2012. Cardiac manifestations of rheumatological conditions: a narrative review. ISRN Rheumatol. 2012, 463620.
Palazzi, C., et al., 2010. Aortitis and periaortitis in ankylosing spondylitis. Jt. Bone Spine 78 (5), 451–455.
Panoulas, V.F., et al., 2008. Hypertension in rheumatoid arthritis. Rheumatology 47 (9), 1286–1298.
Papagoras, C., et al., 2013. Cardiovascular risk profile in patients with spondyloarthritis. Jt. Bone Spine 81 (1), 57–63.
Perrotta, F.M., et al., 2013. Assessment of subclinical atherosclerosis in ankylosing spondylitis: correlations with disease activity indices. Reumatismo 65 (3), 105–112.
Peters, M.J., et al., 2009. Does rheumatoid arthritis equal diabetes mellitus as an independent risk factor for cardiovascular disease? A prospective study. Arthritis Rheum. 61 (11), 1571–1579.
Petri, M.A., et al., 2011. Lupus atherosclerosis prevention study (LAPS). Ann. Rheum. Dis. 70 (5), 760–765.
Pieringer, H., et al., 2014. Will antirheumatic treatment improve cardiovascular outcomes in patients with rheumatoid arthritis? Curr. Pharm. Des. 20 (4), 486–495.
Popa, C., et al., 2005. Influence of anti-tumour necrosis factor therapy on cardiovascular risk factors in patients with active rheumatoid arthritis. Ann. Rheum. Dis. 64 (2), 303–305.
Prasad, M., et al., 2015. Cardiorheumatology: cardiac involvement in systemic rheumatic disease. Nat. Rev. Cardiol. 12 (3), 168–176.
Preusch, M.R., et al., 2008. Critical role of macrophages in glucocorticoid driven vascular calcification in a mouse-model of atherosclerosis. Arterioscler. Thromb. Vasc. Biol. 28 (12), 2158–2164.
Protogerou, A.D., et al., 2011. A pilot study of endothelial dysfunction and aortic stiffness after interleukin-6 receptor inhibition in rheumatoid arthritis. Atherosclerosis 219 (2), 734–736.
Protogerou, A.D., et al., 2013. Arterial hypertension assessed "out-of-office" in a contemporary cohort of rheumatoid arthritis patients free of cardiovascular disease is characterized by high prevalence, low awareness, poor control and increased vascular damage-associated "white coat" phenomenon. Arthritis Res. Ther. 15 (5), R142.

Przywara-Chowaniec, B., et al., 2014. Evaluation of the intima-media complex in patients with systemic lupus erythematosus. Kardiochir. Torakochirurgia Pol. 11 (1), 63–68.

Puato, M., et al., 2010. Atorvastatin reduces macrophage accumulation in atherosclerotic plaques: a comparison of a nonstatin-based regimen in patients undergoing carotid endarterectomy. Stroke 41 (6), 1163–1168.

Puato, M., et al., 2014a. Impact of hypertension on vascular remodeling in patients with psoriatic arthritis. J. Hum. Hypertens. 28 (2), 105–110.

Puato, M., et al., 2014b. Statin treatment and carotid plaque composition: a review of clinical studies. Curr. Vasc. Pharmacol. 12 (3), 518–526.

Qu, B., Qu, T., 2015. Causes of changes in carotid intima-media thickness: a literature review. Cardiovasc. Ultrasound 13 (1), 46.

Rahman, P., et al., 1999. The cholesterol lowering effect of antimalarial drugs is enhanced in patients with lupus taking corticosteroid drugs. J. Rheumatol. 26 (2), 325–330.

Ramonda, R., et al., 2014. Atherosclerosis progression in psoriatic arthritis patients despite the treatment with tumor necrosis factor-alpha blockers: a two-year prospective observational study. Jt. Bone Spine 81 (5), 421–425.

Raterman, H.G., et al., 2013. Increased progression of carotid intima media thickness in thyroid peroxidase antibodies-positive rheumatoid arthritis patients. Eur. J. Endocrinol. 169 (6), 751–757.

Richez, C., et al., 2013. The effect of mycophenolate mofetil on disease development in the gld.apoE (−/−) mouse model of accelerated atherosclerosis and systemic lupus erythematosus. PLoS One 8 (4), e61042.

Roman, M.J., Salmon, J.E., 2007. Cardiovascular manifestations of rheumatologic diseases. Circulation 116 (20), 2346–2355.

Ruiz-Limon, P., et al., 2014. Atherosclerosis and cardiovascular disease in systemic lupus erythematosus: effects of in vivo statin treatment. Ann. Rheum. Dis. 74 (7), 1450–1458.

Sabio, J.M., et al., 2009. Metabolic syndrome is associated with increased arterial stiffness and biomarkers of subclinical atherosclerosis in patients with systemic lupus erythematosus. J. Rheumatol. 36 (10), 2204–2211.

Sacre, K., et al., 2014. Increased arterial stiffness in systemic lupus erythematosus (SLE) patients at low risk for cardiovascular disease: a cross-sectional controlled study. PLoS One 9 (4), e94511.

Sadik, H.Y., et al., 2010. Lack of effect of 8 weeks atorvastatin on microvascular endothelial function in patients with systemic sclerosis. Rheumatology 49 (5), 990–996.

Sahebkar, A., et al., 2015. Statin impact on disease activity and C-reactive protein concentrations in systemic lupus erythematosus patients: a systematic review and meta-analysis of controlled trials. Autoimmun. Rev. 15 (4), 344–353.

Schanberg, L.E., et al., 2012. Use of atorvastatin in systemic lupus erythematosus in children and adolescents. Arthritis Rheum. 64 (1), 285–296.

Schiopu, E., et al., 2014. Prevalence of subclinical atherosclerosis is increased in systemic sclerosis and is associated with serum proteins: a cross-sectional, controlled study of carotid ultrasound. Rheumatology 53 (4), 704–713.

Schoenfeld, S.R., Kasturi, S., Costenbader, K.H., 2013. The epidemiology of atherosclerotic cardiovascular disease among patients with SLE: a systematic review. Semin. Arthritis Rheum. 43 (1), 77–95.

Schroeder, L.L., et al., 2015. Glucocorticoid use is associated with increase in HDL and no change in other lipids in rheumatoid arthritis patients. Rheumatol. Int. 35 (6), 1059–1067.

Senel, S., et al., 2011. Effect of infliximab treatment on QT intervals in patients with ankylosing spondylitis. J. Investig. Med. 59 (8), 1273–1275.
Sharma, A., et al., 2016. Study of endothelial dysfunction in patients of psoriatic arthritis by flow mediated and nitroglycerine mediated dilatation of brachial artery. Int. J. Rheum. Dis. 19 (3), 300–304.
Sherer, Y., et al., 2007. Early atherosclerosis and autoantibodies to heat-shock proteins and oxidized LDL in systemic sclerosis. Ann. N.Y. Acad. Sci. 1108, 259–267.
Skeoch, S., Bruce, I.N., 2015. Atherosclerosis in rheumatoid arthritis: is it all about inflammation? Nat. Rev. Rheumatol. 11 (7), 390–400.
Solomon, D.H., et al., 2013. Cardiovascular risk in rheumatoid arthritis: comparing TNF-alpha blockade with nonbiologic DMARDs. Am. J. Med. 126 (8), 730e9–730e17.
Solomon, D.H., et al., 2015. Disease activity in rheumatoid arthritis and the risk of cardiovascular events. Arthritis Rheumatol. 67 (6), 1449–1455.
Spanakis, E., et al., 2006. Modest but sustained increase of serum high density lipoprotein cholesterol levels in patients with inflammatory arthritides treated with infliximab. J. Rheumatol. 33 (12), 2440–2446.
Stagakis, I., et al., 2012. Anti-tumor necrosis factor therapy improves insulin resistance, beta cell function and insulin signaling in active rheumatoid arthritis patients with high insulin resistance. Arthritis Res. Ther. 14 (3), R141.
Stavropoulos-Kalinoglou, A., et al., 2012. Anti-tumour necrosis factor alpha therapy improves insulin sensitivity in normal-weight but not in obese patients with rheumatoid arthritis. Arthritis Res. Ther. 14 (4), R160.
Sun, S., et al., 2007. TLR7/9 antagonists as therapeutics for immune-mediated inflammatory disorders. Inflamm. Allergy Drug Targets 6 (4), 223–235.
Symmons, D.P., Gabriel, S.E., 2011. Epidemiology of CVD in rheumatic disease, with a focus on RA and SLE. Nat. Rev. Rheumatol. 7 (7), 399–408.
Syngle, A., et al., 2010. Endothelial dysfunction in ankylosing spondylitis improves after tumor necrosis factor-alpha blockade. Clin. Rheumatol. 29 (7), 763–770.
Szabo, S.M., et al., 2011. Increased risk of cardiovascular and cerebrovascular diseases in individuals with ankylosing spondylitis: a population-based study. Arthritis Rheum. 63 (11), 3294–3304.
Szucs, G., et al., 2007. Endothelial dysfunction precedes atherosclerosis in systemic sclerosis—relevance for prevention of vascular complications. Rheumatology 46 (5), 759–762.
Tam, L.S., et al., 2011a. Effects of rosuvastatin on subclinical atherosclerosis and arterial stiffness in rheumatoid arthritis: a randomized controlled pilot trial. Scand. J. Rheumatol. 40 (6), 411–421.
Tam, L.S., et al., 2011b. Tumour necrosis factor alpha blockade is associated with sustained regression of carotid intima-media thickness for patients with active psoriatic arthritis: a 2-year pilot study. Ann. Rheum. Dis. 70 (4), 705–706.
Tam, L.S., Kitas, G.D., Gonzalez-Gay, M.A., 2014. Can suppression of inflammation by anti-TNF prevent progression of subclinical atherosclerosis in inflammatory arthritis? Rheumatology 53 (6), 1108–1119.
Tanay, A., et al., 2007. Vascular elasticity of systemic lupus erythematosus patients is associated with steroids and hydroxychloroquine treatment. Ann. N.Y. Acad. Sci. 1108, 24–34.
Temiz, A., et al., 2015. Epicardial adipose tissue thickness, flow-mediated dilatation of the brachial artery, and carotid intima-media thickness: associations in rheumatoid arthritis patients. Herz 40 (Suppl. 3), 217–224.
Timar, O., et al., 2008. Increased arterial stiffness as the marker of vascular involvement in systemic sclerosis. J. Rheumatol. 35 (7), 1329–1333.

Timar, O., et al., 2013. Rosuvastatin improves impaired endothelial function, lowers high sensitivity CRP, complement and immuncomplex production in patients with systemic sclerosis—a prospective case-series study. Arthritis Res. Ther. 15 (5), R105.

Toms, T.E., et al., 2009. Methotrexate therapy associates with reduced prevalence of the metabolic syndrome in rheumatoid arthritis patients over the age of 60- more than just an anti-inflammatory effect? A cross sectional study. Arthritis Res. Ther. 11 (4), R110.

Toutouzas, K., et al., 2013. Myocardial ischaemia without obstructive coronary artery disease in rheumatoid arthritis: hypothesis-generating insights from a cross-sectional study. Rheumatology 52 (1), 76—80.

Tsifetaki, N., et al., 2010. Subclinical atherosclerosis in scleroderma patients. Scand. J. Rheumatol. 39 (4), 326—329.

Tso, T.K., et al., 2006. A positive correlation between homocysteine and brachial-ankle pulse wave velocity in patients with systemic lupus erythematosus. Clin. Rheumatol. 25 (3), 285—290.

Turiel, M., et al., 2013. Silent cardiovascular involvement in patients with diffuse systemic sclerosis: a controlled cross-sectional study. Arthritis Care Res. 65 (2), 274—280.

Turkyilmaz, A.K., et al., 2013. Relationship between pulse wave velocity and serum YKL-40 level in patients with early rheumatoid arthritis. Rheumatol. Int. 33 (11), 2751—2756.

Urowitz, M.B., et al., 2007. Clinical manifestations and coronary artery disease risk factors at diagnosis of systemic lupus erythematosus: data from an international inception cohort. Lupus 16 (9), 731—735.

Urowitz, M.B., et al., 2008. Accumulation of coronary artery disease risk factors over three years: data from an international inception cohort. Arthritis Rheum. 59 (2), 176—180.

van Breukelen-van der Stoep, D.F., et al., 2015. Association of cardiovascular risk factors with carotid intima media thickness in patients with rheumatoid arthritis with low disease activity compared to controls: a cross-sectional study. PLoS One 10 (10), e0140844.

Van Doornum, S., et al., 2006. Increased case fatality rates following a first acute cardiovascular event in patients with rheumatoid arthritis. Arthritis Rheum. 54 (7), 2061—2068.

Van Doornum, S., et al., 2010. Rheumatoid arthritis patients receive less frequent acute reperfusion and secondary prevention therapy after myocardial infarction compared with the general population. Arthritis Res. Ther. 12 (5), R183.

van Eijk, I.C., et al., 2009. Microvascular function is impaired in ankylosing spondylitis and improves after tumour necrosis factor alpha blockade. Ann. Rheum. Dis. 68 (3), 362—366.

van Sijl, A.M., et al., 2014. Confounding by indication probably distorts the relationship between steroid use and cardiovascular disease in rheumatoid arthritis: results from a prospective cohort study. PLoS One 9 (1), e87965.

van Sijl, A.M., et al., 2015. Tumour necrosis factor blocking agents and progression of subclinical atherosclerosis in patients with ankylosing spondylitis. Ann. Rheum. Dis. 74 (1), 119—123.

Vassilopoulos, D., et al., 2014. Adalimumab decreases aortic stiffness independently of its effect in disease activity in patients with rheumatoid arthritis. Clin. Rheumatol. 34 (2), 359—364.

Vazquez-Del Mercado, M., et al., 2015. Serum levels of anticyclic citrullinated peptide antibodies, interleukin-6, tumor necrosis factor-alpha, and C-reactive protein are associated with increased carotid intima-media thickness: a cross-sectional analysis of a cohort of rheumatoid arthritis patients without cardiovascular risk factors. Biomed. Res. Int. 2015, 342649.

Virdis, A., et al., 2015. Early treatment with hydroxychloroquine prevents the development of endothelial dysfunction in a murine model of systemic lupus erythematosus. Arthritis Res. Ther. 17, 277.

Wang, D.G., et al., 2014. Decreased flow-mediated dilatation in patients with systemic lupus erythematosus: a meta-analysis. Inflammation 37 (6), 2067—2075.

Wang, P., et al., 2015. Increased carotid intima-media thickness in rheumatoid arthritis: an update meta-analysis. Clin. Rheumatol. 35 (2), 315–323.

Watanabe, T., et al., 2014. Clinical significance of brachial flow-mediated dilation in patients with rheumatoid arthritis. Int. J. Rheum. Dis. 17 (1), 26–33.

Wijaya, L.K., et al., 2005. The proportion of dyslipidemia in systemic lupus erythematosus patient and distribution of correlated factors. Acta Med. Indones. 37 (3), 132–144.

Yogasundaram, H., et al., 2014. Hydroxychloroquine-induced cardiomyopathy: case report, pathophysiology, diagnosis, and treatment. Can. J. Cardiol. 30 (12), 1706–1715.

Yu, H.H., et al., 2015. Statin reduces mortality and morbidity in systemic lupus erythematosus patients with hyperlipidemia: a nationwide population-based cohort study. Atherosclerosis 243 (1), 11–18.

Zha, A.M., Di Napoli, M., Behrouz, R., 2015. Prevention of stroke in rheumatoid arthritis. Curr. Neurol. Neurosci. Rep. 15 (12), 77.

Zhu, T.Y., Li, E.K., Tam, L.S., 2012. Cardiovascular risk in patients with psoriatic arthritis. Int. J. Rheumatol. 2012, 714321.

Chapter 5

Atherosclerosis and Autoimmunity

C. Perricone,* F.R. Spinelli* and Y. Shoenfeld[§]
*Rheumatology, Department of Internal Medicine and Medical Speciality, University of la Sapienza Rome, Rome, Italy; [§]Zabludowicz Center for Autoimmune Diseases, Sheba Medical Center, (Affiliated to Tel-Aviv University), Tel-Hashomer, Israel

Key Points

- Autoimmune diseases substantially increase the risk for cardiovascular disease.
- Atherosclerosis seems to occur precociously in autoimmune conditions.
- Autoimmunity and atherosclerosis (AS) share common pathogenic mechanisms.
- Accelerated AS is responsible for an increased morbidity and mortality in autoimmune conditions.
- Accelerated AS is characterized by the activation of immune cells, resulting in the formation of an intravascular plaque that alters the function and structure of the vessels.

1. INTRODUCTION

Despite a decline in mortality rates in several countries, cardiovascular disease (CVD) remains the leading cause of death responsible for approximately half of all deaths on the continent (Szekanecz et al., 2016) (Fig. 5.1). Coronary artery disease (CAD) and stroke are often the result of acute complications of atherosclerosis (AS) and atherothrombosis. AS is a chronic inflammatory disease, which may have an autoimmune background (Wu et al., 2016). Low-density lipoprotein (LDL) infiltrates and accumulates in the intima of the arterial wall leading to an inflammatory process and the formation of atherosclerotic plaques. These contain lipids but also calcified and fibrotic tissue, vascular cells, cellular debris, and both innate and adaptive immune cells recruited into the arterial wall. When the disruption of an atherosclerotic lesion occurs, thrombus may develop leading to atherothrombosis (Frieri and Stampfl, 2016).

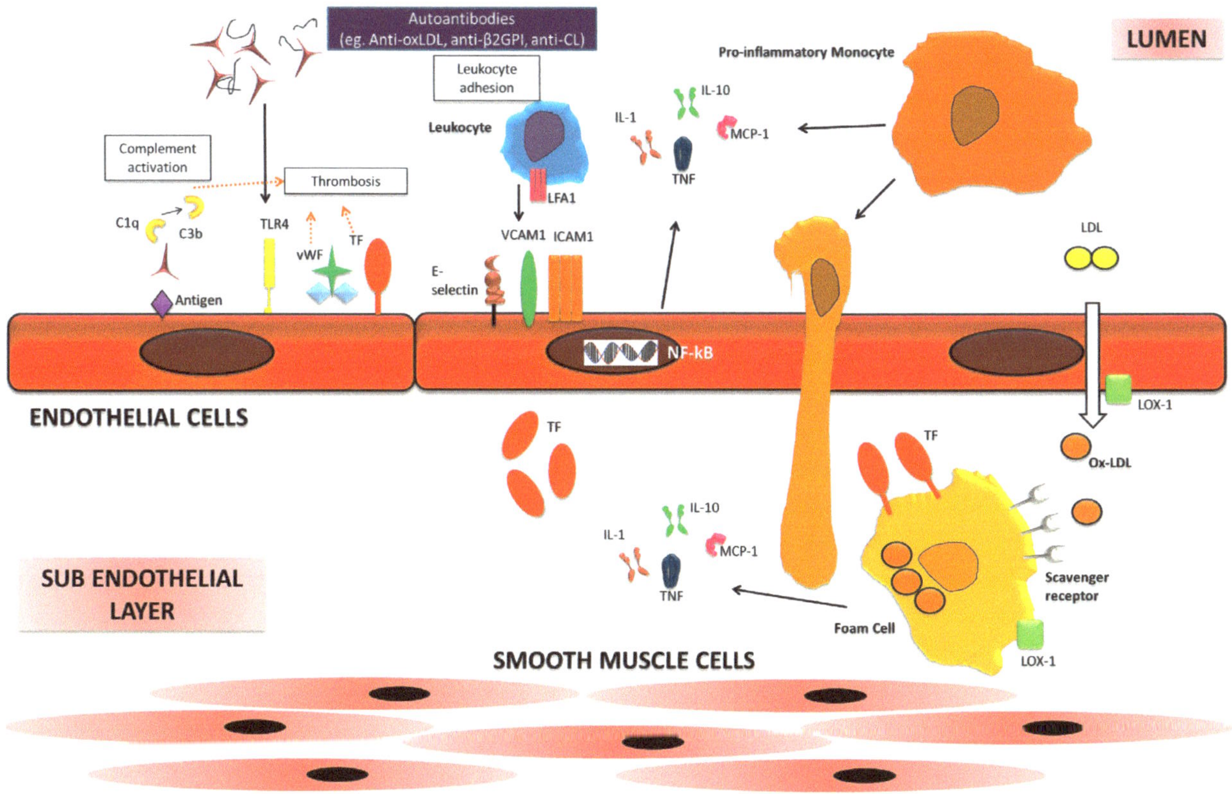

FIGURE 5.1 A synopsis of the possible mechanisms of autoimmune-mediated atherosclerosis. Atherogenesis begins with the recruitment of inflammatory cells to the intima. Autoantibodies (e.g., anti-β2GPI or anticardiolipin), activate components of innate immunity such as complement, endothelial cells and monocytes, as well as the coagulation system (especially through tissue factor). For instance, autoantibodies recognize TLR4 or specific autoantigens such as β2GPI with endothelial cell activation. ICAM-1; VCAM-1; E-selectin IL-1,-6,-8; and TF are expressed changing the phenotype of endothelial cells to a procoagulant form. Moreover, after inflammatory activation, monocytes recruited to the intima express scavenger receptors that permit the uptake of modified low-density lipoprotein (LDL) particles, such as oxidized LDL (oxLDL) leading to the formation of foam cells. These cells can produce proinflammatory mediators, reactive oxygen species, and tissue factor procoagulants that amplify local inflammation and promote thrombotic complications.

It has been recognized that autoimmune diseases substantially increase the risk for CVD. Besides "traditional" risk factors for CVD, including smoking, hypertension, diabetes mellitus, hypercholesterolemia, and family history, other "novel" factors are now considered to be associated with AS and its complications. Indeed, infectious agents, inflammatory processes, and autoimmunity have been suggested to be implicated (Matsuura et al., 2001).

AS seems to occur precociously in autoimmune conditions, suggesting an accelerated process in autoimmune conditions such as rheumatoid arthritis (RA), psoriasis, and systemic lupus erythematosus (SLE). Indeed, AS is a multifactorial disease in which both genetic and environmental factors play a role (Belizna et al., 2007).

Key Points

- CVD remains the leading cause of death in industrialized countries.
- Autoimmune diseases substantially increase the risk for CVD.
- AS seems to occur precociously in autoimmune conditions.

2. PREVALENCE AND EPIDEMIOLOGY

Increased risk of CVD in autoimmunity was first described in SLE 35 years ago. Urowitz et al. suggested a bimodal pattern of SLE mortality with early deaths (<1 year) due to SLE disease activity but later deaths primarily linked with CVD (Rubin et al., 1985). CAD is described in SLE patients with a prevalence ranging from 6% to 10%, and the risk of developing this manifestation is 4–8 times higher than in age-matched healthy subjects. The overall risk of myocardial infarction (MI) in SLE patients is tenfold higher than in the general population, even after accounting for traditional Framingham risk factors (Mazurek et al., 2016). Acute MI seems to be responsible for 3–25% of deaths in SLE patients. Young SLE women (35–44 years old) may be even up to 50 times more likely to have an MI than age-matched women in the Framingham Offspring Study (Frieri and Stampfl, 2016). In antiphospholipid syndrome (APS), the prevalence of asymptomatic AS assessed by ultrasonography is 15% compared to 3% in normal controls (Mazurek et al., 2016). In the Euro-Phospholipid cohort MI appeared during the course of the diseases in 5.5% of patients (Cervera et al., 2015). Thus, not only does AS occur more frequently in SLE patients than in the general population, but also there is epidemiological and clinical evidence that it is accelerated in these patients as well as in patients with diabetes mellitus. Measurement of the intima-media thickness (IMT) of carotid arteries by Doppler ultrasound also represents a quantitative method for detecting preclinical AS (Sharma et al., 2016). Considering carotid ultrasound as a surrogate measure of AS, it was demonstrated that carotid plaque increases more than twofold in SLE patients versus controls showing a more rapid progression pattern in SLE (Kay et al., 2016). Increased IMT has been observed in patients with SLE with a prevalence of focal plaque up to 37% in patients with SLE without previous cardiovascular events (Kisiel et al., 2015a). Patients with SLE display four times more coronary calcifications compared to healthy controls (Liu et al., 2014). Moreover, studies using the dual-isotope single photon emission computed tomographic (SPECT) myocardial perfusion imaging demonstrated that 38% of SLE patients might have perfusion defects indicating subclinical AS (Espinola-Zavaleta et al., 2006). Endothelial dysfunction, on which we will later focus on, measured by flow-mediated dilation (FMD), is accelerated in SLE patients and coronary microvascular function can be observed even in SLE patients with normal coronary arteries (Ramos-Casals, 2014).

Key Points

- CAD is described in SLE patients with a prevalence ranging from 6% to 10%.
- Acute MI seems to be responsible for 3–25% of deaths in SLE patients.
- Carotid plaques increase more than twofold in SLE patients versus controls and show a more rapid progression pattern in SLE.

3. PATHOGENESIS

3.1 Genetic Background

Since both autoimmunity and AS share common pathogenic mechanisms, it is not surprising that they may rely on the same genetic basis.

It was shown that several polymorphisms might influence the susceptibility for both conditions. Pamuk et al. (2014) found that genetic variants of platelet endothelial cell adhesion molecule-1 (PECAM-1) are more frequent in RA and SLE when compared to controls. These PECAM-1 single-nucleotide polymorphisms (SNPs) were also protective against atherosclerotic complications. Chung et al. described polymorphisms in 20 candidate genes (ADAM33, ADIPOQ, CCL5, CCR7, CDKN2B, CSF1, IL4, IL12A, IL23R, INS, IRF5, MIF, MS4A1, PTGS1, PTPN22, RETN, SELE, TNFSF4, TNFRSF11B, and VCAM1) associated with the presence of coronary artery calcium, a measure of AS, in SLE patients (Pamuk et al., 2014).

Another study that compared the expression levels of tumor necrosis factor ligand superfamily member 4 (TNFSF4) and TNF-R–associated factor 2 (TRAF2) mRNAs in peripheral blood mononuclear cells (PBMCs) of patients with SLE found an overexpression of TNFSF4, which correlated with arthritis, AS, and lupus nephritis (Rajabi et al., 2012).

The role of the "interferon signature" in SLE pathogenesis is well known (Ceccarelli et al., 2015). Indeed, interferon (IFN)-α is involved in the development SLE, but also seems to be implicated in SLE-related AS by promoting lipid uptake and macrophage-derived foam cell formation. Li et al.

suggested that IFN-α priming upregulated the expression of Scavenger Receptor class A (SR-A) in human monocyte/macrophages, leading to increased lipid uptake and foam cell formation (Li et al., 2015). It should not be surprising to find an association between Interferon Related Factor (IRF)-5 SNPs and the risk of acute coronary syndrome (Watkins et al., 2015). Indeed, a genetic predisposition to increased type-I IFN production affects the risk of CAD. Using a list of 11 single nucleotide polymorphisms from the results of genome-wide association studies for SLE, Nelson et al. identified a genetic risk score based on three single nucleotide polymorphisms (rs10516487, rs3131379, and rs7574865), which correlated significantly with production of IFN-α by human peripheral leukocytes stimulated with CpG-oligonucleotide (Nelson et al., 2015). Moreover, variant alleles of the mannose-binding lectin gene (MBL2) causing low serum concentrations of functional mannose-binding lectin (MBL) are associated with SLE and development of AS (El-Sherif et al., 2010).

Finally, polymorphisms in genes encoding for mediators of coagulation, such as the coagulation factor II gene (F2), are known to be associated with a higher risk of cardiovascular events in SLE (Demirci et al., 2011), as well as HLA-DRB1*04/*13 alleles seem to be associated with vascular events and an antiphospholipid (aPL) positive immune-phenotype in SLE (Lundström et al., 2013).

Key Points

- Both autoimmunity and AS share common pathogenic mechanisms.
- Expression of TNFSF4 and TRAF2 mRNAs is altered in peripheral blood mononuclear cells from SLE with AS.
- Polymorphisms in the type I interferon pathway are associated with autoimmunity and AS.

3.2 Subclinical Atherosclerosis: Endothelial Dysfunction and Atherosclerotic Plaque Formation

Atherosclerosis is a frequent and precocious event in the course of autoimmune conditions, justifying the increased risk of MI. The accelerated AS is characterized by the activation of immune cells, resulting in the formation of an intravascular plaque that alters the structure and function of the vessels (Szekanecz et al., 2016; Wu et al., 2016). It is evident that the generalized inflammation represents a constant phenomenon of the disease. Disease activity and duration, the use of steroids, hyperhomocysteinemia, and the presence of aPL antibodies can further promote the atherosclerotic process (Nussinovitch and Shoenfeld, 2009).

Several lines of evidence suggest that the early AS is associated with both traditional risk factors and disease-associated risk factors (acute phase reactants, specific autoantibodies, treatment). The measure of the IMT of the carotid arteries by ultrasound is a quantitative method that can identify subclinical AS. Increased IMT has been frequently found in patients with autoimmune conditions such as SLE, with focal plaques even in patients who had not presented cardiovascular events (Fadda et al., 2015). Endothelial dysfunction is the earliest and reversible stage of AS, and the change of FMD at the brachial artery level is widely recognized as a marker of endothelial dysfunction (Mak et al., 2011). Numerous findings have shown an association between elevated plasma concentrations of total and LDL cholesterol and impaired endothelial function. Changes in the structure of lipoprotein, such as the oxidation of LDL, can alter endothelial function. In particular, oxidized LDL alter the phenotype of endothelial cells and monocyte-macrophage in a proatherogenic manner (Mango et al., 2011). The identification of the receptor for oxidized LDL, called lectin like ox-LDL receptor-1 (LOX-1), whose effects are the internalization and degradation of ox-LDL in endothelial cells, has established the importance of these lipoproteins in endothelial dysfunction and then in the early stage of AS (Mango et al., 2003). Several intronic SNPs determine a splice isoform (LOXIN) so that the ratio LOX-1/LOXIN is higher in those patients with a high risk of MI (Vecchione et al., 2007).

Indeed, the "altered-lipoprotein" hypothesis suggests that oxidized LDL (oxLDL) may be responsible for foam cells formation. So far, testing the blood level of LDL cholesterol is the best biomarker for AS (Schoen et al., 2015).

LDL is the ultimate source of cholesterol, which accumulates in foam cells. LDL particles contain hundreds of molecules of phospholipids, free cholesterol, cholesterol esters, and triglycerides (Steinberg et al., 1997). OxLDL, as opposed to native LDL, contains large amounts of lysophosphatidylcholine and can increase adherence and penetration of monocytes. While enhanced oxidation of LDL is considered a proatherogenic step, the nature of the immune reaction against oxLDL regarding its effects on AS is less clear. Elevated levels of anti-oxLDL antibodies usually signify enhanced AS and presence of its manifestations (Sherer et al., 2010). Hence, anti-oxLDL are elevated in patients with early-onset peripheral vascular disease; severe carotid AS; angiographically verified CAD; and are predictive of carotid AS progression, MI occurrence, and mortality (Wu et al., 1997). In addition, patients who underwent PTCA and were positive for the presence of anti-oxLDL antibodies were more likely to develop restenosis within 6 months compared with patients with no subsequent restenosis (George et al., 1999a). As opposed to the earlier-mentioned studies, in animal models of AS, immunization with oxLDL resulted in induction of anti-oxLDL antibodies but suppression rather than aggravation of early atherogenesis (Ameli et al., 1996). These results support the presence of different types of anti-oxLDL antibodies. As oxLDL is a particle rather than an antigen, different autoantibodies against it might have opposite effects. It has been described that autoantibodies against oxLDL and antiidiotypes directed toward these antibodies (namely anti-anti-oxLDL) can be found within commercial preparations of intravenous immunoglobulins (Igs) (Wu et al., 2003). Treatment of animals with intravenous Igs could decrease AS extent. It was speculated that the repertoire of anti-oxLDL in humans include both "protective" and "pathogenic" autoantibodies. Under normal circumstances, anti-oxLDL might help clear oxLDL by immune complexes. However, upon enhanced oxidation of LDL (which can occur due to smoking, lack of antioxidants, etc.), anti-oxLDL with higher affinity or different target epitopes are generated and can enhance AS. In this scenario, the antiidiotypes to anti-oxLDL can have their beneficial effect, similar to their effect in various autoimmune diseases (Sherer et al., 2000).

Nonetheless, during AS, other players may have a fundamental role, including B and T cells, which infiltrate the intima and where the release of several mediators including interleukin-1, tumor necrosis factor alpha, and other proinflammatory cytokines may occur.

Key Points

- Accelerated AS is characterized by the activation of immune cells, resulting in the formation of an intravascular plaque that alters the function and structure of the vessels.
- Early AS is associated with traditional risk factors and disease-associated risk factors.
- The change of FMD in the brachial artery level is widely recognized as a marker of endothelial dysfunction.
- The "altered-lipoprotein" hypothesis suggests that oxLDL may be responsible for foam cells formation.

3.3 Autoantigens and Autoantibodies in Atherosclerosis

The loss of the immunological tolerance to self-antigens represents the first step toward the development of autoimmune phenomena. Susceptible individuals, under the influence of genetic and environmental factors, develop an underlying autoimmunity that manifests as the presence of autoantibodies. Several autoantigens and autoantibodies are also implicated in the pathogenesis of AS (Shoenfeld et al., 2000). Most are considered proatherogenic, whereas some might even have a protective role against AS.

3.4 Cellular Mechanisms

Cells of the immune system can be found within atherosclerotic plaques suggesting a role in the atherogenic process. Migration and activation of immune-competent cells within the plaques can be secondary to various stimuli, including infectious agents. These cells probably aggravate AS. Indeed, both the innate and the adaptive immune systems play important roles in AS (Lewandowski and Kaplan, 2016). It was shown that mice receiving whole B6.SLE CD4(+) T cells, without any other SLE phenotype, had an increased AS of nearly 40%. Dysregulated IL-17 production and reduced frequency of IL-10R expression were present in these B6.SLE regulatory T cells (Treg). Thus, transfer of B6.SLE Teff to LDLr(−/−), Rag(−/−) mice results in accelerated AS independent of the source of Treg (Wilhelm et al., 2015).

It has been shown that $CD4^+$ and $CD8^+$ T-cell depletion reduced fatty streak formation in C57BL/6 mice (Emeson et al., 1996). A particular subset of $CD4^+$ T cells that lacks surface CD28 molecule ($CD4^+CD28^-$) is expanded, probably stimulated by endothelial autoantigens, in the peripheral blood of unstable angina pectoris patients and a subgroup of RA patients (Pingiotti et al., 2007). These cells may infiltrate the atherosclerotic lesions and display a high proinflammatory and tissue-damaging potential that promotes vascular injury. Interestingly, RA patients with $CD4^+CD28^-$cell expansion have a higher degree of endothelial dysfunction and a higher carotid IMT than patients without expansion of these cells. Moreover, cells within AS plaques express CD40 and CD40 ligand. Treatment with antibody against mouse CD40 ligand limited AS in LDL receptor−deficient mice (Mach et al., 1998). A cellular immune response specifically directed against heat-shock proteins (HSPs), oxLDL, and β-glycoprotein-I (β2GPI) has been reported, suggesting a direct involvement of these molecules in AS (Mandal et al., 2005).

Key Points

- Cells of the immune system can be found within atherosclerotic plaques, which suggests that they have a role in the atherogenic process.
- Dysregulated $CD4^+$ T cells from SLE-susceptible mice are sufficient to accelerate AS in LDLr−/− mice.
- A particular subset of $CD4^+$ T cells that lacks surface CD28 molecule ($CD4^+CD28^-$) is expanded in RA and correlates with the development of AS.

3.5 The Role of β2GPI

β2GPI can be found in human atherosclerotic lesions obtained from carotid endarterectomies, is abundantly expressed within the subendothelial regions and the intimal-medial border of human atherosclerotic plaques, and co-localizes with $CD4^+$ lymphocytes (Conti et al., 2014). On transfer of lymphocytes obtained from β2GPI-immunized LDL receptor−deficient mice into syngeneic mice, the recipients exhibited larger fatty streaks compared with mice that received lymphocytes from control mice (Matsuura et al., 2009). β2GPI, or apolipoprotein H, is an abundant plasma glycoprotein that binds to negatively charged phospholipids and is involved in clotting mechanisms and lipid pathways (Aron et al., 1995). In chronic diseases related to endothelial cell dysfunction such as SLE, APS, and AS, β2GPI plays a role as a target antigen for an immune-mediated attack, possibly influencing the progression of disease (Aron et al., 1995; Shoenfeld et al., 2008; Matsuura et al., 2002; Gharavi et al., 1992; Caronti et al., 1999). β2GPI stimulates not only a vigorous adaptive humoral but also a cellular, immune response (Matsuura et al., 1994; Visvanathan and McNeil, 1999; Conti et al., 2003; Sorice et al., 2007). Recently, the presence of autoreactive T cells specific for a cryptic epitope of β2GPI has been described in both patients with APS and healthy subjects (Hattori et al., 2000; Buttari et al., 2005; Kuwana et al., 2005). Moreover, the frequency of these autoreactive cells was found to be significantly increased in patients with APS, suggesting that the production of aPL in patients with APS could be a result of the activation of β2GPI-reactive T cells. Indeed, it was shown that β2GPI is a T cell target in patients with advanced carotid atherosclerotic plaques (Profumo et al., 2010).

The role of β2GPI in the pathogenesis of AS has been demonstrated in humans and in experimental models. In murine models, β2GPI was detected within early atherosclerotic lesions where it was expressed intracellularly and extracellularly. β2GPI has also been detected in human atherosclerotic plaques by immunostaining studies showing that β2GPI and aβ2GPI colocalize with oxLDL (Kobayashi et al., 2003). Furthermore, immunization of Apo-E–deficient mice with β2GPI resulted in an enhancement of AS (George et al., 2000). In an experimental model of LDL receptor–deficient mice, β2GPI-specific cellular immunity showed a central role in promoting atherogenesis (George et al., 1999b). When injected with lymphocytes from β2GPI-immunized animals, mice displayed fatty streaks larger than those shown in mice injected with lymphocytes from albumin-immunized controls. T-cell–depleted splenocytes were unable to promote lesion formation, thus suggesting a primary role for T-lymphocytes in mediating AS (Kobayashi et al., 2003). In response to β2GPI, proliferating PBMC produced higher amount of IFN-γ than nonproliferating ones. By secreting proinflammatory cytokines, such as IFN-γ as well as by facilitating aPL production, β2GPI-specific T cells seem to play a pathogenic role.

It has also been shown that aβ2GPI and anti-oxLDL/β2GPI are associated with an adverse outcome in patients with CAD (Greco et al., 2009). Furthermore, in a previous study, aβ2GPI IgG-oxLDL complexes were suggested to be predictive of IMT in patients with APS (Ames et al., 2006).

Key Points

- β2GPI, or apolipoprotein H, is an abundant plasma glycoprotein that binds to negatively charged phospholipids and is involved in clotting mechanisms and lipid pathways.
- β2GPI can be detected within early atherosclerotic lesions.
- β2GPI and aβ2GPI colocalize with oxLDL.

3.6 Anticardiolipin Antibodies

As earlier mentioned, patients with primary APS have a greater carotid IMT at multiple artery sites than controls. Moreover, aPL levels correlate with increased MI risk even in healthy subjects. Anticardiolipin (aCL) antibodies are the hallmark of the APS. Immunization of LDL receptor–deficient mice with aCL antibodies resulted in the development of high titers of mouse aCL and increased AS compared with controls (Sherer and Shoenfeld, 2003). The presence of high levels of aCL antibodies was found as an independent risk factor for MI or cardiac death in middle-aged men (Bengtsson et al., 2012), and elevated levels of aCL, anti-β2GPI, and anti-oxLDL antibodies were also found in patients having CAD compared with control subjects (Erkkilä et al., 2000). Su et al. reported that the prevalence of low levels of IgM anti-OxCL, and anti-OxPS (both cofactor β2-GPI independent) is associated with the presence of atherosclerotic plaques and in SLE (Su et al., 2013). More recently, Marai et al. described that patients with CVD had endothelial dysfunction and elevated levels of aCL (Marai et al., 2008). In another study, most of young APS patients showed SPECT alterations suggestive of myocardial perfusion defects with coronary calcifications. Right ventricular systolic pressure was elevated in one-third of APS patients. These conditions, well known as cardiovascular risk markers, are combined with elevated levels of aCL and anti-β2GPI antibodies of the IgG class (Espinola-Zavaleta et al., 2006). Thus, in a high percentage of APS patients, clinically silent myocardial ischemia, pulmonary pressure elevation, and coronary AS may be present, and causally related to the presence of aPL antibodies. Interestingly, the prevalence of such adverse outcome was found to be increased especially in patients with two or more positive aPL tests (Mazurek et al., 2016).

Key Points

- aPLs correlate with increased MI risk in healthy subjects.
- aCL antibodies act as an independent risk factor for MI or cardiac death in middle-aged men.
- Patients with CVD have endothelial dysfunction and elevated levels of aCL.

3.7 Anti-oxLDL Antibodies

IgM antibodies recognizing oxLDL are generally considered to be protective against AS in murine models (Cesena et al., 2012); although, paradoxically, the presence of anti-oxLDL antibodies increases risk for AS in SLE patients (Sinicato et al., 2013).

A recent study suggests that anti-oxLDL antibodies develop after the production of antilipoprotein lipase autoantibodies and are responsible for an increased atherosclerotic risk in an SLE cohort with high disease activity (Bassi et al., 2007). The underlying mechanism behind the atherogenicity of anti-oxLDL IgG antibodies is unclear, but decreased immune complex clearing (e.g., lupus nephritis) or the presence of aggregated oxLDL in the subendothelial space could explain the increased atherosclerotic risk (Matsuura et al., 2008). In humans, IgM (and in some studies IgG) antibodies to oxLDL negatively correlate with lesion burden (Ait-Oufella et al., 2010). Some studies suggest that much of the protective antibody activity resides in the IgM compartment. Statin treatment increases levels of oxidized phospholipids and IgM antibodies against oxidized phospholipids in patients with AS suggesting a beneficial effect of these IgM (Soltész et al., 2007).

OxLDL is more likely to undergo uptake by macrophages, which turn into foam cells characterizing atherosclerotic lesions. Anti-oxLDL antibodies are present in patients with AS as well as in those with autoimmune diseases and healthy individuals. Even if anti-oxLDL autoantibodies level seems to be higher in patients with more extensive AS, such positive correlation does not necessarily mean that antibodies are proatherogenic. Indeed, recombinant antibodies to modified LDL were shown to induce regression of AS in mouse models (Schiopu et al., 2007).

Key Points

- IgM antibodies that recognize oxLDL are considered to be protective against AS in murine models.
- The presence of anti-oxLDL antibodies increases risk for AS in humans with SLE.
- Anti-oxLDL autoantibodies tend to be higher in patients with more extensive AS.

3.8 Anti-apoA-1 Antibodies

Anti-apoA-1 antibodies have been detected in 20% of nonautoimmune patients with acute coronary syndromes and in 32.5% of SLE patients and 22.9% of patients with primary APS (Teixeira et al., 2012). Moreover, their presence correlates with more severe disease activity (Abe et al., 2001). ApoA-1 is a major antiinflammatory component of HDL, thus such anti-apoA-1 autoantibodies may lead to the loss of the atheroprotective capabilities of apoA-1 and HDL.

Key Points

- Anti-apoA-1 antibodies can be found in patients with autoimmune diseases.
- Anti-apoA-1 autoantibodies may lead to the loss of the atheroprotective capabilities of apoA-1 and HDL.

3.9 Inflammatory Chemokines and Cytokines in Autoimmune Atherosclerosis

The recruitment of monocytes and lymphocytes in the atherosclerotic plaque is mediated by several molecules released by endothelial cells such as leukocyte adhesion molecules like E-selectin, vascular cell adhesion molecule-1 (VCAM-1), and intercellular adhesion molecule-1 (Hsueh et al., 2016). Their expression is induced by proinflammatory cytokines such as TNF-α and IL-1, and also by the exposition of endothelial cells to lipopolysaccharides of Gram negative bacteria, and oxidized phospholipids such as oxLDL (Jiang et al., 2015).

The migration of the leukocytes through the endothelium into the intima is mediated by other chemotactic proteins including monocyte chemotactic protein-1 (MCP-1) produced by the smooth muscle layer and endothelial cells (Hulsmans et al., 2013).

Again, TNF-α, IL-1, as well as oxLDL can upregulate MCP-1 expression in endothelial cells and smooth muscle cells (Han et al., 2016). Another key molecule is the macrophage migration inhibitory factor (MIF), which seems overexpressed in SLE patients and possess several proinflammatory properties such as the induction of TNF-α, IL-1, IL-6, and matrix metalloproteinases, the activation of T cells, and promotion of angiogenesis (Santos and Morand, 2009).

TNF-α is associated with high triglyceride and low HDL levels and together with IL-1 can enhance the production of macrophage colony-stimulating factor, granulocyte-monocyte colony-stimulating factor, and granulocyte colony-stimulating factor in turn activating monocytes and stimulating their transformation into macrophages and foam cells (López-Pedrera et al., 2010). In addition, IFN-γ can induce the foam cell formation, the adaptive Th1-specific immune response, and plaque development (Sikorski et al., 2011). It was shown that IL-17 and IFN-γ are concomitantly present in patients and clinical specimens of coronary AS (Akhavanpoor et al., 2014), probably playing a synergistic proinflammatory effect.

Key Points

- Several adhesion molecules are implicated in AS including VCAM1 and ICAM1.
- TNF-α, IL-1, as well as oxLDL can upregulate MCP-1 expression in endothelial cells and smooth muscle cells.
- MIF is elevated in SLE patients and possesses several proinflammatory properties such as the induction of TNF-α, IL-1, IL-6, and matrix metalloproteinases.

3.10 Heat-Shock Proteins as Autoantigens in Atherosclerosis

HSPs have important functions in conjugation with the folding and intracellular transport of proteins. They are phylogenetically highly conserved, and thus human HSP60 and mycobacterial HSP65 have 55% homology (Jones et al., 1993). As HSPs are antigenic components of infectious agents, almost all human subjects have immune reactivity against them. Hence, immune cross-reactivity against human HSP60 might arise. Indeed, using sonographic assessment of carotid lesions, subjects with subclinical AS had significantly elevated levels of anti-HSP65 antibodies compared with controls (Xu et al., 1993). This difference was found only in 60–79- year-old patients, but not in younger subjects. Follow-up of these patients disclosed that these antibodies were also associated with increased mortality (Xu et al., 1999).

The association between HSPs and AS is also demonstrated in animal models. Rabbits immunized with material containing HSP65, either in the form of mycobacteria or recombinant HSP65 alone, developed AS lesions (Xu et al., 1992). In another study, C57BL/6 mice were injected with either HSP65, HSP65-rich *Mycobacterium tuberculosis*, or phosphate-buffered saline (PBS). Early AS was significantly enhanced in high-cholesterol diet fed mice that were immunized with HSP65 or *M. tuberculosis*, compared with the PBS-injected mice, and the lesions found in the former two groups were associated with extensive deposits of Igs and infiltration of $CD4^+$ lymphocytes (George et al., 1997). In a similar study, LDL receptor–deficient mice that were immunized with HSP65 developed significantly larger fatty streaks compared with the BSA immunized group (Afek et al., 2000).

Key Points

- HSPs are antigenic components of infectious agents and are associated with the development of AS.
- The association between HSPs and AS is demonstrated in animal models.

3.11 Other Factors: Vitamin D and Obesity

Vitamin D deficiency has been linked to the development of AS, even if the direct demonstration of this phenomenon is still waiting its chance. Yet, vitamin D has been found to have antithrombotic properties improving the risk of CVDs (Liu et al., 2016). In this regard, the fact that a relevant percentage of patients with SLE may also suffer from concomitant APS cannot be disregarded. APS patients show a higher prevalence of vitamin D deficiency compared with a healthy population and lower levels correlate with the occurrence of thrombosis and neurological manifestations (Muniz Caldas and Freire de Carvalho, 2013). Of relevance, active vitamin D is capable of inhibiting the anti-β2GPI antibody-mediated tissue factor expression, thus giving a possible explanation for the hypercoagulability observed in APS (Agmon-Levin et al., 2011).

Obesity is associated to traditional cardiovascular risk factors (hypertension, dyslipidemia) and AS (Fuster et al., 2016). This is a key observation considering the increased prevalence of AS and metabolic syndrome in SLE, and that CVD is a major cause of mortality in SLE patients. High levels of leptin and resistin and low levels of adiponectin were correlated with an increased risk of CVD and metabolic syndrome (Versini et al., 2014). The adipose tissue represents an important source of proinflammatory mediators including TNF and IL-6. These in turn may maintain a state of chronic activation of the innate immune system, perpetuating the systemic inflammatory base of AS. Adipokines are molecules produced by white adipose tissue, which regulate metabolism and energy homeostasis. When considering leptin, it contributes to AS progression and seems elevated in adult and pediatric patients with SLE, especially in those with carotid plaques (Hoffmann et al., 2016; Scotece et al., 2012).

Key Points

- Vitamin D deficiency has been linked to the development of AS.
- Active vitamin D is capable of inhibiting the anti-β2GP I antibody−mediated tissue factor expression.
- Obesity appears to be related to cardiovascular risk factors (hypertension, dyslipidemia) and AS.
- Adipokines and in particular leptin contributes to AS progression and seems elevated in adult and pediatric patients with SLE.

3.12 Systemic Lupus Erythematosus and Atherosclerosis

SLE is a chronic autoimmune disease with a multifactorial pathogenesis including genetic and environmental factors (Conti et al., 2015). The disease is characterized by the production of a wide range of autoantibodies (Yaniv et al., 2015). SLE mainly affects women in their reproductive age, and any organ and system can be involved in the pathological process. Moreover, it is well known that patients with SLE present a higher prevalence of early AS and have a greater risk of developing CVDs than healthy subjects (Sherer et al., 2010). FMD has been consistently reported to be abnormal in subjects affected by AS or presenting cardiovascular risk factors, as well as in patients with SLE (Stalc et al., 2011). In addition, as earlier mentioned, the prevalence of AS seems to be increased among patients with APS (Zinger et al., 2009). Of note, the prevalence of carotid plaque has been reported to be higher in patients with APS secondary to SLE compared with patients with primary APS (Giannakopoulos and Krilis, 2013; Miyakis et al., 2006).

Moreover, in patients with primary APS, the titer of aPL antibodies often represents an independent predictor of IMT (Ames et al., 2002; Medina et al., 2003). This may be consistent with the observation that aCL, mostly those β2GPI-dependent, and anti-β2GPI antibodies are important predictors for cardiovascular events (Brey et al., 2001; Lopez et al., 2004). Furthermore, patients with SLE and APS show a higher prevalence of traditional cardiovascular risk factor such as hypertension, body mass index (BMI), low HDL-cholesterol, and ApoA-1 plasma levels when compared with controls.

Overall, these findings support the role of chronic inflammation in the atherosclerotic vascular damage (Manzi et al., 1999). Some authors have suggested that glucocorticoids could play a role in the development of AS; on the contrary, glucocorticoids are also antiinflammatory molecules that can modulate the disease-related risk factors (Roman et al., 2001).

Key Points

- SLE presents a higher prevalence of early AS and have a greater risk of developing CVDs than healthy subjects.
- In patients with primary APS, the titer of aPL antibodies often represents an independent predictor of IMT.
- Patients with SLE and APS show a higher prevalence of traditional cardiovascular risk factor such as hypertension, BMI, low HDL-cholesterol, and ApoA-1 plasma levels.

3.13 Rheumatoid Arthritis and Atherosclerosis

RA is a systemic inflammatory disease associated with accelerated AS. In this view, coronary heart disease (CHD) still represents a main cause of mortality in these patients (Perricone et al., 2011). The role of inflammation and immunity in the atherosclerotic process offers possible explanations of the increased cardiovascular risk observed in RA patients. In the pathogenesis of RA as well as of AS, posttranslational modifications including citrullination and carbamylation seem to be involved. Citrullination transforms peptide-bound arginine residues into citrulline, a non-natural aminoacid (Sokolove et al., 2013). During the past decade, the immune response to citrullinated peptides has been extensively studied in RA: antibodies directed to citrullinated peptides (ACPA) are now a fundamental for the diagnosis of RA with a specificity of 85–95% and a sensitivity of 68–79% (Aggarwal et al., 2013). ACPA have a predictive role—these antibodies can be detected before the onset of the disease—and a prognostic role too, being associated to a more severe and erosive arthritis (Vander Cruyssen et al., 2007). ACPA are somehow implicated in the pathogenesis of RA: citrullinated peptides bind HLA-DRB1 [the so-called shared epitope (SE)] and ACPA positivity strongly correlates with SE (Ceccarelli et al., 2011). Moreover, smoking habit may induce an immune response to citrullinated peptides, generation of ACPA, and the onset of RA in SE carriers (Perricone et al., 2016). Only few studies investigated the response to citrullinated peptides and the development of atherosclerotic plaque. Sokolove et al. demonstrated a correlation between citrullinated fibrinogen and vimentin with coronary artery calcium score in 134 female patients with RA. Moreover, the authors detected citrullinated proteins and PAD-4 enzyme within the atherosclerotic plaque obtained from non-RA patients and confirmed the ability of ACPA isolated from RA patients to targets these proteins (Sokolove et al., 2013). Citrullinated proteins and PAD enzymes were also detected in the perivascular myocardial interstitium, especially in RA patients (Giles et al., 2012). Cambridge et al. investigated the possible association between antibodies to citrullinated proteins and CHD in 432 healthy subjects without RA followed-up for 5 years. The authors found a significantly higher percentage of ACPA-positive subjects among those who later developed an overt CHD compared to those who did not; the association was still significant even after the adjustment for traditional atherosclerotic risk factors (Cambridge et al., 2013).

Carbamylation is a chemical posttranslational modification consisting of the addition of a cyanate group on self-peptides leading to the production of homocitrulline. Among other factors, tobacco smoke seems to induce protein carbamylation. The immunogenicity of homocitrulline has been recently studied in RA patients. Shi et al. detected antibodies to carbamylated proteins (anti-CarP) in both ACPA positive and ACPA negative patients. In the latter group, anti-CarP positivity was strongly associated to a more erosive disease (Shi et al., 2011). Moreover, the cross-reactivity between antibodies to citrullinated and homocitrullinated proteins seems to be low (Shi et al., 2011). Likewise ACPA and rheumatoid factor, anti-CarP can be detected before the clinical onset of RA suggesting a potential predictive role for these antibodies (Willemze et al., 2013). The exact pathogenic role of carbamylated proteins and the effect of RA treatment on anti-CarP has not been addressed yet. Carbamylation of lipoproteins has been described in patients with CVD. Carbamylated high-density lipoproteins might promote atherogenesis by impairing the balance between macrophage-mediated cholesterol uptake and efflux (Holzer et al., 2011). On the other side, carbamylation of LDL might induce endothelial dysfunction acting via LOX-1 (Speer et al., 2014; Ishikawa et al., 2012). Carbamylated LDL (cLDL) may uncouple endothelial nitric oxide (NO) synthase, thus reducing the NO bioavailability and impairing the endothelium vasodilatation (Speer et al., 2014). Moreover, cLDL seems to promote monocytes adhesion to endothelial cells, damage endothelial cells and progenitor endothelial cells, and induce vascular smooth muscle cells proliferation (Jaisson et al., 2008). Carbamylation of other proteins, not yet clearly elucidated, might further contribute to the pathogenesis of AS.

Evidence of subclinical CVD has been demonstrated in patients with early RA (Kievit et al., 2016). These patients have also been found to have a higher prevalence of atherosclerotic plaques, increased IMT of the carotid arteries (Veselinovic et al., 2012), and significantly impaired endothelial function compared with controls (Yang et al., 2016). The high frequency in RA patients of risk factors like smoking, dyslipidemia, hypertension, diabetes mellitus, and increased BMI only partially accounts for their high cardiovascular morbidity and mortality (Georgiadis et al., 2008). The accelerated AS observed in these patients seems to be due to systemic inflammatory processes (Signorelli et al., 2016). Rheumatoid synovia and atherosclerotic plaques have proinflammatory endothelial phenotypes represented by expression of the same adhesion molecules and cytokines. Increased formation of NO has been shown to improve vascular function, attenuate leukocyte adhesion to endothelial cells, inhibit platelet aggregation, and modulate smooth muscle proliferation (van Zonneveld et al., 2010). Elevated ADMA levels are an independent risk factor for endothelial dysfunction, and they have been associated with hypertension, diabetes, hypercholesterolemia, renal failure, and AS in both experimental models and humans (Inan et al., 2016). Plasma levels of ADMA are increased in a variety of conditions linked with increased risk of CVD. Higher than normal levels have also been found in patients with established CVDs and, more recently, in RA patients as well. Another potential biomarker is apelin, a peptide that causes endothelium-dependent vasorelaxation by triggering the release of NO (Liakos et al., 2016).

The increased risk of CVD observed in RA can be attributed to accelerated, early AS. Using Doppler ultrasound techniques, several groups have documented impaired FMD and IMT in patients with long-standing RA despite chronic DMARDs treatment (Kisiel et al., 2015b). Moreover, an association with the shared epitope has been detected, suggesting that HLA-DRB1 allele status may predict cardiovascular risk in these patients (Gonzalez-Gay et al., 2008).

Key Points

- RA is associated with accelerated AS, and CHD still represents a main cause of mortality in RA patients.
- Common pathogenic mechanisms exist between RA and AS including citrullination and carbamylation.
- In RA patients common risk factors such as smoking, dyslipidemia, hypertension, diabetes mellitus, and increased BMI are more frequent than in general population.
- Elevated ADMA levels are an independent risk factor for endothelial dysfunction in RA.

4. CLINICAL MANIFESTATIONS

The clinical manifestations of AS include various aspects of cardiovascular morbidity and mortality. These include angina pectoris, MI, cardiac arrest, limb claudication, heart failure, transient ischemic attack, stroke, multiinfarct dementia, renal failure, and actually all the clinical manifestations associated with AS, decreased perfusion to target organs or arterial thrombosis. This is true in general population, but is evident also in patients having autoimmune diseases, who are occasionally characterized by enhanced AS (Bentzon et al., 2014). One example for the increased risk of CVDs in SLE, the disease most commonly associated with secondary APS, is that the risk of hospitalization for MI, cerebrovascular accidents, and congestive heart failure was 2.27, 2.03, and 3.01 times, respectively, greater for patients between 18 and 44 years compared with controls (Herity et al., 1999). In a study on 22 patients with SLE and/or APS the carotid ultrasonography and echocardiography showed a 4.5-fold increase in the presence of carotid AS in the patient group compared to healthy controls, and similarly a sixfold increase in the prevalence of left ventricular hypertrophy (Roman et al., 2001). In a study by Doria et al. (2003), the predictors of AS in SLE were not only traditional including age and hypertension, but also the "non-traditional" including cumulative prednisone uptake, renal involvement, and the levels of antioxidized palmitoyl arachidonoyl phosphocholine antibodies.

Key Points

- The clinical manifestations of AS include various aspects of cardiovascular morbidity and mortality.
- These include angina pectoris, MI, cardiac arrest, limb claudication, heart failure, transient ischemic attack, stroke, multiinfarct dementia, and renal failure.

5. DIAGNOSTIC INVESTIGATIONS

Diagnosis of significant AS state is based on patients' symptoms and objective signs detected through the physical examination. All of the earlier-mentioned manifestations of AS have more or less characteristic clinical presentation. Regarding imaging studies, the gold standard for CAD is still the coronary angiography, which can best demonstrate the state of the coronary vessels. Similarly, ultrasound studies can evaluate narrowing and intimal plaques in the carotid arteries, and Doppler studies can aid in the evaluation of renal artery stenosis, for example.

Doppler ultrasonography is the method most widely used to evaluate early, subclinical atherosclerotic modification of arterial wall (i.e., impaired endothelial function and IMT) and it has several advantages, including noninvasiveness, widespread availability, and relative low cost (Lee, 2014). However, while IMT expresses a morphological change of the arterial wall, which increases with disease progression becoming more evident in long-standing autoimmune rheumatic disease, brachial FMD represents an impaired endothelial responsiveness, which indicates a distinct and independent stage of atherosclerotic process.

Barutcu et al. (2015) used transthoracic Doppler echocardiographic (TTE) imaging methods to identify cardiac dysfunction, an indicator of subclinical AS in asymptomatic SLE patients. The authors found several abnormalities including larger left atrium dimension, lower Ssm, and greater E/E′ ratio especially in those patients carrying aCL antibodies suggesting that regular scans with TTE of SLE patients may be important to identify early cardiac involvement (Barutcu et al., 2015).

Nonetheless, in the setting of autoimmunity-associated AS, other less conventional methods can be used for estimation of AS risk or extent, even though their efficacy has not yet been proven. An alternative way to estimate the burden of AS is by noninvasive techniques, such as the dual-helical computerized tomography. This method can assess calcific coronary deposits, which are closely associated with AS. It has been proved as a noninvasive test with a good sensitivity for the detection of coronary wall AS (Budoff et al., 1996). Regarding serologic evaluation of patients, the presence of higher levels of aPL antibodies might indicate an increased risk or presence of enhanced AS.

Surrogate biomarkers have then been suggested. Beside the traditional risk factors for CVD suggested by the Framingham heart studies, including older age, male gender, smoking, high total cholesterol and LDL levels, high systolic blood pressure, diabetes, and left ventricular hypertrophy, there are disease-specific risk factors for AS in autoimmune conditions. For instance, when considering SLE, some authors suggested that higher disease activity was significantly associated with less plaque, but longer disease duration positively correlated with AS. The double proinflammatory role of HDL cannot be disregarded since it must be reminded that, during acute phase, HDL can be converted from their usual antiinflammatory state to proinflammatory, and cause increased LDL oxidation. It was shown that 85% of patients with SLE and carotid plaques had piHDL; moreover, piHDL have been identified as an independent risk factor in RA and APS (McMahon et al., 2014).

Homocysteine should be tested in patients with autoimmune diseases since high levels have been linked to AS in the general population (Bonciani et al., 2016). Homocysteine is toxic to endothelial cells, is prothrombotic, decreases nitric oxide availability, and stimulates foam cell formation (Perna et al., 2010; Mok et al., 2010; Thampi et al., 2008). In SLE, high homocysteine levels are also associated with subclinical AS, and, of course, particular concern should be used when methotrexate is administered (Fijnheer et al., 1998).

Key Points

- Doppler ultrasonography is the method most widely used to evaluate early atherosclerotic modification of arterial wall.
- Regular scans with transthoracic echocardiographic of SLE patients may be important to identify early cardiac involvement.
- Disease-specific risk factors for AS must be considered.

6. TREATMENT

The treatment of the atherosclerotic process should be aimed first at minimizing the Framingham risk factors, then at switching off the inflammatory process, and finally, in case of overt CVD, it should be according to the clinical presentation.

Patients should be at least annually screened for traditional modifiable risk factors for CVD, including smoking status, blood pressure, BMI, diabetes, and serum lipids (including total cholesterol, HDL, LDL, and triglycerides) (Urowitz et al., 2016).

Cessation for tobacco smoking is recommended for SLE patients at the same extent as the control of glycemia, possibly minimizing the glucocorticoid doses in these patients (Kiani et al., 2011). The blood pressure should be maintained within the 130/80 mmHg, and ACE inhibitors should be considered as the first-line therapy in SLE patients with renal involvement as well as in hypertensive patients with inflammatory arthritis because of their potential favorable effects on inflammatory markers and endothelial function in RA (Tselios et al., 2016). On the other hand, β−blockers should be used with caution because they possibly can precipitate Raynaud phenomenon (Mohokum et al., 2012). Statins have several pleiotropic roles. Indeed, besides their lipid-lowering properties, they have a number of antiinflammatory properties such as inhibition of inflammatory cytokines, ROS formation, T-cell activation, and upregulation of nitric oxide synthesis (Levesque and Weinberg, 2004). The antimalarials such as hydroxychloroquine (HCQ), are cardioprotective, although there are isolated reports of HCQ cardiotoxicity (Stojan and Petri, 2013), and HCQ use has been associated with less aortic stiffness (Selzer et al., 2001) and less plaque on carotid ultrasound in SLE. There are reports suggesting that HCQ may reduce the risk of thrombosis in SLE patients. In another study, it was demonstrated that HCQ administration normalized the NO availability in a mouse model of SLE suggesting a role of HCQ in vascular protection via an antioxidant effect (Gómez-Guzmán et al., 2014).

Elevated cumulative glucocorticoid dosage and perpetrated treatment have been associated with AS in SLE patients (Moya et al., 2016). A prednisone dosage higher than 10 mg/day independently predicts high cholesterol levels; thus, the lowest glucocorticoid dosage should be used in autoimmune patients and for the shortest period (Schanberg et al., 2009).

There is evidence that immunosuppressants such as mycophenolate mofetil (MMF) may decrease AS for instance by modulating plaque expression of inflammatory genes and activated T cells with increased numbers of Treg cells (Alpert et al., 2007). In LDLr−/− mice reconstituted with SLE-prone bone marrow, MMF treatment significantly reduced atherosclerotic burden and recruitment of $CD4^+$ T cells to atherosclerotic plaques (van Leuven et al., 2012). Van Leuven et al. found that the reduction of cholesterol levels alone is not atheroprotective in lupus-mediated atherogenesis and that MMF reduces the atherosclerotic burden in a model of lupus-accelerated AS, conversely from atorvastatin (van Leuven et al., 2010).

Despite the pathogenic role of B cells not only in SLE but also in AS, it is known that depletion of B cells from AS-prone mice leads to increased AS (Tsiantoulas et al., 2014). A possible explanation is that subsets of B cells produce atheroprotective molecules such as IL-10 and anti-oxLDL antibodies (Sage and Mallat, 2014). Nonetheless, B-cell−depleting therapies with anti-CD20 antibodies seem to significantly reduce AS in both the ApoE−/− and the LDLr−/− AS-prone mouse models (Kyaw et al., 2012). On the other hand, azathioprine usage was associated with CAD and with increased carotid IMT in a pediatric SLE cohort (Haque et al., 2010). Methotrexate, widely used to treat RA, increases plasma levels of homocysteine, which is a novel, and potentially modifiable, risk factor for CVD in the general population. Concomitant folate supplementation during methotrexate treatment prevents such increase of homocysteine and, more importantly, seem to reduce CVD mortality in RA patients (Kisiel et al., 2015b). Many patients at risk for thrombosis, such as SLE/APS patients, are given aspirin, which can decrease the chance of arterial thrombosis, regardless of the underlying mechanism (the procoagulant activity of autoantibodies, or the enhanced AS state characterizing these diseases). However, one should remember that the best treatment is prevention. Patients having autoimmune diseases are at increased risk for CVDs and enhanced AS not only due to the autoimmune process, but also due to drugs such as steroids, or disease complications such as nephritis leading to hypertension and nephrotic syndrome. Additionally, other classical risk factors might be found in autoimmune diseases. In SLE, there are elevated triglycerides and VLDL cholesterol, decreased HDL cholesterol, and apoA-1 (Borba and Bonfá, 1997), and also elevated levels of homocysteine (Petri et al., 1996). Therefore, patients should receive preventive therapy with education for regular exercise, blood pressure control, and when appropriate use of statins and/or folic acid. Immunomodulation of AS is also an option, even though it is still in the experimental stages (Sherer and Shoenfeld, 2002). It includes use of intravenous Igs, immunosuppression, oral tolerance with autoantigens such as oxLDL, bone-marrow transplantation, cytokine inhibitors, and gene therapy.

Key Points

- Patients should be screened for traditional modifiable risk factors for CVD, including smoking status, blood pressure, BMI, diabetes, and serum lipids (including total cholesterol, HDL, LDL, and triglycerides).
- Glucocorticoids should be used for the shortest period and dosage should be minimized.
- Immunosuppressants, but azathioprine, may improve the inflammatory status thus ameliorating the atherosclerotic process.
- Antimalarials have several antiatherogenic effects also on endothelium.

REFERENCES

Abe, H., Tsuboi, N., Suzuki, S., Sakuraba, H., Takanashi, H., Tahara, K., Tonozuka, N., Hayashi, T., Umeda, M., 2001. Anti-apolipoprotein A-I autoantibody: characterization of monoclonal autoantibodies from patients with systemic lupus erythematosus. J. Rheumatol. 28, 990–995.

Afek, A., George, J., Gilburd, B., Rauova, L., Goldberg, I., Kopolovic, J., Harats, D., Shoenfeld, Y., 2000. Immunization of low-density lipoprotein receptor deficient (LDL-RD) mice with heat shock protein 65 (HSP-65) promotes early atherosclerosis. J. Autoimmun. 14, 115–121.

Aggarwal, A., Srivastava, R., Agrawal, S., 2013. T cell responses to citrullinated self-peptides in patients with rheumatoid arthritis. Rheumatol. Int. 33, 2359–2363.

Agmon-Levin, N., Blank, M., Zandman-Goddard, G., Orbach, H., Meroni, P.L., Tincani, A., Doria, A., Cervera, R., Miesbach, W., Stojanovich, L., Barak, V., Porat-Katz, B.S., Amital, H., Shoenfeld, Y., 2011. Vitamin D: an instrumental factor in the anti-phospholipid syndrome by inhibition of tissue factor expression. Ann. Rheum. Dis. 70, 145–150.

Ait-Oufella, H., Herbin, O., Bouaziz, J.D., Binder, C.J., Uyttenhove, C., Laurans, L., Taleb, S., Van Vré, E., Esposito, B., Vilar, J., Sirvent, J., Van Snick, J., Tedgui, A., Tedder, T.F., Mallat, Z., 2010. B cell depletion reduces the development of atherosclerosis in mice. J. Exp. Med. 207, 1579–1587.

Akhavanpoor, M., Gleissner, C.A., Gorbatsch, S., Doesch, A.O., Akhavanpoor, H., Wangler, S., Jahn, F., Lasitschka, F., Katus, H.A., Erbel, C., 2014. CCL19 and CCL21 modulate the inflammatory milieu in atherosclerotic lesions. Drug Des. Devel Ther. 8, 2359–2371.

Alpert, D., Davis, A., Erkan, D., Roman, M.J., Salmon, J.E., 2007. Subclinical carotid atherosclerosis in a patient with systemic lupus erythematosus. Nat. Clin. Pract. Rheumatol. 3, 473–478.

Ameli, S., Hultgårdh-Nilsson, A., Regnström, J., Calara, F., Yano, J., Cercek, B., Shah, P.K., Nilsson, J., 1996. Effect of immunization with homologous LDL and oxidized LDL on early atherosclerosis in hypercholesterolemic rabbits. Arterioscler Thromb. Vasc. Biol. 16, 1074–1079.

Ames, P.R., Margarita, A., Delgado Alves, J., Tommasino, C., Iannaccone, L., Brancaccio, V., 2002. Anticardiolipin antibody titre and plasma homocysteine level independently predict intima media thickness of carotid arteries in subjects with idiopathic antiphospholipid antibodies. Lupus 11, 208–214.

Ames, P.R., Delgado Alves, J., Lopez, L.R., Gentile, F., Margarita, A., Pizzella, L., Batuca, J., Scenna, G., Brancaccio, V., Matsuura, E., 2006. Antibodies against beta2glycoprotein I complexed with an oxidised lipoprotein relate to intima thickening of carotid arteries in primary antiphospholipid syndrome. Clin. Dev. Immunol. 13, 1–9.

Aron, A.L., Cuellar, R.L., Brey, R.L., Meceown, S., Espinoza, L.R., Shoenfeld, Y., 1995. Early onset of autoimmunity in MLR/++ mice following immunization with beta2-glycoprotein I. Clin. Exp. Immunol. 101, 78–82.

Barutcu, A., Aksu, F., Ozcelik, F., Barutcu, C.A., Umit, G.E., Pamuk, O.N., Altun, A., 2015. Evaluation of early cardiac dysfunction in patients with systemic lupus erythematosus with or without anticardiolipin antibodies. Lupus 24, 1019–1028.

Bassi, N., Ghirardello, A., Iaccarino, L., Zampieri, S., Rampudda, M.E., Atzeni, F., Sarzi-Puttini, P., Shoenfeld, Y., Doria, A., 2007. OxLDL/beta2GPI-anti-oxLDL/beta2GPI complex and atherosclerosis in SLE patients. Autoimmun. Rev. 7, 52–58.

Belizna, C.C., Richard, V., Thuillez, C., Lévesque, H., Shoenfeld, Y., 2007. Insights into atherosclerosis therapy in antiphospholipid syndrome. Autoimmun. Rev. 7, 46–51.

Bengtsson, C., Ohman, M.L., Nived, O., Rantapää Dahlqvist, S., 2012. Cardiovascular event in systemic lupus erythematosus in northern Sweden: incidence and predictors in a 7-year follow-up study. Lupus 21, 452–459.

Bentzon, J.F., Otsuka, F., Virmani, R., Falk, E., 2014. Mechanisms of plaque formation and rupture. Circ. Res. 114, 1852–1866.

Bonciani, D., Antiga, E., Bonciolini, V., Verdelli, A., Del Bianco, E., Volpi, W., Caproni, M., 2016. Homocysteine serum levels are increased and correlate with disease severity in patients with lupus erythematosus. Clin. Exp. Rheumatol. 34, 76–81.

Borba, E.F., Bonfá, E., 1997. Dyslipoproteinemias in systemic lupus erythematosus: influence of disease, activity, and anticardiolipin antibodies. Lupus 6, 533–539.

Brey, R.L., Abbott, R.D., Curb, J.D., Sharp, D.S., Ross, G.W., Stallworth, C.L., Kittner, S.J., 2001. Beta(2)-Glycoprotein 1-dependent anticardiolipin antibodies and risk of ischemic stroke and myocardial infarction: the honolulu heart program. Stroke 32, 1701–1706.

Budoff, M.J., Georgiou, D., Brody, A., Agatston, A.S., Kennedy, J., Wolfkiel, C., Stanford, W., Shields, P., Lewis, R.J., Janowitz, W.R., Rich, S., Brundage, B.H., 1996. Ultrafast computed tomography as a diagnostic modality in the detection of coronary artery disease: a multicenter study. Circulation 93, 898–904.

Buttari, B., Profumo, E., Mattei, V., Siracusano, A., Ortona, E., Margutti, P., Salvati, B., Sorice, M., Riganò, R., 2005. Oxidized beta2-glycoprotein I induces human dendritic cell maturation and promotes a T helper type 1 response. Blood 106, 3880–3887.

Cambridge, G., Acharya, J., Cooper, J.A., Edwards, J.C., Humphries, S.E., 2013. Antibodies to citrullinated peptides and risk of coronary heart disease. Atherosclerosis 228, 243–246.

Caronti, B., Calderaro, C., Alessandri, C., Conti, F., Tinghino, R., Palladini, G., Valesini, G., 1999. Beta2-glycoprotein I (beta2-GPI) mRNA is expressed by several cell types involved in anti-phospholipid syndrome-related tissue damage. Clin. Exp. Immunol. 115, 214–219.

Ceccarelli, F., Perricone, C., Fabris, M., Alessandri, C., Iagnocco, A., Fabro, C., Pontarini, E., De Vita, S., Valesini, G., 2011. Transforming growth factor β 869C/T and interleukin 6 -174G/C polymorphisms relate to the severity and progression of bone-erosive damage detected by ultrasound in rheumatoid arthritis. Arthritis Res. Ther. 13, R111.

Ceccarelli, F., Perricone, C., Borgiani, P., Ciccacci, C., Rufini, S., Cipriano, E., Alessandri, C., Spinelli, F.R., Sili Scavalli, A., Novelli, G., Valesini, G., Conti, F., 2015. Genetic factors in systemic lupus erythematosus: contribution to disease phenotype. J. Immunol. Res. 745647.

Cervera, R., Serrano, R., Pons-Estel, G.J., Ceberio-Hualde, L., Shoenfeld, Y., de Ramón, E., Buonaiuto, V., Jacobsen, S., Zeher, M.M., Tarr, T., Tincani, A., Taglietti, M., Theodossiades, G., Nomikou, E., Galeazzi, M., Bellisai, F., Meroni, P.L., Derksen, R.H., de Groot, P.G., Baleva, M., Mosca, M., Bombardieri, S., Houssiau, F., Gris, J.C., Quéré, I., Hachulla, E., Vasconcelos, C., Fernández-Nebro, A., Haro, M., Amoura, Z., Miyara, M., Tektonidou, M., Espinosa, G., Bertolaccini, M.L., Khamashta, M.A., 2015. Euro-Phospholipid Project Group (European Forum on Antiphospholipid Antibodies). Morbidity and mortality in the antiphospholipid syndrome during a 10-year period: a multicentre prospective study of 1000 patients. Ann. Rheum. Dis. 74, 1011–1018.

Cesena, F.H., Dimayuga, P.C., Yano, J., Zhao, X., Kirzner, J., Zhou, J., Chan, L.F., Lio, W.M., Cercek, B., Shah, P.K., Chyu, K.Y., 2012. Immune-modulation by polyclonal IgM treatment reduces atherosclerosis in hypercholesterolemic apoE-/- mice. Atherosclerosis 220, 59–65.

Conti, F., Sorice, M., Circella, A., Alessandri, C., Pittoni, V., Caronti, B., Calderaro, C., Griggi, T., Misasi, R., Valesini, G., 2003. Beta-2-glycoprotein I expression on monocytes is increased in anti-phospholipid antibody syndrome and correlates with tissue factor expression. Clin. Exp. Immunol. 132, 509–516.

Conti, F., Spinelli, F.R., Alessandri, C., Pacelli, M., Ceccarelli, F., Marocchi, E., Montali, A., Capozzi, A., Buttari, B., Profumo, E., Sorice, M., Arca, M., Valesini, G., Riganò, R., 2014. Subclinical atherosclerosis in systemic lupus erythematosus and antiphospholipid syndrome: focus on β2GPI-specific T cell response. Arterioscler Thromb. Vasc. Biol. 34, 661–668.

Conti, F., Ceccarelli, F., Perricone, C., Massaro, L., Marocchi, E., Miranda, F., Spinelli, F.R., Truglia, S., Alessandri, C., Valesini, G., 2015. Systemic lupus erythematosus with and without anti-dsDNA antibodies: analysis from a large monocentric cohort. Mediators Inflamm. 2015, 328078.

Demirci, F.Y., Dressen, A.S., Kammerer, C.M., Barmada, M.M., Kao, A.H., Ramsey-Goldman, R., Manzi, S., Kamboh, M.I., 2011. Functional polymorphisms of the coagulation factor II gene (F2) and susceptibility to systemic lupus erythematosus. J. Rheumatol. 38, 652–657.

Doria, A., Shoenfeld, Y., Wu, R., Gambari, P.F., Puato, M., Ghirardello, A., Gilburd, B., Corbanese, S., Patnaik, M., Zampieri, S., Peter, J.B., Favaretto, E., Iaccarino, L., Sherer, Y., Todesco, S., Pauletto, P., 2003. Risk factors for subclinical atherosclerosis in a prospective cohort of patients with systemic lupus erythematosus. Ann. Rheum. Dis. 62, 1071–1077.

El-Sherif, W.T., Herdan, O.M., Osman, M.H., Alkady, E.A., 2010. Mannose binding lectin gene polymorphism and preclinical carotid atherosclerosis in patients with systemic lupus erythematosus. Egypt J. Immunol. 17, 131–141.

Emeson, E.E., Shen, M.L., Bell, C.G., Qureshi, A., 1996. Inhibition of atherosclerosis in CD4 T-cell-ablated and nude (nu/nu) C57BL/6 hyperlipidemic mice. Am. J. Pathol. 149, 675–685.

Erkkilä, A.T., Närvänen, O., Lehto, S., Uusitupa, M.I., Ylä-Herttuala, S., 2000. Autoantibodies against oxidized low-density lipoprotein and cardiolipin in patients with coronary heart disease. Arterioscler Thromb. Vasc. Biol. 20, 204–209.

Espinola-Zavaleta, N., Alexanderson-Rosas, E., Granados, N., Elena Soto, M., Amigo, M.C., 2006. Myocardial perfusion defects in patients with autoimmune diseases: a prospective study. Analysis of two diagnostic tests. Lupus 15, 38–43.

Fadda, S., Nassar, H., Gamal, S.M., Al-azizi, H., 2015. Subclinical atherosclerosis in systemic lupus erythematosus patients and its relationship to disease activity and damage indices. Z. Rheumatol. 74, 529–532.

Fijnheer, R., Roest, M., Haas, F.J., De Groot, P.G., Derksen, R.H., 1998. Homocysteine, methylenetetrahydrofolate reductase polymorphism, antiphospholipid antibodies, and thromboembolic events in systemic lupus erythematosus: a retrospective cohort study. J. Rheumatol. 25, 1737–1742.

Frieri, M., Stampfl, H., 2016. Systemic lupus erythematosus and atherosclerosis: review of the literature. Autoimmun. Rev. 15, 16–21.

Fuster, J.J., Ouchi, N., Gokce, N., Walsh, K., 2016. Obesity-induced changes in adipose tissue microenvironment and their impact on cardiovascular disease. Circ. Res. 118, 1786–1807.

George, J., Afek, A., Gilburd, B., Levy, Y., Blank, M., Kopolovic, J., Harats, D., Shoenfeld, Y., 1997. Atherosclerosis in LDL-receptor knockout mice is accelerated by immunization with anticardiolipin antibodies. Lupus 6, 723–729.

George, J., Harats, D., Bakshi, E., Adler, Y., Levy, Y., Gilburd, B., Shoenfeld, Y., 1999a. Anti-oxidized low density lipoprotein antibody determination as a predictor of restenosis following percutaneous transluminal coronary angioplasty. Immunol. Lett. 68, 263–266.

George, J., Harats, D., Gilburd, B., Afek, A., Levy, Y., Schneiderman, J., Barshack, I., Kopolovic, J., Shoenfeld, Y., 1999b. Immunolocalization of beta2-glycoprotein I (apolipoprotein H) to human atherosclerotic plaques: potential implications for lesion progression. Circulation 99, 2227–2230.

George, J., Harats, D., Gilburd, B., Afek, A., Shaish, A., Kopolovic, J., Shoenfeld, Y., 2000. Adoptive transfer of beta(2)-glycoprotein I-reactive lymphocytes enhances early atherosclerosis in LDL receptor-deficient mice. Circulation 102, 1822–1827.

Georgiadis, A.N., Voulgari, P.V., Argyropoulou, M.I., Alamanos, Y., Elisaf, M., Tselepis, A.D., Drosos, A.A., 2008. Early treatment reduces the cardiovascular risk factors in newly diagnosed rheumatoid arthritis patients. Semin. Arthritis Rheum. 38, 13–19.

Gharavi, A.E., Summaritano, L.R., Wen, J., Elkon, E.B., 1992. Induction of antiphospholipid antibodies by immunization with beta2-glycoprotein I (apolipoprotein H). J. Clin. Invest 90, 1105–1111.

Giannakopoulos, B., Krilis, S.A., 2013. The pathogenesis of the antiphospholipid syndrome. N. Engl. J. Med. 368, 1033–1044.

Giles, J.T., Fert-Bober, J., Park, J.K., Bingham 3rd, C.O., Andrade, F., Fox-Talbot, K., Pappas, D., Rosen, A., van Eyk, J., Bathon, J.M., Halushka, M.K., 2012. Myocardial citrullination in rheumatoid arthritis: a correlative histopathologic study. Arthritis Res. Ther. 14, R39.

Gómez-Guzmán, M., Jiménez, R., Romero, M., Sánchez, M., Zarzuelo, M.J., Gómez-Morales, M., O'Valle, F., López-Farré, A.J., Algieri, F., Gálvez, J., Pérez-Vizcaino, F., Sabio, J.M., Duarte, J., 2014. Chronic hydroxychloroquine improves endothelial dysfunction and protects kidney in a mouse model of systemic lupus erythematosus. Hypertension 64, 330–337.

Gonzalez-Gay, M.A., Gonzalez-Juanatey, C., Llorca, J., Ollier, W.E., Martin, J., 2008. Contribution of HLA-DRB1 shared epitope alleles and chronic inflammation to the increased incidence of cardiovascular disease in rheumatoid arthritis: comment on the article by Farragher et al. Arthritis Rheum. 58, 2584.

Greco, T.P., Conti-Kelly, A.M., Greco Jr., T., Doyle, R., Matsuura, E., Anthony, J.R., Lopez, L.R., 2009. Newer antiphospholipid antibodies predict adverse outcomes in patients with acute coronary syndrome. Am. J. Clin. Pathol. 132, 613–620.

Han, X., Han, X., Wang, Z., Shen, J., Dong, Q., 2016. HDAC9 regulates ox-LDL-induced endothelial cell apoptosis by participating in inflammatory reactions. Front Biosci. (Landmark Ed. 21, 907–917.

Haque, S., Gordon, C., Isenberg, D., Rahman, A., Lanyon, P., Bell, A., Emery, P., McHugh, N., The, L.S., Scott, D.G., Akil, M., Naz, S., Andrews, J., Griffiths, B., Harris, H., Youssef, H., McLaren, J., Toescu, V., Devakumar, V., Teir, J., Bruce, I.N., 2010. Risk factors for clinical coronary heart disease in systemic lupus erythematosus: the lupus and atherosclerosis evaluation of risk (LASER) study. J. Rheumatol. 37, 322–329.

Hattori, N., Kuwana, M., Kaburaki, J., Mimori, T., Ikeda, Y., Kawakami, Y., 2000. T cells that are autoreactive to beta2-glycoprotein I in patients with antiphospholipid syndrome and healthy individuals. Arthritis Rheum. 43, 65–75.

Herity, N.A., Ward, M.R., Lo, S., Yeung, A.C., 1999. Review: clinical aspects of vascular remodeling. J. Cardiovasc. Electrophysiol. 10, 1016–1024.

Hoffmann, A., Ebert, T., Klöting, N., Dokas, J., Jeromin, F., Jessnitzer, B., Burkhardt, R., Fasshauer, M., Kralisch, S., 2016. Leptin dose-dependently decreases atherosclerosis by attenuation of hypercholesterolemia and induction of adiponectin. Biochim. Biophys. Acta 1862, 113–120.

Holzer, M., Gauster, M., Pfeifer, T., Wadsack, C., Fauler, G., Stiegler, P., Koefeler, H., Beubler, E., Schuligoi, R., Heinemann, A., Marsche, G., 2011. Protein carbamylation renders high-density lipoprotein dysfunctional. Antioxid. Redox Signal 14, 2337–2346.

Hsueh, T.P., Sheen, J.M., Pang, J.H., Bi, K.W., Huang, C.C., Wu, H.T., Huang, S.T., 2016. The anti-atherosclerotic effect of naringin is associated with reduced expressions of cell adhesion molecules and chemokines through NF-κB pathway. Molecules 21.

Hulsmans, M., Geeraert, B., Arnould, T., Tsatsanis, C., Holvoet, P., 2013. PPAR agonist-induced reduction of Mcp1 in atherosclerotic plaques of obese, insulin-resistant mice depends on adiponectin-induced Irak3 expression. PLoS One 8, e62253.

Inan, B., Ates, I., Ozkayar, N., Kundi, H., Topcuoglu, C., Dede, F., Sennaroglu, E., 2016. Are increased oxidative stress and asymmetric dimethylarginine levels associated with masked hypertension? Clin. Exp. Hypertens. 38, 294–298.

Ishikawa, M., Ito, H., Akiyoshi, M., Kume, N., Yoshitomi, H., Mitsuoka, H., Tanida, S., Murata, K., Shibuya, H., Kasahara, T., Kakino, A., Fujita, Y., Sawamura, T., Yasuda, T., Nakamura, T., 2012. Lectin-like oxidized low-density lipoprotein receptor 1 signal is a potent biomarker and therapeutic target for human rheumatoid arthritis. Arthritis Rheum. 64, 1024–1034.

Jaisson, S., Garnotel, R., Gillery, P., 2008. New evidence to support the clinical and biological relevance of the protein carbamylation process in human pathophysiology. Med. Hypotheses 70, 1070–1071.

Jiang, Y., Jiang, L.L., Maimaitirexiati, X.M., Zhang, Y., Wu, L., 2015. Irbesartan attenuates TNF-α-induced ICAM-1, VCAM-1, and E-selectin expression through suppression of NF-κB pathway in HUVECs. Eur. Rev. Med. Pharmacol. Sci. 19, 3295–3302.

Jones, D.B., Coulson, A.F., Duff, G.W., 1993. Sequence homology between hsp60 and autoantigens. Immunol. Today 14, 115.

Kay, S.D., Poulsen, M.K., Diederichsen, A.C., Voss, A., 2016. Coronary, carotid, and lower-extremity atherosclerosis and their interrelationship in Danish patients with systemic lupus erythematosus. J. Rheumatol. 43, 315–322.

Kiani, A.N., Post, W.S., Magder, L.S., Petri, M., 2011. Predictors of progression in atherosclerosis over 2 years in systemic lupus erythematosus. Rheumatology (Oxford) 50, 2071–2079.

Kievit, W., Maurits, J.S., Arts, E.E., van Riel, P.L., Fransen, J., Popa, C.D. 2016. Cardiovascular screening in patients with rheumatoid arthritis is cost-effective. Arthritis Care Res. (Hoboken).

Kisiel, B., Kruszewski, R., Juszkiewicz, A., Raczkiewicz, A., Bachta, A., Kłos, K., Duda, K., Saracyn, M., Szymański, K., Młozniak-Cieśla, A., Grabowska-Jodkowska, A., Olesińska, M., Bogusławska-Waleck, R., Niemczyk, S., Płoski, R., Tłustochowicz, W., 2015a. Systemic lupus erythematosus: the influence of disease-related and classical risk factors on intima media thickness and prevalence of atherosclerotic plaques—a preliminary report. Beneficial effect of immunosuppressive treatment on carotid intima media thickness. Acta Cardiol. 70, 169–175.

Kisiel, B., Kruszewski, R., Juszkiewicz, A., Raczkiewicz, A., Bachta, A., Tłustochowicz, M., Staniszewska-Varga, J., Kłos, K., Duda, K., Bogusławska-Walecka, R., Płoski, R., Tłustochowicz, W., 2015b. Methotrexate, cyclosporine a, and biologics protect against atherosclerosis in rheumatoid arthritis. J. Immunol. Res. 2015, 759610.

Kobayashi, K., Kishi, M., Atsumi, T., Bertolaccini, M.L., Makino, H., Sakairi, N., Yamamoto, I., Yasuda, T., Khamashta, M.A., Hughes, G.R., Koike, T., Voelker, D.R., Matsuura, E., 2003. Circulating oxidized LDL forms complexes with beta2glycoprotein I: implication as an atherogenic autoantigen. J. Lipid Res. 44, 716–726.

Kuwana, M., Matsuura, E., Kobayashi, K., Okazaki, Y., Kaburaki, J., Ikeda, Y., Kawakami, Y., 2005. Binding of beta 2-glycoprotein I to anionic phospholipids facilitates processing and presentation of a cryptic epitope that activates pathogenic autoreactive T cells. Blood 105, 1552–1557.

Kyaw, T., Tay, C., Hosseini, H., Kanellakis, P., Gadowski, T., MacKay, F., Tipping, P., Bobik, A., Toh, B.H., 2012. Depletion of B2 but not B1a B cells in BAFF receptor-deficient ApoE mice attenuates atherosclerosis by potently ameliorating arterial inflammation. PLoS One 7, e29371.

Lee, W., 2014. General principles of carotid Doppler ultrasonography. Ultrasonography 33, 11–17.

Levesque, M.C., Weinberg, J.B., 2004. The dichotomous role of nitric oxide in the pathogenesis of accelerated atherosclerosis associated with systemic lupus erythematosus. Curr. Mol. Med. 4, 777–786.

Lewandowski, L.B., Kaplan, M.J., 2016. Update on cardiovascular disease in lupus. Curr. Opin. Rheumatol.

Li, C., Tu, Y., Liu, T.R., Guo, Z.G., Xie, D., Zhong, J.K., Fan, Y.Z., Lai, W.Y., 2015. Rosiglitazone attenuates atherosclerosis and increases high-density lipoprotein function in atherosclerotic rabbits. Int. J. Mol. Med. 35, 715–723.

Liakos, C.I., Sanidas, E.A., Perrea, D.N., Grassos, C.A., Chantziara, V., Viniou, N.A., Barbetseas, J.D., Papadopoulos, D.P., 2016. Apelin and visfatin plasma levels in healthy individuals with high normal blood pressure. Am. J. Hypertens. 29, 549–552.

Liu, C.L., Wang, C.Z., Wang, Y., Zhang, L.Z., Liu, L., Bian, X.L., 2014. Early evaluation of carotid elasticity by an instantaneous wave intensity technique in patients with systemic lupus erythematosus. J. Ultrasound Med. 33, 2125–2129.

Liu, M., Li, X., Sun, R., Zeng, Y.I., Chen, S., Zhang, P., 2016. Vitamin D nutritional status and the risk for cardiovascular disease. Exp. Ther. Med. 11, 1189–1193.

Lopez, L.R., Dier, K.J., Lopez, D., Merrill, J.T., Fink, C.A., 2004. Anti-beta 2-glycoprotein I and antiphosphatidylserine antibodies are predictors of arterial thrombosis in patients with antiphospholipid syndrome. Am. J. Clin. Pathol. 121, 142–149.

López-Pedrera, C., Aguirre, M.Á., Barbarroja, N., Cuadrado, M.J., 2010. Accelerated atherosclerosis in systemic lupus erythematosus: role of proinflammatory cytokines and therapeutic approaches. J. Biomed. Biotechnol.

Lundström, E., Gustafsson, J.T., Jönsen, A., Leonard, D., Zickert, A., Elvin, K., Sturfelt, G., Nordmark, G., Bengtsson, A.A., Sundin, U., Källberg, H., Sandling, J.K., Syvänen, A.C., Klareskog, L., Gunnarsson, I., Rönnblom, L., Padyukov, L., Svenungsson, E., 2013. HLA-DRB1*04/*13 alleles are associated with vascular disease and antiphospholipid antibodies in systemic lupus erythematosus. Ann. Rheum. Dis. 72, 1018–1025.

Mach, F., Schönbeck, U., Sukhova, G.K., Atkinson, E., Libby, P., 1998. Reduction of atherosclerosis in mice by inhibition of CD40 signalling. Nature 394, 200–203.

Mak, A., Liu, Y., Ho, R.C., 2011. Endothelium-dependent but not endothelium-independent flow-mediated dilation is significantly reduced in patients with systemic lupus erythematosus without vascular events: a metaanalysis and metaregression. J. Rheumatol. 38, 1296–1303.

Mandal, K., Foteinos, G., Jahangiri, M., Xu, Q., 2005. Role of antiheat shock protein 60 autoantibodies in atherosclerosis. Lupus 14, 742–746.

Mango, R., Clementi, F., Borgiani, P., Forleo, G.B., Federici, M., Contino, G., Giardina, E., Garza, L., Fahdi, I.E., Lauro, R., Mehta, J.L., Novelli, G., Romeo, F., 2003. Association of single nucleotide polymorphisms in the oxidised LDL receptor 1 (OLR1) gene in patients with acute myocardial infarction. J. Med. Genet. 40, 933–936.

Mango, R., Predazzi, I.M., Romeo, F., Novelli, G., 2011. LOX-1/LOXIN: the yin/yang of atheroscleorosis. Cardiovasc. Drugs Ther. 25, 489–494.

Manzi, S., Selzer, F., Sutton-Tyrrell, K., Fitzgerald, S.G., Rairie, J.E., Tracy, R.P., Kuller, L.H., 1999. Prevalence and risk factors of carotid plaque in women with systemic lupus erythematosus. Arthritis Rheum. 42, 51–60.

Marai, I., Shechter, M., Langevitz, P., Gilburd, B., Rubenstein, A., Matssura, E., Sherer, Y., Shoenfeld, Y., 2008. Anti-cardiolipin antibodies and endothelial function in patients with coronary artery disease. Am. J. Cardiol. 101, 1094–1097.

Matsuura, E., Igarashi, Y., Yasuda, T., Triplett, D.A., Koike, T., 1994. Anticardiolipin antibodies recognize beta 2-glycoprotein I structure altered by interacting with an oxygen modified solid phase surface. J. Exp. Med. 179, 457–462.

Matsuura, E., Kobayashi, K., Koike, T., Shoenfeld, Y., 2001. Autoantibody-mediated atherosclerosis. Autoimmun. Rev. 1, 348–353.

Matsuura, E., Kobayashi, K., Koike, T., Shoenfeld, Y., 2002. Autoantibody-mediated atherosclerosis. Autoimmun. Rev. 1, 348–353.

Matsuura, E., Hughes, G.R., Khamashta, M.A., 2008. Oxidation of LDL and its clinical implication. Autoimmun. Rev. 7, 558–566.

Matsuura, E., Kobayashi, K., Lopez, L.R., 2009. Atherosclerosis in autoimmune diseases. Curr. Rheumatol. Rep. 11, 61–69.

Mazurek, A., Iwaniec, T., Olszowska, M., Perricone, C., Widlinska, B., Podolec, P., Musial, J., Plazak, W., 2016. Antiphospholipid and antinuclear antibodies in young patients after myocardial revascularization procedures. Isr. Med. Assoc. J. 18, 228–231.

McMahon, M., Skaggs, B.J., Grossman, J.M., Sahakian, L., Fitzgerald, J., Wong, W.K., Lourenco, E.V., Ragavendra, N., Charles-Schoeman, C., Gorn, A., Karpouzas, G.A., Taylor, M.B., Watson, K.E., Weisman, M.H., Wallace, D.J., Hahn, B.H., 2014. A panel of biomarkers is associated with increased risk of the presence and progression of atherosclerosis in women with systemic lupus erythematosus. Arthritis Rheumatol. 66, 130–139.

Medina, G., Casaos, D., Jara, L.J., Vera-Lastra, O., Fuentes, M., Barile, L., Salas, M., 2003. Increased carotid artery intima-media thickness may be associated with stroke in primary antiphospholipid syndrome. Ann. Rheum. Dis. 62, 607–610.

Miyakis, S., Lockshin, M.D., Atsumi, T., Branch, D.W., Brey, R.L., Cervera, R., Derksen, R.H., De Groot, P.G., Koike, T., Meroni, P.L., Reber, G., Shoenfeld, Y., Tincani, A., Vlachoyiannopoulos, P.G., Krilis, S.A., 2006. International consensus statement on an update of the classification criteria for definite antiphospholipid syndrome (APS). J. Thromb. Haemost 4, 295–306.

Mohokum, M., Hartmann, P., Schlattmann, P., 2012. The association of Raynaud syndrome with β-blockers: a meta-analysis. Angiology 63, 535–540.

Mok, C.C., Poon, W.L., Lai, J.P., Wong, C.K., Chiu, S.M., Wong, C.K., Lun, S.W., Ko, G.T., Lam, C.W., Lam, C.S., 2010. Metabolic syndrome, endothelial injury, and subclinical atherosclerosis in patients with systemic lupus erythematosus. Scand. J. Rheumatol. 39, 42–49.

Moya, F.B., Pineda Galindo, L.F., García de la Peña, M., 2016. Impact of chronic glucocorticoid treatment on cardiovascular risk profile in patients with systemic lupus erythematosus. J. Clin. Rheumatol. 22, 8–12.

Muniz Caldas, C.A., Freire de Carvalho, J., 2013. Cardiovascular comorbidities in antiphospholipid syndrome. Expert Rev. Clin. Immunol. 9, 987–990.

Nelson, C.P., Schunkert, H., Samani, N.J., Erridge, C., 2015. Genetic analysis of leukocyte type-I interferon production and risk of coronary artery disease. Arterioscler Thromb. Vasc. Biol. 35, 1456–1462.

Nussinovitch, U., Shoenfeld, Y., 2009. Autoimmunity and heart diseases: pathogenesis and diagnostic criteria. Arch. Immunol. Ther. Exp. (Warsz) 57, 95–104.

Pamuk, O.N., Tozkir, H., Uyanik, M.S., Gurkan, H., Saritas, F., Duymaz, J., Donmez, S., Yazar, M., Pamuk, G.E., 2014. PECAM-1 gene polymorphisms and soluble PECAM-1 level in rheumatoid arthritis and systemic lupus erythematosus patients: any link with clinical atherosclerotic events? Clin. Rheumatol. 33, 1737–1743.

Perna, M., Roman, M.J., Alpert, D.R., Crow, M.K., Lockshin, M.D., Sammaritano, L., Devereux, R.B., Cooke, J.P., Salmon, J.E., 2010. Relationship of asymmetric dimethylarginine and homocysteine to vascular aging in systemic lupus erythematosus patients. Arthritis Rheum. 62, 1718–1722.

Perricone, C., Ceccarelli, F., Valesini, G., 2011. An overview on the genetic of rheumatoid arthritis: a never-ending story. Autoimmun. Rev. 10, 599–608.

Perricone, C., Versini, M., Ben-Ami, D., Gertel, S., Watad, A., Segel, M.J., Ceccarelli, F., Conti, F., Cantarini, L., Bogdanos, D.P., Antonelli, A., Amital, H., Valesini, G., Shoenfeld, Y., 2016. Smoke and autoimmunity: the fire behind the disease. Autoimmun. Rev. 15, 354–374.

Petri, M., Roubenoff, R., Dallal, G.E., Nadeau, M.R., Selhub, J., Rosenberg, I.H., 1996. Plasma homocysteine as a risk factor for atherothrombotic events in systemic lupus erythematosus. Lancet 348, 1120–1124.

Pingiotti, E., Cipriani, P., Marrelli, A., Liakouli, V., Fratini, S., Penco, M., Giacomelli, R., 2007. Surface expression of fractalkine receptor (CX3CR1) on $CD4^+$/CD28 T cells in RA patients and correlation with atherosclerotic damage. Ann. N. Y Acad. Sci. 1107, 32–41.

Profumo, E., Buttari, B., Alessandri, C., Conti, F., Capoano, R., Valesini, G., Salvati, B., Riganò, R., 2010. Beta2-glycoprotein I is a target of T cell reactivity in patients with advanced carotid atherosclerotic plaques. Int. J. Immunopathol. Pharmacol. 23, 73–80.

Rajabi, P., Alaee, M., Mousavizadeh, K., Samadikuchaksaraei, A., 2012. Altered expression of TNFSF4 and TRAF2 mRNAs in peripheral blood mononuclear cells in patients with systemic lupus erythematosus: association with atherosclerotic symptoms and lupus nephritis. Inflamm. Res. 61, 1347–1354.

Ramos-Casals, M., 2014. The ill endothelium: how atherosclerosis begins in lupus. Rheumatology (Oxford) 53, 583–585.

Roman, M.J., Salmon, J.E., Sobel, R., Lockshin, M.D., Sammaritano, L., Schwartz, J.E., Devereux, R.B., 2001. Prevalence and relation to risk factors of carotid atherosclerosis and left ventricular hypertrophy in systemic lupus erythematosus and antiphospholipid antibody syndrome. Am. J. Cardiol. 87, 663–666. A11.

Rubin, L.A., Urowitz, M.B., Gladman, D.D., 1985. Mortality in systemic lupus erythematosus: the bimodal pattern revisited. Q. J. Med. 55, 87–98.

Sage, A.P., Mallat, Z., 2014. Multiple potential roles for B cells in atherosclerosis. Ann. Med. 46, 297–303.

Santos, L.L., Morand, E.F., 2009. Macrophage migration inhibitory factor: a key cytokine in RA, SLE and atherosclerosis. Clin. Chim. Acta 399, 1–7.

Schanberg, L.E., Sandborg, C., Barnhart, H.X., Ardoin, S.P., Yow, E., Evans, G.W., Mieszkalski, K.L., Ilowite, N.T., Eberhard, A., Levy, D.M., Kimura, Y., von Scheven, E., Silverman, E., Bowyer, S.L., Punaro, L., Singer, N.G., Sherry, D.D., McCurdy, D., Klein-Gitelman, M., Wallace, C., Silver, R., Wagner-Weiner, L., Higgins, G.C., Brunner, H.I., Jung, L., Soep, J.B., Reed, A., Atherosclerosis Prevention in Pediatric Lupus Erythematosus Investigators, 2009. Premature atherosclerosis in pediatric systemic lupus erythematosus: risk factors for increased carotid intima-media thickness in the atherosclerosis prevention in pediatric lupus erythematosus cohort. Arthritis Rheum. 60, 1496–1507.

Schiopu, A., Frendéus, B., Jansson, B., Söderberg, I., Ljungcrantz, I., Araya, Z., Shah, P.K., Carlsson, R., Nilsson, J., Fredrikson, G.N., 2007. Recombinant antibodies to an oxidized low-density lipoprotein epitope induce rapid regression of atherosclerosis in apobec-1(-/-)/low-density lipoprotein receptor(-/-) mice. J. Am. Coll. Cardiol. 50, 2313–2318.

Schoen, M.W., Salas, J., Scherrer, J.F., Buckhold, F.R., 2015. Cholesterol treatment and changes in guidelines in an academic medical practice. Am. J. Med. 128, 403–409.

Scotece, M., Conde, J., Gómez, R., López, V., Pino, J., González, A., Lago, F., Gómez-Reino, J.J., Gualillo, O., 2012. Role of adipokines in atherosclerosis: interferences with cardiovascular complications in rheumatic diseases. Mediators Inflamm. 2012, 125458.

Selzer, F., Sutton-Tyrrell, K., Fitzgerald, S., Tracy, R., Kuller, L., Manzi, S., 2001. Vascular stiffness in women with systemic lupus erythematosus. Hypertension 37, 1075–1082.

Sharma, S.K., Rathi, M., Sahoo, S., Prakash, M., Dhir, V., Singh, S., 2016. Assessment of premature atherosclerosis in systemic lupus erythematosus patients with and without nephritis. Lupus 25, 525–531.

Sherer, Y., Shoenfeld, Y., 2002. Immunomodulation for treatment and prevention of atherosclerosis. Autoimmun. Rev. 1, 21–27.
Sherer, Y., Shoenfeld, Y., 2003. Antiphospholipid antibodies: are they pro-atherogenic or an epiphenomenon of atherosclerosis? Immunobiology 207, 13–16.
Sherer, Y., Levy, Y., Shoenfeld, Y., 2000. Intravenous immunoglobulin therapy of antiphospholipid syndrome. Rheumatology (Oxford) 39, 421–426.
Sherer, Y., Zinger, H., Shoenfeld, Y., 2010. Atherosclerosis in systemic lupus erythematosus. Autoimmunity 43, 98–102.
Shi, J., Knevel, R., Suwannalai, P., van der Linden, M.P., Janssen, G.M., van Veelen, P.A., Levarht, N.E., van der Helm-van Mil, A.H., Cerami, A., Huizinga, T.W., Toes, R.E., Trouw, L.A., 2011. Autoantibodies recognizing carbamylated proteins are present in sera of patients with rheumatoid arthritis and predict joint damage. Proc. Natl. Acad. Sci. U S A 108, 17372–17377.
Shoenfeld, Y., Sherer, Y., George, J., Harats, D., 2000. Autoantibodies associated with atherosclerosis. Ann. Med. 32, 37–40.
Shoenfeld, Y., Twig, G., Katz, U., Sherer, Y., 2008. Autoantibody explosion in antiphospholipid syndrome. J. Autoimmun. 30, 74–83.
Signorelli, S.S., Candido, S., Salemi, R., Fiore, V., Mangiafico, M., Libra, M., 2016. Low levels of inflammation and the absence of subclinical atherosclerosis in rheumatoid arthritis. Mol. Med. Rep. 13, 3521–3524.
Sikorski, K., Czerwoniec, A., Bujnicki, J.M., Wesoly, J., Bluyssen, H.A., 2011. STAT1 as a novel therapeutical target in pro-atherogenic signal integration of IFNγ, TLR4 and IL-6 in vascular disease. Cytokine Growth Factor Rev. 22, 211–219.
Sinicato, N.A., da Silva Cardoso, P.A., Appenzeller, S., 2013. Risk factors in cardiovascular disease in systemic lupus erythematosus. Curr. Cardiol. Rev. 9, 15–19.
Sokolove, J., Brennan, M.J., Sharpe, O., Lahey, L.J., Kao, A.H., Krishnan, E., Edmundowicz, D., Lepus, C.M., Wasko, M.C., Robinson, W.H., 2013. Brief report: citrullination within the atherosclerotic plaque: a potential target for the anti-citrullinated protein antibody response in rheumatoid arthritis. Arthritis Rheum. 65, 1719–1724.
Soltész, P., Szekanecz, Z., Kiss, E., Shoenfeld, Y., 2007. Cardiac manifestations in antiphospholipid syndrome. Autoimmun. Rev. 6, 379–386.
Sorice, M., Longo, A., Capozzi, A., Garofalo, T., Misasi, R., Alessandri, C., Conti, F., Buttari, B., Riganò, R., Ortona, E., Valesini, G., 2007. Anti-beta2-glycoprotein I antibodies induce monocyte release of tumor necrosis factor alpha and tissue factor by signal transduction pathways involving lipid rafts. Arthritis Rheum. 56, 2687–2697.
Speer, T., Owala, F.O., Holy, E.W., Zewinger, S., Frenzel, F.L., Stähli, B.E., Razavi, M., Triem, S., Cvija, H., Rohrer, L., Seiler, S., Heine, G.H., Jankowski, V., Jankowski, J., Camici, G.G., Akhmedov, A., Fliser, D., Lüscher, T.F., Tanner, F.C., 2014. Carbamylated low-density lipoprotein induces endothelial dysfunction. Eur. Heart J. 35, 3021–3032.
Stalc, M., Tomsic, M., Jezovnik, M.K., Poredos, P., 2011. Endothelium-dependent and independent dilation capability of peripheral arteries in patients with systemic lupus erythematosus and antiphospholipid syndrome. Clin. Exp. Rheumatol. 29, 616–623.
Steinberg, H.O., Bayazeed, B., Hook, G., Johnson, A., Cronin, J., Baron, A.D., 1997. Endothelial dysfunction is associated with cholesterol levels in the high normal range in humans. Circulation 96, 3287–3293.
Stojan, G., Petri, M., 2013. Atherosclerosis in systemic lupus erythematosus. J. Cardiovasc. Pharmacol. 62, 255–262.
Su, J., Frostegård, A.G., Hua, X., Gustafsson, T., Jogestrand, T., Hafström, I., Frostegård, J., 2013. Low levels of antibodies against oxidized but not nonoxidized cardiolipin and

phosphatidylserine are associated with atherosclerotic plaques in systemic lupus erythematosus. J. Rheumatol. 40, 1856–1864.

Szekanecz, Z., Kerekes, G., Végh, E., Kardos, Z., Baráth, Z., Tamási, L., Shoenfeld, Y., 2016. Autoimmune atherosclerosis in 3D: how it develops, how to diagnose and what to do. Autoimmun. Rev. 15, 756–769.

Teixeira, P.C., Cutler, P., Vuilleumier, N., 2012. Autoantibodies to apolipoprotein A-1 in cardiovascular diseases: current perspectives. Clin. Dev. Immunol. 868251.

Thampi, P., Stewart, B.W., Joseph, L., Melnyk, S.B., Hennings, L.J., Nagarajan, S., 2008. Dietary homocysteine promotes atherosclerosis in apoE-deficient mice by inducing scavenger receptors expression. Atherosclerosis 197, 620–629.

Tselios, K., Gladman, D.D., Su, J., Urowitz, M.B., 2016. Does renin-angiotensin system blockade protect lupus nephritis patients from atherosclerotic cardiovascular events? A case-control study. Arthritis Care Res. (Hoboken).

Tsiantoulas, D., Diehl, C.J., Witztum, J.L., Binder, C.J., 2014. B cells and humoral immunity in atherosclerosis. Circ. Res. 114, 1743–1756.

Urowitz, M.B., Gladman, D.D., Anderson, N.M., Su, J., Romero-Diaz, J., Bae, S.C., Fortin, P.R., Sanchez-Guerrero, J., Clarke, A., Bernatsky, S., Gordon, C., Hanly, J.G., Wallace, D.J., Isenberg, D., Rahman, A., Merrill, J., Ginzler, E., Alarcón, G.S., Fessler, B.F., Petri, M., Bruce, I.N., Khamashta, M., Aranow, C., Dooley, M., Manzi, S., Ramsey-Goldman, R., Sturfelt, G., Nived, O., Steinsson, K., Zoma, A., Ruiz-Irastorza, G., Lim, S., Kalunian, K.C., İnanç, M., van Vollenhoven, R., Ramos-Casals, M., Kamen, D.L., Jacobsen, S., Peschken, C., Askanase, A., Stoll, T., 2016. Cardiovascular events prior to or early after diagnosis of systemic lupus erythematosus in the systemic lupus international collaborating clinics cohort. Lupus Sci. Med. 3, e000143.

van Leuven, S.I., van Wijk, D.F., Volger, O.L., de Vries, J.P., van der Loos, C.M., de Kleijn, D.V., Horrevoets, A.J., Tak, P.P., van der Wal, A.C., de Boer, O.J., Pasterkamp, G., Hayden, M.R., Kastelein, J.J., Stroes, E.S., 2010. Mycophenolate mofetil attenuates plaque inflammation in patients with symptomatic carotid artery stenosis. Atherosclerosis 211, 231–236.

van Leuven, S.I., Mendez-Fernandez, Y.V., Wilhelm, A.J., Wade, N.S., Gabriel, C.L., Kastelein, J.J., Stroes, E.S., Tak, P.P., Major, A.S., 2012. Mycophenolate mofetil but not atorvastatin attenuates atherosclerosis in lupus-prone LDLr(-/-) mice. Ann. Rheum. Dis. 71, 408–414.

van Zonneveld, A.J., de Boer, H.C., van der Veer, E.P., Rabelink, T.J., 2010. Inflammation, vascular injury and repair in rheumatoid arthritis. Ann. Rheum. Dis. 69, i57–60.

Vander Cruyssen, B., Hoffman, I.E., Peene, I., Union, A., Mielants, H., Meheus, L., De Keyser, F., 2007. Prediction models for rheumatoid arthritis during diagnostic investigation: evaluation of combinations of rheumatoid factor, anti-citrullinated protein/peptide antibodies and the human leucocyte antigen-shared epitope. Ann. Rheum. Dis. 66, 364–369.

Vecchione, L., Gargiulo, E., Borgiani, P., Predazzi, I., Mango, R., Romeo, F., Magnani, M., Novelli, G., 2007. Genotyping OLR1 gene: a genomic biomarker for cardiovascular diseases. Recent Pat Cardiovasc. Drug Discov. 2, 147–151.

Versini, M., Jeandel, P.Y., Rosenthal, E., Shoenfeld, Y., 2014. Obesity in autoimmune diseases: not a passive bystander. Autoimmun. Rev. 13, 981–1000.

Veselinovic, M.V., Zivkovic, V.I., Toncev, S., Tasic, N., Bogdanovic, V., Djuric, D.M., Jakovljevic, V.L.J., 2012. Carotid artery intima-media thickness and brachial artery flow-mediated vasodilatation in patients with rheumatoid arthritis. Vasa 41, 343–351.

Visvanathan, S., McNeil, H.P., 1999. Cellular immunity to beta 2-glycoprotein-1 in patients with the antiphospholipid syndrome. J. Immunol. 162, 6919–6925.

Watkins, A.A., Yasuda, K., Wilson, G.E., Aprahamian, T., Xie, Y., Maganto-Garcia, E., Shukla, P., Oberlander, L., Laskow, B., Menn-Josephy, H., Wu, Y., Duffau, P., Fried, S.K., Lichtman, A.H., Bonegio, R.G., Rifkin, I.R., 2015. IRF5 deficiency ameliorates lupus but promotes atherosclerosis and metabolic dysfunction in a mouse model of lupus-associated atherosclerosis. J. Immunol. 194, 1467–1479.

Wilhelm, A.J., Rhoads, J.P., Wade, N.S., Major, A.S., 2015. Dysregulated CD4^{+} T cells from SLE-susceptible mice are sufficient to accelerate atherosclerosis in LDLr-/- mice. Ann. Rheum. Dis. 74, 778–785.

Willemze, A., Shi, J., Mulder, M., Stoeken-Rijsbergen, G., Drijfhout, J.W., Huizinga, T.W., Trouw, L.A., Toes, R.E., 2013. The concentration of anticitrullinated protein antibodies in serum and synovial fluid in relation to total immunoglobulin concentrations. Ann. Rheum. Dis. 72, 1059–1063.

Wu, R., Nityanand, S., Berglund, L., Lithell, H., Holm, G., Lefvert, A.K., 1997. Antibodies against cardiolipin and oxidatively modified LDL in 50-year-old men predict myocardial infarction. Arterioscler Thromb. Vasc. Biol. 17, 3159–3163.

Wu, R., Shoenfeld, Y., Sherer, Y., Patnaik, M., Matsuura, E., Gilburdm, B., Koike, T., Peter, J.B., 2003. Anti-idiotypes to oxidized LDL antibodies in intravenous immunoglobulin preparations—possible immunomodulation of atherosclerosis. Autoimmunity 36, 91–97.

Wu, G.C., Liu, H.R., Leng, R.X., Li, X.P., Li, X.M., Pan, H.F., Ye, D.Q., 2016. Subclinical atherosclerosis in patients with systemic lupus erythematosus: a systemic review and meta-analysis. Autoimmun. Rev. 15, 22–37.

Xu, Q., Dietrich, H., Steiner, H.J., 1992. Induction of arteriosclerosis in normocholesterolemic rabbits by immunization with heat shock protein 65. Arterioscler. Thromb. 12, 789.

Xu, Q., Willeit, J., Marosi, M., 1993. Association of serum antibodies to heat-shock protein 65 with carotid atherosclerosis. Lancet 341, 255.

Xu, Q., Kiechl, S., Mayr, M., 1999. Association of serum antibodies to heat-shock protein 65 with carotid atherosclerosis: clinical significance determined in a follow-up study. Circulation 100, 1169.

Yang, X., Chang, Y., Wei, W., 2016. Endothelial dysfunction and inflammation: immunity in rheumatoid arthritis. Mediators Inflamm. 2016, 6813016.

Yaniv, G., Twig, G., Shor, D.B., Furer, A., Sherer, Y., Mozes, O., Komisar, O., Slonimsky, E., Klang, E., Lotan, E., Welt, M., Marai, I., Shina, A., Amital, H., Shoenfeld, Y., 2015. A volcanic explosion of autoantibodies in systemic lupus erythematosus: a diversity of 180 different antibodies found in SLE patients. Autoimmun. Rev. 14, 75–79.

Zinger, H., Sherer, Y., Shoenfeld, Y., 2009. Atherosclerosis in autoimmune rheumatic diseases-mechanisms and clinical findings. Clin. Rev. Allergy Immunol. 37, 20–28.

Chapter 6

Inflammasomes and Inflammatory Cytokines in Early Atherosclerosis

E. Matsuura,* X.W. Tan,* L.H. Shen,* N.U. Azmi* and L.R. Lopez[§]
*Collaborative Research Center for Okayama Medical Innovation Center (OMIC) and Department of Cell Chemistry, Okayama University Graduate School of Medicine, Dentistry, and Pharmaceutical Sciences, Okayama, Japan; [§]Corgenix/Orgentec, Broomfield, CO, United States

Key Points

- Chronic dysregulation of early proatherogenic inflammatory pathways may lead to the activation of innate and adaptive immune responses affecting the endothelium, platelets, and arterial wall.
- As with the adaptive immunity, it is now recognized that the innate immune response can cause tissue and organ injury that if left unchecked can progress into chronic inflammatory processes and to disease states.
- Cholesterol crystals and oxidized low-density lipoprotein (oxLDL) can activate endogenous sensors (NLRP3 inflammasomes) to generate proinflammatory IL-1 cytokines.
- OxLDL/β_2-glycoprotein I (β_2GPI) complexes are quickly incorporated into macrophage lysosomes where inflammasome/IL-1 activation is initiated, suggesting a role for β_2GPI in innate immunity and chronic inflammation.
- OxLDL and oxLDL/β_2GPI complexes may initiate an early atherogenic inflammatory response via the innate inflammasome/IL-1 pathway, subsequently may perpetuate it via an adaptive immune response that favors the progression of atherosclerosis.

1. INTRODUCTION

Lipid peroxidation of low-density lipoprotein (LDL) in the arterial intima is a key event in the initiation and progression of atherosclerosis. Oxidized LDL (oxLDL) is a highly inflammatory and immunogenic molecule that promotes a prothrombotic endothelial dysfunction, the synthesis and secretion of proinflammatory and chemotactic cytokines that result in the activation of an atherothrombotic immune response. These abnormalities promote recruitment of macrophages and their subsequent activation and intracellular lipid accumulation within atherosclerotic lesions (Libby, 2002; Hansson, 2005). Most of the research into the autoimmune pathogenesis of atherothrombosis has been directed to the adaptive immune system. However, in the recent years, attention has turned to the fundamentals of inflammatory mechanisms in particular to the role of innate immunity (Hartvigsen et al., 2009; Lundberg and Hansson, 2010).

The innate immune system provides an immediate first-line host defense against a wide variety of pathogens and endogenous danger molecules produced by the damaged tissue, cell irritants, or metabolic by-products such as oxLDL. This may lead to a sustained activation of inflammatory responses and progress into the more specific and memory-bearing adaptive immune response. As with the adaptive immunity, it is now recognized that the innate immune response can cause tissue and organ injury. If such a condition is left unimpeded, it can progress into chronic inflammatory processes and further develop into disease states.

2. LIPID DYSREGULATION IN AUTOIMMUNITY

The underlying metabolic abnormalities associated with atherosclerosis cause a systemic inflammatory background and immune activation that affect the vasculature. The exact mechanisms by which metabolic stress initiates and promotes an inflammatory response and atherogenesis are now better understood (Yin et al., 2013). The oxidative modification of LDL into oxLDL is a significant early inflammatory trigger of atherogenesis associated with the activation of a cytoplasmic system of metabolic sensors referred to as inflammasomes. The activation of inflammasomes requires the upregulation of its components and their posttranslational assembly to convert pro-caspase-1 and IL-1 into proinflammatory active cytokines. Metabolic inflammasome activators causing lysosome damage and reactive oxygen species (ROS) generation have been shown to activate potent inflammatory responses. The chronic metabolic activation of inflammasomes and the proinflammatory background generated will further promote the immune activation of monocyte/macrophage and T-lymphocytes to sustain the progression of the disease. Thus, both the innate inflammatory and adaptive immune responses are important pathologic mechanisms underlying atherosclerosis.

The premature (or accelerated) development of atherosclerosis is now a recognized complication in patients with systemic autoimmune diseases such as systemic lupus erythematosus (SLE) and the antiphospholipid syndrome (APS). The causal relationship between antiphospholipid antibodies and vascular thrombotic events is widely accepted and better understood. In addition to venous thromboembolism, patients with SLE and APS may develop premature atherosclerotic cardiovascular disease associated with significant morbidity and mortality that are not fully explained by the classic risk factors (Schattner and Liang, 2003). Further, the contributory role of an adaptive immune response represented by autoantibodies to β_2-glycoprotein I (β_2GPI) and oxLDL in atherosclerosis is also now widely recognized (Kobayashi et al., 2005).

Systemic autoimmune diseases present chronic dyslipidemia characterized by decreased HDL, high triglycerides, and elevated LDL (Frostegard, 2005; Matsuura et al., 2008). On this background, systemic generation of free radicals by endothelial and circulating mononuclear cells may induce oxidative modifications of LDL (oxLDL). The scavenger receptor-mediated uptake of oxLDL by arterial mononuclear cells results in the release of inflammatory and chemotactic cytokines in the early stages of atherosclerosis, leading to an excessive intracellular accumulation of oxLDL (Hasunuma et al., 1997). Additionally, immunostaining of human atherosclerotic lesions colocalized β_2GPI with oxLDL, suggesting a close relationship of these molecules (Ylä-Herttuala et al., 1989; George et al., 1999). It therefore seems that β_2GPI is strongly implicated in the development of autoimmune arterial and venous thromboembolism, and that oxLDL/β_2GPI are involved in atherogenesis. Hence, these observations support the general concept that autoimmunity plays a role in the development of premature cardiovascular disease (Matsuura et al., 2005).

Moreover, experiments evaluating the intracellular trafficking of β_2GPI within macrophages showed that only complexed β_2GPI (to phosphatidylserine liposomes or to oxLDL) was rapidly transported to lysosomes, to which the addition of antibodies to β_2GPI further accelerated this process (Kajiwara et al., 2007; Kuwana et al., 2005). In this respect, β_2GPI can be viewed as a component of the innate immunity but once bound to oxLDL, the complex may shift to the generation and maintenance of an adaptive immune response that may play an important role in atherogenic inflammation via the inflammasome/IL-1β system.

3. INNATE IMMUNITY AND INFLAMMATORY SIGNALING MECHANISMS

Cells of the innate immune system (neutrophils, macrophages, dendritic, etc.) play key roles in mediating inflammatory responses as they are equipped with an array of signaling receptors that detect foreign substances (pathogens) or altered endogenous molecules generated under stressful situations (Akira et al., 2006) (Fig. 6.1). The innate immune system is an early and perhaps a primitive form of host defense found in all animal species and even plants. It provides an immediate response to harmful agents before the most efficient and specific adaptive immune response becomes activated and turns into action. The innate immune system relies on transmembrane signaling and

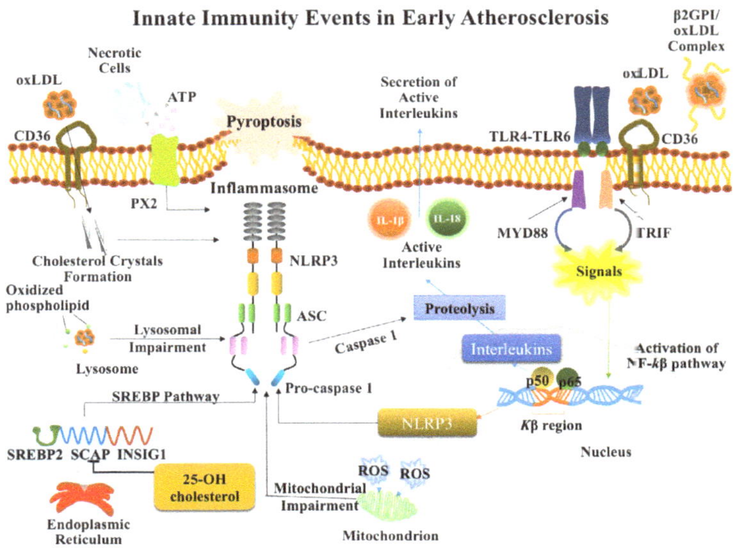

FIGURE 6.1 Multiple signaling pathways of innate immunity-mediated inflammatory responses.

intracellular receptors (danger sensors) that trigger varied biological responses. The receptors of the innate immune system evolved to recognize molecules that are broadly shared by pathogenic microorganisms but distinguishable from host molecules (pathogen-associated molecular patterns or PAMPs). They also recognize damaged tissue and modified self-molecules. Pattern recognition receptors (PRR) include a transmembrane set of toll-like receptors (TLRs) found on macrophages, dendritic cells, and epithelial cells (exogenous sensors) that recognize different types of PAMPs. TLRs turn on the signaling cascades that lead to the expression of various cytokine genes such as tumor necrosis factor α (TNFα), IL-1, and chemokines via activation of NF-κB, which promote inflammation at the site of the interaction (Bauernfeind et al., 2009). It has been recently reported that two oxidized lipids (27-hydroxycholesterol and 4-hydroxynonenal) may contribute to atherosclerotic plaque instability, matrix degradation, and rupture by sustaining the release of inflammatory cytokines and MMP-9 by immune cells through the activation of TLR4 and NK-κB downstream signaling pathway (Gargiulo et al., 2015).

Two families of intracellular receptors (endogenous sensors) have been described: retinoic acid-inducible gene I-like helicases and nucleotide-binding leucine-rich receptors (NLRs) (Gargiulo et al., 2015; Meylan et al., 2006). NLR is a family of intracellular (cytoplasmic) immune receptors with more than 20 members in humans. NLR members are characterized by leucine-rich repeats (LRR) and a nucleotide-binding domain (NBD) by the C-terminal. Differences in their N-terminal subcategorize NLR members. Members of the largest subgroup have an N-terminal pyrin domain (PYD) and are called pyrin-containing NLRs (NLRPs). N-terminal caspase recruitment domain (CARD) characterizes the NLRCs members. NLRP1, NLRP3, and NLRC4 can activate proinflammatory caspases in response to various endogenous stimuli. Activated caspase-1 controls the maturation of IL-1 family of cytokines. As described in the following, multimolecular complexes of NLRs are referred to as inflammasomes because they regulate inflammatory caspases and IL-1 cytokines. NLRP3 activates pro-caspase-1 by recruiting the adapter protein ASC (apoptosis-associated speck-like protein) containing a caspase recruitment (CARD) and PYD domains. ASC and NLRP3 oligomerize with pro-caspase-1 via PYD and CARD terminals to form inflammasomes. In resting cells, caspase-1 is present in an inactive form (pro-caspase-1) (Stutz et al., 2009). Endogenous signals promote polymerization of pro-caspase-1 with NLRP3 inflammasomes. Pro-caspase-1 was previously known as IL-1 converting enzyme. Pro-caspase-1/NLRP3 inflammasome complexes activate caspase-1 to proteolytically cleave pro-IL-1β (35-kDa) into bioactive cytokine IL-1β (17-kDa), a potent pyrogen, initiator of acute-phase response, and activator of mononuclear immune-inflammatory cells (Martinon et al., 2002).

Given these functions, IL-1β is considered a potent proinflammatory cytokine with potential deleterious effects if produced uncontrollably. Caspase-1 can also cleave other proinflammatory members of the IL-1 family like IL-18 and possibly IL-33. Secretion of mature IL-1 cytokines may occur by shedding exosomes from plasma membranes or through unidentified plasma membrane transporters. Release of IL-1 cytokines may precede caspase-1—induced inflammatory cell death seen in response to infections and called pyroptosis with characteristics of both apoptosis and necrosis (Dinarello, 2009). Production of pro-IL-1β and NLRP3 activation can also be mediated through cytokine transmembrane receptors (TNF receptor) or pattern recognition receptors such as TLRs. Released proinflammatory IL-1β cytokines can then activate other cells or self-perpetuate this activation cycle by binding the IL-1R in a feed-forward loop (Ting et al., 2008).

As previously mentioned, NLRP3 inflammasomes can be assembled by stimuli from cytoplasmic proteolytic activity that occurs during lysosomal damage and resulting ROS. NLRPs are thought to act as danger sensors to exogenous but mostly to endogenous signals generated by either infectious or cellular (metabolic) stress. The substances capable of activating NLRP3 inflammasome are manifold and diverse in nature and structure. They include infectious agents (leishmania, *staphylococcus*, *listeria*, influenza A) and toxins (lipopolysaccharide) to particles (microcrystals in gout and pseudogout) and metabolic alterations (low potassium, adenosine triphosphate, hyperglycemia, oxidative stress) (Petrilli et al., 2007; Martinon et al., 2006).

Host-derived oxidation-specific epitopes may be the major activators of innate immunity, recognized by a variety of PRRs (Miller et al., 2011) and therefore can be considered "danger (or damage)-associated molecular patterns." Oxidation-specific epitopes present on apoptotic cells and their cellular debris may have provided the primary evolutionary selection of PRRs. Lipid peroxidation is ubiquitous and represents a major component of the inflammatory state associated with atherosclerosis. Thus, the generation of oxidation-specific epitopes may activate innate immunity through endogenous cytoplasmic sensors such as inflammasomes.

4. INFLAMMASOMES AND IL-1β IN ATHEROGENESIS

Atherosclerosis is a multifactorial low-grade inflammatory disease of the arterial wall that starts with a systemic immune-inflammatory process associated with dyslipidemic and prothrombotic phenotypes that evolves into localized intra-arterial lesions (plaques). No unifying hypothesis has been proposed likely due to the diverse nature and complex interrelationship of these mechanisms (Tall and Yvan-Charvet, 2015). Nonetheless, the search for newer and earlier atherogenic mechanisms such as those related to the innate immunity is gaining popularity. Whether these efforts will provide a unifying view remains as an open question. There is one clinical study showing that IL-1 blockade prevents adverse cardiac remodeling after acute myocardial infarction (Abbate et al., 2010). The recombinant IL-1 receptor antagonist anakinra was safe and favorably affected left-ventricular remodeling in patients with ST-segment elevation myocardial infarction, a condition characterized by an intense inflammatory response mediated in great part by IL-1, suggesting that this therapeutic strategy may prevent heart failure. If mechanisms operating in autoinflammatory diseases also operate in atherosclerosis, they may offer new and perhaps more efficient targets for early intervention or prevention.

Published experimental evidence on the role of inflammasome-induced IL-1β dysregulation in atherosclerotic cardiovascular disease is sparse but very informative (Table 6.1). The effect of proinflammatory cytokines (IL-1β and TNFα) on macrophage foam cells (lipid-loaded THP-1 cells) was studied by Persson et al. (2008). Cells incubated in the absence of cytokines utilized accumulated neutral lipids such as triglycerides. The addition of exogenous IL-1β (and TNFα) resulted in a dose-dependent retention of intracellular cholesterol and triglycerides. The authors concluded that IL-1β and TNFα enhance macrophage foam cell formation, in part by inhibition of intracellular lipid catabolism, and speculated that if these mechanisms are operative in vivo, it will further the proatherogenic role of these two cytokines.

The role of NLRs receptors in pathology was reviewed by Connat (2011), who argued for the role of inflammasomes in the development of cardiovascular diseases. The bioactivation of atherogenic cytokines such as IL-1β and

TABLE 6.1 Evidence for a Role of IL-1β and Pyrin-Containing Nucleotide-Binding Leucine-Rich Receptors (NLRP) Inflammasomes in Atherogenesis

Study Model	Year	Results	Reference
Differentiated primary human macrophages, THP-1 (in vitro)	2008	Intracellular lipid retention in IL-1β and TNF-α enhanced macrophage foam cells	Persson et al. (2008)
Explanted human atherosclerotic arteries. IL-1 receptor antagonist polymorphism	2009	Atherosclerotic arteries exhibited elevated IL-1β and IL-1Ra as compared to normal arteries	Olofsson et al. (2009)
Human macrophages (in vitro)	2010	Cholesterol crystals–mediated release of IL-1β was facilitated by caspase-1–dependent mechanism through the involvement of inflammasome activation pathway	Rajamäki et al. (2010)
Murine atherosclerotic models (in vivo)	2010	Activation of NLRP3 inflammasomes and inflammation (endogenous danger signals) by cholesterol crystals via phagolysosomal damage	Duewell et al. (2010)
Murine diabetic models (in vivo)	2010	Uric acid crystals activated NLPR3 inflammasomes in thioredoxin-dependent conduit	Zhou et al. (2010)
Murine macrophage model (in vitro)	2011	Matured atherogenic cytokines, IL-1β, and IL-18 are discovered in NLRP inflammasomes. Upregulation and activation of plaque NLRP3 inflammasomes in murine macrophages are modulated by oxLDL	Connat (2011)

IL-18 is NLRP inflammasome dependent. Immunocytochemistry showed that NLRP3 inflammasomes are expressed in plaques, upregulated and activated in the CD11b(+)Gr1(high) atherosclerosis-prone monocyte subset and modulated by oxLDL in murine macrophages. He concluded that NLRP3 inflammasome is involved in atherosclerosis.

Human macrophages avidly phagocytose cholesterol crystals and stored the ingested cholesterol as cholesteryl esters (Rajamäki et al., 2010).

Cholesterol crystals induced dose-dependent secretion of mature IL-1β from human monocytes and macrophages. The cholesterol crystal–induced secretion of IL-1β was caspase-1 dependent, suggesting the involvement of an inflammasome-mediated pathway. Silencing the NLRP3 receptor, the crucial component of NLRP3 inflammasome, completely abolished crystal-induced IL-1β secretion, thus identifying NLRP3 inflammasome as the cholesterol crystal–responsive element in macrophages. The crystals were shown to induce leakage of the lysosomal protease cathepsin B into the cytoplasm, and the inhibition of this enzyme reduced cholesterol crystal–induced IL-1β secretion suggesting that NLRP3 inflammasome activation occurred via lysosomal destabilization. The cholesterol crystal–induced inflammasome activation in macrophages may represent an important link between cholesterol metabolism and inflammation in atherosclerotic lesions.

Using a microscopic technique, Duewell et al. (2010) showed that minute cholesterol crystals appear very early in diet-induced atherosclerotic lesions in mice, and that their appearance coincided with the first appearance of inflammatory cells. They showed that cholesterol crystals activate the NLRP3 inflammasome in phagocytes in a process that involves phagolysosomal damage. Similarly, when injected intraperitoneally, cholesterol crystals induced acute inflammation. This response was impaired in mice deficient in components of the NLRP3 inflammasome, cathepsin B, cathepsin L, or IL-1 molecules. Minimally modified LDL can lead to cholesterol crystallization concomitant with NLRP3 inflammasome priming and activation in macrophages. Although there is the possibility that oxidized LDL activates NLRP3 inflammasomes in vivo, these results demonstrate that crystalline cholesterol acts as an endogenous danger signal and its deposition in arteries or elsewhere is an early cause rather than a late consequence of inflammation. These findings provide new insights into the pathogenesis of atherosclerosis and indicate new potential molecular targets for the therapy of this disease.

Zhou et al. (2010) demonstrated that NLRP3 interacted with thioredoxin-interacting protein (TXNIP), a protein linked to insulin resistance. Inflammasome activators such as uric acid crystals induced the dissociation of TXNIP from thioredoxin in an ROS-sensitive manner and allowed it to bind NLRP3. TXNIP deficiency impaired activation of the NLRP3 inflammasome and subsequent secretion of IL-1β. Akin to Txnip(−/−) mice, Nlrp3(−/−) mice showed improved glucose tolerance and insulin sensitivity. The participation of TXNIP in the NLRP3 inflammasome activation may provide a mechanistic link to the observed involvement of IL-1 in the pathogenesis of type 2 diabetes.

IL-1β, IL-1 receptor 1 (IL-1R1), and IL-1 receptor antagonist (IL-1Ra) using TaqMan PCR and ELISA on fresh and endotoxin-stimulated explanted human atherosclerotic and normal arteries were analyzed by Olofsson et al. (2009). Two hundred forty-three survivors of a first myocardial infarction were genotyped for polymorphism of IL-1Ra and their coronary atherosclerosis analyzed by coronary angiography. Levels of IL-1β, IL-1Ra, and IL-1R1 mRNA were significantly increased in atherosclerotic arteries compared to normal arteries. Endotoxin stimulation increased IL-1β levels more than IL-1Ra levels (promoting a proinflammatory state). A polymorphism of IL-1Ra known to increase levels of IL-1Ra was associated with decreased mean coronary artery plaque area. Activation of innate immunity changed the balance between IL-1β and IL-1Ra in atherosclerotic arteries toward a more proinflammatory state. In line with this, the presence of an IL-1Ra intron two polymorphism known to increase IL-1Ra levels, and possibly the IL-1Ra:IL-1β ratio, was associated with reduced coronary atherosclerosis.

5. β_2-GLYCOPROTEIN I IN ATHEROGENIC INNATE IMMUNITY

Once ascertained that β_2GPI was the main antigenic target for antiphospholipid antibodies, the functions of β_2GPI started slowly unraveling; initially described as a natural anticoagulant, β_2GPI has more pleiotropic functions affecting fibrinolysis, angiogenesis, apoptosis as well as atherogenesis due to its interaction with oxLDL (De Groot and Meijers, 2011). In fact, unlike native LDL, β_2GPI binds oxLDL via specific oxidative-derived ligands to form stable and atherogenic oxLDL/β_2GPI complexes (Kobayashi et al., 2001). The interaction between oxLDL and β_2GPI suggest an antioxidant role of β_2GPI by quenching the proinflammatory and proatherogenic effects of oxLDL. But in doing so, oxLDL/β_2GPI complexes also become immunogenic triggering the production of autoantibodies and immune complexes.

Current evidence points toward the atherosclerotic lesions as the primary site of oxLDL/β_2GPI complex formation with subsequent release into the circulation. OxLDL/β_2GPI and immune complexes upregulate the macrophage expression of scavenger and FcγRI receptors and stimulate further oxLDL/β_2GPI uptake and rapid accumulation in lysosomes where danger signals are processed supporting our speculation that in addition to oxLDL, β_2GPI contributes to the activation of inflammasomes. It is possible that β_2GPI-containing complexes mimic crystal structures or aggregated peptides capable of activating inflammasomes. It is also possible that the rapid transportation of β_2GPI to lysosomes is an innocent bystander translocation that nonetheless activates inflammasomes.

Emerging experimental evidence had suggested the occurrence of a low-grade autoinflammatory process and immune activation in thrombotic primary APS and premature atherosclerosis (Ames et al., 2008). Antibodies to β_2GPI derived from patients with primary APS induced the endothelial cell expression of multiple proinflammatory genes, including adhesion molecules and receptors (TNFα, IL-1 receptor 1, IL-18 receptor 1, E-selectin, ICAM, VCAM, etc.) and cytokines/chemokines (IL-6, IL-1β, IL-8) (Hamid et al., 2007). The same markers have been associated with rapidly progressive atherosclerosis in nonautoimmune populations. Outside the autoimmune setting, antiphospholipid antibodies (anti-β_2GPI and anti-oxLDL/β_2GPI) as well as oxLDL/β_2GPI complexes have been demonstrated in patients with type 2 diabetes and cardiovascular disease including acute coronary syndromes (ACS) (Lopez et al., 2005; Ames et al., 2010). The presence of these antibodies in ACS was associated with a 2.9-fold risk of adverse outcomes. Serum levels of oxLDL/β_2GPI complexes in higher quartiles positively correlated with the severity of the disease assessed by angiography and with a 3.5-fold increased risk (Greco et al., 2010). When both antibodies and complexes were present, the risk increased 14-fold, suggesting a synergistic effect between oxLDL/β_2GPI and its antibodies.

6. SUMMARY AND CONCLUSIONS

Endogenous atherogenic danger signals capable of dysregulating an inflammasome-induced IL-1β response may represent an early underlying inflammatory mechanism at play in atherosclerotic cardiovascular diseases. An atherogenic inflammasome/IL-1β response may be driven more by oxLDL than β_2GPI because oxLDL is likely generated before oxLDL/β_2GPI complexes; in either case, these two molecules may represent evolving danger signals that initially stimulate only the innate immunity, but if left unhindered, the latter may progress to an atherogenic adaptive immune response. Whether or not β_2GPI complexed with oxLDL activates the proinflammatory inflammasome/IL-1β pathway seems likely but remains to be verified.

Acute-phase proteins are among the factors that could hamper an atherogenic adaptive response by oxLDL/β_2GPI complexes. C-reactive protein (CRP), serum amyloid A, and components of the complement system are considered soluble PRR innate immunity receptors capable of recognizing distant pathogenic stimulus (exogenous danger signals) and able to activate host inflammatory and phagocytic responses. We have demonstrated that CRP can bind oxLDL or oxLDL/β_2GPI, and reported circulating oxLDL/β_2GPI/CRP (and oxLDL/CRP) complexes in patients with primary APS and type 2 DM (Greco et al., 2010; Tabuchi et al., 2007). An interesting question is whether the interaction between CRP, oxLDL, and β_2GPI indicates an innate immune response developing in the arterial wall. How can inflammasome/IL-1β activation be assessed in the clinical laboratory? Perhaps in addition to measuring IL-1β directly, levels of CRP, oxLDL, oxLDL/β_2GPI, or oxLDL/CRP may point to an inflammasome/IL-1β response.

When high serum levels of oxLDL/β_2GPI are detected, the (cytoplasmic) endogenous process may be so advanced that is already disseminated (systemic) and detectable by other means, i.e., IMT, angiography, imaging, etc. If an antibody response to any of these elements is developed, i.e., anti-oxLDL, anti-β_2GPI, or anti-oxLDL/β_2GPI antibodies, the process had already reached the level of an adaptive immune response pushing toward full clinical disease expression and possibly indicating adverse outcomes. The measurement of these biomarkers could provide more specific information about an underlying atherogenic inflammasome/IL-1β response. Intervention (prevention) at this level may be more effective as has been shown with classical autoinflammatory diseases.

ACKNOWLEDGMENTS

This study was supported in part by grant-in-aid for scientific research from the Ministry of Education, Culture, Sports, Science and Technology (Japan) and the Ministry of Health, Labor and Welfare (Japan).

Disclosures

LRL is an employee (Medical Director) of Corgenix, Inc.

REFERENCES

Abbate, A., Kontos, M.C., Grizzard, J.D., Biondi-Zoccai, G.G., Van Tassell, B.W., Robati, R., Roach, L.M., Arena, R.A., Roberts, C.S., Varma, A., Gelwix, C.C., Salloum, F.N., Hastillo, A., Dinarello, C.A., Vetrovec, G.W., 2010. Interleukin-1 blockade with anakinra to prevent adverse cardiac remodeling after acute myocardial infarction (Virginia Commonwealth University Anakinra Remodeling Trial [VCU-ART] Pilot study). Am. J. Cardiol. 105, 1371.

Akira, S., Uematsu, S., Takeuchi, O., 2006. Pathogen recognition and innate immunity. Cell 124, 783.

Ames, P.R., Antinolfi, I., Ciampa, A., Batuca, J., Scenna, G., Lopez, L.R., Delgado Alves, J., Iannaccone, L., Matsuura, E., 2008. Primary antiphospholipid syndrome: a low-grade autoinflammatory disease? Rheumatology (Oxford) 47, 1832.

Ames, P.R., Ortiz-Cadenas, A., Garcia-De La Torre, I., Nava, A., Oregon-Miranda, A., Batuca, J.R., Kojima, K., Lopez, L.R., Matsuura, E., 2010. Rosuvastatin treatment is associated with a decrease of serum oxidised low-density lipoprotein/beta2-glycoprotein I complex concentration in type 2 diabetes. Br. J. Diabetes Vasc. Dis. 10, 292.

Bauernfeind, F., Horvath, G., Stutz, A., Alnemri, E.S., Macdonald, K., Speert, D., Fernandes-Alnemri, T., Wu, J., Monks, B.G., Fitzgerald, K.A., Hornung, V., Latz, E., 2009. NF-kB activating pattern recognition and cytokine receptors license NLRP3 inflammasome activation by regulating NLRP3 expression. J. Immunol. 183, 787.

Connat, J.L., 2011. Inflammasome and cardiovascular diseases. Ann. Cardiol. Angeiol. 60, 48.

Dinarello, C.A., 2009. Immunological and inflammatory functions of the interleukin-1 family. Annu. Rev. Immunol. 27, 519.

Duewell, P., Kono, H., Rayner, K.J., Sirois, C.M., Vladimer, G., Bauernfeind, F.G., Abela, G.S., Franchi, L., Nuñez, G., Schnurr, M., Espevik, T., Lien, E., Fitzgerald, K.A., Rock, K.L., Moore, K.J., Wright, S.D., Hornung, V., Latz, E., 2010. NLRP3 inflamasomes are required for atherogenesis and activated by cholesterol crystals that form early in disease. Nature 464, 1357.

Frostegard, J., 2005. Atherosclerosis in patients with autoimmune disorders. Arterioscler. Thromb. Vasc. Biol. 25, 1776.

Gargiulo, S., Gamba, P., Testa, G., Rossin, D., Biasi, F., Poli, G., Leonarduzzi, G., 2015. Relation between TLR4/NF-kappaB signaling pathway activation by 27-hydroxycholesterol and 4-hydroxynonenal, and atherosclerotic plaque instability. Aging Cell 14, 569.

George, J., Harats, D., Gilburd, B., Afek, A., Levy, Y., Schneiderman, J., Barshack, I., Kopolovic, J., Shoenfeld, Y., 1999. Immunolocalization of β_2-glycoprotein I (Apolipoprotein H) to human atherosclerotic plaques. Circulation 99, 2227.

Greco, T.P., Conti-Kelly, A.M., Anthony, J.R., Greco Jr., T., Doyle, R., Boisen, M., Kojima, K., Matsuura, E., Lopez, L.R., 2010. Oxidized-LDL/beta(2)-glycoprotein I complexes are associated with disease severity and increased risk for adverse outcomes in patients with acute coronary syndromes. Am. J. Clin. Pathol. 133, 737.

De Groot, P.G., Meijers, J.C., 2011. beta(2)-Glycoprotein I: evolution, structure and function. J. Thromb. Haemost 9, 1275.

Hamid, C., Norgate, K., D'cruz, D.P., Khamashta, M.A., Arno, M., Pearson, J.D., Frampton, G., Murphy, J.J., 2007. Anti-β(2)GPI-antibody-induced endothelial cell gene expression profiling reveals induction of novel pro-inflammatory genes potentially involved in primary antiphospholipid syndrome. Ann. Rheum. Dis. 66, 1000.

Hansson, G.K., 2005. Inflammation, atherosclerosis, and coronary artery disease. N. Engl. J. Med. 352, 1685.

Hartvigsen, K., Chou, M.Y., Hansen, L.F., Shaw, P.X., Tsimikas, S., Binder, C.J., Witztum, J.L., 2009. The role of innate immunity in atherogenesis. J. Lipid Res. 50 (Suppl.), S388.

Hasunuma, Y., Matsuura, E., Makita, Z., Katahira, T., Nishi, S., Koike, T., 1997. Involvement of beta 2-glycoprotein I and anticardiolipin antibodies in oxidatively modified low-density lipoprotein uptake by macrophages. Clin. Exp. Immunol. 107, 569.

Kajiwara, T., Yasuda, T., Matsuura, E., 2007. Intracellular trafficking of beta2-glycoprotein I complexes with lipid vesicles in macrophages: implications on the development of antiphospholipid syndrome. J. Autoimmun. 29, 164.

Kobayashi, K., Matsuura, E., Liu, Q., Furukawa, J.-I., Kaihara, K., Inagaki, J., Atsumi, T., Sakairi, N., Yasuda, T., Voelker, D.R., Koike, T., 2001. A specific ligand for β_2-glycoprotein I mediates autoantibody-dependent uptake of oxidized low density lipoprotein by macrophages. J. Lipid Res. 42, 697.

Kobayashi, K., Lopez, L.R., Shoenfeld, Y., Matsuura, E., 2005. The role of innate and adaptive immunity to oxidized low-density lipoprotein in the development of atherosclerosis. Ann. N. Y. Acad. Sci. 1051, 442.

Kuwana, M., Matsuura, E., Kobayashi, K., Okazaki, Y., Kaburaki, J., Ikeda, Y., Kawakami, Y., 2005. Binding of β_2-glycoprotein I to anionic phospholipids facilitates processing and presentation of a cryptic epitope that activates pathogenic autoreactive T cells. Blood 105, 1552.

Libby, P., 2002. Inflammation in atherosclerosis. Nature 420, 868.

Lopez, L.R., Hurley, B.L., Simpson, D.F., Matsuura, E., 2005. Oxidized low-density lipoprotein/beta2-glycoprotein I complexes and autoantibodies in patients with type 2 diabetes mellitus. Ann. N. Y. Acad. Sci. 1051, 97.

Lundberg, A.M., Hansson, G.K., 2010. Innate immune signals in atherosclerosis. Clin. Immunol. 134, 5.

Martinon, F., Burns, K., Tschopp, J., 2002. The inflammasome: a molecular platform triggering activation of inflammatory caspases and processing of proIL-β. Mol. Cell 10, 417.

Martinon, F., Petrilli, V., Mayor, A., Tardivel, A., Tschopp, J., 2006. Gout-associated uric acid crystals activate the NALP3 inflammasome. Nature 440, 237.

Matsuura, E., Kobayashi, K., Inoue, K., Lopez, L.R., Shoenfeld, Y., 2005. Oxidized LDL/β_2-glycoprotein I complexes: new aspects in atherosclerosis. Lupus 14, 736.

Matsuura, E., Kobayashi, K., Lopez, L.R., 2008. Preventing autoimmune and infection triggered atherosclerosis for an enduring healthful lifestyle. Autoimmun. Rev. 7, 214.

Meylan, E., Tschopp, J., Karin, M., 2006. Intracellular pattern recognition receptors in the host response. Nature 442, 39.

Miller, Y.I., Choi, S.H., Wiesner, P., Fang, L., Harkewicz, R., Hartvigsen, K., Boullier, A., Gonen, A., Diehl, C.J., Que, X., Montano, E., Shaw, P.X., Tsimikas, S., Binder, C.J., Witztum, J.L., 2011. Oxidation-specific epitopes are danger-associated molecular patterns recognized by pattern recognition receptors of innate immunity. Circ. Res. 108, 235.

Olofsson, P.S., Sheikine, Y., Jatta, K., Ghaderi, M., Samnegard, A., Eriksson, P., Sirsjo, A., 2009. A functional interleukin-1 receptor antagonist polymorphism influences atherosclerosis development. The interleukin-1beta:interleukin-1 receptor antagonist balance in atherosclerosis. Circ. J. 73, 1531.

Persson, J., Nilsson, J., Lindholm, M.W., 2008. Interleukin-1beta and tumour necrosis factor-alpha impede neutral lipid turnover in macrophage-derived foam cells. BMC Immunol. 9, 70.

Petrilli, V., Papin, S., Dostert, C., Mayor, A., Martinon, F., Tschopp, J., 2007. Activation of the NALP3 inflammasome is triggered by low intracellular potassium concentration. Cell Death Differ 14, 1583.

Rajamäki, K., Lappalainen, J., Öörni, K., Välimäki, E., Matikainen, S., Kovanen, P.T., Eklund, K.K., 2010. Cholesterol crystals activate the NLRP3 inflammasome in human macrophages: a novel link between cholesterol metabolism and inflammation. PLoS One 5, e11765.

Schattner, A., Liang, M.H., 2003. The cardiovascular burden of lupus: a complex challenge. Arch. Intern. Med. 163, 1507.

Stutz, A., Golenbock, D.T., Latz, E., 2009. Inflammasomes: too big to miss. J. Clin. Invest. 119, 3502.

Tabuchi, M., Inoue, K., Usui-Kataoka, H., Kobayashi, K., Teramoto, M., Takasugi, K., Shikata, K., Yamamura, M., Ando, K., Nishida, K., Kasahara, J., Kume, N., Lopez, L.R., Mitsudo, K., Nobuyoshi, M., Yasuda, T., Kita, T., Makino, H., Matsuura, E., 2007. The association of C-reactive protein with an oxidative metabolite of LDL and its implication in atherosclerosis. J. Lipid Res. 48, 768.

Tall, A.R., Yvan-Charvet, L., 2015. Cholesterol, inflammation and innate immunity. Nat. Rev. Immunol. 15, 104.

Ting, J.P., Willingham, S.B., Bergstralh, D.T., 2008. NLRs at the intersection of cell death and immunity. Nat. Rev. Immunol. 8, 372.

Yin, Y., Pastrana, J.L., Li, X., Huang, X., Mallilankaraman, K., Choi, E.T., Madesh, M., Wang, H., Yang, X.F., 2013. Inflammasomes: sensors of metabolic stresses for vascular inflammation. Front. Biosci. (Landmark Ed) 18, 638.

Ylä-Herttuala, S., Palinski, W., Rosenfeld, M.E., Parthasarathy, S., Carew, T.E., Butler, S., Witztum, J.L., Steinberg, D., 1989. Evidence for the presence of oxidatively modified low density lipoprotein in atherosclerotic lesions of rabbit and man. J. Clin. Invest. 84, 1086.

Zhou, R., Tardivel, A., Thorens, B., Choi, I., Tschopp, J., 2010. Thioredoxin-interacting protein links oxidative stress to inflammasome activation. Nat. Immunol. 11, 136.

Chapter 7

Treatment of Lipid Metabolism Disturbances in Autoimmune Diseases

N. Ronda* and P.L. Meroni[§,¶]
*Department of Pharmacy, University of Parma, Parma, Italy; [§]University of Milan, Milan, Italy; [¶]IRCCS Istituto Auxologico Italiano, ASST G. Pini, Milan, Italy

Key Points

- Autoimmune diseases are associated with increased cardiovascular risk due to inflammatory and immune processes adding to traditional risk factors also affecting lipid metabolism.
- Proatherogenic lipid metabolism disturbances in autoimmune conditions differ from disease to disease and vary with disease activity and drug treatment.
- Lipoprotein serum levels alone have a limited value in cardiovascular risk evaluation.
- Both lipoprotein level and function modifications in autoimmune diseases are important for cardiovascular disease development and are currently object of investigation.
- Treatment of lipid disturbances in autoimmune diseases is based on:
  - control of disease activity, which should be obtained through a careful choice of the less atherogenic drugs as possible;
  - modulation of serum lipoprotein levels with healthy lifestyle/diet, nutraceuticals, and drugs;
  - modulation of lipoprotein functions with healthy lifestyle/diet, nutraceuticals, and drugs.

1. INTRODUCTION

Autoimmune diseases are associated with increased cardiovascular (CV) risk (Table 7.1), not only in consequence of specific disease-driven autoimmune

The Heart in Systemic Autoimmune Diseases.

TABLE 7.1 Reported Cardiovascular (CV) Risk Values Are From Literature on the Basis of CV Events or of Carotid Plaques/Stenosis Detection. Accelerated Atherosclerosis Markers Include Increased Carotid Intima-Media Thickness, Reduced Flow-Mediated Dilation, Increased Pulse Wave Velocity

Autoimmune Disease	CV Risk (OR)	ATH Markers
Rheumatoid arthritis	3–5	↑
Systemic lupus erythematosus	2–10	↑
Psoriatic arthritis	1.3–3	↑
Systemic sclerosis	2–3	↑
Dermatomyositis-polymyositis	2.2–3	↑
Ankylosing spondilitis	1.2–1.5	↑
Sjögren syndrome	2–3	↑
Systemic vasculitides	2–4	↑

processes targeting the vessels and the heart, but also because of accelerated atherosclerosis (ATH). The latter itself is a complex multifactorial process influenced by both classical and autoimmune disease–associated risk factors. Since the first reports of atherosclerotic lesions and ischemic heart disease in young systemic lupus erythematosus (SLE) patients more than 40 years ago, research has largely demonstrated that ATH plays a major role in the premature CV disease (CVD) development, reported for most if not all chronic autoimmune disorders (Shoenfeld et al., 2005).

Notwithstanding the increasing awareness of the problem, CVD prevention and management in autoimmune disorders are still insufficient. This is probably due to the lack of tailored algorithms or criteria for risk evaluation, the complexity of CVD pathogenesis, and the paucity of controlled trials on efficacy and safety of various treatment approaches in this patient population (Hollan et al., 2015). For example, Corrales recently reported that more than 60% RA patients with an mSCORE between 2 and 4, corresponding to moderate CV risk, present carotid artery plaques (Corrales et al., 2014), instrumental finding considered equivalent to a previous CV event in CVD prevention guidelines (Perk et al., 2012). In particular, the complex and peculiar lipid metabolism disturbances demonstrated in autoimmune patients raise uncertainty on the use of the classical lipid indexes for CV risk calculation and on the usefulness of lipid-lowering drugs.

2. LIPID METABOLISM DISTURBANCES RELEVANT FOR ATHEROSCLEROSIS AND CARDIOVASCULAR RISK IN AUTOIMMUNE DISEASES

A wide spectrum of lipid metabolism abnormalities has been reported in patients with autoimmune diseases, from classical dyslipidemia to unexpectedly low cholesterolemia and/or disturbances in circulating lipoprotein functions.

Classic dyslipidemia can be the result of genetic milieu, incorrect diet and lifestyle, or drugs such as glucocorticoids. Its prevalence differs among diseases, being for example more frequent in SLE (Tselios et al., 2016; Ahmad et al., 2014; Durcan et al., 2016) and in psoriatic arthritis (PA) (Patel et al., 2011) than in rheumatoid arthritis (RA) (Lee et al., 2016) and showing significant variability among patients with the same disease. High, normal, or low total cholesterol (TC) and low-density lipoprotein cholesterol (LDL-C) levels have been reported in different studies on SLE, RA, and systemic sclerosis (SSc). This is possibly due, at least in part, to the fact that TC and LDL-C levels generally fluctuate according to disease activity, being lower during disease relapses as an effect of inflammation (Robertson et al., 2013) and raising after treatment. Moreover, it has been demonstrated that TC and LDL-C levels are inversely rather than directly associated to CV risk in active RA, phenomenon called "RA lipid paradox" (Myasoedova et al., 2011). Similarly, data on serum high-density lipoprotein cholesterol (HDL-C) levels in autoimmune diseases are very much conflicting, including reports of both normal and low HDL-C in active diseases and normal, low, and high values in drug-induced disease remission (Akiyama et al., 2015).

The issue of lipid disturbances in autoimmune diseases is complicated by the fact that intrinsic proatherogenic LDL potential may vary according to its composition/oxidation and the occurrence of specific antibodies. For example, circulating concentration of oxidized LDL (oxLDL) correlates with ATH markers and CVD events and is increased in autoimmune diseases (Ahmad et al., 2014). Anti-oxLDL antibodies may be either protective or proatherogenic, depending on their characteristics, promoting oxLDL clearance via the reticuloendothelial system or increasing oxLDL uptake in macrophages and foam cell formation (de Carvalho et al., 2007).

There is established evidence that the antiatherogenic properties of HDL are due to their capacity to induce antiinflammatory effects and promote macrophage cholesterol efflux leading to cholesterol body disposal, both activities being dependent on composition (Hahn and McMahon, 2008) and not necessarily correlated to their measured circulating levels (Klancic et al., 2016). Impaired cholesterol efflux capacity has been demonstrated in SLE and RA (Ronda et al., 2014), in PA (Holzer et al., 2012), and in ankylosing spondylitis (AS) (Gkolfinopoulou et al., 2015).

For example, changes in antioxidant enzymes carried by HDL (Podrez, 2010) reduced sphingosine-1-phosphate HDL content (Levkau, 2015) and serum anti-HDL antibodies (El-Lebedy et al., 2016; Rodríguez-Carrio et al., 2016) might affect HDL function.

We can conclude that, for the time being, the use of TC and LDL-C serum levels to evaluate CVD risk in autoimmune patients does not appear entirely appropriate, unless the disease is steadily controlled. Only during disease remission, in fact, it seems likely that the rule "the lower the better," accepted for the general population with respect to LDL-C, can be applied in autoimmune populations. Even stronger is the uncertainty on the utility of HDL-C levels for CV risk evaluation in autoimmune diseases. It seems reasonable considering very low HDL-C levels during disease remission as a risk factor, while normal or high HDL-C levels should not necessarily be reckoned as protective in autoimmune patients, until tests for HDL function evaluation will be available in clinical practice.

Lipid metabolism management can be based at present on two kinds on tools. The first one is using diet, nutraceuticals, and lipid-lowering drugs to control serum TC, LDL-C, and HDL-C levels. In this regard, guidelines recommending LDL-C target in autoimmune diseases are lacking, and clinicians still refer to expert opinion in most cases. For example, a proposal for LDL-C desirable levels in RA, according to the extent of disease aggressiveness and comorbidities, has been recently released (Hollan et al., 2015). The second available kind of tool to manage lipid metabolism in autoimmune diseases is the amelioration of lipoprotein functions by nutraceutical/drug use or by controlling the disease itself. However, as the various drugs used to this last aim have different effects on lipid metabolism and CV risk, it is important to establish the best pharmacologic treatment for each autoimmune disease with respect to cardiovascular protection.

3. SERUM LIPID LEVEL CONTROL IN AUTOIMMUNE DISEASES

3.1 Diet and Nutraceuticals

CVD prevention and treatment through a healthy lifestyle and diet is largely recommended for the general population and for patients with proatherogenic conditions such as diabetes mellitus and chronic renal failure. As physical exercise and a healthy diet have antiinflammatory effects, these tools appear to be particularly useful in autoimmune diseases and indeed many papers report their beneficial effects in clinical studies. However, physical activity, diet regimens, and available nutraceutical preparations include a huge spectrum of possibilities and strong definitive evidence for each of them is lacking in most cases. In general, there is agreement on the concept that hypercaloric Western-style diets, characterized by high salt, animal fat, red meat, sugar-sweetened drinks, fried food, and low fiber, upregulate cellular proinflammatory pathways, promote a switch of gut microbiota toward a pattern affecting unfavorably host metabolism, induce dyslipidemia, alter intestinal immunity, and cause low-grade chronic systemic inflammation. On the contrary, low-calorie diets rich in vegetables, fruit, legumes, fish, prebiotics, and probiotics act on nuclear receptors and enzymes that downregulate the synthesis of proinflammatory molecules and restore or maintain a healthy symbiotic gut microbiota (Riccio and Rossano, 2015).

Particular diet components and nutraceutical preparations have been suggested to be beneficial for CVD prevention as well as for disease control in autoimmune diseases, because of lipid-regulating, antioxidant, and anti-inflammatory properties (Laev & Salakhutdinov 2015). Among these are: vitamin D (Yang et al., 2013; Terrier et al., 2012; Lin et al., 2016); resveratrol (Diaz-Gerevini et al., 2016); oil flavonoids such as terpenes, quinones, and catechins; polyphenols (Laev & Salakhutdinov 2015); propolis (Schmitz et al., 2015); omega-3 fatty acids (Ebrahimi et al., 2009); and fibers (Hartley et al., 2016). Oral intake of probiotics (adequate amount of selected live microorganisms) modulate the enteric flora and gut immune functions (Kang and Im, 2015), leading to beneficial effects not only on inflammatory bowel diseases but also on systemic autoimmune disorders such as RA (Zamani et al., 2016), type 1 diabetes mellitus (Uusitalo et al., 2016), or eczematous dermatitis (Kalliomaki et al., 2007). There is increasing evidence that probiotics modulate particularly T cells phenotype and functions (Kang and Im, 2015; Owaga et al., 2015). Indeed, gut microbiota is at present considered a pivotal element connecting immune functions, lipid metabolism, and diet components.

In summary, low fat-high fiber diet and many nutraceuticals may reduce TC and LDL-C serum levels (Rumawas et al., 2009). Conversely, diet seems to have little (Rumawas et al., 2009) or no effect (Fogli-Cawley et al., 2007) on HDL-C levels. In a recent study with a 16-year follow up, diet showed some correlation with higher HDL-C levels based on a low sucrose intake (Sonestedt et al., 2016). HDL-C levels are more clearly positively affected by regular physical exercise (Kodama et al., 2007). However, as discussed earlier, studies to establish the influence of diet and nutraceuticals on lipoprotein functions would be very important.

It should be noted that randomized controlled trials aimed at establishing the efficacy of diet and nutraceuticals on lipid metabolism modulation specifically in autoimmune diseases are lacking.

3.2 Total Cholesterol- and Low-Density Lipoprotein Cholesterol-Lowering Drugs: Statins

Statins appear to be the drugs of choice to lower TC and LDL-C levels in autoimmune patients for their multiple effects on inflammation and immune cells functions. They inhibit HMG-CoA reductase, the enzyme catalyzing the conversion of 3-hydroxy-3-methylglutaryl-coenzyme A to L-mevalonic acid, the rate-limiting step in cholesterol synthesis. The inhibition of cholesterol synthesis increases LDL receptor expression in the liver, thus promoting serum LDL-C clearance. However, mevalonate is a precursor of important isoprenoid intermediates, such as farnesyl pyrophosphate and geranylgeranyl pyrophosphate, involved in posttranslational modification of a range of proteins, including small GTPases (Ras, Rho, Rac) (Cai et al., 2015). These, in turn, regulate endothelial nitric oxide synthase expression, vascular smooth muscle cells migration and proliferation, reactive oxygen species generation, inflammatory cells infiltration, and foam cells formation (Cai et al., 2015). Thus, statins modulate many intracellular processes potentially involved in both immune system functions and CVD.

3.2.1 Potential and Proven Benefits of Statin Use in Patients With Autoimmune Diseases

3.2.1.1 Effects on the Autoimmune Disease

Antiinflammatory and immune-regulating effects of statins have been related to several intracellular mechanisms: inhibition of small GTPases (Cai et al., 2015) as well as of the pathways dependent on peroxisome proliferator-activated receptor α/γ and phosphatidylinositol 3-kinase (PI3K)/Akt (Yano et al., 2007); isoprenoid depletion (Jantzen et al., 2007); lipoprotein-associated phospholipase A2 reduction (Zalewski and Macphee, 2005); and inhibition of NF-κB (Meroni et al., 2001) and nicotinamide adenine dinucleotide phosphate oxidase (Al-Shabrawey et al., 2008). The modulation of these signal transduction pathways by statins in endothelial cells, vascular smooth muscle cells, immune cells, and fibroblasts is the recognized mechanism of a large number of effects on disease-related mechanisms. With respect to immune cell functions, the final results are inhibition of differentiation, activation and Fc receptor-mediated phagocytosis of macrophages, reduction of toll-like receptor 4 and adhesion molecules expression, reactive oxygen species production, and cytokine secretion. Statins inhibit T-cell activation and proliferation through disruption of T-cell receptor and blockade of the signaling cascade. They modulate Th1/Th2 differentiation; antagonize Th17-mediated response; and inhibit IL-2, IL-4, and IFN-γ production. Statins inhibit the proliferation and differentiation of lipopolysaccharide-stimulated B cells.

In contrast to the large in vitro evidence pointing to a role for statins in modulating autoimmune disease processes, the results from in vivo studies are much more conflicting. Overall beneficial effects of statins on inflammation and disease manifestations result from recent metaanalyses for RA (Xing et al., 2015; Lv et al., 2015), SSc (Ladak and Pope, 2015), SLE (Sahebkar et al., 2016), and PA (Mosiewicz et al., 2013). However, single studies often report variable results, likely due to the differences in statin molecule and treatment regimens used, patient populations, concomitant pharmacologic treatment, and considered parameters (Tselios et al., 2016).

3.2.1.2 Effects on Lipid Metabolism and Cardiovascular Disease

The efficacy of statins in controlling dyslipidemia and reducing CVD manifestations has been reported for RA (Danninger et al., 2014; Sheng et al., 2012), PA, and AS (Semb et al., 2012). Improvement has been reported also on various vessel function parameters used as ATH estimates in RA (Paraskevas, 2008). More conflicting results have been published on carotid intima-media thickness and other instrumental parameters after statin therapy in SLE patients, recently revised by Tselios (Tselios et al., 2016). It is important to consider that results may be influenced by many confounding factors such as the concomitant use of proatherogenic drugs, inhomogeneous populations with respect to serum lipid levels, or relatively low statin dosage in the various studies.

Until clear and specific international guidelines are available, the clinical indication for statin use in autoimmune diseases should be established based on the patient general profile in terms of disease activity, lipid levels, comorbidities, and drug use, considering that the autoimmune disease itself is a strong ATH risk factor. Suggestions for LDL-C targets have been given for RA (Hollan et al., 2015) and SLE (Soubrier et al., 2013). In any case, statin treatment should be added to a healthy diet and adequate physical exercise, and attention should be paid to possibly use the less atherogenic drugs available for the control of each disease. For example, high-dose and/or long-term glucocorticoids induce dyslipidemia and promote macrophage cholesterol accumulation (Greco et al., 2014); their use is an independent ATH risk factor in autoimmune diseases (Wei and MacDonald, 2004; Amaya—Amaya et al., 2013; Karp et al., 2008; Roubille et al., 2015). Nonsteroidal antiinflammatory drugs are associated with increased CV risk (Garcí Rodríguez et al., 2011). The increase in serum levels of TC and LDL-C induced by methotrexate and anti-TNFα or anti-IL6 agents has raised concern about a possible proatherogenic action of these drugs. However, in most cases they appear to reduce CV risk, possibly due to the predominance of the positive effect of the antiinflammatory activity (Mäki-Petäjä et al., 2012; Bili et al., 2014; Provan et al., 2015) and due to the amelioration of lipoprotein functions (Ronda et al., 2015). Hydroxychloroquine has also been shown to reduce CV risk in patients with RA (Sharma et al., 2016), as it was expected on the basis of its antiinflammatory, immunoregulatory, and lipid-lowering properties (Rainsford et al., 2015).

A number of plant-derived substances are currently used for their ability to inhibit HMG-CoA reductase, the so-called natural statins, and for additional antiinflammatory, lipid-regulating (Zimetti et al., 2015), and cell function—modulating activities (Patel, 2016) considered beneficial for ATH (Pirro et al., 2016; Jin et al., 2016). Among these are monacolin K and berberine, the latter tested on a mouse model of collagen-induced arthritis (Yang et al., 2004). However, specific studies are needed to assess their efficacy for CVD prevention and safety in autoimmune diseases.

3.2.2 *Potential Harms of Statin Use in Patients With Autoimmune Diseases*

Among the potential adverse effects of statins, particularly worrying for autoimmune prone patients, is the reported association of statin treatment with autoimmune disorders. For example, drug-induced lupus and the appearance of antinuclear and anti-dsDNA antibodies have been described (Tselios et al., 2016), with a latency of 12–18 months. Myasthenia gravis occurrence has also been reported (Gale and Danesh-Meyer, 2014), as well as pemphigus erythematosus relapse (Schiavo et al., 2014), dermatomyositis (Zaraa et al., 2011), and anti-HMGCoA reductase antibody-positive autoimmune myositis (Kennedy et al., 2016). The latter develops in genetically predisposed individuals (Mammen et al., 2013) most often but not always (Allenbach et al., 2014) after statin treatment. It does not recede with statin withdrawal alone, but requires immunosuppressive treatment (Selva-O'Callaghan et al., 2015).

3.3 Total Cholesterol- and Low-Density Lipoprotein Cholesterol-Lowering Drugs: Fibrates

Fibrates target and activate the nuclear receptor peroxisome proliferator-activated receptor alpha (predominantly expressed in liver, kidney, heart, and muscle), inducing many effects on lipid metabolism (Barter and Rye, 2016): reduction of serum triglyceride levels by inhibiting synthesis and stimulating hydrolysis; reduction of very low-density lipoproteins and chylomicrons production; reduction of apolipoprotein C-III synthesis; and increase in serum HDL-C. With respect to LDL, fibrates promote a shift toward larger, more buoyant particles that are less susceptible to oxidation and have an increased affinity for the LDL receptor (Fazio and Linton, 2004). This results in LDL-C serum reduction between 6% and 35% (Irvin et al., 2016).

Clinical trials to demonstrate the effect of fibrates on CVD manifestations in patients without autoimmune diseases have given conflicting results, but post hoc analyses indicate that major benefits in terms of CV events reduction are obtained in patients with hypertriglyceridemia and low HDL-C serum levels (Barter and Rye, 2016). No data are available on CV risk reduction by fibrates in autoimmune patients. Because of lack of information and substantial side effects, including autoimmune thrombocytopenia (Agapakis and Massa, 2015), fibrate use in autoimmune diseases is limited to patients with severe hypertriglyceridemia. However, interest is arising on the possible combined effects of these molecules on lipid metabolism and on inflammation (van Eekeren et al., 2013). In fact, studies in humans and in animal models have shown the potential benefit of fibrates both on systemic (Shirinsky et al., 2013) and articular manifestations of RA and osteoarthritis (van Eekeren et al., 2013; Koufany et al., 2014).

3.4 High-Density Lipoprotein Cholesterol Increasing Drugs

HDL-C increasing drugs have been object of great interest in the attempt to lower the so-called residual CV risk, still present despite optimal LDL-C control. Fibrates and niacin have been demonstrated to increase HDL-C together with decreasing CV risk (Birjmohun et al., 2005). However, later reports showed more uncertain results (Remaley et al., 2014; Gomaraschi et al., 2015); these agents also lower proatherogenic serum lipoproteins, rendering conclusive information on the specific clinical impact of HDL-C raising effect difficult to obtain (Kingwell et al., 2014). Moreover, studies with these agents in most cases are performed in addition to statin treatment, with a masking effect as a possible consequence. Cholesteryl ester transfer protein (CETP) inhibitors have been shown to increase HDL-C and apolipoprotein A-I levels as monotherapy and combined with statins (Nicholls et al., 2015), but strong differences exist between the effects of the various molecules, revised by Kingwell (Kingwell et al., 2014). Future studies should clarify the possible benefits of this approach in autoimmune patients.

4. LIPOPROTEIN FUNCTION MODULATION IN AUTOIMMUNE DISEASES

No specific pharmacological tool to ameliorate LDL or HDL functions is available at present for generalized clinical practice. However, since the importance of lipoprotein function for CVD development has been widely recognized, data from in vitro and in vivo studies are emerging. For example, some nutraceuticals, such as resveratrol (Voloshyna et al., 2016) or berberine (Zimetti et al., 2015) have been shown to ameliorate cholesterol efflux capacity of HDL. CETP inhibitors increase cholesterol efflux capacity of HDL through lipoprotein remodeling (Kingwell et al., 2014; Brownell and Rohatgi, 2016). Available data on fibrates differ with respect to the considered molecule, ciprofibrate, fenofibrate, or bezafibrate, and the cell cholesterol transporter involved in cholesterol efflux, indicating however an effect on HDL structure and function (Brownell and Rohatgi, 2016). Apo AI, apo AI Milano, and reconstituted HDL are currently under study as tools to increase cell cholesterol efflux, as well as drugs stimulating apo AI synthesis (Remaley et al., 2014; Brownell and Rohatgi, 2016; Kempen et al., 2016). Again, most of the available data on humans are from studies performed in nonautoimmune subjects.

The choice of specific treatment protocols to control the autoimmune disease may have consequences not only on lipoprotein levels, as discussed earlier, but also on lipoprotein functions. For example, methotrexate and the anti-TNFα adalimumab have been shown to improve circulating LDL and HDL functions relevant for cell cholesterol homeostasis (Ronda et al., 2015), while glucocorticoids may affect negatively macrophage expression of receptors involved in the interaction with serum lipoprotein (Greco et al., 2014).

REFERENCES

Agapakis, D., Massa, E., 2015. A case of fenofibrate-induced immune thrombocytopenia: first report. P. R. Health Sci. J. 34 (3), 170–173.

Ahmad, H.M., Sarhan, E.M., Komber, U., 2014. Higher circulating levels of OxLDL % of LDL are associated with subclinical atherosclerosis in female patients with systemic lupus erythematosus. Rheumatol. Int. 34 (5), 617–623.

Akiyama, M., et al., 2015. Prevalence of dyslipidemia in Japanese patients with rheumatoid arthritis and effects of atorvastatin treatment. Clin. Rheumatol. 34 (11), 1867–1875.

Allenbach, Y., et al., 2014. Anti-HMGCR autoantibodies in European patients with autoimmune necrotizing myopathies: inconstant exposure to statin. Medicine 93 (3), 150–157.

Al-Shabrawey, M., et al., 2008. Role of NADPH oxidase and Stat3 in statin-mediated protection against diabetic retinopathy. Invest. Ophthalmol. Vis. Sci. 49 (7), 3231–3238.

Amaya-Amaya, J., et al., 2013. Novel risk factors for cardiovascular disease in rheumatoid arthritis. Immunol. Res. 56 (2–3), 267–286.

Barter, P.J., Rye, K., 2016. New era of lipid-lowering drugs. Pharmacol. Rev. 68 (2), 458–475.

Bili, A., et al., 2014. Tumor necrosis factor α inhibitor use and decreased risk for incident coronary events in rheumatoid arthritis. Arthritis Care Res. 66, 355–363.

Birjmohun, R.S., et al., 2005. Efficacy and safety of high-density lipoprotein cholesterol-increasing compounds: a meta-analysis of randomized controlled trials. J. Am. Coll. Cardiol. 45 (2), 185–197.

Brownell, N., Rohatgi, A., May 20, 2016. Modulating cholesterol efflux capacity to improve cardiovascular disease. Curr. Opin. Lipidol. 27 (4), 398–407 [Epub ahead of print].

Cai, A., Zhou, Y., Li, L., 2015. Rho-GTPase and atherosclerosis: pleiotropic effects of statins. J. Am. Heart Assoc. 4 (7), e002113.

de Carvalho, J.F., Sherer, Y., Shoenfeld, Y., 2007. The fine-tuning of anti-oxidized low-density lipoprotein antibodies in cardiovascular disease and thrombosis. Thromb. Haemost. 98 (6), 1157–1159.

Corrales, A., et al., 2014. Carotid ultrasound is useful for the cardiovascular risk stratification of patients with rheumatoid arthritis: results of a population-based study. Ann. Rheum. Dis. 73 (4), 722–727.

Danninger, K., Hoppe, U.C., Pieringer, H., 2014. Do statins reduce the cardiovascular risk in patients with rheumatoid arthritis? Int. J. Rheum. Dis. 17 (6), 606–611.

Diaz-Gerevini, G.T., et al., 2016. Beneficial action of resveratrol: how and why? Nutrition 32 (2), 174–178.

Durcan, L., et al., 2016. Longitudinal evaluation of lipoprotein variables in systemic lupus erythematosus reveals adverse changes with disease activity and prednisone and more favorable profiles with hydroxychloroquine therapy. J. Rheum. 43 (4), 745–750.

Ebrahimi, M., et al., 2009. Omega-3 fatty acid supplements improve the cardiovascular risk profile of subjects with metabolic syndrome, including markers of inflammation and auto-immunity. Acta Cardiol. 64 (3), 321–327.

van Eekeren, I.C.M., et al., 2013. Fibrates as therapy for osteoarthritis and rheumatoid arthritis? A systematic review. Ther. Adv. Musculoskelet. Dis. 5 (1), 33–44.

El-Lebedy, D., et al., 2016. Anti-apolipoprotein A-1 autoantibodies as risk biomarker for cardiovascular diseases in type 2 diabetes mellitus. J. Diabetes Complications 30 (4), 580–585.

Fazio, S., Linton, M., 2004. The role of fibrates in managing hyperlipidemia: mechanisms of action and clinical efficacy. Curr. Atheroscler. Rep. 6 (2), 148–157.

Fogli-Cawley, J.J., et al., 2007. The 2005 Dietary Guidelines for Americans and risk of the metabolic syndrome. Am. J. Clin. Nutr. 86 (4), 1193–1201.

Gale, J., Danesh-Meyer, H.V., 2014. Statins can induce myasthenia gravis. J. Clin. Neurosci. 21 (2), 195–197.

García Rodríguez, L.A., et al., 2011. NSAID use selectively increases the risk of non-fatal myocardial infarction: a systematic review of randomised trials and observational studies. PLoS One 6 (2), e16780.

Gkolfinopoulou, C., et al., 2015. Impaired antiatherogenic functions of high-density lipoprotein in patients with ankylosing spondylitis. J. Rheumatol. 42 (9), 1652–1660.

Gomaraschi, M., et al., 2015. Effects of established hypolipidemic drugs on HDL concentration, subclass distribution, and function. Handb. Exp. Pharmacol. 224, 593–615.

Greco, D., et al., 2014. Hydrocortisone directly promotes cholesterol accumulation in macrophages. Ann. Rheum. Dis. 73 (6), 1274–1276.

Hahn, B.H., McMahon, M., 2008. Atherosclerosis and systemic lupus erythematosus: the role of altered lipids and of autoantibodies. Lupus 17 (5), 368–370.

Hartley, L., May Michael, D., Rees, K., January 7, 2016. Dietary fibre for the primary prevention of cardiovascular disease. Cochrane Database Sys. Rev. 1, CD011472.

Hollan, I., et al., 2015. Prevention of cardiovascular disease in rheumatoid arthritis. Autoimmun. Rev. 14 (10), 952–969.

Holzer, M., et al., 2012. Psoriasis alters HDL composition and cholesterol efflux capacity. J. Lipid Res. 53 (8), 1618–1624.

Irvin, M.R., et al., March 21, 2016. A genome-wide study of lipid response to fenofibrate in Caucasians: a combined analysis of the GOLDN and ACCORD studies. Pharmacogenet. Genomics 26 (7), 324–333 [Epub ahead of print].

Jantzen, F., et al., 2007. Isoprenoid depletion by statins antagonizes cytokine-induced down-regulation of endothelial nitric oxide expression and increases no synthase activity in human umbilical vein endothelial cells. J. Physiol. Pharmacol. 58 (3), 503–514.

Jin, Y., Khadka, D.B., Cho, W.-J., 2016. Pharmacological effects of berberine and its derivatives: a patent update. Expert Opin. Ther. Pat. 26 (2), 229–243.

Kalliomaki, M., et al., 2007. Probiotics during the first 7 years of life: a cumulative risk reduction of eczema in a randomized, placebo-controlled trial. J. Allergy Clin. Immunol. 119 (4), 1019–1021.

Kang, H.-J., Im, S.-H., 2015. Probiotics as an immune modulator. J. Nutr. Sci. Vitaminol. 61, S103–S105.

Karp, I., et al., 2008. Recent corticosteroid use and recent disease activity: independent determinants of coronary heart disease risk factors in systemic lupus erythematosus? Arthritis Rheum. 59 (2), 169–175.

Kempen, H.J., et al., 2016. Persistent changes in lipoprotein lipids after a single infusion of ascending doses of MDCO-216 (apoA-IMilano/POPC) in healthy volunteers and stable coronary artery disease patients. Atherosclerosis 255, 17–24.

Kennedy, N., Keating, P., O'Donnell, J., 2016. HMGCR-associated myositis: a New Zealand case series and estimate of incidence. Int. Med. J. 46 (5), 622–625.

Kingwell, B.A., et al., 2014. HDL-targeted therapies: progress, failures and future. Nat. Rev. Drug Discov. 13 (6), 445—464.

Klancic, T., et al., 2016. High density lipoprotein and metabolic disease: potential benefits of restoring its functional properties. Mol. Metab. 5 (5), 321—327.

Kodama, S., et al., 2007. Effect of aerobic exercise training on serum levels of high-density lipoprotein cholesterol: a meta-analysis. Arch. Intern. Med. 167 (10), 999—1008.

Koufany, M., Jouzeau, J., Moulin, D., 2014. Fenofibrate vs pioglitazone: comparative study of the anti-arthritic potencies of PPAR-alpha and PPAR-gamma agonists in rat adjuvant-induced arthritis. Biomed. Mater. Eng. 24 (1 Suppl.), 81—88.

Ladak, K., Pope, J.E., 2015. A review of the effects of statins in systemic sclerosis. Semin. Arthritis Rheum. 45 (6), 1—8.

Laev, S.S., Salakhutdinov, N.F., 2015. Anti-arthritic agents: progress and potential. Bioorg. Med. Chem. 23 (13), 3059—3080.

Lee, S., et al., 2016. Relationship between metabolic syndrome and rheumatoid arthritis. Korean J. Fam. Med. 37 (1), 44—50.

Levkau, B., 2015. HDL-S1P: cardiovascular functions, disease-associated alterations, and therapeutic applications. Front. Pharmacol. 6, p243.

Lin, J., et al., 2016. Serum vitamin D level and rheumatoid arthritis disease activity: review and meta-analysis. PLoS One 11 (1), e0146351.

Lv, S., et al., 2015. The impact of statins therapy on disease activity and inflammatory factor in patients with rheumatoid arthritis: a meta-analysis. Clin. Exp. Rheumatol. 33 (1), 69—76.

Mäki-Petäjä, K.M., et al., 2012. Anti-tumor necrosis factor-α therapy reduces aortic inflammation and stiffness in patients with rheumatoid arthritis. Circulation 126 (21), 2473—2480.

Mammen, A.L., et al., 2013. Increased frequency of DRB1*11:01 in anti-HMG-CoA reductase-associated autoimmune myopathy. Arthritis Care Res. (Hoboken) 64 (8), 1233—1237.

Meroni, P., et al., 2001. Statins prevent endothelial cell activation induced by antiphospholipid (anti-beta2-glycoprotein I) antibodies: effect on the proadhesive and proinflammatory phenotype. Arthritis Rheum. 44 (12), 2870—2878.

Mosiewicz, J., et al., 2013. Rational for statin use in psoriatic patients. Arch. Dermatol. Res. 305 (6), 467—472.

Myasoedova, E., et al., 2011. Lipid paradox in rheumatoid arthritis: the impact of serum lipid measures and systemic inflammation on the risk of cardiovascular disease. Ann. Rheum. Dis. 70 (3), 482—487.

Nicholls, S.J., et al., 2015. Cholesterol efflux capacity and pre-beta-1 HDL concentrations are increased in dyslipidemic patients treated with evacetrapib. J. Am. Coll. Cardiol. 66 (20), 2201—2210.

Owaga, E., et al., 2015. Th17 cells as potential probiotic therapeutic targets in inflammatory bowel diseases. Int. J. Mol. Sci. 16 (9), 20841—20858.

Paraskevas, K.I., 2008. Statin treatment for rheumatoid arthritis: a promising novel indication. Clin. Rheumatol. 27 (3), 281—287.

Patel, R.V., et al., 2011. Psoriasis and vascular disease-risk factors and outcomes: a systematic review of the literature. J. Gen. Inter. Med. 26 (9), 1036—1049.

Patel, S., 2016. Functional food red yeast rice (RYR) for metabolic syndrome amelioration: a review on pros and cons. World J. Microbiol. Biotechnol. 32 (5), 87.

Perk, J., et al., 2012. European Guidelines on cardiovascular disease prevention in clinical practice (version 2012). Eur. Heart J. 33 (13), 1635—1701.

Pirro, M., et al., 2016. The effects of a nutraceutical combination on plasma lipids and glucose: a systematic review and meta-analysis of randomized controlled trials. Pharmacol. Res. 110, 76—88.

Podrez, E.A., 2010. Anti-oxidant properties of high-density lipoprotein and atherosclerosis. Clin. Exp. Pharmacol. Physiol. 37 (7), 719–725.

Provan, S.A., et al., 2015. The impact of newer biological disease modifying anti-rheumatic drugs on cardiovascular risk factors: a 12-month longitudinal study in rheumatoid arthritis patients treated with rituximab, abatacept and tociliziumab. PLoS One 10 (6), e0130709.

Rainsford, K.D., et al., 2015. Therapy and pharmacological properties of hydroxychloroquine and chloroquine in treatment of systemic lupus erythematosus, rheumatoid arthritis and related diseases. Inflammopharmacology 23 (5), 231–269.

Remaley, A.T., Norata, G.D., Catapano, A.L., 2014. Novel concepts in HDL pharmacology. Cardiovasc. Res. 103 (3), 423–428.

Riccio, P., Rossano, R., 2015. Nutrition facts in multiple sclerosis. ASN Neuro. 7 (1), 1–20.

Robertson, J., et al., 2013. Changes in lipid levels with inflammation and therapy in RA: a maturing paradigm. Nat. Rev. Rheumatol. 9 (9), 513–523.

Rodríguez-Carrio, J., et al., 2016. PON activity is modulated by rs662 polymorphism and IgG anti-HDL antibodies in rheumatoid arthritis patients: potential implications for CV disease. Arthritis Rheumatol. 68 (6), 1367–1376.

Ronda, N., et al., 2014. Impaired serum cholesterol efflux capacity in rheumatoid arthritis and systemic lupus erythematosus. Ann. Rheum. Dis. 73 (3), 609–615.

Ronda, N., et al., 2015. Newly identified antiatherosclerotic activity of methotrexate and adalimumab: complementary effects on lipoprotein function and macrophage cholesterol metabolism. Arthritis Rheumatol. 67 (5), 1155–1164.

Roubille, C., et al., 2015. The effects of tumour necrosis factor inhibitors, methotrexate, non-steroidal anti-inflammatory drugs and corticosteroids on cardiovascular events in rheumatoid arthritis, psoriasis and psoriatic arthritis: a systematic review and meta-analysis. Ann. Rheum. Dis. 74 (3), 480–489.

Rumawas, M.E., et al., 2009. Mediterranean-style dietary pattern, reduced risk of metabolic syndrome traits, and incidence in the framingham offspring cohort. Am. J. Clin. Nutr. 90 (6), 1608–1614.

Lo Schiavo, A., et al., 2014. Pemphigus erythematosus relapse associated with atorvastatin intake. Drug Des. Devel. Ther. 8, 1463–1465.

Sahebkar, A., et al., 2016. Statin impact on disease activity and C-reactive protein concentrations in systemic lupus erythematosus patients: a systematic review and meta-analysis of controlled trials. Autoimmun. Rev. 15 (4), 344–353.

Schmitz, K., et al., 2015. "Disease modifying nutricals" for multiple sclerosis. Pharmacol. Ther. 148, 85–113.

Selva-O'Callaghan, A., et al., 2015. Statins and myositis: the role of anti-HMGCR antibodies. Expert Rev. Clin. Immunol. 11 (12), 1277–1279.

Semb, A.G., et al., 2012. Effect of intensive lipid-lowering therapy on cardiovascular outcome in patients with and those without inflammatory joint disease. Arthritis Rheum. 64 (9), 2836–2846.

Sharma, T.S., et al., 2016. Hydroxychloroquine use is associated with decreased incident cardiovascular events in rheumatoid arthritis patients. J. Am. Heart Assoc. 5 (1), e002867.

Sheng, X., et al., 2012. Effectiveness of statins on total cholesterol and cardiovascular disease and all-cause mortality in osteoarthritis and rheumatoid arthritis. J. Rheumatol. 39 (1), 32–40.

Shirinsky, I., et al., 2013. The effects of fenofibrate on inflammation and cardiovascular markers in patients with active rheumatoid arthritis: a pilot study. Rheumatol. Int. 33 (12), 3045–3048.

Shoenfeld, Y., et al., 2005. Accelerated atherosclerosis in autoimmune rheumatic diseases. Circulation 112 (21), 3337–3347.

Sonestedt, E., et al., 2016. Diet quality and change in blood lipids during 16 years of follow-up and their interaction with genetic risk for dyslipidemia. Nutrients 8 (5), 274.

Soubrier, M., et al., 2013. Do all lupus patients need statins? Joint Bone Spine 80 (3), 244–249.

Terrier, B., et al., 2012. Restoration of regulatory and effector T cell balance and B cell homeostasis in systemic lupus erythematosus patients through vitamin D supplementation. Arthritis Res. Ther. 14 (5), R221.

Tselios, K., et al., 2016. Dyslipidemia in systemic lupus erythematosus: Just another comorbidity? Semin. Arthritis Rheum. 45 (5), 604–610.

Uusitalo, U., et al., 2016. Association of early exposure of probiotics and islet autoimmunity in the TEDDY study. JAMA Pediatr. 170 (1), 20–28.

Voloshyna, I., et al., April 27, 2016. Resveratrol counters systemic lupus erythematosus-associated atherogenicity by normalizing cholesterol efflux. Exp. Biol. Med. 241 (14), 1611–1619 [Epub ahaed of print].

Wei, L., MacDonald, M.D.,F., 2004. Taking glucocorticoids by prescription is associated with subsequent cardiovascular disease. Ann. Intern. Med. 141 (10), 764–771.

Xing, B., et al., 2015. Effect of 3-hydroxy-3-methylglutaryl-coenzyme a reductase inhibitor on disease activity in patients with rheumatoid arthritis: a meta-analysis. Medicine 94 (8), e572.

Yang, C.Y., et al., 2013. The implication of vitamin D and autoimmunity: a comprehensive review. Clin. Rev. Allergy Immunol. 45 (2), 217–226.

Yang, L., et al., 2004. Enhancement of human ACAT1 gene expression to promote the macrophage-derived foam cell formation by dexamethasone. Cell Res. 14 (4), 315–323.

Yano, M., et al., 2007. Statins activate peroxisome proliferator-activated receptor gamma through extracellular signal-regulated kinase 1/2 and p38 mitogen-activated protein kinase-dependent cyclooxygenase-2 expression in macrophages. Circ. Res. 100, 1442–1451.

Zalewski, A., Macphee, C., 2005. Role of lipoprotein-associated phospholipase A2 in atherosclerosis: biology, epidemiology, and possible therapeutic target. Arterioscler. Thromb. Vasc. Biol. 25 (5), 923–931.

Zamani, B., et al., May 2, 2016. Clinical and metabolic response to probiotic supplementation in patients with rheumatoid arthritis: a randomized, double-blind, placebo-controlled trial. Int. J. Rheum. Dis. 19 (9), 869–879 [Epub ahead of print].

Zaraa, I.R., et al., March 29, 2011. Simvastatin-induced dermatomyositis in a 50-year-old man. BMJ Case Rep. http://dx.doi.org/10.1136/bcr.02.2011.3832.

Zimetti, F., et al., 2015. The natural compound berberine positively affects macrophage functions involved in atherogenesis. Nutr. Metab. Cardiovasc. Dis. 25 (2), 195–201.

Chapter 8

Cardiac Imaging Techniques in Systemic Autoimmune Diseases

M. Turiel,* L. Gianturco,* F. Atzeni,[§,¶] P. Sarzi-Puttini,[¶] M. Porcu[||] and M. Corda[||]

*Cardiology Unit, IRCCS Galeazzi Orthopedic Institute, Milan, Italy; [§]IRCCS Galeazzi Orthopedic Institute, Milan, Italy; [¶]Rheumatology Unit, L. Sacco University Hospital, Milan, Italy; [||]Cardiology Unit, Brotzu Hospital, Cagliari, Italy

Key Points

- In comparison with the general population, patients affected by systemic autoimmune diseases (SADs) are at significantly increased risk of cardiovascular (CV) risk factors, CV events, and mortality.
- Various authors have favored the use of noninvasive tests to detect suspected or known coronary artery disease, and/or study the valve lesions and other structural and/or morphological abnormalities induced by SADs.
- CV imaging is a reliable means of screening, diagnosing, and following-up CV involvement in patients with SADs, but new technologies such as speckle tracking echocardiography and/or 3D ultrasonography are diagnostically more accurate.
- In addition to using instrumental diagnostic investigations, there is growing evidence that plasma asymmetric dimethylarginine levels closely correlate with CV disease in patients with autoimmune disorders.

1. INTRODUCTION

The most frequent systemic autoimmune diseases (SADs) are rheumatoid arthritis (RA), systemic lupus erythematosus (SLE), primary antiphospholipid syndrome (APS), systemic sclerosis, and systemic vasculitis. Patients with SADs are at risk of increased cardiovascular (CV) morbidity and mortality that is mainly due to enhanced atherosclerosis and only partially related to traditional CV risk factors (Knockaert, 2007; Riboldi et al., 2002). In particular, the

CV disease occurs at a younger age than in the general population, and often remains asymptomatic at least in the early stages (Tanasescu et al., 2009).

The excess CV morbidity and mortality (Gianturco et al., 2015) may be explained by specific risk factors strictly related to autoimmune diseases, such as chronic inflammation, disease duration and activity, and immunosuppressive therapy with glucocorticoids, methotrexate, or antitumor necrosis factor α (TNFα) (van Zonneveld et al., 2010). All of the components of the heart can be affected by various pathogenetic mechanisms involving the valves, coronary arteries, conduction system, myocardium, endocardium, and pericardium, which lead to a wide range of clinical manifestations, including pericarditis, myocarditis and myocardial fibrosis, rhythm and conduction disturbances, coronaritis with ischemic heart disease, valvular diseases, pulmonary hypertension, syncope, and diastolic or systolic heart failure (Turiel et al., 2009a,b).

A number of studies have shown that chronic inflammation plays an important role in the development of atherosclerotic plaque (Sattar et al., 2003) and endothelial dysfunction, a process in which a reduction in the bioavailability of nitric oxide (NO) seems to be the *primum movens* (Arosio et al., 2007). Asymmetric dimethylarginine (ADMA) is widely recognized as the major endogenous inhibitor of NO-synthase and is considered an emerging CV risk factor. High plasma ADMA levels have been found in patients affected by SADs such as RA (Kiani et al., 2007; Turiel et al., 2009a,b).

Various authors have favored the use of noninvasive tests (Lee and Boucher, 2001; Turiel et al., 2009a,b) to detect suspected or known coronary artery disease (CAD), and/or study the valve lesions and other structural and/or morphological abnormalities induced by SADs (Kerekes et al., 2012) (Table 8.1). Furthermore, as underlined by international referral societies such as EULAR, it is necessary to have guidelines for the diagnosis and management of SAD patients in specialized and multidisciplinary centers (EULAR Task Force, 2016) as an early diagnosis can significantly improve management and provide insights into the prognosis. The choice of imaging technique should be based on that which is considered to be the most reliable of the techniques available at a given institution.

A wide range of cardiac manifestations have been described in RA patients (Braunwald, 1997; Shoenfeld et al., 2005), and it is well known that their incidence is also high in patients with SLE and APS (Cervera et al., 1992). Two-dimensional (2D) echocardiography studies have shown that 57% of SLE patients have valvular, myocardial, or pericardial abnormalities (Nihoyannopoulos et al., 1990; Omdal et al., 2001). In order to detect early disease, other authors have also used stress echocardiography to investigate coronaries abnormalities. Turiel's group has conducted a number of studies of RA patients using transthoracic dipyridamole stress echocardiography with an evaluation of coronary flow reserve (CFR), defined as the ratio between peak diastolic velocity in the distal left anterior descending coronary artery (LAD) during stress and at baseline. Hirata et al. (2007) have also used transthoracic

TABLE 8.1 Diagnostic and Imaging Techniques for Assessing Cardiovascular Involvement in Systemic Autoimmune Diseases

Evaluation of Sub-clinical Accelerated Atherosclerosis

1. Inflammatory risk factors: C-reactive protein (CRP), cytokines (TNFα; interleukin (IL) 1; IL-6; IL-18), etc.
2. Platelet and endothelial markers: fibrinogen, homocysteine, etc.
3. Vascular homeostasis and lipid metabolism: asymmetric dimethylarginine, circulating endothelial cells, circulating endothelial progenitor cells, etc.

Measurement of Endothelial Function

1. Coronary arteries
   Invasive: Assessment of coronary diameter by means of quantitative coronarography or intravascular ultrasound
   Noninvasive: Assessment of CFR by means of transthoracic or transesophageal ultrasonography (US), magnetic resonance imaging (MRI), and positron emission tomography (PET) after endothelium-dependent vasodilatory provocation
2. Peripheral circulation
   Invasive: Strain gage plethysmography of an upper extremity after the intraarterial infusion of an endothelium-dependent vasodilator
   Noninvasive: Flow-mediated vasodilation (FMD) of the brachial artery measured by means of US or MRI

Evaluation of General Atherosclerotic Burden

1. Arterial stiffness parameters
   Pulse wave analysis: augmentation index (AIx)
   Pulse wave velocity
2. Common carotid intima-media thickness (ccIMT) and carotid plaque analysis
3. Determination of coronary calcium content

dipyridamole stress echocardiography to study SLE patients, and found that their coronary vasomotor function is impaired, thus supporting the view that many of these young patients have subclinical coronary artery disease.

As CV damage in patients with autoimmune diseases is associated with adverse outcomes, it is important to identify the patients at higher risk early in order to improve their long-term prognosis. CV imaging is a reliable means of screening, diagnosing, and following-up CV involvement in patients with SADs, but new technologies such as speckle tracking echocardiography (STE) and/or 3D ultrasonography (Fig. 8.1) are diagnostically more accurate.

This chapter will review the role of the cardiac imaging techniques frequently used in patients with SADs.

2. TRANSTHORACIC ECHOCARDIOGRAPHY

This reliable, inexpensive, and noninvasive technique allows an accurate evaluation of valve abnormalities, pericardial diseases, and ventricular wall motion defects, whereas Doppler analysis is useful for studying left ventricular diastolic filling, valve function, and pulmonary pressures.

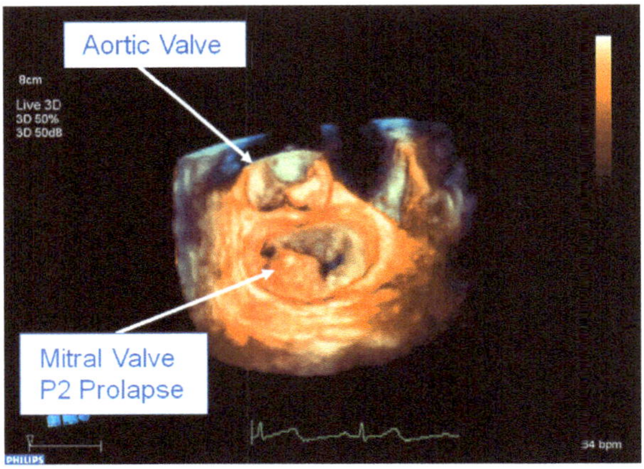

FIGURE 8.1 **Tridimensional view of mitral valve prolapse (P2).**

Rexhepaj et al. (2006) found significant differences in early diastolic flow velocity (E), atrial flow velocity (A), and E/A ratios between RA patients and a control group, thus suggesting that the former have subclinically impaired left and right ventricular function when left ventricular thickness, size, and myocardial performance indexes are still normal.

Interestingly, most studies have related valvulopathy to the presence of antiphospholipid (aPL) antibody (Khamashta et al., 1990; Brenner et al., 1991; Cervera et al., 1991; Galve et al., 1992); a number of TTE studies have shown that cardiac involvement is also frequent in patients with primary APS (Giunta et al., 1993; Metz et al., 1994).

There have been reports of a 32–38% prevalence of valve lesions, most frequently involving left-sided valves, valvular rings, the chordae tendinae or other parts of the ventricular or atrial endocardium (Hojnik et al., 1996). The valvular lesions are characterized by diffuse leaflet thickening, sometimes to the point of valve stenosis; these lesions are often associated with valvular regurgitation.

The unusual manifestations of APS include intracardiac thrombosis (Cervera, 2000), which can occur in both primary and secondary APS, and is usually seen in the clinical setting of left ventricular dysfunction. The thrombus can be found in any of the chambers of the heart, but it may rarely be present as an intracardiac mass simulating myxoma, and diagnosis can only be made by histology.

Noninfective endocarditis has been reported in many patients with SLE and primary APS (Cervera, 2000), who may present with fever, cardiac murmurs, valve vegetations, negative blood cultures and high aPL levels. It is difficult to exclude infective endocarditis in these patients, but CRP, a white blood cell count, and echocardiography findings may be helpful in differentiating the two conditions.

Historically, left ventriclcular (LV) diastolic filling could only be determined on the basis of Doppler-derived mitral and pulmonary venous flow velocities, but now the most widely used parameter for assessing diastolic function is E/E′, a form of integration between the old indices derived from transmitral pulsed-wave (PW) Doppler analysis and the new parameters assessed by means of tissue Doppler imaging.

An impaired relaxation pattern (grade 1 diastolic dysfunction) identifies patients with early-stage heart disease, and appropriate therapy may avert progression and functional disability. A pseudonormalized pattern (grade 2) is a transitional phase between abnormal relaxation and restrictive physiology and signifies increased filling pressures and decreased compliance. In this phase, it is clinically helpful to reduce preload, optimize afterload, and treat the underlying disease. A restrictive physiological pattern (grade 3−4) identifies advanced, usually symptomatic disease with a poor prognosis. Therapy is aimed at normalizing loading conditions and improving the restrictive filling pattern (grade 3 when reversible), although this may not be feasible in certain heart diseases (grade 4 when irreversible).

Many patients have LV filling patterns that appear indeterminate or mixed. In these cases, clinical information, left artrial (LA) and LV size, pulmonary venous flow velocity, and altering preload by means of the Valsalva maneuver help assess diastolic function and estimate diastolic filling pressure.

Patients with APS can also have isolated diastolic dysfunction. In a Doppler echocardiography study of 10 consecutive patients with APS, Hasnie et al. (1995) found a decrease in peak early filling velocity, the peak early to atrial filling velocity ratio, and the mean deceleration time of early filling velocity in comparison with the control group, although the patients' LV mass, systolic function, and ejection fractions were normal. These findings may represent subclinical myocardial damage.

The prevalence of echocardiographic evidence of pericardial effusion is about 15−20%, but its underlying mechanism, prognosis, and sequelae are not yet known. Cardiac tamponade may rarely be observed in RA patients (Yousuf et al., 2015), but is more likely in patients with SLE (Buppajamrntham et al., 2014). It may also be a pediatric manifestation (Maharaj and Chang, 2015), and various authors have used noninvasive imaging to study pediatric patients (Mavrogeni et al., 2015).

Predominantly mitral and aortic valve abnormalities have been found in 61% of SLE patients (Roldan et al., 1996); the most frequent was valve thickening, but the type of lesion frequently changes over time.

3. TRANSESOPHAGEAL ECHOCARDIOGRAPHY

Another very useful application of echocardiography in systemic autoimmune diseases is the transesophageal approach, which is widely recognized as being more sensitive than TTE in detecting valve lesions (Turiel et al., 2000) and identifying intracardiac masses. Turiel et al. (2005) observed a large 61% prevalence of valvular thickening or vegetations and/or potential embolic sources using a TEE in 56 patients with primary APS followed-up for 5 years. The recent development of 3D TEE makes it possible to visualize cross-sections of the mitral, aortic, and tricuspid valves, thus improving diagnostic sensitivity in comparison with traditional 2D imaging (Plastiras et al., 2009). The main advantages of the clinical applications of 3D echocardiography include more accurate and reproducible assessments of LV volume, mass, and ejection fraction; the more precise identification of wall motion abnormalities; the possibility of studying the right ventricle; and a better understanding of valvular and subvalvular abnormalities (Marsan et al., 2009).

The usefulness of TEE in identifying minimal cardiac abnormalities or vegetations and intracardiac embolic sources is well known (Jafar et al., 1994; Asherson and Cervera, 1991; Espinola-Zavaleta et al., 1999). Turiel et al. (2000) found cardiac involvement (valvular thickening and/or regurgitation, vegetations or masses, and potential embolic sources) in 33 out of 40 APS patients (82%); the most frequent abnormality (63%) was mitral valve thickening. They also demonstrated embolic sources in ten of the patients (25%): seven showed marked spontaneous echocontrast (three of whom had mitral stenosis) and noninfective vegetations (Libman-Sacks endocarditis) were found in three (one on the aortic and two on tricuspid valves with severe tricuspid regurgitation). The number of associated and/or recurrent thromboembolic events was highest in the patients with anticardiolipin antibody titers of >40 GPL units, who also presented more potential embolic sources revealed by TEE than patients with anticardiolipin antibody titers of <40 GPL units ($\chi^2 = 10.03$, $p < .01$).

The use of TEE should therefore be recommended in APS patients with clinical findings and/or a high anticardiolipin antibody titer in order to define their cardiac abnormalities more precisely, detect embolic sources (Black et al., 1991), and establish appropriate antiplatelet and/or anticoagulant therapy.

A recent TEE study of 30 unselected RA patients has shown that cardiac involvement is extremely common, including echo-generating nodules on mitral or aortic valves, frequent aortic atheromas, and mitral or aortic regurgitation (Guedes et al., 2001).

A number of authors now prefer real-time 3D TEE.

4. STRESS ECHOCARDIOGRAPHY

A pharmacological stress test is indicated for patients who cannot exercise adequately because of rheumatological, orthopedic, vascular, or pulmonary conditions.

There are various ways of evaluating CFR in such patients, of which transthoracic stress echocardiography with dipyridamole is a simple, noninvasive, and inexpensive method (Gaibazzi et al., 2010; Chiribiri et al., 2013; Nakazato et al., 2013). CFR is assessed in the distal left anterior

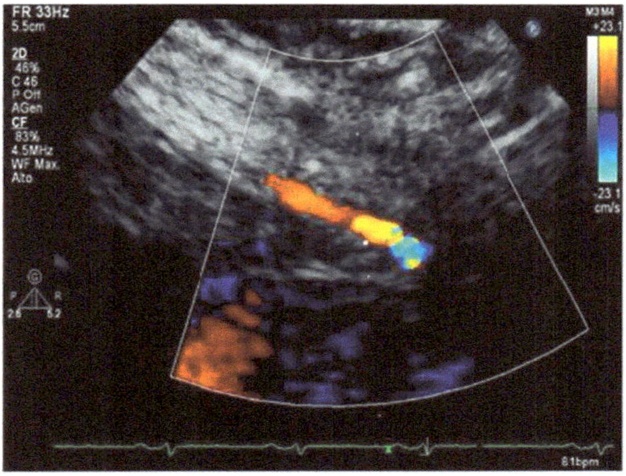

FIGURE 8.2 Color Doppler signal in the distal left anterior descending coronary artery.

descending coronary artery and defined as the ratio between peak diastolic velocity during stress and at baseline (Figs. 8.2 and 8.3). It is a highly sensitive (>90%) diagnostic marker of CAD (Caiati et al., 1999; Hozumi et al., 1998) and, when associated with regional wall motion analysis, it is also highly specific (Rigo et al., 2003). It has been shown that a CFR value of <2 accurately predicts the presence of coronary stenosis (Hozumi et al., 1998). In the absence of epicardial coronary stenosis, an abnormal CFR may reflect impaired coronary microcirculation in patients with a

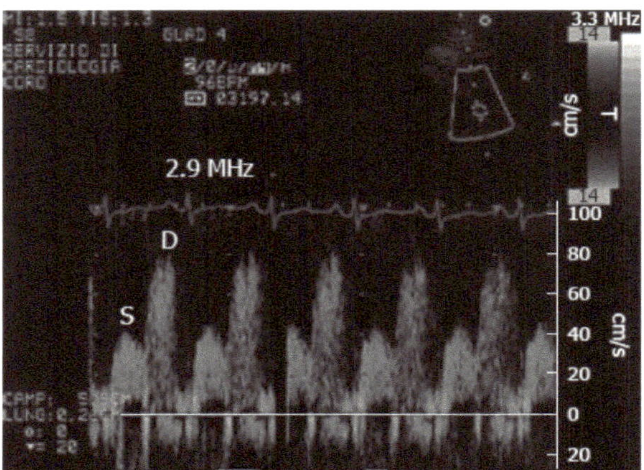

FIGURE 8.3 **Example of coronary flow Doppler signal during dypiridamole-induced hyperaemia.** *D*, diastolic flow; *S*, systolic flow.

reperfused myocardial infarction, arterial hypertension with or without left ventricular hypertrophy, diabetes mellitus, hypercholesterolemia, syndrome X, hypertrophic cardiomyopathy, and other diseases (Dimitrow, 2002). CFR also has prognostic value insofar as a reduced CFR correlates with a negative prognosis (Rigo et al., 2006), and it has been shown that not only a binary (normal/abnormal) response in CFR, but also the continuous spectrum of CFR values is a strong independent prognostic predictor in patients with known or suspected CAD (Cortigiani et al., 2010).

Hirata et al. (2007) found a significant reduction in CFR in premenopausal women with SLE compared with age- and gender-matched controls, and concluded that microvascular impairment in SLE could be explained by the functional endothelial alteration responsible for the decrease in vasodilation in response to pharmacological stress. Turiel et al. (2009a,b) detected significantly impaired CFR in 25 untreated patients with early RA (disease duration <1 year and without antirheumatic therapy): the reduced CFR in the absence of wall motion abnormalities at rest and during pharmacological stress showed that coronary microcirculation involvement is present in early RA (ERA) and associated with endothelial dysfunction. CFR cannot distinguish micro- and macrovascular coronary disease, but it is important to assess its additional diagnostic value over conventional wall motion analysis.

Ciftci et al. (2008) showed that RA patients have increased IMT and a reduced CFR. Chung et al. found that patients with long-standing RA have a higher prevalence of more severe coronary calcifications than those with ERA, and Del Rincon et al. (2007) demonstrated that they are also more likely to have ATS than healthy controls. The importance of recognizing and treating patients in the early stages of RA is due to the risk that active disease may lead to progressive joint and CV damage. Turiel et al. (2010) studied 25 ERA patients before and after treatment with disease-modifying antirheumatic drugs (DMARDs) and 25 healthy volunteers with no history or current signs of CAD or other traditional risk factors. CFR was evaluated by means of dipyridamole transthoracic stress echocardiography, and the IMT of the common carotid arteries by means of carotid ultrasonography; ADMA levels were also measured. CFR was significantly reduced in the ERA patients (six of whom had a CFR of <2, which is consistent with potentially dangerous coronary impairment), who also showed greater IMT and had higher plasma ADMA levels. When the patients' CFR was measured again after 18 months of DMARD treatment, it had significantly improved, probably because of the drugs' antiinflammatory effects. RA patients are at higher risk of developing CV diseases than the general population and the noninvasive echo-Doppler evaluation of CFR can be used to detect early functional damage (Sitia et al., 2010; Kerekes et al., 2012). Consequently, careful screening for impaired coronary microcirculation is essential from the earliest stages of RA even in the absence of any signs or symptoms of CV involvement (Turiel et al., 2000).

A number of published studies have shown that PsA patients without conventional CV risk factors or clinically evident CV disease have endothelial dysfunction and a higher prevalence of increased carotid artery IMT than controls (Kimhi et al., 2007), and it was found subclinical cardiac involvement in a group of 22 outpatients satisfying the ClASsification of Psoriatic ARthritis study group criteria for PsA without a history of CV disease, who were compared with 35 controls (Atzeni et al., 2011a,b). Although the patients did not have any signs of, or risk factors for, CV disease; they had higher ADMA levels and a significantly reduced CFR. The significant correlation between the reduced CFR and increased ADMA levels may be indicative of endothelial dysfunction and impaired coronary microcirculation and confirm that active PsA is a risk factor for CV disease as recently demonstrated by Wakkee and de Jong (2013).

Ahlehoff et al. (2010) conducted a cohort study of the entire Danish population, including 34,371 subjects with mild psoriasis, 2621 with severe disease, and 607 with PsA. CV events were more frequent in the psoriasis patients, and the rate increased with disease severity and decreased with age at the time of onset. The risk was similar in the subjects with severe skin affection alone and those with PsA. Given the high CV burden mainly related to endothelial dysfunction and ATS, an early diagnosis is clearly fundamental in patients with PsA (Atzeni et al., 2011a,b).

Systemic sclerosis (SSc) is a multisystem disease characterized by vasculopathy typically affecting the small vessels, although macrovascular involvement has also been demonstrated, and there is still controversy concerning the predominant mechanism (Veale et al., 1995). In 2003, Montisci et al. used the new noninvasive method of contrast (Levovist)-enhanced transthoracic Doppler echocardiography during adenosine infusion in 27 SSc pts without any evidence of ischemic heart disease and 23 controls and found that LAD CFR was severely reduced in 14 of the patients.

Turiel et al. (2013) recently enrolled 20 patients fulfilling the American College of Rheumatology criteria for SSc without any signs or history of coronary artery disease, and 20 healthy volunteers, all of whom underwent dypiridamole echocardiography and the calculation of CFR. The SSc patients had a significantly lower CFR than controls, which seems to support the hypothesis of subclinical CV involvement in subjects with diffuse SSc.

Finally, Vacca et al. (2013) confirmed these data in a group of 41 patients with SSc who were asymptomatic for CAD using transthoracic Doppler echocardiography with adenosine infusion to study the microcirculation, and dobutamine stress echocardiography to search for LV wall motion abnormalities. CFR was reduced in 19 SSc patients, and 16 showed wall motion abnormalities.

All of the earlier findings confirm the importance of using noninvasive methods to detect abnormal coronary microcirculation at a subclinical stage. CFR may be a useful marker of subclinical cardiac damage in SAD patients and allows the early detection of any preclinical involvement of the coronary microcirculation.

In conclusion, as SAD patients are at higher risk of developing CV diseases than the general population, it is essential to detect endothelial dysfunction and impaired coronary microcirculation especially in asymptomatic subjects. Coronary angiography remains the gold standard for diagnosing coronary stenosis, but new, noninvasive, and more reliable diagnostic techniques have been introduced into clinical practice to detect subclinical abnormalities in the microcirculation. Echocardiography and its many variables (including CFR) seems to be the most appropriate screening technique as it noninvasively, reliably, sensitively, and specifically identifies preclinical cardiac involvement in patients with SADs. Common carotid IMT measured by means of carotid ultrasonography can provide additional information that is useful for stratifying CV risk in SAD patients, but increased IMT reflects a later stage of the atherosclerotic process when anatomical changes have already occurred, whereas impaired CFR is an earlier marker identifying functional damage. It is therefore important to stress that a functional injury is potentially reversible, and this allows a better prevention strategy than a later diagnosis made after the occurrence of anatomical abnormalities. Its relatively low cost means that measuring CFR can be considered a modern gold-standard for detecting and controlling ATS in SADs patients even in this time of economic constraint.

5. TISSUE DOPPLER IMAGING

Tissue Doppler imaging (TDI) is a new modality that allows myocardial velocities to be measured. It has so far been considered a reliable means of assessing myocardial deformations, but this is limited by the fact that its angle dependency means that only deformations along the ultrasound beam can be derived from velocities, whereas the myocardium deforms simultaneously in three dimensions (Dandel and Hetzer, 2009). Birdane et al. (2007) demonstrated that RA patients showed significant impairment of TDI biventricular diastolic functional parameters in comparison with healthy controls, depending on age and use of steroids.

TDI makes it possible to record the low Doppler shift frequencies of high energy generated by ventricular wall motion that are purposely filtered out in standard Doppler blood flow studies. It can be performed using pulsed Doppler, 2D color Doppler, and M-mode color mode Doppler. Pulsed Doppler tissue imaging offers a high level of temporal resolution and can therefore be used to analyze the temporal relationship between myocardium systolic and diastolic velocity waves. Color 2D Doppler provides a good level of spatial resolution that allows the differentiation of the velocity profiles of the subendocardial and subepicardial layers, but is limited by its poor temporal resolution. M-mode color-coded tissue imaging is characterized by a high level of spatial–temporal resolution, but only samples a single line. Both 2D and

M-mode color-coded tissue imaging require specific modifications of current ultrasound machines.

Extensive work has been done over the last few years to demonstrate the potential of TDI for assessing both systolic and diastolic function, and its use with advanced analysis of left ventricular Doppler inflow will probably further extend the frontiers of Doppler echocardiography assessment of diastolic function.

6. SPECKLE TRACKING ECHOCARDIOGRAPHY

In order to overcome the limitations of TDI, STE has been introduced to evaluate myocardial strain along the longitudinal, circumferential, and radial axes (Sitia et al., 2010a,b). This is a new technique that allows studies of regional myocardial deformation (Leitman et al., 2004) expressed by means of a dimensionless parameter, strain (ε), which is defined by the Lagrangian formula as the percent change from the original dimension (Pislaru et al., 2002). Furthermore, displacement reflects myocardial motion: if all parts of a myocardial segment have the same motion over a defined period of time, the segment will change position (displacement) but not shape (deformation) but, when different parts of a segment move differently, it becomes deformed. The study of both ε and displacement therefore makes it possible to discriminate the passive movement and active contraction of each myocardial segment (Pavlopoulos and Nihoyannopoulos, 2008) (Fig. 8.4). As described for the first time by Heimdal et al.

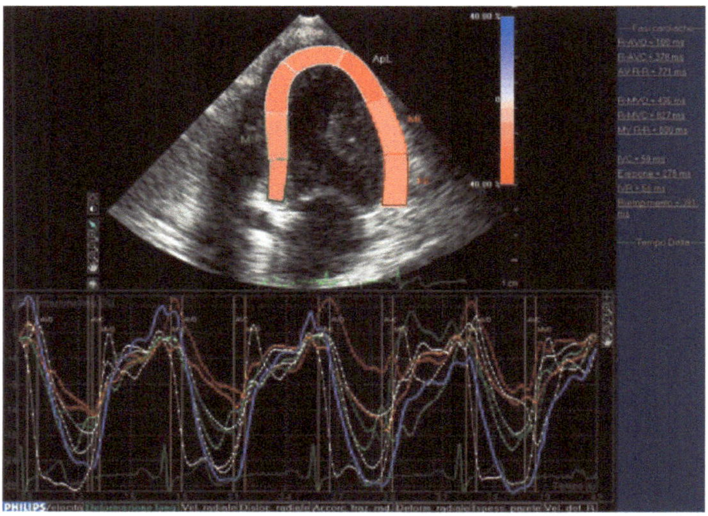

FIGURE 8.4 **Systolic myocardial deformation after electromechanical activation.** Left ventriclcular longitudinal strain from the apical four-chamber view: time strain curves show a negative end-systolic strain representing myocardial shortening during systole.

(1998), tissue deformation occurs over time during the cardiac cycle, and the rate of this deformation (the strain rate, SR) is equivalent to the velocity gradient. Myocardial ε can be determined by both TDI and STE but, unlike TDI, STE is angle independent and allows an accurate assessment of segmental myocardial deformation using grayscale-based frame-by-frame image analysis. Furthermore, myocardial ε can be tracked in two dimensions along the direction of the wall and not along the ultrasound beam (Dandel and Hetzer, 2009), which means myocardial ε can be analyzed along the three spatial axes of cardiac muscle physiology. After electromechanical activation, systolic myocardial deformation takes the form of longitudinal and circumferential shortening, and radial thickening, thus making STE a reliable means of detecting early subtle cardiac involvement in various clinical settings such as connective tissue diseases (Sitia et al., 2009).

To the best of our knowledge, the study of Sitia is the first evaluating LA function in SSc by means of STE strain analysis, although a number of papers had previously described subclinical LV and right ventricle (RV) abnormalities in SSc patients, using TDI parameters and strain rate imaging (Meune et al., 2008; Mele et al., 2008; Kepez et al., 2008; Spethmann et al., 2012). Mele et al. (2008) showed that TDI-derived myocardial systolic deformation indices based on strain and strain rate analysis and the E/E′ ratio are valuable for detecting cardiac involvement in asymptomatic SSc patients. D'Andrea et al. (2005) further confirmed that STE imaging can detect early RV and LV involvement, as well as CFR and brachial artery flow-mediated dilatation, as signs of early vascular impairment in SSc. In another study, Schattke et al. (2010) used isovolumetric acceleration, a new tissue Doppler parameter, to detect early RV systolic impairment in SSc patients without pulmonary hypertension. Kepez et al. (2008) found that SSc patients without pulmonary hypertension or overt clinical cardiac involvement had reduced myocardial strain and strain rate despite normal 2D, conventional Doppler and TDI parameters. Interestingly, Yiu et al. (2011) showed that subtle LV dysfunction assessed by means of STE strain analysis is related to lower functional capacity and rhythm disturbances in patients with SSc, and Spethmann et al. (2012) found that LV systolic impairment assessed by strain imaging is primarily due to alterations in the basal LV segments in SSc patients with a preserved LVEF.

None of the previous speckle tracking studies of SSc patients ever addressed LA function or dimensions because they were focused on LV or RV function. It is true that assessing LV and RV dysfunction is the main target of cardiac assessment and represents the final result of all potential pathophysiological impairments, but many of these alterations can be intercepted earlier by detecting changes in LA regional mechanical characteristics and function. A few previous studies had evaluated LA characteristics in SSc patients: Dimitroulas et al. (2010) showed that LA volume may be a useful noninvasive marker for predicting high pulmonary artery pressure. Furthermore, impaired electromechanical LA function, including prolonged intra-/interatrial electromechanical delay and greater P-wave dispersion in comparison with controls, has confirmed their greater risk of developing supraventricular arrhythmias.

7. MYOCARDIAL CONTRAST ECHOCARDIOGRAPHY

Myocardial contrast echocardiography (MCE) is an emerging technique in which microbubble contrast agents are visualized in the coronary microvasculature. MCE is an ideal means of noninvasive evaluation of acute coronary syndromes (ACS) because it allows the portable, simultaneous assessment of regional wall motion and myocardial perfusion. Recent advances in microbubble contrast agents and ultrasound imaging technology have allowed new clinical applications, and studies suggest it can play a promising role in evaluating chest pain, establishing the diagnosis and prognosis of acute myocardial infarction, assessing the success of reperfusion, and differentiating myocardial stunning and myocardial necrosis. Potential future applications of MCE in ACS include the detection of inflammation and ultrasound-induced thrombolysis.

8. USEFULNESS OF BIOMARKERS OF ENDOTHELIAL DYSFUNCTION

In the field of systemic autoimmune disease, a new challenge for cardiologists is the early diagnosis of subtle cardiac abnormalities at a preclinical stage. In addition to using instrumental diagnostic investigations, there is growing evidence that plasma ADMA levels closely correlate with CV disease in patients with autoimmune disorders. Increased levels have been demonstrated in a number of pathological conditions characterized by a high CV risk, such as hypercholesterolemia (Böger et al., 1998), hypertriglyceridemia (Lundman et al., 2001), peripheral arterial disease (Böger et al., 1997), hypertension (Surdacki et al., 1999), type 2 diabetes mellitus (Stühlinger et al., 2002), ACS (Bae et al., 2005), and end-stage renal disease (MacAllister et al., 1996). Kiani et al. (2007) have described higher ADMA levels among SLE patients, in whom they seemed to be associated with coronary calcium and poor prognosis. Turiel et al. (2009a,b) also found that increased plasma ADMA levels in early RA patients free of antirheumatic therapy were associated with a subclinical impairment of the coronary microcirculation. Interestingly, the same authors (Turiel et al., 2010) observed that the improvement in inflammatory status and better control of disease activity induced by 18 months of treatment with MTX or anti-TNFα agents significantly improved CFR. An evaluation of arterial distensibility and stiffness represent good indices of endothelial dysfunction and preclinical atherosclerosis: reduced arterial distensibility disturbs coronary perfusion and has been related to an increased CV risk (Wang and Fitch, 2004). Yildiz (2010) has reported subclinical impairment of aortic pulse wave velocity in patients with chronic inflammatory rheumatic disorders such as SLE, RA, psoriasis, and systemic sclerosis, which is mainly due to their chronic inflammatory status.

9. CAROTID ULTRASONOGRAPHY

9.1 Carotid Atherosclerosis

Elastic arteries, such as carotid arteries, are close to the skin and easily accessible for ultrastructural investigation. Wall abnormalities can be assessed using a 7 MHz linear array transducer for B-mode ultrasonography. The ccIMT measured in the far wall is one of the most relevant indicators of vascular aging(Virmani et al., 1991), and an IMT of >1 mm rather than localized carotid atherosclerosis is considered to be a reliable indicator of generalized atherosclerosis (Fig. 8.4) (Bots et al., 1997). Increased ccIMT indicates a higher risk of myocardial infarction, peripheral arterial disease, and stroke (Bots et al., 1996) but is only moderately sensitive in predicting future cardiovascular events (Simon et al., 2007). The site of measurement is a crucial element for standardization and reliability (Nambi et al., 2012) but, although ccIMT assessments are considered to be quantitative, they do not allow a fine ultrastructural analysis of the whole extra-cranial carotid system (Stein et al., 2008). The presence of plaque in the carotid system or the determination of total plaque area are considered to be better predictors of future myocardial and cerebrovascular events than ccIMT (Spence 2002) (Fig. 8.5), and the combined assessment of ccIMT and plaque detection is

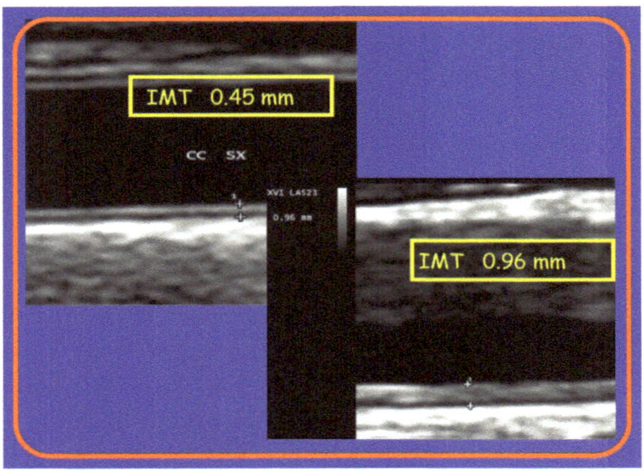

FIGURE 8.5 **Different intima-media thickness (IMT) measurements.**

recommended in asymptomatic adults at intermediate risk of cardiovascular events (Greenland et al., 2010; Stein et al., 2008).

Increased ccIMT indicating atherosclerosis has been described in RA (Shoenfeld et al., 2005; Gerli et al., 2005; Kumeda et al., 2002), and ccIMT has become the most widely used indicator of subclinical atherosclerosis in rheumatic diseases. Numerous cross-sectional studies have showed increased ccIMT indicating accelerated atherosclerosis (Kerekes et al., 2011; Kerekes et al., 2009a,b; Kramer and Giles, 2011; Gonzalez-Gay et al., 2008) in patients with RA or AS (Bodnar et al., 2011; Gonzalez-Juanatey et al., 2009a,b; Peters et al., 2009), and subclinical atherosclerosis has been detected in patients with PsA, SLE, and SSc (Szücs et al., 2007; Gonzalez-Juanatey et al., 2006; Salmon and Roman 2008). One small follow-up cohort study has supported the long-term predictive power of ccIMT for future cardiovascular events in patients with RA (Gonzalez-Juanatey et al., 2009a,b). As RA is an important risk factor for atherosclerosis according to current guidelines, ccIMT might be a useful for screening this patient population.

The reported effects of biological agents (primarily TNF blockers and rituximab) on carotid atherosclerosis are inconsistent, depending on the type of drug, treatment duration, and its clinical efficacy (Kitas and Gabriel, 2011; Kerekes et al., 2009a,b, 2011; Sidiropoulos et al., 2009).

A number of studies have assessed early endothelial dysfunction in RA patients by measuring FMD or nitroglycerine-mediated vasodilatation (NMD) (Shoenfeld et al., 2005; Bergholm et al., 2002; Vaudo et al., 2004). FMD and NMD respectively indicate endothelium-dependent and endothelium-independent vasodilation (Lekakis et al., 1998; Corretti et al., 2002), and both impaired (Bergholm et al., 2002) and normal FMD (Van Doornum et al., 2003) have been reported in patients with rheumatic diseases.

Early endothelial dysfunction has been assessed by means of high-resolution ultrasonography measurements of brachial artery FMD and NMD (Corretti et al., 2002): the percentage increase from baseline in FMD induced by reactive hyperemia was significantly lower in RA patients (5.3%) than in healthy subjects (8.3%), whereas there was no difference in the percentage increase in NMD after the administration of nitroglycerine in the patients (18.3%) and controls (17.5%). Impaired FMD has been detected in young RA patients with low disease activity (Bergholm et al., 2002). Similar observations have been made in patients with SSc (impaired FMD% associated with normal NMD%) (Szamosi et al., 2009), whereas both FMD% and NMD% are impaired in SLE patients (Szekanecz and Shoenfeld, 2006; Kiss et al., 2006).

In terms of imaging, high ccIMT values are associated with impaired FMD%. The early endothelial dysfunction indicated by FMD% may precede the manifest atherosclerosis indicated by ccIMT, and more pronounced endothelial dysfunction may lead to more accelerated atherosclerosis in RA (Shoenfeld et al., 2005; Giles et al., 2006). High ccIMT values also correlate with age and total cholesterol levels.

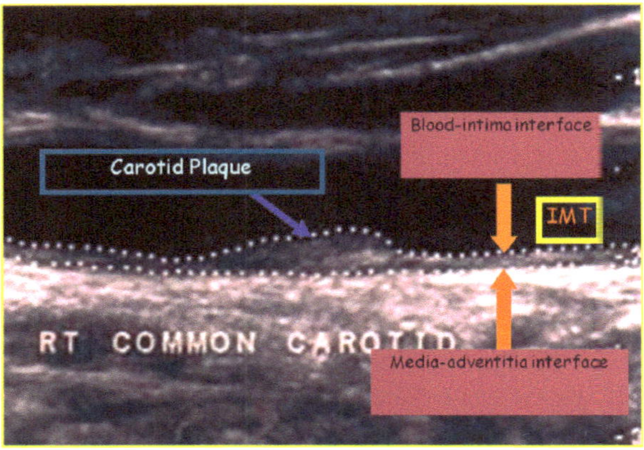

FIGURE 8.6 **Carotid plaque.**

Disease duration is significantly associated with impaired FMD%, and there is a tendency for higher ccIMT values to be found in RA patients with a longer disease duration. The role of age and disease duration in RA-associated atherosclerosis has been confirmed by Peters et al. (2008), Stamatelopoulos et al. (2009), Protogerou et al. (2008), and Vanhoutte (2009).

The measurement of ccIMT is a standard method of assessing overt atherosclerosis (Kerekes et al., 2008; Sherer et al., 2007; Kanters et al., 1997); PW velocity and the augmentation index (AIx) are parameters of arterial stiffness and wave reflection.

There is a need for new diagnostic techniques that can predict early endothelial dysfunction and overt atherosclerosis preclinically (Kerekes et al., 2008; Corretti et al., 2002; Soltesz et al., 2009; Kerekes et al., 2012; Szekanecz et al., 2016) (Fig. 8.6). These need to be rapid, reproducible, and applicable to

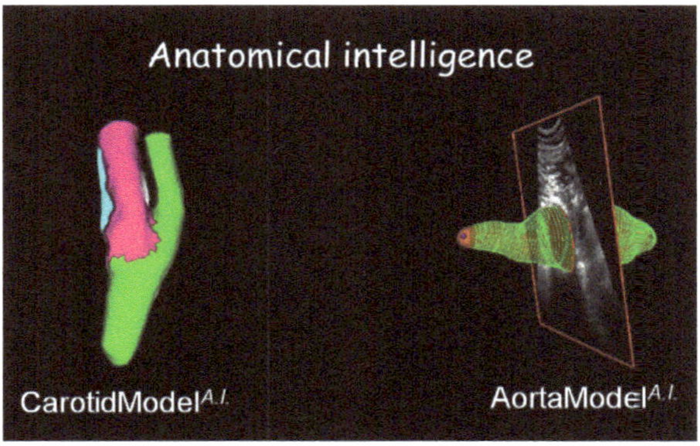

FIGURE 8.7 **3D carotid and aorta models.**

a relatively large number of patients, and should be able to identify patients at high risk of CV morbidity and mortality easily and cost-effectively. The new 3D carotid and aortic approach will improve the likelihood of detecting preclinical atherosclerosis (Fig. 8.7).

10. CONCLUSION

CV mortality and morbidity is increased in patients with SADs; invasive and noninvasive imaging is a reliable means of screening, diagnosing, and following-up CV involvement in patients with SADs.

REFERENCES

Ahlehoff, O., Gislason, G.H., Skov, L., Hansen, P.R., 2010. Psoriasis and atherothrombotic disease. Ugeskr. Laeger 172, 1983.

Arosio, E., De Marchi, S., Rigoni, A., 2007. Forearm haemodynamics, arterial stiffness and microcirculatory reactivity in rheumatoid arthritis. J. Hypertens. 25, 1273.

Asherson, R.A., Cervera, R., 1991. Antiphospholipid antibodies and heart. Lessons Pitfalls Cardiol. Circ. 84, 920.

Atzeni, F., Sarzi-Puttini, P., Sitia, S., 2011a. Coronary flow reserve and asymmetric dimethylarginine levels: new measurements for identifying subclinical atherosclerosis in patients with psoriatic arthritis. J. Rheumatol. 38, 1661.

Atzeni, F., Turiel, M., Boccassini, L., 2011b. Cardiovascular involvement in psoriatic arthritis. Reumatismo 63, 148.

Bae, S.W., Stühlinger, M.C., Yoo, H.S., et al., 2005. Plasma asymmetric dimethylarginine concentrations in newly diagnosed patients with acute myocardial infarction or unstable angina pectoris during two weeks of medical treatment. Am. J. Cardiol. 95, 729.

Bergholm, R., Leirisalo-Repo, M., Vehkavaara, S., et al., 2002. Impaired responsiveness to NO in newly diagnosed patients with rheumatoid arthritis. Arterioscler. Thromb. Vasc. Biol. 22, 1637.

Birdane, A., Korkmaz, C., Ata, N., Cavusoglu, Y., 2007. Tissue Doppler imaging in the evaluation of the left and right ventricular diastolic functions in rheumatoid arthritis. Echocardiography 24, 485.

Black, I.W., Hopkins, A.P., Lee, L.C.L., 1991. Left atrial spontaneous echo contrast: a clinical and echocardiographic analysis. J. Am. Coll. Cardiol. 18, 398.

Bodnar, N., et al., 2011. Assessment of subclinical vascular disease associated with ankylosing spondylitis. J. Rheumatol. 38, 723.

Böger, R.H., Bode-Böger, S.M., Szuba, A., et al., 1998. Asymmetric dimethylarginine (ADMA): a novel risk factor for endothelial dysfunction: its role in hypercholesterolemia. Circulation 98, 1842.

Böger, R.H., Bode-Böger, S.M., Thiele, W., et al., 1997. Biochemical evidence for impaired nitric oxide synthesis in patients with peripheral arterial occlusive disease. Circulation 95, 2068.

Bots, M.L., Hofman, A., De Jong, P.T., Grobbee, D.E., 1996. Common carotid intima-media thickness as an indicator of atherosclerosis at other sites of the carotid artery. The Rotterdam study. Ann. Epidemiol. 6, 147.

Bots, M.L., Hofman, A., Grobbee, D.E., 1997. Increased common carotid intima-media thickness. Adaptive response or a reflection of atherosclerosis? Findings from the Rotterdam study. Stroke 28, 2442.

Braunwald, E., 1997. Heart Disease: A Textbook of Cardiovascular Medicine fifth ed. Saunders, London, p. 1776.

Brenner, B., Blumenfeld, Z., Markiewicz, W., 1991. Cardiac involvement in patients with primary antiphospholipid syndrome. J. Am. Coll. Cardiol. 18, 931.

Buppajamrntham, T., Palavutitotai, N., Katchamart, W., 2014. Clinical manifestation, diagnosis, management, and treatment outcome of pericarditis in patients with systemic lupus erythematosus. J. Med. Assoc. Thai. 97 (12), 1234.

Caiati, C., Zedda, N., Montaldo, C., 1999. Contrast-enhanced transthoracic second harmonic echo Doppler with adenosine: a noninvasive, rapid and effective method for coronary flow reserve assessment. J. Am. Coll. Cardiol. 34, 122.

Cervera, R., Font, J., Paré, C., 1992. Cardiac disease in systemic lupus erythematosus. Prospective study of 70 patients. Ann. Rheum. Dis. 51, 156.

Cervera, R., Khamashta, A., Font, J., 1991. High prevalence of significant heart valve lesion in patients with the primary antiphospholipid syndrome. Lupus 1, 43.

Cervera, R., 2000. Recent advances in antiphospholipid antibody-related valvulopathies. J. Autoimmun. 15, 123.

Chiribiri, A., Hautvast, G.L., Lockie, T., et al., 2013. Assessment of coronary artery stenosis severity and location: quantitative analysis of transmural perfusion gradients by high-resolution MRI versus FFR. JACC Cardiovasc. Imaging 6 (5), 600.

Ciftci, O., Yilmaz, S., Topcu, S., 2008. Impaired coronary microvascular function and increased intima-media thickness in rheumatoid arthritis. Atherosclerosis 198, 332.

Corretti, M.C., Anderson, T.J., Benjamin, E.J., et al., 2002. Guidelines for the ultrasound assessment of endothelial-dependent flow-mediated vasodilation of the brachial artery: a report of the International Brachial Artery Reactivity Task Force. J. Am. Coll. Cardiol. 39, 257.

Cortigiani, L., Rigo, F., Gherardi, S., 2010. Implication of the continuous prognostic spectrum of Doppler echocardiographic derived coronary flow reserve on left anterior descending artery. Am. J. Cardiol. 105 (2), 158.

Dandel, M., Hetzer, R., 2009. Echocardiographic strain and strain rate imaging—clinical applications. Int. J. Cardiol. 132, 11.

D'Andrea, A., Stisi, S., Bellissimo, S., et al., 2005. Eur. J. Echocardiogr. 6 (6), 407–418.

Del Rincón, I., O'Leary, D.H., Freeman, G.L., Escalante, A., 2007. Acceleration of atherosclerosis during the course of rheumatoid arthritis. Atherosclerosis 195, 354.

Dimitroulas, T., Giannakoulas, G., Papadopoulou, K., et al., 2010. Early detection of cardiac involvement in systemic sclerosis assessed by tissue-doppler echocardiography: relationship with neurohormonal activation and endothelial dysfunction. J. Rheumatol. 37 (5), 993–999.

Dimitrow, P.P., 2002. Coronary Flow Reserve-Measurement and Application: Focus on Transthoracic Doppler Echocardiography. Kluwer Academic Publishers, Boston, Dordrecht, London.

Espinola-Zavaleta, N., Vargas-Barracòn, J., Colmenares-Galvis, T., 1999 Echocardiographic evaluation of patients with primary antiphospholipid syndrome. Am. Heart J. 137, 973.

EULAR Task Force, 2016.

Gaibazzi, N., Rigo, F., Reverberi, C., 2010. Detection of coronary artery disease by combined assessment of wall motion, myocardial perfusion and coronary flow reserve: a multiparametric contrast stress-echocardiography study. J. Am. Soc. Echocardiogr. 23 (12), 1242–1250.

Galve, E., Ordi, J., Barquinero, J., 1992. Valvular heart disease in the primary antiphospholipid syndrome. Ann. Intern. Med. 116, 293.

Gerli, R., Sherer, Y., Vaudo, G., et al., 2005. Early atherosclerosis in rheumatoid arthritis. Effects of smoking on thickness of the carotid intima media. Ann. NY Acad. Sci. 1051, 281.

Gianturco, L., Bodini, B.D., Atzeni, F., et al., 2015. Cardiovascular and autoimmune diseases in females: the role of microvasculature and dysfunctional endothelium. Atherosclerosis 241 (1), 259.
Giles, J.T., Post, W., Blumenthal, R.S., Bathon, J.M., 2006. Therapy insight: managing cardiovascular risk in patients with rheumatoid arthritis. Nat. Clin. Pract. Rheumatol. 2, 320.
Giunta, A., Picillo, U., Maione, S., 1993. Spectrum of cardiac involvement in systemic lupus erythematosus: echocardiographic, echo-Doppler observations and immunological investigation. Acta Cardiol. 2, 183.
Gonzalez-Gay, M.A., Gonzalez-Juanatey, C., Vazquez-Rodriguez, T.R., et al., 2008. Endothelial dysfunction, carotid intima-media thickness, and accelerated atherosclerosis in rheumatoid arthritis. Semin. Arthritis Rheum. 38, 67.
Gonzalez-Juanatey, C., Llorca, J., Garcia-Porrua, C., et al., 2006. Effect of anti-tumor necrosis factor alpha therapy on the progression of subclinical atherosclerosis in severe rheumatoid arthritis. Arthritis Rheum. 55, 150.
Gonzalez-Juanatey, C., et al., 2009a. The high prevalence of subclinical atherosclerosis in patients with ankylosing spondylitis without clinically evident cardiovascular disease. Medicine 88, 358.
Gonzalez-Juanatey, C., Llorca, J., Martin, J., Gonzalez-Gay, M.A., 2009b. Carotid intima-media thickness predicts the development of cardiovascular events in patients with rheumatoid arthritis. Semin. Arthritis Rheum. 38, 366.
Greenland, P., Alpert, J., Beller, G., et al., December 21, 2010. ACCF/AHA guideline for assessment of cardiovascular risk in asymptomatic adults: executive summary. A report of the American College of Cardiology Foundation/American Heart Association Task Force on Practice Guidelines. Circulation 122 (25), 2748–2764.
Guedes, C., Bianchi-Fior, P., Cormier, B., 2001. Cardiac manifestations of rheumatoid arthritis: a case-control transesophageal echocardiography study in 30 patients. Arthritis Rheum. 45, 129.
Hasnie, A.M., Stoddard, M.F., Gleason, C.B., 1995. Diastolic dysfunction is a feature of the antiphospholipid syndrome. Am. Heart J. 129, 1009.
Heimdal, A., Støylen, A., Torp, H., et al., 1998. Real-time strain rate imaging of the left ventricle by ultrasound. J. Am. Soc. Echocardiogr. 11, 1013.
Hirata, K., Kadirvelu, A., Kinjo, M., et al., 2007. Altered coronary vasomotor function in young patients with systemic lupus erythematosus. Arthritis Rheum. 56, 1904.
Hojnik, M., George, J., Ziporen, L., 1996. Heart valve involvement (Libman-Sacks endocarditis) in the antiphospholipid syndrome. Circulation 93, 1579.
Hozumi, T., Yoshida, K., Ogata, Y., 1998. Noninvasive assessment of significant left anterior descending coronary artery stenosis by coronary flow velocity reserve with transthoracic color Doppler echocardiography. Circulation 97, 1557.
Jafar, M.Z., Morgan, M.C., Gorcsan III, J., 1994. Transesophageal echocardiographic detection of multiple mitral valve masses in primary antiphospholipid syndrome with stroke. Am. Heart J. 127, 445.
Kanters, S.D.J.M., Algra, A., van Leeuwen, M.S., et al., 1997. Reproducibility of in vivo carotid intima–media thickness measurements. Stroke 28, 665.
Kepez, A., Akdogan, A., Sade, L.E., et al., 2008. Detection of subclinical cardiac involvement in systemic sclerosis by echocardiographic strain imaging. Echocardiography 25, 191–197.
Kerekes, G., Szekanecz, Z., Dér, H., et al., 2008. Endothelial dysfunction and atherosclerosis in rheumatoid arthritis: a multiparametric analysis using imaging techniques and laboratory markers of inflammation and autoimmunity. J. Rheumatol. 35, 398.
Kerekes, G., et al., 2009a. Effects of biologics on vascular function and atherosclerosis associated with rheumatoid arthritis. Ann. NY Acad. Sci. 1173, 814.

Kerekes, G., et al., 2009b. Effects of rituximab treatment on endothelial dysfunction, carotid atherosclerosis, and lipid profile in rheumatoid arthritis. Clin. Rheumatol. 28, 705.

Kerekes, G., et al., 2011. Effects of adalimumab treatment on vascular disease associated with early rheumatoid arthritis. Isr. Med. Assoc. J. 13, 147.

Kerekes, G., Soltész, P., Nurmohamed, M.T., et al., 2012. Validated methods for assessment of subclinical atherosclerosis in rheumatology. Nat. Rev. Rheumatol. 8 (4), 224.

Khamashta, M.A., Cervera, R., Asherson, R.A., 1990. Association of antibodies against phospholipids with heart valve disease in systemic lupus erythematosus. Lancet 335, 1541.

Kiani, A.N., Mahoney, J.A., Petri, M., 2007. Asymmetric dimethylarginine is a marker of poor prognosis and coronary calcium in systemic lupus erythematosus. J. Rheumatol. 34, 1502.

Kimhi, O., Caspi, D., Bornstein, N.M., 2007. Prevalence and risk factors of atherosclerosis in patients with psoriatic arthritis. Semin. Arthritis Rheum. 36, 203.

Kiss, E., Soltesz, P., Der, H., et al., 2006. Reduced flow-mediated vasodilation as a marker for cardiovascular complications in lupus patients. J. Autoimmun. 27, 211.

Kitas, G.D., Gabriel, S.E., 2011. Cardiovascular disease in rheumatoid arthritis: state of the art and future perspectives. Ann. Rheum. Dis. 70, 8.

Knockaert, D.C., 2007. Cardiac involvement in systemic inflammatory diseases. Eur. Heart J. 28, 1797.

Kramer, H.R., Giles, J.T., 2011. Cardiovascular disease risk in rheumatoid arthritis: progress, debate, and opportunity. Arthritis Care Res. 63, 484.

Kumeda, Y., Inaba, M., Goto, H., et al., 2002. Increased thickness of the arterial intima-media detected by ultrasonography in patients with rheumatoid arthritis. Arthritis Rheum. 46, 1489.

Lee, T.H., Boucher, C.A., 2001. Noninvasive tests in patients with stable coronary artery disease. N. Engl. J. Med. 344, 1840.

Leitman, M., Lysyansky, P., Sidenko, S., et al., 2004. Two-dimensional strain-a novel software for real-time quantitative echocardiographic assessment of myocardial function. J. Am. Soc. Echocardiogr. 17, 1021.

Lekakis, J., Mavrikakis, M., Papamichael, C., et al., 1998. Short-term estrogen administration improves abnormal endothelial function in women with systemic sclerosis and Raynaud's phenomenon. Am. Heart J. 136, 905.

Lundman, P., Eriksson, M.J., Stühlinger, M., et al., 2001. Mild-to-moderate hypertriglyceridemia in young men is associated with endothelial dysfunction and increased plasma concentrations of asymmetric dimethylarginine. J. Am. Coll. Cardiol. 38, 111.

MacAllister, R.J., Rambausek, M.H., Vallance, P., et al., 1996. Concentration of dimethyl-L-arginine in the plasma of patients with end-stage renal failure. Nephrol. Dial Transplant. 11, 2449.

Maharaj, S.S., Chang, S.M., 2015. Cardiac tamponade as the initial presentation of systemic lupus erythematosus: a case report and review of the literature. Pediatr. Rheumatol. Online J. 13, 9.

Marsan, N.A., Tops, L.F., Nihoyannopoulos, P., 2009. Real-time three dimensional echocardiography: current and future clinical applications. Heart 95, 1881.

Mavrogeni, S., Servos, G., Smerla, R., et al., 2015. Cardiovascular involvement in pediatric systemic autoimmune diseases: the emerging role of noninvasive cardiovascular imaging. Inflamm. Allergy Drug Targets 13 (6), 371.

Mele, D., Censi, S., La Corte, R., et al., 2008. Abnormalities of left ventricular function in asymptomatic patients with systemic sclerosis using Doppler measures of myocardial strain. J. Am. Soc. Echocardiogr. 21, 1257−1264.

Metz, D., Jolly, D., Graciet-Richard, J., 1994. Prevalence of valvular involvement in systemic lupus erythematosus and association with antiphospholipid syndrome: a matched echocardiographic study. Cardiology 85, 129.

Meune, C., Avouac, J., Wahbi, K., et al., 2008. Cardiac involvement in systemic sclerosis assessed by tissue-doppler echocardiography during routine care: a controlled study of 100 consecutive patients. Arthritis Rheum. 58, 1803–1809.

Montisci, R., Vacca, A., Garau, P., 2003. Detection of early impairment of coronary flow reserve in patients with systemic sclerosis. Ann. Rheum. Dis. 62, 890.

Nakazato, R., Berman, D.S., Alexanderson, E., et al., 2013. Myocardial perfusion imaging with PET. Imaging Med. 5 (1), 35.

Nambi, V., et al., 2012. Common carotid artery intima-media thickness is as good as carotid intima-media thickness of all carotid artery segments in improving prediction of coronary heart disease risk in the Atherosclerosis Risk in Communities (ARIC) study. Eur. Heart J. 33 (2), 183.

Nihoyannopoulos, P., Gomez, P.M., Joshi, J., 1990. Cardiac abnormalities in systemic lupus erythematosus. Circulation 82, 369.

Omdal, R., Lunde, P., Rasmussen, K., 2001. Transesophageal and transthoracic echocardiography and Doppler-examinations in systemic lupus erythematosus. Scand. J. Rheumatol. 30, 275.

Pavlopoulos, H., Nihoyannopoulos, P., 2008. Strain and strain rate deformation parameters: from tissue Doppler to 2D speckle tracking. Int. J. Cardiovasc. Imaging 24, 479–491.

Peters, M.J., et al., 2008. Relations between autoantibodies against oxidized low-density lipoprotein, inflammation, subclinical atherosclerosis, and cardiovascular disease in rheumatoid arthritis. J. Rheumatol. 35, 1495.

Peters, M.J., et al., 2009. Signs of accelerated preclinical atherosclerosis in patients with ankylosing spondylitis. J. Rheumatol. 37, 161.

Pislaru, C., Abraham, T.P., Belohlavek, M., 2002. Strain and strain rate echocardiography. Curr. Opin. Cardiol. 17, 443.

Plastiras, S.C., Pamboucas, C.A., Tzelepis, G.E., 2009. Assessing mitral valve stenosis by real-time 3-dimensional echocardiography in systemic lupus erythematosus: a look inside the heart. J. Rheumatol. 36, 1843.

Protogerou, A.D., Stergiou, G.S., Lourida, P., et al., 2008. Arterial stiffness and orthostatic blood pressure changes in untreated and treated hypertensive subjects. J. Am. Soc. Hypertens. 2 (5), 372–377.

Rexhepaj, N., Bajraktari, G., Berisha, I., 2006. Left and right ventricular diastolic functions in patients with rheumatoid arthritis without clinically evident cardiovascular disease. Int. J. Clin. Pract. 60, 683.

Riboldi, P., Gerosa, M., Luzzana, C., 2002. Cardiac involvement in systemic autoimmune diseases. Clin. Rev. Allergy Immunol. 23, 247.

Rigo, F., Richieri, M., Pasanisi, E., 2003. Usefulness of coronary flow reserve over regional wall motion when added to dual-imaging dipyridamole echocardiography. Am. J. Cardiol. 91, 269.

Rigo, F., Gherardi, S., Galderisi, M., 2006. The prognostic impact of coronary flow-reserve assessed by Doppler echocardiography in non-ischaemic dilated cardiomyopathy. Eur. Heart J. 27, 1319.

Roldan, C.A., Shively, B.K., Crawford, M.H., 1996. An echocardiographic study of valvular heart disease associated with systemic lupus erythematosus. N. Engl. J. Med. 335, 1424.

Salmon, J.E., Roman, M.J., 2008. Subclinical atherosclerosis in rheumatoid arthritis and systemic lupus erythematosus. Am. J. Med. 121 (10 Suppl. 1), S3–S8.

Sattar, N., McCarey, D.W., Capell, H., 2003. Explaining how "high-grade" systemic inflammation accelerates vascular risk in rheumatoid arthritis. Circulation 108, 2957–2963.

Schattke, S., Knebel, F., Grohmann, A., et al., 2010. Early right ventricular systolic dysfunction in patients with systemic sclerosis without pulmonary hypertension: a Doppler Tissue and Speckle Tracking echocardiography study. Cardiovasc. Ultrasound 8, 3.

Sherer, Y., Gerli, R., Gilburd, B., et al., 2007. Thickened carotid artery intima–media in rheumatoid arthritis is associated with elevated anticardiolipin antibodies. Lupus 16, 259.
Shoenfeld, Y., Gerli, R., Doria, A., et al., 2005. Accelerated atherosclerosis in autoimmune rheumatic diseases. Circulation 112, 3337.
Sidiropoulos, P.I., et al., 2009. Sustained improvement of vascular endothelial function during anti-TNFalpha treatment in rheumatoid arthritis patients. Scand. J. Rheumatol. 38, 6.
Simon, A., Chironi, G., Levenson, J., 2007. Comparative performance of subclinical atherosclerosis tests in predicting coronary heart disease in asymptomatic individuals. Eur. Heart J. 28, 2967.
Sitia, S., Tomasoni, L., Criseo, M., et al., 2009. Speckle tracking echocardiography for detection of subclinical cardiac involvement in rheumatoid arthritis. Eur. J. Echocardiogr. 10, S131.
Sitia, S., Gianturco, L., Tomasoni, L., 2010a. Role of cardiovascular imaging in systemic autoimmune diseases. World J. Cardiol. 2, 237.
Sitia, S., Tomasoni, L., Turiel, M., 2010b. Speckle tracking echocardiography: a new approach to myocardial function. World J. Cardiol. 2, 1.
Soltész, P., Dér, H., Kerekes, G., et al., 2009. Comparative study of arterial stiffness, flow-mediated vasodilation of the brachial artery, and the thickness of the carotid artery intima-media in patients with systemic autoimmune diseases. Clin. Reumatol. 28, 655.
Spence, J.D., 2002. Ultrasound measurement of carotid plaque as a surrogate outcome for coronary artery disease. Am. J. Cardiol. 10–15.
Spethmann, S., Dreger, H., Schattke, S., et al., 2012. Eur. Heart J. Cardiovasc. Imaging 13 (10), 863–870.
Stamatelopoulos, K.S., Kitas, G.D., Papamichael, C.M., et al., 2009. Atherosclerosis in rheumatoid arthritis versus diabetes: a comparative study. Arterioscler. Thromb. Vasc. Biol. 29 (10), 1702–1708.
Stein, J.H., et al., 2008. Use of carotid ultrasound to identify subclinical vascular disease and evaluate cardiovascular disease risk: a consensus statement from the American Society of Echocardiography Carotid Intima-Media Thickness Task Force. Endorsed by the Society for Vascular Medicine. J. Am. Soc. Echocardiogr. 21, 93.
Stühlinger, M.C., Abbasi, F., Chu, J.W., et al., 2002. Relationship between insulin resistance and an endogenous nitric oxide synthase inhibitor. JAMA 287, 1420.
Surdacki, A., Nowicki, M., Sandmann, J., et al., 1999. Reduced urinary excretion of nitric oxide metabolites and increased plasma levels of asymmetric dimethylarginine in men with essential hypertension. J. Cardiovasc. Pharmacol. 33, 652.
Szamosi, S., Csiki, Z., Szomják, E., et al., 2009. Plasma homocysteine levels, the prevalence of tetrahydrofolate reductase gene C677T polymorphism and macrovascular disorders in systemic sclerosis: risk factors for accelerated macrovascular damage? J. Rheumatol. 36, 145.
Szekanecz, Z., Shoenfeld, Y., 2006. Lupus and cardiovascular disease: the facts. Lupus 15 (Suppl. 1), 3.
Szücs, G., Szekanecz, Z., Zilahi, E., et al., 2007. Systemic sclerosis–rheumatoid arthritis overlap syndrome: a unique combination of features suggests a distinct genetic, serological and clinical entity. Rheumatology (Oxford) 46 (6), 989–993.
Szekanecz, Z., Kerekes, G., Végh, E., et al., 2016. Autoimmune atherosclerosis in 3D: how it develops, how to diagnose and what to do. Autoimmun. Rev. pii:S1568–9972(16)30062-3 http://dx.doi.org/10.1016/j.autrev.2016.03.014.
Tanasescu, C., Jurcut, C., Jurcut, R., 2009. Vascular disease in rheumatoid arthritis: from subclinical lesions to cardiovascular risk. Eur. J. Intern. Med. 20, 348.
Turiel, M., Muzzupappa, S., Gottardi, B., 2000. Evaluation of cardiac abnormalities and embolic sources in primary antiphospholipid syndrome by transesophageal echocardiography. Lupus 9, 406–412.

Turiel, M., Sarzi-Puttini, P., Peretti, R., 2005. Five-year follow-up by transesophageal echocardiographic studies in primary antiphospholipid syndrome. Am. J. Cardiol. 96, 574.
Turiel, M., Atzeni, F., Tomasoni, L., et al., 2009a. Non-invasive assessment of coronary flow reserve and ADMA levels: a case-control study of early rheumatoid arthritis patients. Rheumatology 48, 834.
Turiel, M., Sitia, S., Tomasoni, L., 2009b. Cardiac involvement in rheumatoid arthritis. Reumatismo 61, 244.
Turiel, M., Tomasoni, L., Sitia, S., 2010. Effects of long-term disease-modifying antirheumatic drugs on endothelial function in patients with early rheumatoid arthritis. Cardiovasc. Ther. 28, e53.
Turiel, M., Gianturco, L., Ricci, C., 2013. Silent cardiovascular involvement in patients with diffuse systemic sclerosis: a controlled cross-sectional study. Arthritis Care Res. 65, 274.
Vacca, A., Montisci, R., Garau, P., 2013. Prognostic impact of coronary microcirculation abnormalities in systemic sclerosis: a prospective study to evaluate the role of non-invasive tests. Arthritis Res. Ther. 15, R8.
Van Doornum, S., McColl, G., Jenkins, A., et al., 2003. Screening for atherosclerosis in patients with rheumatoid arthritis: comparison of two in vivo tests for vascular function. Arthritis Rheum. 48, 72.
Vanhoutte, P.M., 2009. Endothelial dysfunction: the first step toward coronary arteriosclerosis. Circ. J. 73 (4), 595–601.
van Zonneveld, A.J., de Boer, H.C., van der Veer, E.P., 2010. Inflammation, vascular injury and repair in rheumatoid arthritis. Ann. Rheum. Dis. 69 (Suppl. 1), i57.
Vaudo, G., Marchesi, S., Gerli, R., et al., 2004. Endothelial dysfunction in young patients with rheumatoid arthritis and low disease activity. Ann. Rheum. Dis. 63, 31.
Veale, D.J., Collidge, T.A., Belch, J.J., 1995. Increased prevalence of symptomatic macrovascular disease in systemic sclerosis. Ann. Rheum. Dis. 54, 853.
Virmani, R., et al., 1991. Effect of aging on aortic morphology in populations with high and low prevalence of hypertension and atherosclerosis. Comparison between occidental and Chinese communities. Am. J. Pathol. 139, 1119.
Wakkee, M., de Jong, E.M., 2013. Is psoriasis a dependent cardiovascular risk factor? Ned. Tijdschr. Geneeskd. 157, A5417.
Wang, Y.X., Fitch, R.M., 2004. Vascular stiffness: measurements, mechanisms and implications. Curr. Vasc. Pharmacol. 2, 379.
Yildiz, M., 2010. Arterial distensibility in chronic inflammatory rheumatic disorders. Open Cardiovasc. Med. J. 4, 83.
Yiu, K.H., Schouffoer, A.A., Marsan, N.A., et al., 2011. Left ventricular dysfunction assessed by speckle-tracking strain analysis in patients with systemic sclerosis: relationship to functional capacity and ventricular arrhythmias. Arthritis Rheum. 63, 3969–3978.
Yousuf, T., Kramer, J., Kopiec, A., et al., 2015. A rare case of cardiac tamponade induced by chronic rheumatoid arthritis. J. Clin. Med. Res. 7 (9), 720.

FURTHER READING

Atzeni, F.,, Sarzi-Puttini, P., Delfino, L., et al., 2004. Decreased coronary flow reserve in patients with rheumatoid arthritis. Ann. Rheum. Dis. 63, S196.
Baillet, A., et al., 2016. Points to consider for reporting, screening for and preventing selected comorbidities in chronic inflammatory rheumatic diseases in daily practice: a EULAR initiative. Ann. Rheum. Dis. 75, 965.
Bijl, M.,, Brouwer, J., Kallemberg, G.G.M., 2000. Grand rounds from international lupus centres. Cardiac abnormalities in SLE: pancarditis. Lupus 9, 236.

Candell-Riera, J.,, Armadans-Gil, L., Simeon, C.P., 1996. Comprehensive noninvasive assessment of cardiac involvement in limited systemic sclerosis. Arthritis Rheum. 39, 1138.

Chung, C.P.,, Oeser, A., Raggi, P., et al., 2005. Increased coronary artery atherosclerosis in rheumatoid arthritis: relationship to disease duration and cardiovascular risk factors. Arthritis Rheum. 52, 3045.

Daza, L.,, Aguirre, M., Jimenez, M., et al., 2007. Common carotid intima-media thickness and von Willebrand factor serum levels in rheumatoid arthritis female patients without cardiovascular risk factors. Clin. Rheumatol. 26, 533.

del Rincon, I.,, Williams, K., Stern, M.P., 2001. High incidence of cardiovascular events in a rheumatoid arthritis cohort not explained by traditional cardiac risk factors. Arthritis Rheum. 44, 2737.

Del Rincon, I.,, Williams, K., Stern, M.P., et al., 2003. Association between carotid atherosclerosis and markers of inflammation in rheumatoid arthritis patients and healthy subjects. Arthritis Rheum. 48, 1833.

Deswall, A., Follansbee, W.P., 1996. Cardiac involvement in scleroderma. Rheum. Dis. Clin. North Am. 22, 841.

Eichenberger, A.C.,, Schuiki, E., Kochli, D.V., 1994. Ischaemic heart disease: assessment with gadolinium-enhanced ultrafast MR imaging and dipyridamole stress. J. Magn. Reson. Imag. 4, 425.

Ferri, C.,, Di Bello, V., Martini, A., 1998. Heart involvement in systemic sclerosis: an ultrasonic tissue characterisation study. Ann. Rheum. Dis. 57, 296.

Ferri, C.,, Bernini, L., Bongiorni, M.G., 1985. Noninvasive evaluation of cardiac dysrhythmias, and their relationship with systemic symptoms, in progressive systemic sclerosis. Arthritis Rheum. 28, 1259.

Follansbee, W.P.,, Curtiss, E.I., Rahko, P.S., 1985. The electrocardiogram in systemic sclerosis (scleroderma). Study of 102 consecutive cases with functional correlations and review of the literature. Am. J. Med. 79, 183.

Gerli, R., et al., 2007. Precocious atherosclerosis in rheumatoid arthritis: role of traditional and disease-related cardiovascular risk factors. Ann. NY Acad. Sci. 1108, 372.

Ghaffary, S., 1999. Detection and management of coronary artery disease in patients with rheumatological disorders. Rheum. Dis. Clin. North Am. 25, 657.

Gonzalez-Juanatey, C.,, Llorca, J., Testa, A., et al., 2003. Increased prevalence of severe subclinical atherosclerotic findings in long-term treated rheumatoid arthritis patients without clinically evident atherosclerotic disease. Medicine 82, 407.

Goodson, N., 2002. Coronary artery disease and rheumatoid arthritis. Curr. Opin. Rheumatol. 14, 115.

Hannawi, S.,, Haluska, B.,, Marwick, T.H., Thomas, R., 2007. Atherosclerotic disease is increased in recent-onset rheumatoid arthritis: a critical role for inflammation. Arthritis Res. Ther. 9, R116.

Ishida, R.,, Murata, Y., Sawada, Y., 2000. Thallium-201 myocardial SPET in patients with collagen disease. Nucl. Med. Commun. 21, 729.

Jiménez, S.,, Ramos-Casals, M., Cervera, R., 2001. Atherosclerosis in systemic lupus erythematosus: clinical relevance. In: Shoenfeld, Y., Harats, D., Wick, G. (Eds.), Atherosclerosis and Autoimmunity. Elsevier, Amsterdam, p. 255.

Johns, J.P.,, Abraham, S.A., Eagle, K.A., 1995. Dipyridamol-thallium versus dobutamine echocardiographic stress testing: a clinician's view point. Am. Heart J. 130, 373.

Kahan, A.,, Devaux, J., Amor, B., 1990. The effect of captopril on thallium 201 myocardial perfusion in systemic sclerosis. Clin. Pharmacol. Ther. 47, 483.

Lanza, G.A.,, Camici, P.G., Galiuto, L., et al., 2013. Methods to investigate coronary microvascular function in clinical practice. J. Cardiovasc. Med. 14 (1), 1.

Legrand, V.,, Raskinet, B., Laarman, G., 1997. Diagnostic value of exercise electrocardiography and angina after coronary artery stenting. Benestent Study Group. Am. Heart J. 133, 240.

Manzi, S.,, Kuller, L.H., Edmundowicz, D., 2000. Vascular imaging: changing the face of cardiovascular research. Lupus 9, 176.

Maradit-Kremers, H.,, Crowson, C.S., Nicola, P.J., et al., 2005. Increased unrecognized coronary heart disease and sudden deaths in rheumatoid arthritis: a population-based cohort study. Arthritis Rheum. 52, 402.

Matura, et al., 2014. Is atherosclerosis an autoimmune disease? BMC Med. 12, 47.

Moser, D.K.,, Stevenson, W.G., Woo, M.A., 1991. Frequency of late potentials in systemic sclerosis. Ann. Cardiol. 67, 541.

Park, Y.B.,, Ahn, C.W., Choi, H.K., et al., 2002. Atherosclerosis in rheumatoid arthritis: morphologic evidence obtained by carotid ultrasound. Arthritis Rheum. 46, 1714.

Plazak, W.,, Zabinska-Plazak, E., Wojas-Pelc, A., 2002. Heart structure and function in systemic sclerosis. Eur. J. Dermatol. 12, 257.

Sherer, Y., Shoenfeld, Y., 2006. Mechanisms of disease: atherosclerosis in autoimmune diseases. Nat. Clin. Pract. Rheumatol. 2, 1.

Solomon, D.H.,, Karlson, E.W., Rimm, E.B., et al., 2003. Cardiovascular morbidity and mortality in women diagnosed with rheumatoid arthritis. Circulation 107, 1303.

Solomon, D.H.,, Curhan, G.C., Rimm, E.B., et al., 2004. Cardiovascular risk factors in women with and without rheumatoid arthritis. Arthritis Rheum. 50, 3444.

Szekanecz, Z., et al., 2007. Accelerated atherosclerosis in rheumatoid arthritis. Ann. NY Acad. Sci. 1108, 349.

Szekanecz, Z.,, Kerekes, G., Soltesz, P., 2009. Vascular effects of biologic agents in RA and spondyloarthropathies. Nat. Rev. Rheumatol. 5, 677.

Watson, D.J.,, Rhodes, T., Guess, H.A., 2003. All-cause mortality and vascular events among patients with rheumatoid arthritis, osteoarthritis, or no arthritis in the UK General Practice Research Database. J. Rheumatol. 30, 1196.

Chapter 9

New Cardiac Imaging Tools and Invasive Techniques in Systemic Autoimmune Diseases (Part II)

M. Corda,* M. Porcu,* F. Atzeni,[§] L. Gianturco,[¶] P. Sarzi-Puttini[||] and M. Turiel[¶]

*Cardiology Unit, Brotzu Hospital, Cagliari, Italy; [§]IRCCS Galeazzi Orthopedic Institute, Milan, Italy; [¶]Cardiology Unit, IRCCS Galeazzi Orthopedic Institute, Milan, Italy; [||]Rheumatology Unit, L. Sacco University Hospital, Milan, Italy

Key Points

- Cardiovascular involvement in systemic inflammatory diseases is highly heterogeneous, with manifestations affecting different heart structures. New instruments now allow an early diagnosis and prompt treatment.
- Cardiac magnetic resonance imaging has emerged as a noninvasive means of accurately and reproducibly assessing myocardial anatomy and function.
- Computed tomography is a noninvasive tool, which is highly sensitive in detecting coronary artery disease and evaluating pericardial disease.
- Right heart catheterization is a fundamental means to confirm a diagnosis of pulmonary arterial hypertension in patients with SADs.
- Endomyocardial biopsy is still the gold standard for the diagnosis of myocarditis.

1. INTRODUCTION

Systemic inflammatory diseases are associated with an increase in cardiovascular (CV) morbidity and mortality. The relationship between systemic inflammatory diseases and heart disease can only partially be explained by traditional CV risk factors, which are highly prevalent among subjects with inflammatory diseases. That prominent role is played by the immuno-mediated

The Heart in Systemic Autoimmune Diseases.

inflammatory pattern, which is activated in systemic inflammatory diseases, and the potentially unfavorable CV and metabolic effects caused by steroidal and nonsteroidal antiinflammatory drugs. Cardiovascular involvement in systemic inflammatory diseases is highly heterogeneous, with manifestations affecting the pericardium, cardiac muscle, endocardium and valves, conduction system, coronary arteries, pulmonary arterioles, great and small vessels of the systemic circulation, with an increased risk of major cardiovascular and cerebral complications.

The advances made in increasingly accurate instruments now allow an early diagnosis and prompt treatment. This chapter will describe the current role of two noninvasive [cardiac magnetic resonance imaging (CMRI) and coronary computed tomography (CT)] and two invasive methods (right heart catheterization and endomyocardial biopsy).

2. CARDIAC MAGNETIC RESONANCE IMAGING

Over the last 15 years, CMRI has emerged as a noninvasive means of accurately and reproducibly assessing myocardial anatomy and function and has become the gold standard for measuring the ejection fraction and left and right ventricular volumes (Gosh-Dastidar et al., 2016; Semelka et al., 1990). It can reveal myocardial lesions in patients with mixed connective tissue disease (CTD) and cardiac symptoms requiring further cardiac investigation and/or treatment, including myocardial infarction, inflammation, widespread subendocardial fibrosis, and perfusion defects (Mavrogeni et al., 2015). It can also be used to assess myocardial viability in patients with ischemic cardiomyopathies, to detect intraventricular thrombi and constrictive pericarditis, to quantify valve dysfunction and iron overload (T2*), to diagnose congenital heart disease and interstitial fibrosis in dilated and infiltrative cardiomyopathies, and to assess patients with suspected arrhythmogenic right ventricular dysplasia/cardiomyopathy.

2.1 Cardiac Magnetic Resonance Imaging Techniques

2.1.1 Cine Imaging

Steady-state free precession is the sequence of choice for cine imaging because of its clear definition of endocardial and epicardial borders.

2.1.2 T2-Weighted Imaging

T2-weighted (T2W) short-tau inversion recovery (STIR) imaging is a sequence sensitive to increased myocardial water content and thus allows the delineation of areas of myocardial edema. The increased mobile water content associated with edema appears hyperintense on T2W-STIR images (Abdel-Aty and Schulz-Menger, 2007) and it has been shown that the quantification of myocardial edema using tissue signal thresholds closely correlates with ischemic time (Aletras et al., 2006; Abdel-Aty and Schulz-Menger,, 2007). Myocardial edema may be present after any form of myocardial injury, including myocardial ischemia, acute infarction, myocarditis, sarcoidosis, and trauma (Abdel-Aty et al., 2007).

2.1.3 First-Pass Myocardial Perfusion Imaging

This technique tracks the transit of a contrast agent through the cardiac chambers and its perfusion in the myocardium (McAlindon et al., 2015). It is mainly used in conjunction with a stressor to evaluate the presence of inducible perfusion defects (a surrogate for inducible myocardial ischemia), which appear as hypointense areas lacking contrast perfusion because of significant coronary stenosis. The images are often acquired at the time of peak stress and during rest for purposes of comparison. The most widely used stressors are vasodilators such as adenosine and dypyridamole. In patients with acute coronary syndromes, resting first-pass perfusion can be used to assess the presence of early microvascular obstruction as a marker of microvascular damage.

2.1.4 Late Gadolinium Enhancement Imaging

One of the unique properties of CMRI is its ability to characterize tissue by means of late gadolinium enhancement imaging (LGE) because of the inherent relative differences in the distribution volume of gadolinium (Gd) in normal and abnormal myocardium (Arheden et al., 1999; Rolf et al., 2009). Gd is normally confined to the extracellular and interstitial space (e.g., it does not penetrate intact myocardial cell membranes) but changes in the interstitium, such as infiltration or fibrosis, do increase its volume of distribution and allow a larger amount of Gd to penetrate into the tissue. T1-weighted (T1W) CMRI early after Gd administration is used to assess myocardial perfusion during its "first-pass" entry into the myocardial microcirculation, whereas late imaging (10−20 min after Gd administration) allows washout from the myocardial circulation. The myocardial signal is nullified by the use of an inversion pulse, leaving the normal myocardium looking black and areas of abnormal myocardium appearing relatively bright due to the residual Gd in the tissue (Kim et al., 2003; Weaver and McCrohon, 2008). Myocyte necrosis leads to the loss of cell membrane integrity, thus allowing the intracellular accumulation of Gd as occurs in the LGE imaging of patients with myocardial infarction (Thygesen et al., 2007) (Fig. 9.1).

2.2 Clinical Role and Indications for Cardiac Magnetic Resonance Imaging

2.2.1 Ischemic Cardiomyopathy

CMRI is now considered the gold standard for assessing myocardial viability. Numerous studies have shown that left ventricular (LV) dysfunction in patients

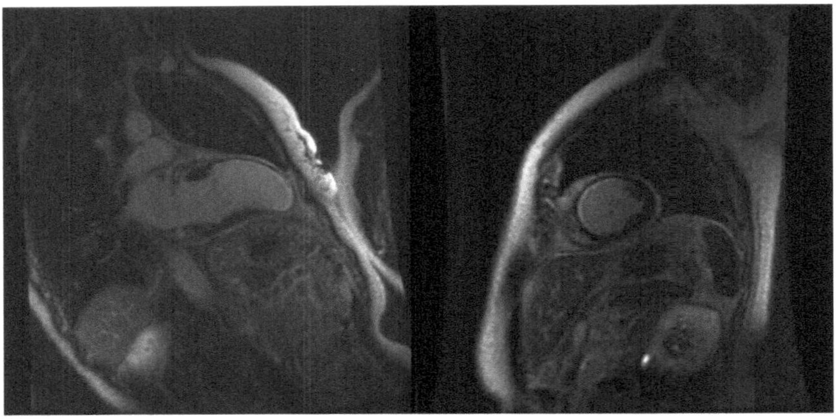

FIGURE 9.1 Cardiac magnetic resonance. A patient with a nonrecent anterior myocardial infarction. Late enhancement imaging shows transmural infarction in the left anterior descending artery territory.

with coronary artery disease (CAD) may be a reversible phenomenon related to myocardial stunning or myocardial hibernation, thus establishing that not all dysfunctional myocardium in ischemic heart disease is irreversible (Bucciarelli-Ducci et al., 2006). LGE CMRI allows the differentiation of viable and nonviable myocardium and identifies the segments that could benefit from revascularization. It has recently been demonstrated that CMRI in patients with symptomatic CTD and normal echocardiography findings can assess disease acuity and identify vasculitis, myocarditis, and myocardial infarction (Mavrogeni et al., 2014).

2.2.2 Interstitial Fibrosis

Diffuse interstitial or replacement myocardial fibrosis is a common feature of a many cardiomyopathies. Myocardial fibrosis leads to impaired diastolic and systolic function and is associated with adverse cardiovascular events. CMRI can characterize the extent of replacement fibrosis and may have prognostic value in various cardiomyopathies.

2.2.3 Infiltrative Cardiomyopathies

Infiltrative cardiomyopathies, which may present with systolic or diastolic heart failure, arrhythmias or sudden cardiac death, can be difficult to diagnose. CMRI accurately assesses ventricular morphology and allows the imaging of abnormal areas of myocardium with particular LGE patterns that correlate with the underlying infiltrative diagnosis (Mahrholdt et al., 2005). Such conditions include sarcoidosis, CTD, endomyocardial fibrosis, and amyloid infiltration (Ichinose et al., 2008; Hamilton-Craig et al., 2008) (Fig. 9.2).

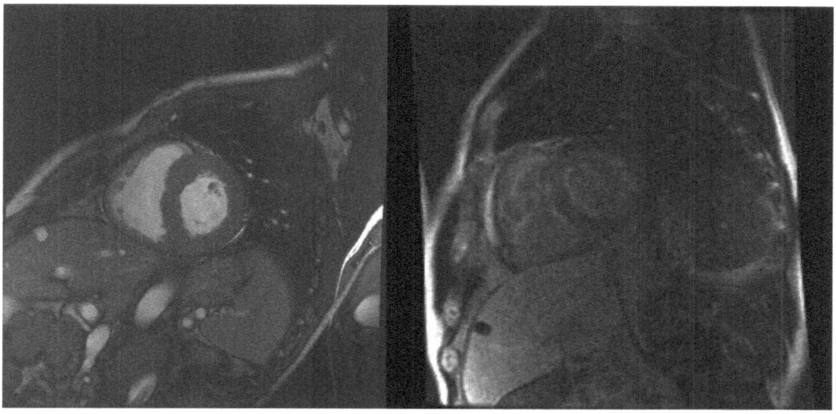

FIGURE 9.2 Cardiac magnetic resonance. Cardiac amyloidosis before and after Gadolinium administration.

2.2.4 Valve Dysfunction

CMRI can assess anatomical mechanisms and quantify severity. Echocardiographic measurements of regurgitation may be inaccurate, particularly in dilated ventricles (Schwammenthal et al., 1994), but the 3-dimensional volumetric nature of CMRI helps to overcome the heterogeneity and eccentricity of regurgitant jets (D'Ancona et al., 2008).

2.2.5 Arrhythmogenic Right Ventricular Dysplasia

CMRI is the best imaging technique for assessing RV free wall contraction abnormalities, and is particularly valuable in patients with suspected arrhythmogenic RV dysplasia (Jain et al., 2008; Sen-Chowdhry et al., 2006).

2.2.6 Constrictive Pericarditis

This condition is notoriously difficult to diagnose as the echocardiographic and invasive hemodynamic findings are often subtle. CMRI accurately assesses pericardial thickness using double and triple inversion recovery sequences and can noninvasively demonstrate ventricular interdependence (Fig. 9.3).

2.2.7 Inflammatory Vasculitis

Vasculitis (as in the case of giant cell arteritis, Takayasu arteritis, idiopathic aortitis, polyarteritis nodosa, Behçet diseasem and Churg-Strauss syndrome) can lead to devastating complications, including blindness, renal failure, aortic rupture, and heart failure as a result of a variety of end-organ effects. A delayed diagnosis significantly contributes to poor outcomes, but CMRI (with and without exogenous contrast medium) offers various noninvasive

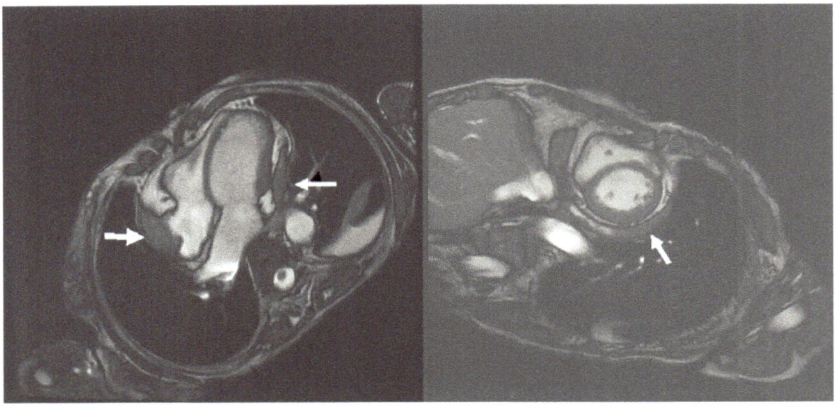

FIGURE 9.3 Cardiac magnetic resonance. On the left is a four chamber view of the ventricles showing a thickened pericardium (*arrows*). On the right is a short axis view of the same patient.

angiography and vessel wall imaging techniques. The usefulness of these techniques in patients with inflammatory vasculitis comes from the fact that they can accurately delineate the presence and extent of the disease at the time of initial presentation and they allow ongoing dialogue between CMRI specialists and the clinicians responsible for its diagnosis and long-term management (Raman et al., 2012).

3. COMPUTED TOMOGRAPHY

CT has evolved into such a potent means of diagnosis that it is now impossible to imagine clinical practice without it. It has become very important for cardiologists as it is widely available, easy to use, noninvasive, and highly sensitive in detecting coronary artery disease and evaluating pericardial diseases, pericardial fluid, and pericardial neoplasms. As coronary arteries are small, high resolution is critical for assessing their lumens, but the spatial and temporal resolution of modern multidetector row CT systems (and their volume coverage) are sufficient to allow their robust imaging in many patients (Halliburton et al., 2012).

Radiation doses are a matter of concern and special measures need to be taken to avoid unnecessarily high doses when CT is used for coronary artery imaging (Hausleiter et al., 2010). Recent advances in scanner technology and image sequencing have addressed this issue in randomized clinical trials, which indicate that coronary CT angiography (CTA) will play a greater role in assessing CAD in the years to come (Markham et al., 2016). Coronary artery CT can be performed without using contrast (coronary calcium scoring) or after an intravenous injection of an iodinated contrast agent (coronary CTA).

3.1 Coronary Calcium Scoring

Multidetector row CT without contrast can detect calcified coronary lesions, which are usually quantified using the "Agatston score" (Agatston et al., 1990). With the exception of patients with renal failure (who may have medial calcification), coronary calcium is exclusively due to coronary atherosclerosis, and correlates with its extent (O'Rourke et al., 2000), although its correlation with the degree of luminal narrowing is poor. Even severe calcification may not cause luminal stenosis, which therefore cannot be ruled out on the grounds of a low calcium score in symptomatic subjects, especially when they are young and the symptoms are acute (Marwan et al., 2009).

3.2 Coronary Computed Tomography Angiography

After the intravenous injection of a contrast agent, CT can visualize the coronary artery lumen provided that it is at least 64-slice CT, and the patients are carefully selected and prepared (Fig. 9.4). Coronary CTA should only be considered in the case of nonobese patients with a favorable calcium score who are in sinus rhythm, have a heart rate ≤65 b.p.m. (preferably ≤60 b.p.m.), and can hold their breath adequately (Abbara et al., 2009). If necessary, the use of short-acting β-blockers or other heart rate–lowering medication is recommended. As the specificity of coronary CTA decreases with increasing amounts of coronary calcium (Budoff et al., 2008; Brodoefel et al., 2008; Chen et al., 2011), and it has been found that the prevalence of coronary artery stenosis is high in symptomatic subjects with an Agatston score of >400

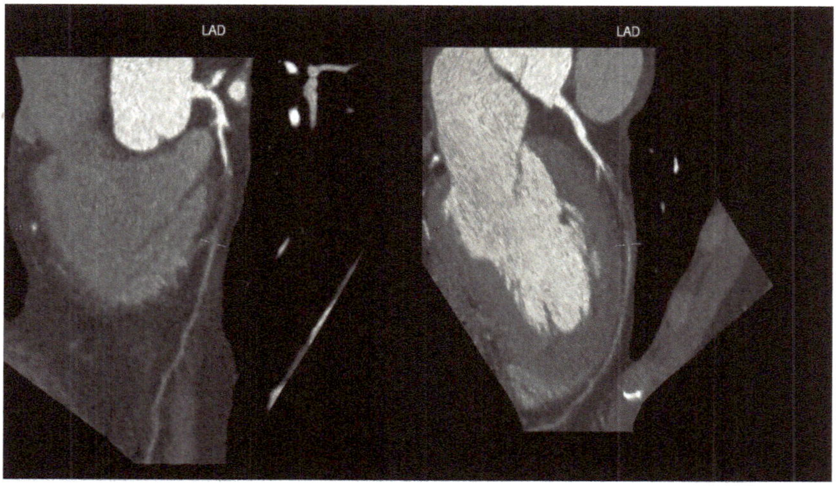

FIGURE 9.4 Cardiac computed tomography: a severe left anterior descending artery stenosis.

(van Werkhoven et al., 2010), it is reasonable not to proceed with coronary CTA if the score is >400 (Meijs et al., 2009). However, at individual patient level, per segment calcification affects diagnostic accuracy more than calcium (Vavere et al., 2011), and the effect calcium on the accuracy of coronary CTA is less pronounced in patients with low heart rates and when modern CT systems are used (Alkadhi et al., 2008; Westwood et al., 2013). If no calcium score is obtained and calcifications are only seen on the completed coronary CTA scan, it may be prudent to refrain from trying to quantify stenosis in areas of extensive calcifications and call the test "unclear."

Multicenter studies using 64-slice CT have found a sensitivity of 95–99% and a specificity of 64–83% in patients with suspected CAD, as well as negative predictive values of 97–99% for the identification of subjects with at least one coronary artery stenosis revealed by invasive coronary angiography (Budoff et al., 2008; Meijboom et al., 2008). Meta-analyses of smaller trials confirm the high sensitivity (98–99%) and negative predictive values (99–100%), and the lower specificity (82–89%) and positive predictive values (91–93%) (Paech and Weston, 2011). Severe coronary calcium negatively affects the accuracy of coronary CTA (Brodoefel et al., 2008; Vavere et al., 2011). The role of the imaging in coronary stents has been demonstrated, but partial volume effects and artifacts caused by metal frequently prevent adequate visualization of the coronary lumen inside them. The assessment of coronary artery bypass grafts is highly accurate, but there are limitations concerning the detection of stenosis at the site of the anastomosis to the coronary artery and in the peripheral run-off vessels (Ropers et al., 2006; Weustink et al., 2009). Registry data confirm an excellent prognosis if coronary CTA demonstrates the absence of coronary artery stenosis (Min et al., 2011; Chow et al., 2011).

The diagnostic performance of coronary CTA is very accurate in subjects in the lower range of intermediate pretest probability for the disease (Paech and Weston, 2011; Meijboom et al., 2007) and so it may be useful in ruling out coronary stenosis in such patients. If they have the characteristics described earlier, good image quality and reasonably low radiation exposure can be expected if appropriate technology and expertise are available. However, coronary CTA cannot rule out functional CAD.

The developments in coronary CTA, such as CT-FFR (fractional flow reserve) need further validation (Min et al., 2012).

3.3 Pericardial Disease

Pericardial disease is frequently encountered in clinical practice and may be present alone or associated with other systemic disorders such as autoimmune

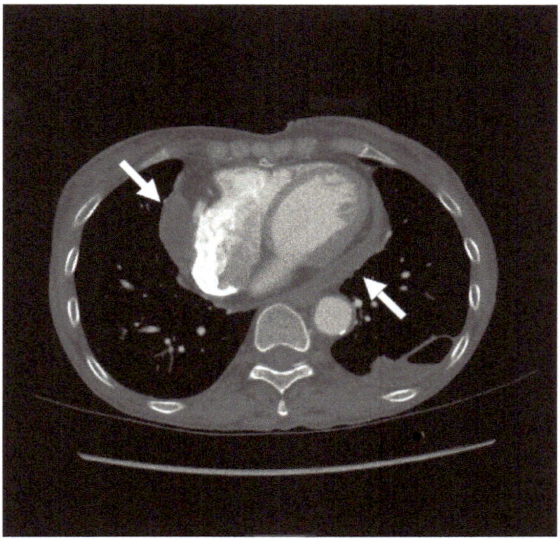

FIGURE 9.5 Cardiac computed tomography: thickened pericardium (*arrows*).

diseases. Recognizing pericardial disease can be relatively easy, particularly if the clinical manifestation is typical (e.g., acute pericarditis and an audible friction rub, reported retrosternal pain exacerbated by inspiration, or being in the supine position). However, pericardial disease can also be associated with nonspecific symptoms and equivocal physical findings that can be difficult to diagnose. In this setting, CT may be very useful as it is the most accurate means of imaging to detect the calcified tissue that is very frequent in chronic pericarditis (Cosyns et al., 2014) (Fig. 9.5).

The more common diagnostic CT findings in pericardial disease are:

- thickened pericardial layers becoming enhanced after the administration of contrast medium;
- abnormalities involving the entire pericardium;
- variable amounts of pericardial fluid;
- thickened pericardial layers and pericardial calcification (Fig. 9.6);
- possible extension of the fibrocalcific process to the adjacent myocardium;
- compression of cardiac contents by a rigid, deformed pericardium;
- fluid accumulation in the pericardial sac and/or pericardial sinuses; and
- a pericardial width of >4 mm, regarded as an abnormal amount of fluid.

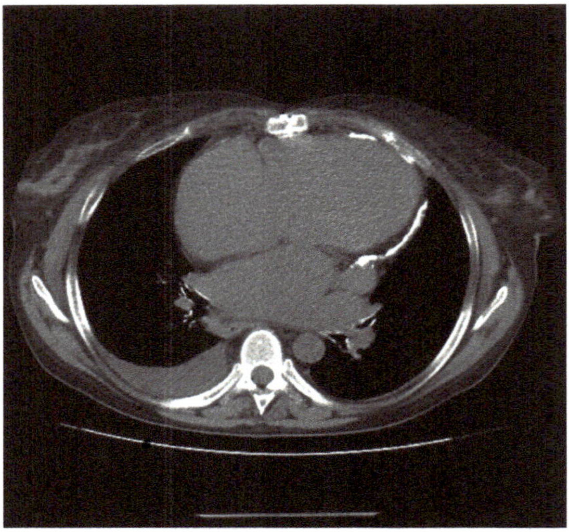

FIGURE 9.6 Cardiac computed tomography: pericardial calcification.

4. RIGHT HEART CATHETERIZATION

Pulmonary hypertension (PH) is defined as an increase in mean resting pulmonary arterial pressure (PAPm) ≥25 mmHg as assessed by means of right heart catheterization (RHC) (Hoeper et al., 2013). Normal resting PAPm is 14 ± 3 mmHg, with an upper limit of 20 mmHg (Kovacs et al., 2009); the clinical significance of PAPm values of between 21 and 24 mmHg is not clear (Hoeper et al., 2013).

Pulmonary arterial hypertension (PAH) is one of the major complications of CTDs such as systemic sclerosis (SSc), systemic lupus erythematosus, and mixed CTD (Khanna et al., 2013; Hao et al., 2014), and PAH associated with CTD is the second most prevalent type of PAH after idiopathic PAH in Western countries (Coghlan, 2013). SSc (particularly its limited variant) is the main CTD associated with PAH in Europe and the USA (Khanna et al., 2013; Hao et al., 2014) and the prevalence of precapillary PH in SSc patients ranges from 5% to 12% (Khanna et al., 2013; Hachulla et al., 2009, 2005; Avouac et al., 2010). In such patients, PH may occur in association with interstitial lung disease or be due to an isolated pulmonary vascular disease, which may affect the precapillary arterioles (PAH) and postcapillary venules as in pulmonary veno-occlusive disease (Humbert and Hassoun, 2014; Gunther et al., 2012). These patients may also have pulmonary venous hypertension due to left heart disease (Humbert and Hassoun, 2014; Fox et al., 2013; Hoeper et al., 2006). It is therefore essential to determine which hemodynamic mechanism is involved in each patient because precapillary PH [pulmonary artery wedge pressure (PAWP) ≤15 mmHg] alone must be treated with specific drugs: endothelin receptor antagonists; phosphodiesterase type 5 inhibitors and guanylate cyclase stimulators; prostacyclin analogues; and prostacyclin receptor agonists (Galie et al., 2015).

RHC allows the hemodynamic evaluation of the right heart and pulmonary artery circulation, including capillary wedge pressures. It allows to measure the cardiac output and the pulmonary vascular resistances and to detect intracardiac shunts.

It is a fundamental tool to confirm a diagnosis of PAH and to assess the risk. When performed at dedicated centers, this invasive procedure is associated with low morbidity and mortality rates (1.1% and 0.055%, respectively) (Hoeper et al., 2006). RHC is carried out antegrade through the inferior or superior vena cava, with percutaneous entry through the femoral, subclavian, jugular, or antecubital vein. The widely used balloon flotation (Swan-Ganz) catheter (Fig. 9.7) is between 50 and 125 cm long and has proximal and distal hubs, a balloon inflation valve with a syringe, and a thermistor connector. The distal tip is equipped with a balloon and end-hole, while the proximal injection port is 30 cm from the distal lumen and the thermistor just proximal to the balloon. It is both flexible and flow directed but, when the femoral approach is used, fluoroscopic guidance is almost always necessary to advance into the pulmonary artery and obtain pulmonary capillary wedge position. It is also important to measure LV end-diastolic pressure to avoid the misclassification of patients with high PAWP when this is unexpected and may be incorrect (age<65 years; no left heart disease or valvulopathy; no risk factors for heart failure with preserved ejection fraction; a normal sized left atrium and absence of echocardiographic markers of high LV filling pressures).

The most frequent complications of RHC are nonsustained atrial and ventricular arrhythmias. Major complications are infrequent but include

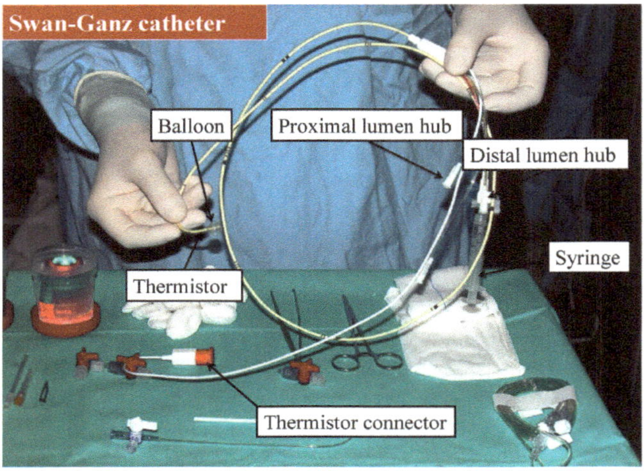

FIGURE 9.7 Swan-Ganz catheter.

pulmonary infarction, pulmonary artery, or right ventricle perforation and infection.

5. ENDOMYOCARDIAL BIOPSY

Myocarditis is an inflammatory disease of the myocardium caused by various infectious and noninfectious triggers. Systemic autoimmune diseases such as Churg-Strauss syndrome (Vinit et al., 2010) or hypereosinophilic syndrome (Loeffler disease) (Corssmit et al., 1999) can be associated with eosinophilic myocarditis. In the case of cardiac sarcoidosis (Nunes et al., 2010) and giant cell myocarditis (Cooper, 2005), which are rare causes of inflammatory myocardial disease, early diagnosis and treatment significantly improve prognosis. The diagnostic gold standard is still the endomyocardial biopsy (EMB).

5.1 Biopsy Technique

An EMB is mainly performed via the internal jugular or, less frequently, subclavian vein, although the advent of long, flexible bioptome devices permits a femoral venous approach with similar efficacy. An LV biopsy is rarely performed, but can be obtained via an arterial approach, and is indicated in the case of suspected cardiac sarcoidosis or myocarditis with primary LV involvement (Ardehali et al., 2005). It can be performed using disposable or reusable bioptomes (Figs. 9.8 and 9.9). Monitoring should include electrocardiographic rhythm, blood pressure, and pulse oximetry. The most widely used devices for the internal jugular vein approach are the stiff-shafted Caves-Schulz Stanford bioptome and the floppy-shafted King bioptome. EMB usually is performed safely under fluoroscopic guidance, but echocardiographic guidance can help visualize the biopsy location, which is important to confirm that the same site is not repeatedly biopsied (Copeland et al., 1984; Miller et al., 1988).

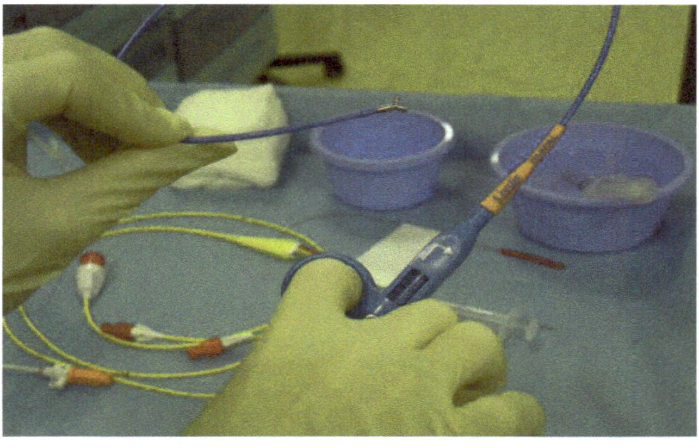

FIGURE 9.8 *Cordis* disposable bioptome. Forceps jaws (*arrow*).

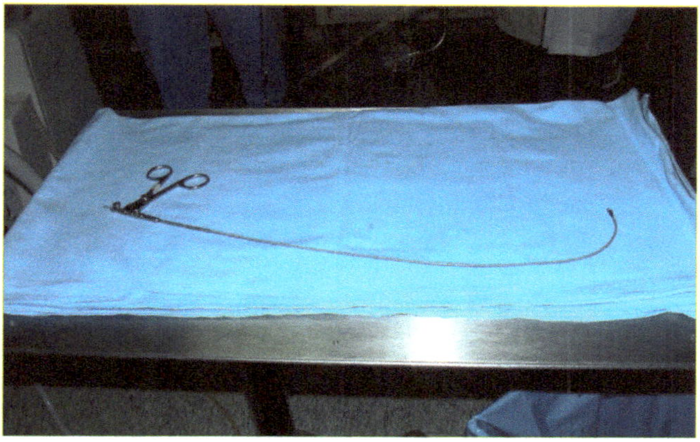

FIGURE 9.9 Stanford Caves-Shulz reusable bioptome.

First of all, a 7−9F sheath is introduced using Seldinger technique. Then a 7−9F bioptome is advanced to reach the right atrium and then, using counterclockwise rotation, the right ventricle through the tricuspid valve. The presence of ventricular premature beats and the absence of further advance indicates that the bioptome has reached the myocardium. The bioptome is then withdrawn slightly from the endocardium and the forceps jaws are opened, after which the bioptome is readvanced to the endocardium and the forceps are closed. Slight traction is felt when the device is removed. Because the right ventricular free wall is thin, obtaining biopsy specimens from this area is dangerous; consequently, biopsy samples should be taken from the interventricular septum (Ardehali et al., 2005). Between four and six samples should be taken for pathological analysis.

5.2 Complications

All decisions regarding an EMB should consider the complications associated with the procedure. The risks include myocardial perforation with pericardial tamponade, arrhythmias, heart block, pneumothorax, arterial puncture, pulmonary embolization, nerve block or injury, hematoma, damage to the tricuspid valve, the creation of an arteriovenous fistula, and deep venous thrombosis. The reported complication rates vary from <1% to as much as 6% (Yilmaz et al., 2010; Chimenti and Frustaci, 2013). The overall safety of EMB was validated in a series of nearly 6800 patients (Sekiguchi and Take, 1980): the incidence of complications was 1.2%, with perforation occurring in 0.42% and death in 0.03% of cases. Myocardial perforation can usually be managed conservatively with careful clinical and echocardiographic monitoring, although pericardiocentesis and/or thoracotomy may be required in rare cases.

6. CONCLUSION

CV complications are rather frequent in patients with SADs and may significantly increase mortality and morbidity. These invasive and noninvasive techniques are reliable means for screening, diagnosing, and following up CV manifestations in this complex group of patients. All these tools must be used keeping in mind the probability to obtain significant clinical information, balancing the usefulness and the potential procedural risks, particularly when radiological or invasive procedures are planned.

ACKNOWLEDGMENT

We would like to thank Gildo Matta, Radiology Unit of Brotzu Hospital of Cagliari, for the MRI and CT images.

REFERENCES

Abbara, S., Arbab-Zadeh, A., Callister, T.Q., et al., 2009. SCCT guidelines for performance of coronary computed tomographic angiography: a report of the Society of Cardiovascular Computed Tomography Guidelines Committee. J. Cardiovasc. Comput. Tomogr. 3, 190.

Abdel-Aty, H., Schulz-Menger, J., January 2007. Cardiovascular magnetic resonance T2-weighted imaging of myocardial edema in acute myocardial infarction. Recent Pat. Cardiovasc. Drug Discov. 2 (1), 63–68 (Review).

Abdel-Aty, H., Simonetti, O., Friedrich, M.G., 2007. T2-weighted cardiovascular magnetic resonance imaging. J. Magn. Reson. Imaging 26, 452.

Agatston, A.S., Janowitz, W.R., Hildner, F.J., et al., 1990. Quantification of coronary artery calcium using ultrafast computed tomography. J. Am. Coll. Cardiol. 15, 827.

Aletras, A.H., Tilak, G.S., Natanzon, A., et al., 2006. Retrospective determination of the area at risk for reperfused acute myocardial infarction with T2-weighted cardiac magnetic resonance imaging: histopathological and displacement encoding with stimulated echoes (DENSE) functional validations. Circulation 113, 1865.

Alkadhi, H., Scheffel, H., Desbiolles, L., et al., 2008. Dualsource computed tomography coronary angiography: influence of obesity, calcium load, and heart rate on diagnostic accuracy. Eur. Heart J. 29, 766.

Ardehali, H., Howard, D.L., Hariri, A., et al., 2005. A positive endomyocardial biopsy result for sarcoid is associated with poor prognosis in patients with initially unexplained cardiomyopathy. Am. Heart J. 150, 459.

Arheden, H., Saeed, M., Higgins, C.B., et al., 1999. Measurement of the distribution volume of gadopentetate dimeglumine at echo-planar MR imaging to quantify myocardial infarction: comparison with 99m Tc-DTPA autoradiography in rats. Radiology 211, 698.

Avouac, J., Airo, P., Meune, C., et al., 2010. Prevalence of pulmonary hypertension in systemic sclerosis in European Caucasians and metaanalysis of 5 studies. J. Rheumatol. 37, 2290.

Brodoefel, H., Burgstahler, C., Tsiflikas, I., et al., 2008. Dual-source CT: effect of heart rate, heart rate variability, and calcification on image quality and diagnostic accuracy. Radiology 247, 346.

Bucciarelli-Ducci, C., Wu, E., Lee, D.C., et al., 2006. Contrast enhanced cardiac magnetic resonance in the evaluation of myocardial infarction and myocardial viability in patients with ischemic heart disease. Curr. Probl. Cardiol. 31 (2), 128.

Budoff, M.J., Dowe, D., Jollis, J.G., et al., 2008. Diagnostic performance of 64-multidetector row coronary computed tomographic angiography for evaluation of coronary artery stenosis in individuals without known coronary artery disease: results from the prospective multicenter ACCURACY (Assessment by Coronary Computed Tomographic Angiography of Individuals Undergoing Invasive Coronary Angiography) trial. J. Am. Coll. Cardiol. 52, 1724.

Chen, C.C., Chen, C.C., Hsieh, I.C., et al., 2011. The effect of calcium score on the diagnostic accuracy of coronary computed tomography angiography. Int. J. Cardiovasc. Imaging 27 (Suppl. 1), 37.

Chimenti, C., Frustaci, A., 2013. Contribution and risks of left ventricular endomyocardial biopsy in patients with cardiomyopathies: a retrospective study over a 28-year period. Circulation 128, 1531.

Chow, B.J., Small, G., Yam, Y., et al., 2011. Incremental prognostic value of cardiac computed tomography in coronary artery disease using CONFIRM: COroNary computed tomography angiography evaluation for clinical outcomes: an InteRnational Multicenter registry. Circ. Cardiovasc. Imaging 4, 463.

Coghlan, G., 2013. Does left heart disease cause most systemic sclerosis associated pulmonary hypertension? Eur. Respir. J. 42, 888.

Cooper Jr., L.T., 2005. Giant cell and granulomatous myocarditis. Heart Fail. Clin. 1, 431.

Copeland, J.G., Valdes-Cruz, L., Sahn, D.J., 1984. Endomyocardial biopsy with fluoroscopic and two-dimensional echocardiographic guidance: case report of a patient suspected of having multiple cardiac tumors. Clin. Cardiol. 7, 449.

Corssmit, E.P., Trip, M.D., Durrer, J.D., 1999. Loeffler's endomyocarditis in the idiopathic hypereosinophilic syndrome. Cardiology 91, 272.

Cosyns, B., Plein, S., Nihoyanopoulos, P., Smiseth, O., et al., 2014. On behalf of the European Association of Cardiovascular Imaging (EACVI) and European Society of Cardiology Working Group (ESC WG) on Myocardial and Pericardial diseases. European Association of Cardiovascular Imaging (EACVI) position paper: multimodality imaging in pericardial disease. Eur. Heart J. Cardiovasc. Imaging 16, 12.

D'Ancona, G., Biondo, D., Mamone, G., et al., 2008. Ischemic mitral valve regurgitation in patients with depressed ventricular function: cardiac geometrical and myocardial perfusion evaluation with magnetic resonance imaging. Eur. J. Cardiothorac. Surg. 34, 964.

Fox, B.D., Shimony, A., Langleben, D., et al., 2013. High prevalence of occult left heart disease in scleroderma-pulmonary hypertension. Eur. Respir. J. 42, 1083.

Galie, N., Humbert, M., Vachiery, J.L., et al., 2015. ESC/ERS guidelines for the diagnosis and treatment of pulmonary hypertension: the joint task force for the diagnosis and treatment of pulmonary hypertension of the European Society of Cardiology (ESC) and the European Respiratory Society (ERS): endorsed by: Association for European Paediatric and Congenital Cardiology (AEPC), International Society for Heart and Lung Transplantation (ISHLT). Eur. Respir. J. 46, 903.

Gosh-Dastidar, A., Rodrigues, J., Baritussio, A., et al., 2016. Magnetic resonance imaging in the assessment of ischaemic heart disease. Heart 102 (3), 239.

Gunther, S., Jaïs, X., Maitre, S., et al., 2012. Computed tomography findings of pulmonary venoocclusive disease in scleroderma patients presenting with precapillary pulmonary hypertension. Arthritis Rheum. 64, 2995.

Hachulla, E., Carpentier, P., Gressin, V., et al., 2009. ItinerAIR-Sclerodermie Study Investigators. Risk factors for death and the 3-year survival of patients with systemic sclerosis: the French ItinerAIR-Sclerodermie study. Rheumatology 48, 304.

Hachulla, E., Gressin, V., Guillevin, L., et al., 2005. Early detection of pulmonary arterial hypertension in systemic sclerosis: a French nationwide prospective multicenter study. Arthritis Rheum. 52, 3792.

Halliburton, S., Arbab-Zadeh, A., Dey, D., et al., 2012. State-of-the-art in CT hardware and scan modes for cardiovascular CT. J. Cardiovasc. Comput. Tomogr. 6, 154.

Hamilton-Craig, C.R., Harker, J., Strugnell, W.E., et al., 2008. Diagnostic features of endomyocardial fibrosis by cardiac MRI. Heart Lung Circ. 17, S52.

Hao, Y.J., Jiang, X., Zhou, W., 2014. Connective tissue disease-associated pulmonary arterial hypertension in Chinese patients. Eur. Respir. J. 44, 963.

Hausleiter, J., Martinoff, S., Hadamitzky, M., 2010. Image quality and radiation exposure with a low tube voltage protocol for coronary CT angiography results of the PROTECTION II Trial. JACC Cardiovasc. Imaging 3, 1113.

Hoeper, M.M., Bogaard, H.J., Condliffe, R., et al., 2013. Definitions and diagnosis of pulmonary hypertension. J. Am. Coll. Cardiol. 62 (Suppl.), D42.

Hoeper, M.M., Lee, S.H., Voswinckel, R., et al., 2006. Complications of right heart catheterization procedures in patients with pulmonary hypertension in experienced centers. J. Am. Coll. Cardiol. 48, 2546.

Humbert, M., Hassoun, P.M., 2014. Update in systemic sclerosis-associated pulmonary arterial hypertension. Presse Med. 43, e293.

Ichinose, A., Otani, H., Oikawa, M., et al., 2008. MRI of cardiac sarcoidosis: basal and subepicardial localization of myocardial lesions and their effect on left ventricular function. AJR Am. J. Roentgenol. 191, 862.

Jain, A., Tandri, H., Calkins, H., et al., 2008. Role of cardiovascular magnetic resonance imaging in arrhythmogenic right ventricular dysplasia. J. Cardiovasc. Magn. Reson. 10, 32.

Khanna, D., Gladue, H., Channick, R., et al., 2013. Recommendations for screening and detection of connective tissue disease-associated pulmonary arterial hypertension. Arthritis Rheum. 65, 3194.

Kim, R.J., Choi, K., Judd, R.M., et al., 2003. Assessment of Myocardial Viability by Contrast Enhancement. Cardiovascular MRI and MRA. Lippincot Williams and Wilkins, Philadelpia, PA, p. 209.

Kovacs, G., Berghold, A., Scheidl, S., et al., 2009. Pulmonary arterial pressure during rest and exercise in healthy subjects. A systematic review. Eur. Respir. J. 34, 888.

Mahrholdt, H., Wagner, A., Judd, R.M., et al., 2005. Delayed enhancement cardiovascular magnetic resonance assessment of non-ischaemic cardiomyopathies. Eur. Heart J. 26, 1461.

Markham, R., et al., 2016. Coronary computed tomography angiography and its increasing application in day to day cardiology practice. Intern. Med. J. 46 (1), 29.

Marwan, M., Ropers, D., Pflederer, T., et al., 2009. Clinical characteristics of patients with obstructive coronary lesions in the absence of coronary calcification: an evaluation by coronary CT angiography. Heart 95, 1056.

Mavrogeni, S., et al., 2014. Cardiac tissue characterization and the diagnostic value of cardiovascular magnetic resonance in systemic connective tissue diseases. Arthritis Care Res. 66 (1), 104.

Mavrogeni, S., et al., 2015. Imaging patterns of cardiovascular involvement in mixed connective tissue disease evaluated by cardiovascular magnetic resonance. Inflamm. Allergy Drug Targets 14 (2), 111.

McAlindon, E.J., Pufulete, M., Harris, J.M., et al., 2015. Measurement of myocardium at risk with cardiovascular MR: comparison of techniques for edema imaging, 275 (1), 61.

Meijboom, W.B., Meijs, M.F., Schuijf, J.D., et al., 2008. Diagnostic accuracy of 64-slice computed tomography coronary angiography: a prospective, multicenter, multivendor study. J. Am. Coll. Cardiol. 52, 2135.

Meijboom, W.B., van Mieghem, C.A., Mollet, N.R., et al., 2007. 64-slice computed tomography coronary angiography in patients with high, intermediate, or low pretest probability of significant coronary artery disease. J. Am. Coll. Cardiol. 50, 1469.

Meijs, M.F., Meijboom, W.B., Prokop, M., et al., 2009. Is there a role for CT coronary angiography in patients with symptomatic angina? Effect of coronary calcium score on identification of stenosis. Int. J. Cardiovasc. Imaging 25, 847.

Miller, L.W., Labovitz, A.J., McBride, L.A., et al., 1988. Echocardiography-guided endomyocardial biopsy: a 5-year experience. Circulation 78 (5 pt 2), III−99.

Min, J.K., Dunning, A., Lin, F.Y., et al., 2011. Age- and sex-related differences in all-cause mortality risk based on coronary computed tomography angiography findings results from the International Multicenter CONFIRM (Coronary CTAngiography Evaluation for Clinical Outcomes: an International Multicenter Registry) of 23,854 patients without known coronary artery disease. J. Am. Coll. Cardiol. 58, 849.

Min, J.K., Leipsic, J., Pencina, M.J., et al., 2012. Diagnostic accuracy of fractional flow reserve from anatomic CT angiography. JAMA 308, 1237.

Nunes, H., Freynet, O., Naggara, N., et al., 2010. Cardiac sarcoidosis. Semin. Respir. Crit. Care Med. 31, 428.

O'Rourke, R.A., Brundage, B.H., Froelicher, V.F., et al., 2000. American College of Cardiology/American Heart Association Expert Consensus document on electron-beam computed tomography for the diagnosis and prognosis of coronary artery disease. Circulation 102, 126.

Paech, D.C., Weston, A.R., 2011. A systematic review of the clinical effectiveness of 64-slice or higher computed tomography angiography as an alternative to invasive coronary angiography in the investigation of suspected coronary artery disease. BMC Cardiovasc. Disord. 11, 32.

Raman, et al., 2012. CMR in inflammatory vasculitis. J. Cardiovasc. Magn. Reson. 14, 82.

Rolf, A., Nef, H.M., Mollmann, H., et al., 2009. Immunohistological basis of the late gadolinium enhancement phenomenon in tako-tsubo cardiomyopathy. Eur. Heart J. 30, 1635.

Ropers, D., Pohle, F.K., Kuettner, A., et al., 2006. Diagnostic accuracy of noninvasive coronary angiography in patients after bypass surgery using 64-slice spiral computed tomography with 330-ms gantry rotation. Circulation 114, 2334.

Schwammenthal, E., Chen, C., Benning, F., et al., 1994. Dynamics of mitral regurgitant flow and orifice area. Physiologic application of the proximal flow convergence method: clinical data and experimental testing. Circulation 90, 307.

Sekiguchi, M., Take, M., 1980. World survey of catheter biopsy of the heart. In: Sekiguchi, M., Olsen, E.G. (Eds.), Cardiomyopathy: Clinical, Pathological and Theoretical Aspects. University Park Press, Baltimore.

Semelka, R.C., Tomei, E., Wagner, S., et al., 1990. Interstudy reproducibility of dimensional and functional measurements between cine magnetic resonance studies in the morphologically. Am. Heart J. 119 (6), 1367.

Sen-Chowdhry, S., Prasad, S.K., Syrris, P., et al., 2006. Cardiovascular magnetic resonance in arrhythmogenic right ventricular cardiomyopathy revisited: comparison with task force criteria and genotype. J. Am. Coll. Cardiol. 48, 2132.

Thygesen, K., Alpert, J.S., White, H.D., 2007. On behalf of the Joint ESC/ACCF/AHA/WHF Task Force for the Redefinition of Myocardial Infarction. Universal definition of myocardial infarction. J. Am. Coll. Cardiol. 50, 2173.

van Werkhoven, J.M., de Boer, S.M., Schuijf, J.D., et al., 2010. Impact of clinical presentation and pretest likelihood on the relation between calcium score and computed tomographic coronary angiography. Am. J. Cardiol. 106, 1675.

Vavere, A.L., Arbab-Zadeh, A., Rochitte, C.E., et al., 2011. Coronary artery stenoses: accuracy of 64-detector row CT angiography in segments with mild, moderate, or severe calcification: a sub analysis of the CORE-64 trial. Radiology 261, 100.

Vinit, J., Bielefeld, P., Muller, G., et al., 2010. Heart involvement in Churg-Strauss syndrome: retrospective study in French Burgundy population in past 10 years. Eur. J. Intern. Med. 21, 341.

Weaver, J.C., McCrohon, J.A., 2008. Contrast-enhanced cardiac MRI in myocardial infarction. Heart Lung Circ. 17, 290.

Westwood, M.E., Raatz, H.D., Misso, K., et al., 2013. Systematic review of the accuracy of dual-source cardiac CT for detection of arterial stenosis in difficult to image patient groups. Radiology 267 (2), 387.

Weustink, A.C., Nieman, K., Pugliese, F., et al., 2009. Diagnostic accuracy of computed tomography angiography in patients after bypass grafting: comparison with invasive coronary angiography. JACC Cardiovasc. Imaging 2, 816.

Yilmaz, A., Kindermann, I., Kindermann, M., et al., 2010. Comparative evaluation of left and right ventricular endomyocardial biopsy: differences in complication rate and diagnostic performance. Circulation 122, 900.

Chapter 10

Cardiac Diseases in Rheumatoid Arthritis

R. Agca, M. Heslinga and M. Nurmohamed
Amsterdam Rheumatology and Immunology Center and Reade, Amsterdam, The Netherlands

Key Points

- Rheumatoid arthritis (RA) is a chronic systemic autoinflammatory disorder that is associated with an increased cardiovascular (CV) morbidity and mortality, mainly caused by atherosclerotic disease, but nonatherosclerotic traditional rheumatic heart disease also contributes.
- In patients with RA, traditional risk factors for cardiovascular disease (CVD) are more often present.
- Inflammation substantially contributes to the increased CV risk, independent of traditional CV risk factors.
- Awareness of the heightened CV risk and timely initiation of CV risk management, next to optimal control of inflammation with antiinflammatory therapy, is necessary to reduce the occurrence of CVD in patients with RA.
- CV risk assessment should be performed regularly in these patients according to existing recommendations for prevention and management of CVD in the general population and in patients with inflammatory joint disorders.

1. INTRODUCTION

1.1 Rheumatoid Arthritis

Rheumatoid arthritis (RA) is the prototype systemic autoimmune disease. It affects approximately 1% of the general population worldwide (Gabriel and Michaud, 2009). The prevalence varies across different populations and increases with age. Disease onset is typically in the fourth, fifth, or sixth decade of life, with a predominance in women (i.e., female to male ratio

The Heart in Systemic Autoimmune Diseases.

2–3:1). RA is characterized by a chronic symmetric inflammation of synovial joints leading to severe pain, major disability, and premature death. The systemic inflammation of RA can involve extraarticular tissues including the skin, bowels, lungs, kidneys, nervous system, and also the cardiovascular system (Gabriel and Michaud, 2009). The etiology of RA is unknown. The interplay between several genetic and environmental risk factors is suggested to play a role in susceptibility, development, and progression of this disease (Symmons, 2002). It is suggested that the incidence and severity of RA has declined over the past few decades (Doran et al., 2002; Silman, 2002), but some studies report an increased incidence and prevalence in women in the last decennium (Cross et al., 2014; Myasoedova et al., 2010). Possible explanations are the use of new-generation oral contraceptives with lower doses of synthetic estrogen, a slower decline of smoking rate in women and vitamin D deficiency (Myasoedova et al., 2010). Early and optimal antiinflammatory therapy is expected to decrease the extraarticular effects of RA. Nonetheless, mortality rates remain high and cardiovascular disease (CVD) is thought to be one of the major contributing factors.

1.2 Mortality in Rheumatoid Arthritis

RA is associated with progressive joint damage, functional disability, increased mortality rates, and decreased quality of life. The majority of studies from around the world report increased standardized mortality ratios (SMRs) in RA ranging from 0.9 to 2.7 in comparison with the general population (Table 10.1). A large proportion of these deaths is attributable to CVD (Solomon et al., 2003; Sparks et al., 2015; Turesson et al., 2004). A recent metaanalysis of 14 observational cohort studies showed a relative risk of 1.48 (95% CI 1.36–1.62) for a first ever cardiovascular (CV) event in RA patients, predominantly caused by an increased risk of myocardial infarction (MI), cerebrovascular accidents (CVA), and congestive heart failure (CHF) (Avina-Zubieta et al., 2012). A small proportion of RA patients dies of other causes, such as pulmonary disease, infection, renal disease, gastrointestinal disorders, lymphoproliferative disorders, and lung cancer (Naz and Symmons, 2007) more frequently than the general population. Some studies suggest that the disease course of RA has become milder in recent years as a result of advances in (earlier) therapeutic treatment, but CVD-related mortality has remained equally elevated over the past 5 decades (Meune et al., 2009). Cardiac involvement in RA can be of atherosclerotic or non-atherosclerotic origin (Fig. 10.1). As both types of CVD have clinical implications for these patients, an understanding and awareness of these extraarticular manifestations of RA is vital for clinicians to timely initiate CV risk management in these patients in daily clinical practice. In this chapter, an overview of the recent literature regarding both atherosclerotic and non-atherosclerotic cardiovascular manifestations of RA will be presented.

TABLE 10.1 Mortality Studies in Rheumatoid Arthritis

Study/Reference	Inclusion Period	*n*	SMR	CV Mortality
England et al. (2016)/England et al. (2015)	2003–2013	1652 (men)	1.97	Excess CV death
Sparks et al. (2015)	1976 –2012	964 (women)	1.40	Excess CV death
Humphreys et al. (2014)	1990–2011	2517	1.22 (overall) 1.39 (antibody-positives)	Excess CV death in antibody-positive subgroup
Kuo et al. (2013)	2002–2007	15,967	1.25	No excess CVD deaths
Lassere et al. (2012)/Lassere et al. (2013)	1990–1994	608	1.65	Excess CV death
Gonzalez et al. (2007)	1955–1995	822	1.35	Not reported
Young et al. (2006)/Young et al. (2007)	1986–2004	1429	1.27	Excess CV death
Goodson et al. (2005)	1981–2002	1010	1.45 (males) 1.84 (females)	Excess CV death
Pincus et al. (2004)	1985–1995	1378	1.6	Not reported
Thomas et al. (2003)	1981–2000	33,318	2.07 (males) 1.97 (females)	Excess CV death
Gabriel et al. (2003)	1955–1994	609	1.27	Not reported
Wolfe et al. (2003) (Stanford)	1965–1990	886	3.08	Excess CVD deaths
Mikuls et al. (2002)	1986–1997	158	1.52[a]	Excess CVD deaths
Peltomaa et al. (2002)	1986–1989	87	0.93	No excess CVD deaths

Continued

TABLE 10.1 Mortality Studies in Rheumatoid Arthritis—cont'd

Study/Reference	Inclusion Period	*n*	SMR	CV Mortality
Bjornadal et al. (2002)	1964–1995	46,917	2.03	Excess CVD deaths
Riise et al. (2001)	1978–1982	187	2.0	No excess CVD deaths
Chehata et al. (2001)	1981–1985	309	1.65	Not reported
Martinez et al. (2001)	1989–1998	182	1.85	Excess CV death
Kroot et al. (2000)/Kroot et al. (2001)	1985–1997	622	No increased mortality	No excess CVD deaths
Kvalvik et al. (2000)	1977	147	1.49	Excess CV deaths in females
Lindqvist and Eberhardt (1999)	1985–1989	183	0.87	No excess CVD deaths
Sokka et al. (1999)	1983–1989	135	1.28	No excess CVD deaths
Symmons et al. (1998)	1968–1974	448	2.7	Excess CVD deaths
Wållberg-Jonsson et al. (1997)	1979	606	1.57	Excess CVD deaths
Callahan et al. (1996)	1980–1990	1384	1.54	Not reported
Wolfe et al. (1994) (Santa Clara)	1978–1979	305	2.18	Excess CVD deaths
Wolfe et al. (1994) (Saskatoon)	1966–1974	905	2.24	Excess CVD deaths
Wolfe et al. (1994) (Wichita)	1973–1990	1405	1.98	Excess CVD deaths
Jacobsson et al. (1993)	1965–1989	2979	1.28	Excess CVD deaths
van Schaardenburg et al. (1993)	1980–1986	130	1.69	Excess CVD deaths
Reilly et al. (1990)	1957–1963	100	1.4	Excess CVD deaths

[a]*Relative risk of mortality is described in this study instead of SMR.*

2. ATHEROSCLEROTIC CARDIOVASCULAR DISEASE IN RHEUMATOID ARTHRITIS

2.1 Introduction

In the last decade inflammation has been linked to atherogenesis and the development of atherosclerotic lesions (Blake and Ridker, 2001). Nowadays, atherosclerosis itself is regarded as an inflammatory process with inflammatory cells involved in all its stages (Libby et al., 2002; Ross, 1999). In this section a literature overview will be presented of atherosclerotic cardiovascular disease in RA. The role of traditional and novel CV risk factors and the inflammation inherent to RA will be discussed.

2.2 Epidemiology

The magnitude of the increased CV risk in RA has been investigated in several studies. A recent metaanalysis of observational cohort studies comprising over 40,000 patients from different parts of the world showed an overall 48% (pooled RR 1.48, 95% CI 1.36–1.62) increased risk of a first ever CV event in RA patients, mainly caused by an increased risk of MI (pooled RR 1.68, 95% CI 1.40–2.03), CVA (pooled RR 1.41, 95% CI 1.14–1.74), and CHF (pooled RR 1.87, 95% CI 1.47–2.39) (Avina-Zubieta et al., 2012). In this metaanalysis, RA patients had a higher risk of MI (overall 68%) than stroke (overall 41%) when compared to the general population, while there are also studies that report a nonsignificant trend for an increased stroke risk in these patients (Levy et al., 2008; Solomon et al., 2003; Turesson et al., 2004). Only one study described a significant increased risk of CHF in RA patients when compared to controls, most evident in rheumatoid-factor positive patients (Nicola et al., 2005). Heterogeneity was statistically significant for the included studies in this metaanalysis, with no statistically significant increased risk of CVD in the included inception cohorts, most probably due to a shorter RA duration, less severe disease, and a shorter follow-up. A prospective Dutch study from 2009 also demonstrated a two-fold increased risk of CV events in RA independent of traditional CV risk factors (Peters et al., 2009). The CV risk was equal to that in diabetes mellitus (DM) type 2 (Peters et al., 2009). Similar results were found in a Danish nationwide study in 2011 (Lindhardsen et al., 2011). Several studies suggest that the disease course of RA has become milder in recent years as a result of developments in therapeutic strategies, but CVD-related mortality has remained high in RA patients when compared to the general population (Meune et al., 2009; Widdifield et al., 2015). Under-recognition and undertreatment of CV risk factors or a lack of optimal disease control by medication might be the reason for this. Another plausible explanation is that the favorable effects of antiinflammatory therapy on CV risk may only be evident after decades of treatment. It is presumed that control of inflammation with optimal antirheumatic therapy should reduce CV risk in

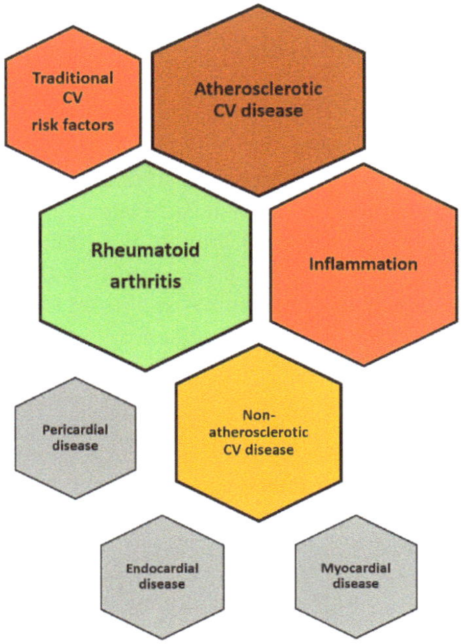

FIGURE 10.1 Factors contributing to cardiovascular diseases in rheumatoid arthritis.

these patient. Recently published cohort studies with extended follow-up investigating incident CVD are lacking. There is a need for continuous high-quality large population-based studies on CV morbidity and mortality in RA patients over time to investigate the prevalence/incidence of CVD in RA.

2.3 Etiology of Ischaemic Heart Disease in Rheumatoid Arthritis

The development of CVD is associated with several risk factors in the general population (Dawber, 1980). These risk factors are shown in Table 10.2. The conventional CV risk factors are more often present in patients with RA, but cannot fully explain the excess morbidity and mortality found in RA populations. The chronic inflammation inherent to RA is suggested to play an important role in the development and progression of atherosclerosis and might explain the excess CV risk in these patients. In addition, some novel risk factors have been associated to CVD development in recent years.

2.3.1 Traditional Cardiovascular Risk Factors

Traditional risk factors for CVD (Table 10.2) are more often present in patients with RA (Peters et al., 2009). These modifiable and nonmodifiable risk factors

TABLE 10.2 Traditional Risk Factors for Cardiovascular Diseases

Nonmodifiable	Age
	(male) Gender
	Family history of CVD
Modifiable	Smoking
	Physical inactivity
	Obesity
	Hypertension
	Dyslipidemia
	Insulin resistance/diabetes mellitus

contribute to the excess CV risk in RA, but for some risk factors this contribution is different than in the general population. In this section, we discuss the effects of these risk factors in RA.

2.3.1.1 Hypertension

A cross-sectional study of 400 second-care patients with RA identified hypertension in 70.5% of these patients, but only 60.6% were receiving antihypertensive therapy (Panoulas et al., 2007). Most of them had suboptimal blood pressure control and hypertension was undiagnosed and untreated in the remaining 39.6%. The international COMORA study reported a hypertension prevalence of 40.4% in RA patients, but there was no control group in this study (Dougados et al., 2014). A metaanalysis from 2011 reported no significant difference in blood pressure between RA patients and the general population (Boyer et al., 2011). However, some studies published after this metaanalysis did report an increased prevalence of hypertension in patients with RA (Protogerou et al., 2013; van Halm et al., 2009). This disparity in study results might be due to underrecognition and undertreatment of hypertension in patients with RA, or due to differences in the definition of hypertension (Boyer et al., 2011; Gonzalez et al., 2008; Panoulas et al., 2007). A possible explanation for an elevated blood pressure in RA might be the use of certain antiinflammatory agents, such as corticosteroids and nonsteroidal antiinflammatory drugs (NSAIDs). Also, inflammatory cells involved in the etiology of RA itself might cause endothelial dysfunction and peripheral vascular resistance (Wong et al., 2003). Currently, there is some evidence suggesting that certain antirheumatic agents, such as TNF-α inhibitors (TNFi) can have positive effect on blood pressure in these patients (Sandoo et al., 2011a).

2.3.1.2 Smoking

Smoking is acknowledged as a risk factor for CVD development. This risk is dose and duration dependent without a lower limit for detrimental effects in the general population (Perk et al., 2012). It is suggested that smoking increases CV risk by affecting endothelial function, platelet function, and vasomotor function through reactive oxygen species triggering inflammatory processes in the arterial wall (Perk et al., 2012). Any type of smoking is a risk factor for the development of RA (Costenbader et al., 2006; Sugiyama et al., 2010; Wolfe, 2000) and the amount of duration seems to be associated with severity (Saag et al., 1997). Smoking is more prevalent in RA patients compared to controls (Boyer et al., 2011; Solomon et al., 2003; Stolt et al., 2003). However, the contribution of smoking to CV risk in RA is less well-established (Gonzalez et al., 2008). Smoking is associated with RA-related factors that are associated with CV outcomes themselves, such as rheumatoid factor (RF) and anti-citrullinated protein anibody (ACPA) positivity (Klareskog et al., 2011; Wolfe, 2000), rheumatoid nodules (Wolfe, 2000), response to TNFi (Abhishek et al., 2010; Hyrich et al., 2006), and rheumatoid cachexia (Stavropoulos-Kalinoglou et al., 2008). These interactions make it difficult to determine the exact contribution of smoking to CV risk in RA.

2.3.1.3 Lipids

In the general population high serum levels of total cholesterol (TC), low-density lipoprotein cholesterol (LDLc), and triglycerides (TG) and low serum levels of high-density lipoprotein cholesterol (HDLc) are associated with an increased CV risk. RA patients with active disease have low TC and LDLc levels, while their CV risk is increased (Boyer et al., 2012; Myasoedova et al., 2011). Simultaneously, HDLc decreases during disease flares in these patients, with possible negative effects of inflammation on the antiatherogenic properties of HDLc and LDLc (Boyer et al., 2012). This proatherogenic change in lipids might be a possible explanation of the increased CV risk in these patients. In addition, certain lipid particles are capable of influencing inflammatory pathways; for example, HDLc is able to intervene in the interaction between T-cell lymphocytes and macrophages. Thus, in certain circumstances HDLc becomes a modifier of inflammation (Burger and Dayer, 2002). Antirheumatic therapy decreases inflammation and generally normalizes the lipid profile in RA. HDLc levels generally improve with treatment (Navarro-Millan et al., 2013), but LDLc and TC levels generally also increase in serum. However, it is unlikely that the increase in TC and LDLc levels after antiinflammatory treatment translates into an increased CV risk in these patients due to a concomitant increase of HDLc. This increase in lipids is thus a reflection of a good response to therapy. Moreover, HDL efflux function may improve with antiinflammatory therapy even in the absence of quantitative changes in lipids. Still, the clinical relevance of short-term changes in lipid particles protein content on CV outcomes remains to be determined. Dyslipidemia can effectively be treated with statins to reduce CV risk in RA equal to the general population (Rollefstad et al., 2015; Schoenfeld et al., 2015). In addition, statins have antiinflammatory effects and may reduce CV risk even further in RA when combined with antirheumatic therapy (Maki-Petaja et al., 2007). Another important issue to acknowledge is that the earlier mentioned changes in lipids in active RA could lead to a possible underestimation of CV risk in these patients. Thus, lipid levels should be assessed in periods of remission and if that is not possible when the disease activity is low or stable. If this is also not possible, the total cholesterol HDLc ratio is recommended for CV-risk estimation as this is a more stable lipid marker under inflammatory conditions (Peters et al., 2010b; Toms et al., 2011). The TC/HDLc ratio correlates better with C-reactive protein levels and the subsequent CV event risk in comparison to TC or HDLc alone (Peters et al., 2010b; Toms et al., 2011).

2.3.1.4 Insulin Resistance and Diabetes Mellitus

Insulin resistance (IR) is increased in RA when compared to the general population and associated with elevated serum levels of C-reactive protein (CRP), erythrocyte sedimentation rate (ESR), interleukin-6, and tumor necrosis factor α (Liao and Solomon, 2013). However, data regarding the prevalence of type 2 DM in RA are conflicting. It is not clear whether DM and RA are associated in a pathophysiological way. The association of both IR and DM with CV risk in RA appears to be similar to that in the general population (Baghdadi et al., 2015).

2.3.1.5 Physical Activity

Patients with RA are more physically inactive on average when compared to controls and this is associated with an increased CV risk (van den Berg et al., 2007). Exercise reduces CV risk in the general population, possibly through reduction of inflammation. One study described beneficial effects of exercise on serum CRP levels in the general population (Ford, 2002). Although there are not many studies investigating the effects of exercise on CV risk in RA, it is presumable that exercise might also have beneficial effects on the CV risk in these patients. There is no evidence that the effects of exercise would differ in patients with RA when compared to the general population. A recent study indeed shows beneficial effects of exercise therapy on vascular function, cardiorespiratory fitness, and CV risk in RA (Stavropoulos-Kalinoglou et al., 2013).

2.3.1.6 Body Weight and Composition

It is unclear whether body mass index (BMI) differs between patients with RA and the general population. A high BMI is associated with an increased CV risk. In the same manner, a low BMI is also associated with an increased CV risk in RA (van Halm et al., 2009). Patients with RA have more body fat for a given BMI when compared to controls (Giles et al., 2010). In active RA, lean body mass or muscle mass is commonly lost while fat mass is preserved or increased (Summers et al., 2010). This is also known as rheumatoid cachexia. One study in patients with RA with active disease reported lower BMI and fat-free mass in patients with disease flares when compared to healthy controls, which disappeared after treatment (Binymin et al., 2011). In most patients with RA the BMI remains stable over the course of the disease while fat-free mass is lost and fat mass is increased. Therefore, BMI may not give an accurate assessment of the CV risk in these patients. Restoring lean body mass in these patients has been shown to be possible with high-intensity resistance training and this has beneficial effects on the CV risk (Lemmey et al., 2009).

2.3.2 Other Cardiovascular Risk Factors

Several other risk factors have been associated with CVD risk in recent years such as high-sensitivity CRP, fibrinogen, homocysteine, and lipoprotein-associated phospholipase. Although these risk markers have shown to be independently associated with CV risk, they have only limited additional value when they are added to CV risk assessment tools such as the SCORE algorithm (Perk et al., 2012) together with high costs in general. The most recent European Cardiology guideline for CVD prevention in clinical practice advises to use these biomarkers only for refined risk assessment in patients with an unusual or moderate CV risk.

Next to these biomarkers of CVD, thyroid disease has been identified as another contributor to CV risk. Autoimmune hypothyroidism is a common disease with an estimated prevalence of up to 2% in the general population (Canaris et al., 2000; Vanderpump et al., 1995). The prevalence of hypothyroidism is increased in RA (Raterman et al., 2012). Autoimmune hypothyroidism and RA often coexist and this has been associated with an increased CV risk in females compared to euthyroid RA females (Raterman et al., 2008). Hypothyroidism and inflammatory arthritis are independently associated with an elevated CV risk and this CV risk is amplified in patients when both rheumatoid arthritis and hypothyroidism are present (Raterman et al., 2012). This might be due to detrimental effects of inflammation on endothelial function, leading to oxidative stress and accelerated atherosclerosis. Assessment of thyroid function and consequent treatment of thyroid disorders might improve CV risk in patients with RA.

Another new area of interest is that of lipidomics. Hyperlipidemia is a well-recognized risk factor for CVD in the general population. In RA, the "classic" hyperlipidaemic phenotype is rarely observed. Therefore, other lipid measurements such as HDL lipid and protein composition and HDL size distribution but also measurements of HDL functionality reflected by the capacity to efflux cholesterol from different tissue depots might be a better reflection of the pro- or antiatherogenic status of these molecules, leading to an improved risk assessment in RA populations. Lipoproteins comprise a continuum of particles that have different sizes, densities, and apolipoprotein and lipid composition. The distribution of these subfractions differs between individuals, even if their conventional lipid profiles (i.e., TC, HDLc and LDLc levels) are similar and this might translate into different cardiovascular risk profiles. For example, reduced levels of large HDL2 subfractions are thought to be associated with CVD. HDLc is known for its atheroprotective properties, which rely directly on its capacity to promote cholesterol transport from the peripheral tissues, including macrophages, to the liver for excretion into the faeces via the bile. Recently, the capacity of HDLc to efflux cholesterol has been linked to CV risk. Additionally, a cross-sectional study evaluated HDLc function in the context of disease activity in RA and found that RA patients with a high level of disease activity had impaired HDL efflux (Charles-Schoeman et al., 2012). The most prominent difference is the presence of SAA on HDL, which interferes with normal efflux capacity. Contemplating these results, it has been proposed that HDL efflux capacity might be a good marker for CVD prediction, especially in RA.

2.4 Inflammation and Cardiovascular Disease in Rheumatoid Arthritis

Traditional CV risk factors are important contributors to the CV risk in RA patients. Despite this fact, adjustment for these risk factors still results in an increased absolute CV risk in patients with RA when compared to the general population (Gonzalez et al., 2008). The increased CV morbidity and mortality found in RA cannot be explained by traditional CV risk factors alone. Indeed, a study from 2009 demonstrated that RA is associated with an increased risk of CV events, independent of traditional risk factors (Peters et al., 2009). A plausible explanation is the inflammatory pathogenesis of both RA and atherosclerosis. Atherosclerosis is regarded as an inflammatory process, with inflammatory cells involved in all its stages (Libby et al., 2002; Ross, 1999). The mechanisms behind formation, progression, instability, and rupture of an atherosclerotic plaque resemble the mechanisms behind the development of synovitis. High-grade systemic inflammation appears central to the CV risk in patients with RA (Sattar et al., 2003) and a higher inflammatory burden with an increased number of disease flares has been associated with an increased CV risk in patients with RA (Myasoedova et al., 2016). Chronic inflammation enhances endothelial dysfunction and induces maladaptive remodeling of the vascular wall, resulting in plaque instability and rupture (van Sijl et al., 2012). The link between inflammation and atherosclerosis was first established in the general population where CRP levels are associated with CV risk (Kaptoge et al., 2010). In RA patients, markers of active inflammation, including levels of CRP, erythrocyte sedimentation rates, number of involved joints and disease activity scores, as well as disease severity or cumulative inflammation (estimated by radio-graphic scores), have all been linked to cardiovascular risk (Kremers et al., 2008; Liang et al., 2009; Maradit-Kremers et al., 2007; Rho et al., 2009). The endothelium plays a central role in vascular function by producing vasoactive factors and regulating interactions between the vessel wall and circulating blood cells and homeostasis. In this respect nitric oxide is one of the most important mediators, and its regulation can be disrupted by inflammation (Lerman and Zeiher, 2005). Studies assessing peripheral vascular function and morphology, which correlate with coronary circulation, showed that both vascular function and morphology are altered in patients with RA (Sandoo et al., 2011b). Not only blood vessel function can be affected in RA, the composition of the atherosclerotic plaque also has a role in the incidence of cardiovascular disease in patients with RA. In patients with RA coronary plaques are more frequent, more severe, and more prone to rupture (Karpouzas et al., 2014). Higher rheumatic disease activity is associated with increased plaque vulnerability (Semb et al., 2013). Additionally, patients with RA have worse outcomes after acute coronary syndrome, with increased and earlier recurrence of MI and an increased risk of death (Douglas et al., 2006). These histological features of coronary artery disease in patients with RA suggest that the mechanisms responsible for cardiovascular morbidity and mortality are different in patients with RA compared with the general population.

Another possible link between inflammation and increased risk of cardiovascular disease is a hypercoagulable state, as the immune and coagulation systems are linked: inflammation can lead to activation of coagulation, but coagulation also considerably affects the inflammatory activity (Zoller et al., 2012). The inflammatory cytokine network induces several prothrombotic conditions like insulin resistance, dyslipidaemia, endothelial dysfunction, activation of the extrinsic coagulation system, and the impairment of the fibrinolytic pathway. In addition, the inflammatory response is augmented and perpetuated by these alterations in coagulation. This two-way reciprocity has been established in several pathologic conditions, including atherosclerosis. Previous studies have reported several blood parameters reflecting a protrombotic state in RA (Beinsberger et al., 2014). These include platelet mass, markers of platelet activation, markers of inflammation and leukocyte activation, and markers of coagulation and fibrinolysis. In normal hemostasis, the vessel-wall prevents adhesion of platelets and leukocytes to the endothelium by the production of inhibitory mediators and the absence of cellular adhesion molecules (Versteeg et al., 2013). Inflammation causes damage to the vessel wall, exposing the subendothelial collagen and tissue factor, leading to platelet activation and formation of fibrin, which leads to formation of a thrombus. Platelets are considered important mediators in the process of vascular inflammation and atherosclerosis, as they interact with leukocytes by producing a range of thrombotic and inflammatory molecules; the adhesion and aggregation of platelets play a central role in the development of MI after plaque rupture. Increased platelet mass is associated with cardiovascular disease, and several studies have shown an increased platelet count in patients with RA. In RA patients with active disease, enhanced expression of expression platelet activation markers (i.e., platelet aggregation, activation of integrin αIIbβ3, and increased expression of CD63 and P-selectin) had been reported, as well as elevated markers of thrombin generation and fibrin turnover (Beinsberger et al., 2014). Elevated plasma levels of fibrinogen, von Willebrand factor, thrombin generation markers such as thrombin-antithrombin complexes, prothrombin fragments 1 + 2 (F1+2), tissue plasminogen activator, plasminogen activator inhibitor-1, and D-dimer have been demonstrated in RA patients. Increased antithrombin levels accompanied by attenuated fibrinolysis have also been reported in RA. In conclusion, RA can be considered as a prothrombotic state, which explains partly why patients with RA are at an increased risk of thromboembolic cardiovascular events (Chung et al., 2014).

2.5 Cardiovascular Risk Assessment in Rheumatoid Arthritis

The CV risk is elevated in patients with RA compared to the general population due to both traditional CV risk factors as well as the detrimental effects of chronic inflammation. The CV risk is even comparable to the risk excess found in patients with type 2 DM. This necessitates implementation of optimal CV risk assessment and management methods as part of routine usual care in these patients. The European League Against Rheumatism (EULAR) convened a task force in 2009 to critically appraise the existing literature on CV risk in inflammatory joint disorders, including RA, and to formulate CV risk management recommendations for these patients (Peters et al., 2010a). The key elements of CV risk management in RA are the identification of CV risk factors, determining a 10-year risk with available CV risk algorithms such as the SCORE (Conroy et al., 2003) or Framingham (D'Agostino, Sr. et al., 2008) prompt treatment of modifiable risk factors for CVD when the calculated CV risk exceeds a certain value and optimal reduction of RA disease activity. CV risk estimation in RA should be done according to existing guidelines, such as the ESC guideline for CVD prevention in clinical practice (Perk et al., 2012). This guideline describes the use of earlier-mentioned risk algorithm SCORE for the calculation of a first ever CV event in the general population. The SCORE algorithm includes age, gender, smoking status, blood pressure, and total cholesterol or TC/HDLc ratio (Perk et al., 2012). However, these commonly used risk estimation tools for the general population usually produce an inaccurate estimation of CV risk in patients with RA (Arts et al., 2015a; Gomez-Vaquero et al., 2013). Therefore, in 2009 the EULAR task force recommended a multiplication factor of 1.5 when using existing risk estimation algorithms for patients with RA. This recommendation was based on the available literature at that time (Peters et al., 2010a). It was argued that this multiplication factor also did not accurately reclassify patients into more appropriate risk categories, but alternative methods have not produced better estimations of the CV risk in these patients (Corrales et al., 2013; Gomez-Vaquero et al., 2013). Therefore, with the lack of superior prediction models for this population, the most evidence-based method of calculating the CV risk in these patients is the use of a multiplication factor of 1.5. There is still a lack of validated RA-specific CV risk algorithms with a proven efficacy.

There are some issues with risk assessment in patients with active disease or a disease flare as some risk factors are influenced by inflammation as well as antiinflammatory therapy. Therefore, risk estimation during active disease produces distorted results. Lipid measurements, for example should ideally be performed during disease remission or low disease activity. When this is not possible, the TC/HDLc ratio is the best parameter for CV risk estimation in these patients. During periods of high-grade inflammation this value is the most stable and it has a better correlation with CRP levels than TC or HDLc individually (Peters et al., 2010b; Toms et al., 2011). Also, risk assessment should be repeated after major changes in antirheumatic therapy as this influences both CV risk and CV risk factors.

2.5.1 Added Value of Novel Biomarkers and Imaging

Several novel and RA specific disease markers, such as ACPA and RF positivity, functional disability, and severe extraarticular manifestations have been associated with CVD risk (Cambridge et al., 2013; Goodson et al., 2002; Heliovaara et al., 1995; Radovits et al., 2010), but their additional value to existing risk estimation models remains to be determined. In a large registry study consisting of 10,156 RA patients with established disease with a median follow-up of 22 months markers of RA disease severity did not improve the predictive value of CV risk estimation tools (Solomon et al., 2010). Also, adding new risk factors to the SCORE algorithm did not improve the predictive capacity for patients with RA (Arts et al., 2015b). The QRISK2, a CV risk assessment calculator for the general population, does include RA as an independent risk factor, but tends to overestimate the CV risk in RA (Arts et al., 2015a). The Reynolds risk score has CRP levels incorporated in the algorithm (Ridker et al., 2007), but it is not clear whether the CRP levels of patients with coexistent RA can be incorporated and regarded as a prognostic marker in the same way as in the general population.

Several imaging modalities are available for the detection of coronary artery disease (CAD) in symptomatic patients. The performance of these tests depends on the clinicians pretest estimates of disease, the pretest probability (PTP), which is influenced by the prevalence of the disease in a certain population and the clinical features of the patient (Montalescot et al., 2013). The post-test probability will be the most accurate when this method is used for an individual patient. The presence of coronary atherosclerosis in symptomatic patients can be objectified by the use of invasive techniques like the invasive coronary angiography (golden standard) and noninvasive techniques such as exercise electrocardiogram testing, stress echocardiography, or radionuclide scintigraphy (Montalescot et al., 2013). In patients with a low PTP for CAD, other causes for the complaints should be investigated. Patients with symptoms of unstable angina or a high PTP of disease have established disease and should be treated accordingly. In patients with an intermediate or moderate PTP for CAD noninvasive testing is useful to establish whether CAD is significant or nonsignificant. In addition to the earlier-mentioned modalities that are used in standard care, several other tests are available for this purpose.

Magnetic resonance imaging is a promising tool for detecting coronary atherosclerosis, but the sensitivity and specificity of this technique is still not high enough for screening. Calcification in the coronary arteries as an indication of atherosclerosis can also be measured by means of a coronary calcium score (CAC-score) detected on a computed tomography scan. However, a CAC-score gives an indication of neither the stability of an atherosclerotic plaque nor the degree of stenosis in the diseased artery, as the specificity for the presence of a >50% stenosis is only 50%. The CAC-score does have a very high negative predictive value, thus a low CAC-score rules out significant CAD. However, it is possible to have a significant stenosis in the absence of calcifications in the coronary arteries, especially in unstable angina or non-ST elevation MI and in younger patients. Arterial disease can also be detected by a carotid ultrasound. Severe atherosclerosis in one arterial territory has been associated with atherosclerosis in other arteries in the general population (O'Leary et al., 1999). With carotid ultrasound the intima-media thickness (IMT) of the carotid artery can be measured and significant atherosclerosis could be detected early in seemingly healthy individuals. An increased IMT is associated with CV risk and value of 0.9 mm is considered as abnormal (Perk et al., 2012). RA patients with bilateral carotid plaques have an increased risk of a future acute coronary syndrome (4.3 per 100 person years, 95% CI 2.9−6.3) when compared to RA patients without carotid plaques (1.1 per 100 person years, 95% CI 0.6−1.7) (Ajeganova et al., 2012; Evans et al., 2011). Carotid artery disease is considered to be equivalent to CAD and lipid lowering therapy is recommended (Perk et al., 2012). In addition, carotid ultrasound has been shown to reclassify a considerable proportion of patients with RA into a more appropriate CV risk category (Corrales et al., 2014; Perk et al., 2012). However, screening for carotid plaques is currently not routinely recommended for patients with RA.

2.6 Treatment

There is increasing evidence that cumulative disease activity as well as the number of disease flares over time contribute to CV risk in RA (Myasoedova et al., 2016; Zhang et al., 2014). In addition, both inflammation and antirheumatic therapy modify certain CV risk factors. In this section, we will discuss antiinflammatory therapy and its influence on CV risk and CV risk factors in patients with RA.

2.6.1 Antiinflammatory Therapy and Cardiovascular Risk

Antirheumatic therapy of RA starts with disease-modifying antirheumatic drugs (DMARDs). These medications are capable of reducing disease symptoms by interfering with the systemic inflammatory process in RA. Several types of DMARDs are used in the treatment of RA, including conventional synthetic DMARDs (csDMARDs), targeted synthetic DMARDs (tsDMARDs), and biological DMARDs (bDMARDs). An overview of DMARDs is presented in Table 10.3. Antiinflammatory therapy starts with csDMARDs, usually with methotrexate alone or combined with sulfasalazine or hydroxychloroquine or (bridging) glucocorticosteroids. If

TABLE 10.3 Medications Used in the Treatment of Rheumatoid Arthritis

Group	Examples
NSAIDs	Diclofenac
	Ibuprofen
	Naproxen
	Meloxicam
	Nabumetone
	Celecoxib
	Etoricoxib
Conventional synthetic DMARDs	Methotrexate
	Hydroxychloroquine
	Sulfasalazine
	Leflunomide
Tumor necrosis factor alpha inhibitors*	Infliximab (i.v)
	Etanercept
	Adalimumab
	Golimumab

TABLE 10.3 Medications Used in the Treatment of Rheumatoid Arthritis—cont'd

Group	Examples
	Certoluzumab pegol
T cell costimulation inhibitor*	Abatacept
Anti-B cell agent*	Rituximab (i.v.)
Interleukin-6 receptor blocking monoclonal antibody*	Tocilizumab i.v. or s.c.
Interleukin-1 inhibitor*	Anakinra
Targeted synthetic DMARDs	Tofacitinib
Glucocorticosteroids, oral, or intraarticular	Prednis(ol)on
	Methylprednisolon
	Triamcinolon
	Dexamethason

*biological disease-modifying antirheumatic drugs (bDMARDs).

within 6 months remission according to the ACR-EULAR criteria is not achieved (Smolen et al., 2014), a different csDMARD combination is tried or bDMARDs, generally TNFi, are initiated. Proper randomized clinical trials on CV outcomes have not yet been published in RA patients groups but observational studies have shown beneficial effects of csDMARDs and TNFi on lipid profile, insulin resistance, metabolic syndrome, and IMT in patients with RA (Ristic et al., 2010). Treatment with csDMARDs and TNFi generally increases all lipid components in the serum (i.e., TC, HDLc, LDLc, TG), but predominantly HDLc. This results in a beneficial TC/HDLc-ratio (Peters et al., 2007). Treatment with tocilizumab and tofacitinib may cause sustained elevations of lipids, probably die to interleukin-6 inhibition, which can be reduced effectively with statin therapy (Souto et al., 2015). Glucocorticosteroids are known to rapidly and effectively reduce the inflammation of RA, but they are known to induce side-effects like impaired glucose tolerance, dyslipidaemia, obesity, and hypertension. Indeed, studies have described a dose-dependent increase in CV risk with corticosteroid therapy (Ajeganova et al., 2014; Avina-Zubieta et al., 2013; del Rincon et al., 2014). Still, reducing high-grade inflammation in patients with RA who have active disease may reverse this negative effect. Also, the role of low daily doses of corticosteroids in the development of CV events is not clear. In view of CVD prevention, the lowest dose possible should be prescribed for the shortest duration in accordance with the EULAR recommendation on management of glucocorticoid therapy in this respect (Duru et al., 2013). NSAIDs are also used in the treatment of some RA symptoms. A recent metaanalysis reports that overall NSAIDs have a negative effect on CV outcomes in patients with RA (Roubille et al., 2015), but these results were mainly observed due to the use of rofecoxib in this study. Rofecoxib has been withdrawn from the market in 2004. There is some evidence that NSAIDs might have a less pronounced CV risk increasing effect in patient with RA when compared to the general population (Lindhardsen et al., 2013). NSAIDs have antiinflammatory properties and they might improve physical function in patient with RA. Therefore, they might have some beneficial effects on CV risk. Thus, NSAIDs can be prescribed as recommended in national guidelines for the general population in patients with RA. Generally, this means that NSAIDs should be used with caution or that they are contraindicated in this population, may be with the exception of naproxen. Diclofenac and ibuprofen are contraindicated in patients with a history of CHF (NYHA class II−IV), ischemic heart disease, cerebrovascular disease, or peripheral arterial disease (EMA PRAC Recommendation Diclofenac, 2013; EMA PRAC Recommendation Ibuprofen, 2015). Some observational studies suggest that paracetamol is associated with a dose-dependent increase in CV risk, but this needs to be further investigated (Roberts et al., 2016). An increased intake of paracetamol might just be a reflection of a higher degree of pain due to the underlying disease, which is the actual cause of the higher CV risk. A recent study from 2015 suggests that proton-pump inhibitors (PPIs) might also be associated with adverse cardiovascular outcomes, but further research is needed to confirm this effect of PPIs (Shah et al., 2015).

2.6.2 Treatment of Cardiovascular Risk Factors and Cardiovascular Disease in Rheumatoid Arthritis

In the general population CV risk is calculated with risk algorithms, which estimate a 10-year risk of a first ever CV event using values like gender, age, smoking status, blood pressure, and total cholesterol and/or other lipids. Patients who exceed a certain threshold of CV risk and patients with established CVD should be treated for all CV risk factors that are present according to existing national guidelines, just like in the general population. Next to prompt treatment of CV risk factors, reduction of inflammation by optimal antiinflammatory therapy is necessary to reduce CV risk in these patients. The presence of CV risk factors such as blood pressure, lipid levels, and insulin resistance should be checked regularly. At the very least, some form of CV screening should be done at the diagnosis of RA and it should be repeated after major changes in antiinflammatory therapy. Also, CV risk assessment should be performed every few years according to available guidelines on prevention and management of CVD. Antihypertensive agents can be used as in the general population and there is no evidence for a preferred antihypertensive agent in patients with RA. Statins are also as effective as in the general population and should be used according to general population guidelines (Rollefstad et al., 2015; Schoenfeld et al., 2015). There is no evidence that statins may be less effective in patient with RA and during certain types of antiinflammatory treatment. Indeed, statins have antiinflammatory effects and may reduce CV risk even further in RA when combined with antirheumatic therapy (Maki-Petaja et al., 2007). In addition, patients should be informed about lifestyle changes that can lower CV risk. Smoking cessation should be advised and where possible patients should be referred to centers where evidence-based smoking cessation programs are available, even if they have failed previously. As physical inactivity is common in RA with adverse CV effects (Hernandez-Hernandez et al., 2014; Metsios et al., 2009; van den Berg et al., 2007), patients should be advised to exercise. High-intensity exercise is not contraindicated in RA and should be encouraged (Lemmey et al., 2009). Physical activity that is enjoyable for the patients and that can be sustained should be recommended. Finally, a healthy diet should be recommended as part of a healthy lifestyle following national guidelines available on this subject. The Mediterranean diet appears to be the healthiest diet in cardiovascular terms, and it is characterized by a high intake of vegetables, legumes, fruits, cereals, and fish, while consumption of red meat is limited. Olive oil is the most important source of fat in this diet. The Mediterranean diet is associated with a reduction in the incidence of CV events in the general population (Estruch et al., 2013). In addition, this diet may have a suppressive effect on disease activity in RA patients (Skoldstam et al., 2003). In which way lifestyle interventions can best be advocated to patients remains elusive. Generally, the most effective way to communicate lifestyle interventions to patients is to link the provided information with behavioral education (Iversen et al., 2010). If such an approach is effective regarding lifestyle modifications in patients with RA is to be determined, although a randomized controlled trial evaluating this approach showed improved behavioral intentions in RA patients receiving cognitive behavioral patient education compared to those that did only receive information (John et al., 2013).

3. NONATHEROSCLEROTIC CARDIOVASCULAR DISEASE

Recent reports of studies in the field of cardiovascular disease in RA have mainly focused on the incidence of atherosclerotic and ischaemic events rather than nonischaemic CVD. However, patients with RA and other inflammatory joint disorders are not just at increased risk for ischaemic CV events, nonischaemic cardiac involvement is also common, and RA can affect nearly all components of the heart. A range of cardiac manifestations can present during the course of RA, although cardiac manifestations often remain clinically silent (Kitas et al., 2001).

In the past, data on traditional rheumatoid heart disease have been generated from autopsy and imaging (mostly echocardiographic) studies, and some of these were carried out decades ago. Traditional and clinically overt rheumatoid heart disease is rare nowadays, possibly related with the introduction of improved RA treatment strategies. However, recent developments in cardiac imaging suggest that microvascular disease and myocarditis are still common, as is cardiac autonomic neuropathy, particularly during active phases of the disease (Mavrogeni et al., 2009).

Traditional cardiac manifestations include pericarditis, cardiomyopathy, myocarditis, cardiac amyloidosis, arrhythmia, and valve diseases, but also vasculitis of the coronary arteries and CHF (Table 10.4). This section discusses the epidemiological aspects of these traditional rheumatoid heart diseases in more detail.

3.1 Pericardial Disease

3.1.1 Introduction

Pericarditis is the most common form of cardiac involvement in RA, although clinically evident cases are rare as pericardial involvement in RA is usually clinically silent. It is observed secondary to the underlying inflammatory process and patients with active RA and other extraarticular manifestations are affected most frequently (Voskuyl, 2006).

3.1.2 Prevalence

As rheumatoid pericarditis rarely causes clinically overt disease, the true prevalence is difficult to establish and varies according to the method of assessment. Pericarditis is mostly an incidental discovery on autopsy or by echocardiography as clinical evidence of pericarditis is considerably less frequent than prevalences reported by autopsy or echocardiographic findings.

Clinically evident RA pericarditis generally affects ≤10% of patients with severe RA, including patients with asymptomatic pericardial effusions

TABLE 10.4 Traditional Cardiac Manifestations of Rheumatoid Arthritis

Pericardium
Myocardium
Endocardium and heart valves
Conducting system and autonomic nervous system
Coronary arteries and vascular tree

(Gordon et al., 1973). In autopsy and echocardiographic studies (Table 10.5), a higher prevalence of pericardial disease in RA is reported. Autopsy studies report prevalence ranging up to 50%, although a trend towards lower rates is seen in most recent studies (Bely et al., 1992; Bonfiglio and Atwater, 1969; Cathcart and Spodick, 1962; Koivuniemi et al., 2013). Almost all studies include small number of patients and thus carry a risk of selection bias, as patients are usually selected from a hospital setting, pointing to more severe disease. Numerous echocardiographic studies have been carried out in RA cohorts and the reported prevalence of echocardiographic pericardial effusion ranges from 1% to 30% (Dawson et al., 2000; Guedes et al., 2001; Maione et al., 1993; Mody et al., 1987; Nomeir et al., 1979; Tlustochowicz et al., 1997; Wislowska et al., 1999).

It is worth mentioning that the majority of studies have been performed decades ago, and the prevalence nowadays is not exactly known. It is likely that the prevalence of pericarditis in RA is reducing as a result of improved treatment strategies.

TABLE 10.5 **Pericardial Disease in Rheumatoid Arthritis**

	Method of Assessment	N	Reported Prevalence
Bonfiglio and Atwater (1969)	Autopsy		50%
Bely et al. (1992)	Autopsy	169	2%
Cathcart and Spodick (1962)	Autopsy		
Koivuniemi et al. (2013)	Autopsy	369	27%
Guedes et al. (2001)	Echocardiography (trans-oesophageal)	30	13%
Nomeir et al. (1979)	Echocardiography	30	20%
Mody et al. (1987)	Echocardiography	101	6%
Maione et al. (1993)	Echocardiography	39	7%
Tlustochowicz (1997)	Echocardiography	100	26%
Wislowska et al. (1999)	Echocardiography	70	4%
Dawson et al. (2000)	Echocardiography	143	1%
Mavrogeni et al. (2013)	MRI	20	6/13
Turesson et al. (2007)	Medical records	81 (severe extraarticular RA)	16%

3.1.3 Etiology of Pericardial Involvement in Rheumatoid Arthritis

RA pericarditis occurs most frequently in seropositive patients with severely destructive and nodular RA, as is the case with other extraarticular features of RA(Voskuyl et al., 1996). It has also been reported to occur more frequent in male patients; however, results from different studies have been contradictory. In the majority of RA patients pericarditis develops during the course of RA, but it may also proceed the onset of arthritis and be the first symptom of an autoimmune disease (Voskuyl et al., 1996). Therefore, establishing the etiology of pericarditis in patients presenting with pericardial effusion may aid in diagnosing RA at early stage.

Other potential etiologies of pericarditis are infection, acute MI, use of certain medications, and trauma, and must be ruled out.

3.1.4 Mortality

As pericarditis in RA is usually asymptomatic, it does not seem to significantly contribute to excess mortality. However, in patients with extraarticular manifestations and more severe disease mortality is markedly increased compared to patients with milder disease (Turesson et al., 2002). Pericarditis itself is associated with a high morbidity and mortality in patients with constrictive pericarditis or rapidly progressive effusive pericarditis, but these cases are rare. The prognosis of RA patients with clinical pericarditis appears to be mostly impaired in the first year after diagnosis (Hara et al., 1990).

3.1.5 Pathology

Normal pericardium consists of a two-layered sac that folds over the surface of the heart. The visceral pericardium is the thin visceral inner layer and lies adherent to the myocardium. The parietal pericardium, the thicker outer layer, is contiguous with the inner layer and both layers are separated by pericardial fluid that is secreted by the inner layer. The most prominent feature of pericarditis is the accumulation of (usually exudative) pericardial fluid in the sac, resulting in pericardial effusion: usually a clear exudate containing neutrophils with a high protein and low glucose content (Hara et al., 1990). Long-standing effusions may contain cholesterol crystals. Persistent chronic inflammation thickens the pericardium, which ultimately may result in constrictive pericarditis leading to restriction of cardiac filling, although this is rarely seen. Pericardial calcification is also a seldomly observed consequence of chronic pericarditis.

3.1.6 Clinical Manifestations

Pericarditis is often clinically silent as only a small fraction of patients have symptoms. The most common symptom is a pleuritic chest pain: an acute and sharp pain that is relieved by leaning forward. In constrictive disease cardiac tamponade, signs of hemodynamic compromise or even shock can develop and require immediate intervention. A pericardial friction rub occurs in up to 40% of patients (Kitas et al., 2001).

3.1.7 Diagnostic Investigations

Electrocardiographic changes are present in approximately 90% of patients with acute pericarditis, and include ST-segment elevation and depression in the PR-segment (Troughton et al., 2004). Laboratory evaluation should include markers of inflammation, cardiac markers as creatine, and troponin-I. Pericardial effusion and thickening may be seen on echocardiographic evaluation and transthoracic echocardiography should always be performed. Pericardial effusion can also be diagnosed by chest radiography.

In some cases, pericardiocentesis is indicated: in cases with refractory effusion that show signs of hemodynamic compromise, or if the effusion is suspected to be purulent, tuberculous, or neoplastic.

3.1.8 Differential Diagnosis and Management

In all patients who present with acute chest pain, other causes of chest pain should be ruled out, including MI and pulmonary embolism. In RA patients pericarditis is most likely to be autoinflammatory, but infective causes of pericardial effusion should be considered and cultures may be necessary.

Most cases of pericarditis can be treated in the outpatient clinic. If there is any doubt on the etiology, or if refractory or severe disease is present, a cardiologist consultation is recommended.

NSAIDs are usually first-line treatment, as it relieves pain and dampens inflammation. Colchicine is often used in the treatment of pericarditis in non-RA patients. Glucocorticosteroids can also be used, especially in more severe cases and in autoreactive causes (Adler et al., 2015).

It is important that in RA, pericarditis is a manifestation of active disease. Thus, RA treatment should be intensified to control the active disease.

3.2 Endocardial Involvement in Rheumatoid Arthritis

3.2.1 Valvular Disease

Echocardiographic and autopsy studies show a high prevalence of valvular involvement in RA, although clinically overt disease is rare (Bacon and Gibson, 1974). Endocardial involvement is thought to be a consequence of systemic aspecific inflammation, and all valves may be involved. Thickening and calcification of valves occur mainly at the base of the valves and granulomatous lesions may develop, leading to valve regurgitation. As this is a slowly developing process it does not cause any symptoms in most patients as the ventricles adapt without decompensating.

3.2.2 Coronary Arteritis

Coronary arteritis is another cardiac manifestation that rarely presents as clinical disease but is frequently reported in RA autopsy studies, affecting up to 20% of cases (Bonfiglio and Atwater, 1969). Small and medium intramyocardial vessels are usually affected, and this may lead to small infarctions causing patchy myocardial necrosis. Epicardial vessel arteritis has also been reported as a nonocclusive arteritis, and if this leads to MI is not known (Morris et al., 1986).

3.3 Myocardial Involvement and Conduction System Abnormalities in Rheumatoid Arthritis

Myocarditis in RA can be focal or diffuse, granulomatous, and nonspecific. Nonspecific myocarditis is frequently asymptomatic and its clinical significance is not known. The conduction system may be affected leading to conduction abnormalities. Several types of conduction abnormalities have been reported in RA patients, ranging from cardiac arrhythmias to complete heart block possibly due to disruption of the atrioventricular node by rheumatoid granulomata (Ahern et al., 1983; Goldeli et al., 1998).

4. CONCLUSION

RA is associated with an increased risk of mortality with SMRs ranging from 0.9 to 2.7 as compared to the general population. CVD is the main reason for premature death in these patients, which is mostly of atherosclerotic origin. Nonatherosclerotic traditional rheumatic heart disease also contributes, although clinically overt and severe cases are rare nowadays, presumably related to the development of improved RA treatment strategies. The excess CV risk in patients with RA is accounted to both an increased prevalence of traditional CV risk factors as well as the detrimental effects of chronic systemic inflammation. Early diagnosis of RA could lower CV risk. More importantly, awareness of this heightened CV risk is vital for clinicians as well as patients with RA to timely initiate CV risk management in daily clinical practice, next to optimal treatment of inflammation with antiinflammatory therapy. CV risk assessment and management should be performed in accordance to existing guidelines for the general population and for patients with inflammatory joint diseases, including RA, to reduce CV risk.

REFERENCES

Abhishek, A., Butt, S., Gadsby, K., Zhang, W., Deighton, C.M., 2010. Anti-TNF-alpha agents are less effective for the treatment of rheumatoid arthritis in current smokers. J. Clin. Rheumatol. 16 (1), 15–18. Available from: PM: 20051749.

Adler, Y., Charron, P., Imazio, M., Badano, L., Baron-Esquivias, G., Bogaert, J., Brucato, A., Gueret, P., Klingel, K., Lionis, C., Maisch, B., Mayosi, B., Pavie, A., Ristic, A.D., Sabate, T.M., Seferovic, P., Swedberg, K., Tomkowski, W., Achenbach, S., Agewall, S., Al-Attar, N., Angel, F.J., Arad, M., Asteggiano, R., Bueno, H., Caforio, A.L., Carerj, S., Ceconi, C., Evangelista, A., Flachskampf, F., Giannakoulas, G., Gielen, S., Habib, G., Kolh, P., Lambrinou, E., Lancellotti, P., Lazaros, G., Linhart, A., Meurin, P., Nieman, K., Piepoli, M.F., Price, S., Roos-Hesselink, J., Roubille, F., Ruschitzka, F., Sagrista, S.J., Sousa-Uva, M., Uwe, V.J., Luis, Z.J., 2015. 2015 ESC guidelines for the diagnosis and management of pericardial diseases: the task force for the diagnosis and management of pericardial diseases of the European Society of Cardiology (ESC) endorsed by: the European Association for Cardio-Thoracic Surgery (EACTS). Eur. Heart J. 36 (42), 2921–2964. Available from: PM: 26320112.

Ahern, M., Lever, J.V., Cosh, J., 1983. Complete heart block in rheumatoid arthritis. Ann. Rheum. Dis. 42 (4), 389–397. Available from: PM: 6882034.

Ajeganova, S., de, F.U., Jogestrand, T., Frostegard, J., Hafstrom, I., 2012. Carotid atherosclerosis, disease measures, oxidized low-density lipoproteins, and atheroprotective natural antibodies for cardiovascular disease in early rheumatoid arthritis—an inception cohort study. J. Rheumatol. 39 (6), 1146–1154. Available from: PM: 22589258.

Ajeganova, S., Svensson, B., Hafstrom, I., 2014. Low-dose prednisolone treatment of early rheumatoid arthritis and late cardiovascular outcome and survival: 10-year follow-up of a 2-year randomised trial. BMJ Open. 4 (4), e004259. Available from: PM: 24710131.

Arts, E.E., Popa, C., Den Broeder, A.A., Semb, A.G., Toms, T., Kitas, G.D., van Riel, P.L., Fransen, J., 2015a. Performance of four current risk algorithms in predicting cardiovascular events in patients with early rheumatoid arthritis. Ann. Rheum. Dis. 74 (4), 668–674. Available from: PM: 24389293.

Arts, E.E., Popa, C.D., Den Broeder, A.A., Donders, R., Sandoo, A., Toms, T., Rollefstad, S., Ikdahl, E., Semb, A.G., Kitas, G.D., van Riel, P.L., Fransen, J., 2015b. Prediction of cardiovascular risk in rheumatoid arthritis: performance of original and adapted SCORE algorithms. Ann. Rheum. Dis. Available from: PM: 25691119.

Avina-Zubieta, J.A., Abrahamowicz, M., De Vera, M.A., Choi, H.K., Sayre, E.C., Rahman, M.M., Sylvestre, M.P., Wynant, W., Esdaile, J.M., Lacaille, D., 2013. Immediate and past cumulative effects of oral glucocorticoids on the risk of acute myocardial infarction in rheumatoid arthritis: a population-based study. Rheumatology (Oxford) 52 (1), 68–75. Available from: PM: 23192907.

Avina-Zubieta, J.A., Thomas, J., Sadatsafavi, M., Lehman, A.J., Lacaille, D., 2012. Risk of incident cardiovascular events in patients with rheumatoid arthritis: a meta-analysis of observational studies. Ann. Rheum. Dis. 71 (9), 1524–1529. Available from: PM: 22425941.

Bacon, P.A., Gibson, D.G., 1974. Cardiac involvement in rheumatoid arthritis. An echocardiographic study. Ann. Rheum. Dis. 33 (1), 20–24. Available from: PM: 4821378.

Baghdadi, L.R., Woodman, R.J., Shanahan, E.M., Mangoni, A.A., 2015. The impact of traditional cardiovascular risk factors on cardiovascular outcomes in patients with rheumatoid arthritis: a systematic review and meta-analysis. PLoS One 10 (2), e0117952. Available from: PM: 25689371.

Beinsberger, J., Heemskerk, J.W., Cosemans, J.M., 2014. Chronic arthritis and cardiovascular disease: altered blood parameters give rise to a prothrombotic propensity. Semin. Arthritis Rheum. 44 (3), 345–352. Available from: PM: 25077842.

Bely, M., Apathy, A., Beke-Martos, E., 1992. Cardiac changes in rheumatoid arthritis. Acta Morphol. Hung. 40 (1–4), 149–186. Available from: PM: 1365761.

Binymin, K., Herrick, A., Carlson, G., Hopkins, S., 2011. The effect of disease activity on body composition and resting energy expenditure in patients with rheumatoid arthritis. J. Inflamm. Res. 4, 61–66. Available from: PM: 22096370.

Bjornadal, L., Baecklund, E., Yin, L., Granath, F., Klareskog, L., Ekbom, A., 2002. Decreasing mortality in patients with rheumatoid arthritis: results from a large population based cohort in Sweden, 1964–95. J. Rheumatol. 29 (5), 906–912. Available from: PM: 12022348.

Blake, G.J., Ridker, P.M., 2001. Novel clinical markers of vascular wall inflammation. Circ. Res. 89 (9), 763–771. Available from: PM: 11679405.

Bonfiglio, T., Atwater, E.C., 1969. Heart disease in patients with seropositive rheumatoid arthritis; a controlled autopsy study and review. Arch. Intern. Med. 124 (6), 714–719. Available from: PM: 4901063.

Boyer, J.F., Bongard, V., Cantagrel, A., Jamard, B., Gottenberg, J.E., Mariette, X., Davignon, J.L., Ferrieres, J., Ruidavets, J.B., Dallongeville, J., Arveiler, D., Cambon-Thomsen, A., Constantin, A., 2012. Link between traditional cardiovascular risk factors and inflammation in patients with early arthritis: results from a French multicenter cohort. Arthritis Care Res. (Hoboken) 64 (6), 872–880. Available from: PM: 22275176.

Boyer, J.F., Gourraud, P.A., Cantagrel, A., Davignon, J.L., Constantin, A., 2011. Traditional cardiovascular risk factors in rheumatoid arthritis: a meta-analysis. Joint Bone Spine 78 (2), 179–183. Available from: PM: 20851020.

Burger, D., Dayer, J.M., 2002. High-density lipoprotein-associated apolipoprotein A-I: the missing link between infection and chronic inflammation? Autoimmun. Rev. 1 (1–2), 111–117. Available from: PM: 12849067.

Callahan, L.F., Cordray, D.S., Wells, G., Pincus, T., 1996. Formal education and five-year mortality in rheumatoid arthritis: mediation by helplessness scale score. Arthritis Care Res. 9 (6), 463–472. Available from: PM: 9136290.

Cambridge, G., Acharya, J., Cooper, J.A., Edwards, J.C., Humphries, S.E., 2013. Antibodies to citrullinated peptides and risk of coronary heart disease. Atherosclerosis 228 (1), 243–246. Available from: PM: 23474125.

Canaris, G.J., Manowitz, N.R., Mayor, G., Ridgway, E.C., 2000. The Colorado thyroid disease prevalence study. Arch. Intern. Med. 160 (4), 526–534. Available from: PM: 10695693.

Cathcart, E.S., Spodick, D.H., 1962. Rheumatoid heart disease. A study of the incidence and nature of cardiac lesions in rheumatoid arthritis. N. Engl. J. Med. 266, 959–964. Available from: PM: 13877345.

Charles-Schoeman, C., Lee, Y.Y., Grijalva, V., Amjadi, S., FitzGerald, J., Ranganath, V.K., Taylor, M., McMahon, M., Paulus, H.E., Reddy, S.T., 2012. Cholesterol efflux by high density lipoproteins is impaired in patients with active rheumatoid arthritis. Ann. Rheum. Dis. 71 (7), 1157–1162. Available from: PM: 22267330.

Chehata, J.C., Hassell, A.B., Clarke, S.A., Mattey, D.L., Jones, M.A., Jones, P.W., Dawes, P.T., 2001. Mortality in rheumatoid arthritis: relationship to single and composite measures of disease activity. Rheumatology (Oxford) 40 (4), 447–452. Available from: PM: 11312385.

Chung, W.S., Peng, C.L., Lin, C.L., Chang, Y.J., Chen, Y.F., Chiang, J.Y., Sung, F.C., Kao, C.H., 2014. Rheumatoid arthritis increases the risk of deep vein thrombosis and pulmonary thromboembolism: a nationwide cohort study. Ann. Rheum. Dis. 73 (10), 1774–1780. Available from: PM: 23926057.

Conroy, R.M., Pyorala, K., Fitzgerald, A.P., Sans, S., Menotti, A., De, B.G., De, B.D., Ducimetiere, P., Jousilahti, P., Keil, U., Njolstad, I., Oganov, R.G., Thomsen, T., Tunstall-Pedoe, H., Tverdal, A., Wedel, H., Whincup, P., Wilhelmsen, L., Graham, I.M., 2003.

Estimation of ten-year risk of fatal cardiovascular disease in Europe: the SCORE project. Eur. Heart J. 24 (11), 987–1003. Available from: PM: 12788299.

Corrales, A., Gonzalez-Juanatey, C., Peiro, M.E., Blanco, R., Llorca, J., Gonzalez-Gay, M.A., 2014. Carotid ultrasound is useful for the cardiovascular risk stratification of patients with rheumatoid arthritis: results of a population-based study. Ann. Rheum. Dis. 73 (4), 722–727. Available from: PM: 23505241.

Corrales, A., Parra, J.A., Gonzalez-Juanatey, C., Rueda-Gotor, J., Blanco, R., Llorca, J., Gonzalez-Gay, M.A., 2013. Cardiovascular risk stratification in rheumatic diseases: carotid ultrasound is more sensitive than Coronary Artery Calcification Score to detect subclinical atherosclerosis in patients with rheumatoid arthritis. Ann. Rheum. Dis. 72 (11), 1764–1770. Available from: PM: 23852762.

Costenbader, K.H., Feskanich, D., Mandl, L.A., Karlson, E.W., 2006. Smoking intensity, duration, and cessation, and the risk of rheumatoid arthritis in women. Am. J. Med. 119 (6), 503–509. Available from: PM: 16750964.

Cross, M., Smith, E., Hoy, D., Carmona, L., Wolfe, F., Vos, T., Williams, B., Gabriel, S., Lassere, M., Johns, N., Buchbinder, R., Woolf, A., March, L., 2014. The global burden of rheumatoid arthritis: estimates from the global burden of disease 2010 study. Ann. Rheum. Dis. 73 (7), 1316–1322. Available from: PM: 9517761.

D'Agostino Sr., R.B., Vasan, R.S., Pencina, M.J., Wolf, P.A., Cobain, M., Massaro, J.M., Kannel, W.B., 2008. General cardiovascular risk profile for use in primary care: the Framingham Heart Study. Circulation 117 (6), 743–753. Available from: PM: 18212285.

Dawber, T., 1980. The Framingham Study: The Epidemiology of Atherosclerotic Disease. Harvard University Press, Cambridge, MA.

Dawson, J.K., Goodson, N.G., Graham, D.R., Lynch, M.P., 2000. Raised pulmonary artery pressures measured with Doppler echocardiography in rheumatoid arthritis patients. Rheumatology (Oxford) 39 (12), 1320–1325. Available from: PM: 11136873.

del Rincon, I., Battafarano, D.F., Restrepo, J.F., Erikson, J.M., Escalante, A., 2014. Glucocorticoid dose thresholds associated with all-cause and cardiovascular mortality in rheumatoid arthritis. Arthritis Rheumatol. 66 (2), 264–272. Available from: PM: 24504798.

Doran, M.F., Pond, G.R., Crowson, C.S., O'Fallon, W.M., Gabriel, S.E., 2002. Trends in incidence and mortality in rheumatoid arthritis in Rochester, Minnesota, over a forty-year period. Arthritis Rheum. 46 (3), 625–631. Available from: PM: 11920397.

Dougados, M., Soubrier, M., Antunez, A., Balint, P., Balsa, A., Buch, M.H., Casado, G., Detert, J., El-Zorkany, B., Emery, P., Hajjaj-Hassouni, N., Harigai, M., Luo, S.F., Kurucz, R., Maciel, G., Mola, E.M., Montecucco, C.M., McInnes, I., Radner, H., Smolen, J.S., Song, Y.W., Vonkeman, H.E., Winthrop, K., Kay, J., 2014. Prevalence of comorbidities in rheumatoid arthritis and evaluation of their monitoring: results of an international, cross-sectional study (COMORA). Ann. Rheum. Dis. 73 (1), 62–68. Available from: PM: 24095940.

Douglas, K.M., Pace, A.V., Treharne, G.J., Saratzis, A., Nightingale, P., Erb, N., Banks, M.J., Kitas, G.D., 2006. Excess recurrent cardiac events in rheumatoid arthritis patients with acute coronary syndrome. Ann. Rheum. Dis. 65 (3), 348–353. Available from: PM: 16079169.

Duru, N., van der Goes, M.C., Jacobs, J.W., Andrews, T., Boers, M., Buttgereit, F., Caeyers, N., Cutolo, M., Halliday, S., Da Silva, J.A., Kirwan, J.R., Ray, D., Rovensky, J., Severijns, G., Westhovens, R., Bijlsma, J.W., 2013. EULAR evidence-based and consensus-based recommendations on the management of medium to high-dose glucocorticoid therapy in rheumatic diseases. Ann. Rheum. Dis. 72 (12), 1905–1913. Available from: PM: 23873876.

England, B.R., Sayles, H., Michaud, K., Caplan, L., Davis, L.A., Cannon, G.W., Sauer, B.C., Solow, E.B., Reimold, A.M., Kerr, G.S., Schwab, P., Baker, J.F., Mikuls, T.R., 2015. Cause-specific mortality in US veteran men with rheumatoid arthritis. Arthritis Care Res. (Hoboken). Available from: PM: 26097231.

Estruch, R., Ros, E., Salas-Salvado, J., Covas, M.I., Corella, D., Aros, F., Gomez-Gracia, E., Ruiz-Gutierrez, V., Fiol, M., Lapetra, J., Lamuela-Raventos, R.M., Serra-Majem, L., Pinto, X., Basora, J., Munoz, M.A., Sorli, J.V., Martinez, J.A., Martinez-Gonzalez, M.A., 2013. Primary prevention of cardiovascular disease with a Mediterranean diet. N. Engl. J. Med. 368 (14), 1279–1290. Available from: PM: 23432189.

Evans, M.R., Escalante, A., Battafarano, D.F., Freeman, G.L., O'Leary, D.H., del Rincon, I., 2011. Carotid atherosclerosis predicts incident acute coronary syndromes in rheumatoid arthritis. Arthritis Rheum. 63 (5), 1211–1220. Available from: PM: 21305526.

Ford, E.S., 2002. Does exercise reduce inflammation? Physical activity and C-reactive protein among U.S. adults. Epidemiology 13 (5), 561–568. Available from: PM: 12192226.

Gabriel, S.E., Crowson, C.S., Kremers, H.M., Doran, M.F., Turesson, C., O'Fallon, W.M., Matteson, E.L., 2003. Survival in rheumatoid arthritis: a population-based analysis of trends over 40 years. Arthritis Rheum. 48 (1), 54–58. Available from: PM: 12528103.

Gabriel, S.E., Michaud, K., 2009. Epidemiological studies in incidence, prevalence, mortality, and comorbidity of the rheumatic diseases. Arthritis Res. Ther. 11 (3), 229. Available from: PM: 19519924.

Giles, J.T., Allison, M., Blumenthal, R.S., Post, W., Gelber, A.C., Petri, M., Tracy, R., Szklo, M., Bathon, J.M., 2010. Abdominal adiposity in rheumatoid arthritis: association with cardiometabolic risk factors and disease characteristics. Arthritis Rheum. 62 (11), 3173–3182. Available from: PM: 20589684.

Goldeli, O., Dursun, E., Komsuoglu, B., 1998. Dispersion of ventricular repolarization: a new marker of ventricular arrhythmias in patients with rheumatoid arthritis. J. Rheumatol. 25 (3), 447–450. Available from: PM: 9517761.

Gomez-Vaquero, C., Corrales, A., Zacarias, A., Rueda-Gotor, J., Blanco, R., Gonzalez-Juanatey, C., Llorca, J., Gonzalez-Gay, M.A., 2013. SCORE and REGICOR function charts underestimate the cardiovascular risk in Spanish patients with rheumatoid arthritis. Arthritis Res. Ther. 15 (4), R91. Available from: PM: 9517761.

Gonzalez, A., Maradit, K.H., Crowson, C.S., Ballman, K.V., Roger, V.L., Jacobsen, S.J., O'Fallon, W.M., Gabriel, S.E., 2008. Do cardiovascular risk factors confer the same risk for cardiovascular outcomes in rheumatoid arthritis patients as in non-rheumatoid arthritis patients? Ann. Rheum. Dis. 67 (1), 64–69. Available from: PM: 17517756.

Gonzalez, A., Maradit, K.H., Crowson, C.S., Nicola, P.J., Davis III, J.M., Therneau, T.M., Roger, V.L., Gabriel, S.E., 2007. The widening mortality gap between rheumatoid arthritis patients and the general population. Arthritis Rheum. 56 (11), 3583–3587. Available from: PM: 17968923.

Goodson, N., Marks, J., Lunt, M., Symmons, D., 2005. Cardiovascular admissions and mortality in an inception cohort of patients with rheumatoid arthritis with onset in the 1980s and 1990s. Ann. Rheum. Dis. 64 (11), 1595–1601. Available from: PM: 9517761.

Goodson, N.J., Wiles, N.J., Lunt, M., Barrett, E.M., Silman, A.J., Symmons, D.P., 2002. Mortality in early inflammatory polyarthritis: cardiovascular mortality is increased in seropositive patients. Arthritis Rheum. 46 (8), 2010–2019. Available from: PM: 12209502.

Gordon, D.A., Stein, J.L., Broder, I., 1973. The extra-articular features of rheumatoid arthritis. A systematic analysis of 127 cases. Am. J. Med. 54 (4), 445–452. Available from: PM: 4348718.

Guedes, C., Bianchi-Fior, P., Cormier, B., Barthelemy, B., Rat, A.C., Boissier, M.C., 2001. Cardiac manifestations of rheumatoid arthritis: a case-control transesophageal echocardiography study in 30 patients. Arthritis Rheum. 45 (2), 129–135. Available from: PM: 11324775.

Hara, K.S., Ballard, D.J., Ilstrup, D.M., Connolly, D.C., Vollertsen, R.S., 1990. Rheumatoid pericarditis: clinical features and survival. Medicine (Baltimore) 69 (2), 81–91. Available from: PM: 2319940.

Heliovaara, M., Aho, K., Knekt, P., Aromaa, A., Maatela, J., Reunanen, A., 1995. Rheumatoid factor, chronic arthritis and mortality. Ann. Rheum. Dis. 54 (10), 811–814. Available from: PM: 7492219.

Hernandez-Hernandez, V., Ferraz-Amaro, I., Diaz-Gonzalez, F., 2014. Influence of disease activity on the physical activity of rheumatoid arthritis patients. Rheumatology (Oxford) 53 (4), 722–731. Available from: PM: 24369410.

Humphreys, J.H., Warner, A., Chipping, J., Marshall, T., Lunt, M., Symmons, D.P., Verstappen, S.M., 2014. Mortality trends in patients with early rheumatoid arthritis over 20 years: results from the Norfolk Arthritis Register. Arthritis Care Res. (Hoboken) 66 (9), 1296–1301. Available from: PM: 24497371.

Hyrich, K.L., Watson, K.D., Silman, A.J., Symmons, D.P., 2006. Predictors of response to anti-TNF-alpha therapy among patients with rheumatoid arthritis: results from the British Society for Rheumatology Biologics Register. Rheumatology (Oxford) 45 (12), 1558–1565. Available from: PM: 16705046.

Iversen, M.D., Hammond, A., Betteridge, N., 2010. Self-management of rheumatic diseases: state of the art and future perspectives. Ann. Rheum. Dis. 69 (6), 955–963.

Jacobsson, L.T., Knowler, W.C., Pillemer, S., Hanson, R.L., Pettitt, D.J., Nelson, R.G., del, P.A., McCance, D.R., Charles, M.A., Bennett, P.H., 1993. Rheumatoid arthritis and mortality. A longitudinal study in Pima Indians. Arthritis Rheum. 36 (8), 1045–1053. Available from: PM: 8343181.

John, H., Hale, E.D., Treharne, G.J., Kitas, G.D., Carroll, D., 2013. A randomized controlled trial of a cognitive behavioural patient education intervention vs a traditional information leaflet to address the cardiovascular aspects of rheumatoid disease. Rheumatology (Oxford) 52 (1), 81–90.

Kaptoge, S., Di, A.E., Lowe, G., Pepys, M.B., Thompson, S.G., Collins, R., Danesh, J., 2010. C-reactive protein concentration and risk of coronary heart disease, stroke, and mortality: an individual participant meta-analysis. Lancet 375 (9709), 132–140. Available from: PM: 20031199.

Karpouzas, G.A., Malpeso, J., Choi, T.Y., Li, D., Munoz, S., Budoff, M.J., 2014. Prevalence, extent and composition of coronary plaque in patients with rheumatoid arthritis without symptoms or prior diagnosis of coronary artery disease. Ann. Rheum. Dis. 73 (10), 1797–1804. Available from: PM: 23887286.

Kitas, G., Banks, M.J., Bacon, P.A., 2001. Cardiac involvement in rheumatoid disease. Clin. Med. (Lond) 1 (1), 18–21. Available from: PM: 11358070.

Klareskog, L., Malmstrom, V., Lundberg, K., Padyukov, L., Alfredsson, L., 2011. Smoking, citrullination and genetic variability in the immunopathogenesis of rheumatoid arthritis. Semin. Immunol. 23 (2), 92–98. Available from: PM: 21376627.

Koivuniemi, R., Paimela, L., Suomalainen, R., Leirisalo-Repo, M., 2013. Cardiovascular diseases in patients with rheumatoid arthritis. Scand. J. Rheumatol. 42 (2), 131–135. Available from: PM: 23244227.

Kremers, H.M., Crowson, C.S., Therneau, T.M., Roger, V.L., Gabriel, S.E., 2008. High ten-year risk of cardiovascular disease in newly diagnosed rheumatoid arthritis patients: a population-based cohort study. Arthritis Rheum. 58 (8), 2268–2274. Available from: PM: 18668561.

Kroot, E.J., van Gestel, A.M., Swinkels, H.L., Albers, M.M., van de Putte, L.B., van Riel, P.L., 2001. Chronic comorbidity in patients with early rheumatoid arthritis: a descriptive study. J. Rheumatol. 28 (7), 1511–1517. Available from: PM: 11469455.

Kuo, C.F., Luo, S.F., See, L.C., Chou, I.J., Chang, H.C., Yu, K.H., 2013. Rheumatoid arthritis prevalence, incidence, and mortality rates: a nationwide population study in Taiwan. Rheumatol. Int. 33 (2), 355–360. Available from: PM: 22451027.

Kvalvik, A.G., Jones, M.A., Symmons, D.P., 2000. Mortality in a cohort of Norwegian patients with rheumatoid arthritis followed from 1977 to 1992. Scand. J. Rheumatol. 29 (1), 29–37. Available from: PM: 9517761.

Lassere, M.N., Rappo, J., Portek, I.J., Sturgess, A., Edmonds, J.P., 2013. How many life years are lost in patients with rheumatoid arthritis? Secular cause-specific and all-cause mortality in rheumatoid arthritis, and their predictors in a long-term Australian cohort study. Intern. Med. J. 43 (1), 66–72. Available from: PM: 22289054.

Lemmey, A.B., Marcora, S.M., Chester, K., Wilson, S., Casanova, F., Maddison, P.J., 2009. Effects of high-intensity resistance training in patients with rheumatoid arthritis: a randomized controlled trial. Arthritis Rheum. 61 (12), 1726–1734. Available from: PM: 19950325.

Lerman, A., Zeiher, A.M., 2005. Endothelial function: cardiac events. Circulation 111 (3), 363–368. Available from: PM: 15668353.

Levy, L., Fautrel, B., Barnetche, T., Schaeverbeke, T., 2008. Incidence and risk of fatal myocardial infarction and stroke events in rheumatoid arthritis patients. A systematic review of the literature. Clin. Exp. Rheumatol. 26 (4), 673–679. Available from: PM: 18799105.

Liang, K.P., Kremers, H.M., Crowson, C.S., Snyder, M.R., Therneau, T.M., Roger, V.L., Gabriel, S.E., 2009. Autoantibodies and the risk of cardiovascular events. J. Rheumatol. 36 (11), 2462–2469. Available from: PM: 19833748.

Liao, K.P., Solomon, D.H., 2013. Traditional cardiovascular risk factors, inflammation and cardiovascular risk in rheumatoid arthritis. Rheumatology (Oxford) 52 (1), 45–52. Available from: PM: 22986289.

Libby, P., Ridker, P.M., Maseri, A., 2002. Inflammation and atherosclerosis. Circulation 105 (9), 1135–1143. Available from: PM: 11877368.

Lindhardsen, J., Ahlehoff, O., Gislason, G.H., Madsen, O.R., Olesen, J.B., Torp-Pedersen, C., Hansen, P.R., 2011. The risk of myocardial infarction in rheumatoid arthritis and diabetes mellitus: a Danish nationwide cohort study. Ann. Rheum. Dis. 70 (6), 929–934. Available from: PM: 21389043.

Lindhardsen, J., Gislason, G.H., Jacobsen, S., Ahlehoff, O., Olsen, A.M., Madsen, O.R., Torp-Pedersen, C., Hansen, P.R., 2013. Non-steroidal anti-inflammatory drugs and risk of cardiovascular disease in patients with rheumatoid arthritis: a nationwide cohort study. Ann. Rheum. Dis. Available from: PM: 23749610.

Lindqvist, E., Eberhardt, K., 1999. Mortality in rheumatoid arthritis patients with disease onset in the 1980s. Ann. Rheum. Dis. 58 (1), 11–14. Available from: PM: 10343534.

Maione, S., Valentini, G., Giunta, A., Tirri, R., Giacummo, A., Lippolis, C., Arnese, M., de, P.A., Marone, G., Tirri, G., 1993. Cardiac involvement in rheumatoid arthritis: an echocardiographic study. Cardiology 83 (4), 234–239. Available from: PM: 8281539.

Maki-Petaja, K.M., Booth, A.D., Hall, F.C., Wallace, S.M.L., Brown, J., McEniery, C.M., Wilkinson, I.B., 2007. Ezetimibe and simvastatin reduce inflammation, disease activity, and aortic stiffness and improve endothelial function in rheumatoid arthritis. J. Am. Coll. Cardiol. 50 (9), 852–858. Available from: PM: 17719471.

Maradit-Kremers, H., Nicola, P.J., Crowson, C.S., Ballman, K.V., Jacobsen, S.J., Roger, V.L., Gabriel, S.E., 2007. Raised erythrocyte sedimentation rate signals heart failure in patients with rheumatoid arthritis. Ann. Rheum. Dis. 66 (1), 76–80. Available from: PM: 16818462.

Martinez, M.S., Garcia-Monforte, A., Rivera, J., 2001. Survival study of rheumatoid arthritis patients in Madrid (Spain). A 9-year prospective follow-up. Scand. J. Rheumatol. 30 (4), 195–198. Available from: PM: 11578012.

Mavrogeni, S., Spargias, K., Markussis, V., Kolovou, G., Demerouti, E., Papadopoulou, E., Stavridis, G., Kaklamanis, L., Douskou, M., Constantoulakis, P., Cokkinos, D.V., 2009. Myocardial inflammation in autoimmune diseases: investigation by cardiovascular magnetic resonance and endomyocardial biopsy. Inflamm. Allergy Drug Targets 8 (5), 390–397. Available from: PM: 20025587.

Mavrogeni, S., Bratis, K., Sfendouraki, E., Papadopoulou, E., Kolovou, G., 2013. Myopericarditis, as the first sign of rheumatoid arthritis relapse, evaluated by cardiac magnetic resonance. Inflamm. Allergy Drug Targets 12 (3), 206–211. PMID: 23547732.

Metsios, G.S., Stavropoulos-Kalinoglou, A., Panoulas, V.F., Wilson, M., Nevill, A.M., Koutedakis, Y., Kitas, G.D., 2009. Association of physical inactivity with increased cardiovascular risk in patients with rheumatoid arthritis. Eur. J. Cardiovasc. Prev. Rehabil. 16 (2), 188–194. Available from: PM: 19238083.

Meune, C., Touze, E., Trinquart, L., Allanore, Y., 2009. Trends in cardiovascular mortality in patients with rheumatoid arthritis over 50 years: a systematic review and meta-analysis of cohort studies. Rheumatology (Oxford) 48 (10), 1309–1313. Available from: PM: 19696061.

Mikuls, T.R., Saag, K.G., Criswell, L.A., Merlino, L.A., Kaslow, R.A., Shelton, B.J., Cerhan, J.R., 2002. Mortality risk associated with rheumatoid arthritis in a prospective cohort of older women: results from the Iowa Women's Health Study. Ann. Rheum. Dis. 61 (11), 994–999. Available from: PM: 12379522.

Mody, G.M., Stevens, J.E., Meyers, O.L., 1987. The heart in rheumatoid arthritis—a clinical and echocardiographic study. Q. J. Med. 65 (247), 921–928. Available from: PM: 3455547.

Montalescot, G., Sechtem, U., Achenbach, S., Andreotti, F., Arden, C., Budaj, A., Bugiardini, R., Crea, F., Cuisset, T., Di, M.C., Ferreira, J.R., Gersh, B.J., Gitt, A.K., Hulot, J.S., Marx, N., Opie, L.H., Pfisterer, M., Prescott, E., Ruschitzka, F., Sabate, M., Senior, R., Taggart, D.P., van der Wall, E.E., Vrints, C.J., Zamorano, J.L., Achenbach, S., Baumgartner, H., Bax, J.J., Bueno, H., Dean, V., Deaton, C., Erol, C., Fagard, R., Ferrari, R., Hasdai, D., Hoes, A.W., Kirchhof, P., Knuuti, J., Kolh, P., Lancellotti, P., Linhart, A., Nihoyannopoulos, P., Piepoli, M.F., Ponikowski, P., Sirnes, P.A., Tamargo, J.L., Tendera, M., Torbicki, A., Wijns, W., Windecker, S., Knuuti, J., Valgimigli, M., Bueno, H., Claeys, M.J., Donner-Banzhoff, N., Erol, C., Frank, H., Funck-Brentano, C., Gaemperli, O., Gonzalez-Juanatey, J.R., Hamilos, M., Hasdai, D., Husted, S., James, S.K., Kervinen, K., Kolh, P., Kristensen, S.D., Lancellotti, P., Maggioni, A.P., Piepoli, M.F., Pries, A.R., Romeo, F., Ryden, L., Simoons, M.L., Sirnes, P.A., Steg, P.G., Timmis, A., Wijns, W., Windecker, S., Yildirir, A., Zamorano, J.L., 2013. 2013 ESC guidelines on the management of stable coronary artery disease: the task force on the management of stable coronary artery disease of the European Society of Cardiology. Eur. Heart J. 34 (38), 2949–3003. Available from: PM: 23996286.

Morris, P.B., Imber, M.J., Heinsimer, J.A., Hlatky, M.A., Reimer, K.A., 1986. Rheumatoid arthritis and coronary arteritis. Am. J. Cardiol. 57 (8), 689–690. Available from: PM: 3953457.

Myasoedova, E., Chandran, A., Ilhan, B., Major, B.T., Michet, C.J., Matteson E.L., Crowson, C.S., 2016. The role of rheumatoid arthritis (RA) flare and cumulative burden of RA severity in the risk of cardiovascular disease. Ann. Rheum. Dis. 75 (3), 560–565. Available from: PM: 25637001.

Myasoedova, E., Crowson, C.S., Kremers, H.M., Roger, V.L., Fitz-Gibbon, P.D., Therneau, T.M., Gabriel, S.E., 2011. Lipid paradox in rheumatoid arthritis: the impact of serum lipid measures and systemic inflammation on the risk of cardiovascular disease. Ann. Rheum. Dis. 70 (3), 482–487. Available from: PM: 21216812.

Myasoedova, E., Crowson, C.S., Kremers, H.M., Therneau, T.M., Gabriel, S.E., 2010. Is the incidence of rheumatoid arthritis rising?: results from Olmsted County, Minnesota, 1955-2007. Arthritis Rheum. 62 (6), 1576–1582. Available from: PM: 20191579.

Navarro-Millan, I., Charles-Schoeman, C., Yang, S., Bathon, J.M., Bridges Jr., S.L., Chen, L., Cofield, S.S., Dell'Italia, L.J., Moreland, L.W., O'Dell, J.R., Paulus, H.E., Curtis, J.R., 2013. Changes in lipoproteins associated with methotrexate or combination therapy in early rheumatoid arthritis: results from the treatment of early rheumatoid arthritis trial. Arthritis Rheum. 65 (6), 1430–1438. Available from: PM: 23460074.

Naz, S.M., Symmons, D.P., 2007. Mortality in established rheumatoid arthritis. Best Pract. Res. Clin. Rheumatol. 21 (5), 871–883. Available from: PM: 17870033.

Nicola, P.J., Maradit-Kremers, H., Roger, V.L., Jacobsen, S.J., Crowson, C.S., Ballman, K.V., Gabriel, S.E., 2005. The risk of congestive heart failure in rheumatoid arthritis: a population-based study over 46 years. Arthritis Rheum. 52 (2), 412–420. Available from: PM: 15692992.

Nomeir, A.M., Turner, R.A., Watts, L.E., 1979. Cardiac involvement in rheumatoid arthritis. Followup study. Arthritis Rheum. 22 (6), 561–564. Available from: PM: 454495.

O'Leary, D.H., Polak, J.F., Kronmal, R.A., Manolio, T.A., Burke, G.L., Wolfson Jr., S.K., 1999. Carotid-artery intima and media thickness as a risk factor for myocardial infarction and stroke in older adults. Cardiovascular Health Study Collaborative Research Group. N. Engl. J. Med. 340 (1), 14–22. Available from: PM: 9878640.

Panoulas, V.F., Douglas, K.M., Milionis, H.J., Stavropoulos-Kalinglou A., Nightingale, P., Kita, M.D., Tselios, A.L., Metsios, G.S., Elisaf, M.S., Kitas, G.D., 2007. Prevalence and associations of hypertension and its control in patients with rheumatoid arthritis. Rheumatology (Oxford) 46 (9), 1477–1482. Available from: PM: 17704521.

Peltomaa, R., Paimela, L., Kautiainen, H., Leirisalo-Repo, M., 2002. Mortality in patients with rheumatoid arthritis treated actively from the time of diagnosis. Ann. Rheum. Dis. 61 (10), 889–894. Available from: PM: 12228159.

Perk, J., De, B.G., Gohlke, H., Graham, I., Reiner, Z., Verschuren, M., Albus, C., Benlian, P., Boysen, G., Cifkova, R., Deaton, C., Ebrahim, S., Fisher, M., Germano, G., Hobbs, R., Hoes, A., Karadeniz, S., Mezzani, A., Prescott, E., Ryden, L., Scherer, M., Syvanne, M., Scholte op Reimer, W.J., Vrints, C., Wood, D., Zamorano, J.L., Zannad, F., 2012. European guidelines on cardiovascular disease prevention in clinical practice (version 2012). The fifth joint task force of the European Society of Cardiology and Other Societies on cardiovascular disease prevention in clinical practice (constituted by representatives of nine societies and by invited experts). Eur. Heart J. 33 (13), 1635–1701. Available from: PM: 22555213.

Peters, M.J., van Halm, V.P., Voskuyl, A.E., Smulders, Y.M., Boers, M., Lems, W.F., Visser, M., Stehouwer, C.D., Dekker, J.M., Nijpels, G., Heine, R., Dijkmans, B.A., Nurmohamed, M.T., 2009. Does rheumatoid arthritis equal diabetes mellitus as an independent risk factor for cardiovascular disease? A prospective study. Arthritis Rheum. 61 (11) 1571–1579. Available from: PM: 19877093.

Peters, M.J., Vis, M., van Halm, V.P., Wolbink, G.J., Voskuyl, A.E., Lems, W.F., Dijkmans, B.A., Twisk, J.W., de Koning, M.H., van de Stadt, R.J., Nurmohamed, M.T., 2007. Changes in lipid profile during infliximab and corticosteroid treatment in rheumatoid arthritis. Ann. Rheum. Dis. 66 (7), 958–961. Available from: PM: 17314120.

Peters, M.J.L., Symmons, D.P.M., McCarey, D., Dijkmans, B.A.C., Nicola, P., Kvien, T.K., McInnes, I.B., Haentzschel, H., Gonzalez-Gay, M.A., Provan, S., Semb, A., Sidiropoulos, P., Kitas, G., Smulders, Y.M., Soubrier, M., Szekanecz, Z., Sattar, N., Nurmohamed, M.T., 2010a. EULAR evidence-based recommendations for cardiovascular risk management in patients with rheumatoid arthritis and other forms of inflammatory arthritis. Ann. Rheum. Dis. 69 (2), 325–331. Available from: PM: 19773290.

Peters, M.J.L., Voskuyl, A.E., Sattar, N., Dijkmans, B.A.C., Smulders, Y.M., Nurmohamed, M.T., 2010b. The interplay between inflammation, lipids and cardiovascular risk in rheumatoid arthritis: why ratios may be better. Int. J. Clin. Pract. 64 (10), 1440–1443. Available from: PM: 20716150.

Pharmacovigilance Risk Assessment Committee (PRAC). New Safety Advice for Diclofenac – CMDh Endorses PRAC Recommendation. http://www.ema.europa.eu/ema/index.jsp?curl=pages/news_and_events/news/2013/06/news_detail_001830.jsp&mid=WC0b01ac058004d5c1.

Pharmacovigilance Risk Assessment Committee (PRAC). PRAC Recommends Updating Advice on Use of High-dose Ibuprofen. http://www.ema.europa.eu/ema/index.jsp?curl=pages/news_and_events/news/2015/04/news_detail_002306.jsp&mid=WC0b01ac058004d5c1.

Pincus, T., Keysor, J., Sokka, T., Krishnan, E., Callahan, L.F., 2004. Patient questionnaires and formal education level as prospective predictors of mortality over 10 years in 97% of 1416 patients with rheumatoid arthritis from 15 United States private practices. J. Rheumatol. 31 (2), 229–234. Available from: PM: 14760789.

Protogerou, A.D., Panagiotakos, D.B., Zampeli, E., Argyris, A.A., Arida, K., Konstantonis, G.D., Pitsavos, C., Kitas, G.D., Sfikakis, P.P., 2013. Arterial hypertension assessed "out-of-office" in a contemporary cohort of rheumatoid arthritis patients free of cardiovascular disease is characterized by high prevalence, low awareness, poor control and increased vascular damage-associated "white coat" phenomenon. Arthritis Res. Ther. 15 (5), R142. Available from: PM: 24286134.

Radovits, B.J., Fransen, J., Al, S.S., Eijsbouts, A.M., van Riel, P.L., Laan, R.F., 2010. Excess mortality emerges after 10 years in an inception cohort of early rheumatoid arthritis. Arthritis Care Res. (Hoboken) 62 (3), 362–370. Available from: PM: 20391482.

Raterman, H.G., Nielen, M.M., Peters, M.J., Verheij, R.A., Nurmohamed, M.T., Schellevis, F.G., 2012. Coexistence of hypothyroidism with inflammatory arthritis is associated with cardiovascular disease in women. Ann. Rheum. Dis. 71 (7), 1216–1218. Available from: PM: 22419774.

Raterman, H.G., van Halm, V.P., Voskuyl, A.E., Simsek, S., Dijkmans, B.A., Nurmohamed, M.T., 2008. Rheumatoid arthritis is associated with a high prevalence of hypothyroidism that amplifies its cardiovascular risk. Ann. Rheum. Dis. 67 (2), 229–232. Available from: PM: 17557891.

Reilly, P.A., Cosh, J.A., Maddison, P.J., Rasker, J.J., Silman, A.J., 1990. Mortality and survival in rheumatoid arthritis: a 25 year prospective study of 100 patients. Ann. Rheum. Dis. 49 (6), 363–369. Available from: PM: 2383059.

Rho, Y.H., Chung, C.P., Oeser, A., Solus, J., Asanuma, Y., Sokka, T., Pincus, T., Raggi, P., Gebretsadik, T., Shintani, A., Stein, C.M., 2009. Inflammatory mediators and premature coronary atherosclerosis in rheumatoid arthritis. Arthritis Rheum. 61 (11), 1580–1585. Available from: PM: 19877084.

Ridker, P.M., Buring, J.E., Rifai, N., Cook, N.R., 2007. Development and validation of improved algorithms for the assessment of global cardiovascular risk in women: the Reynolds Risk Score. JAMA 297 (6), 611–619. Available from: PM: 17299196.

Riise, T., Jacobsen, B.K., Gran, J.T., Haga, H.J., Arnesen, E., 2001. Total mortality is increased in rheumatoid arthritis. A 17-year prospective study. Clin. Rheumatol. 20 (2), 123–127. Available from: PM: 11346224.

Ristic, G.G., Lepic, T., Glisic, B., Stanisavljevic, D., Vojvodic, D., Petronijevic, M., Stefanovic, D., 2010. Rheumatoid arthritis is an independent risk factor for increased carotid intima-media thickness: impact of anti-inflammatory treatment. Rheumatology (Oxford) 49 (6), 1076–1081. Available from: PM: 20208070.

Roberts, E., Delgado, N.V., Buckner, S., Latchem, S., Constanti, M., Miller, P., Doherty, M., Zhang, W., Birrell, F., Porcheret, M., Dziedzic, K., Bernstein, I., Wise, E., Conaghan, P.G., 2016. Paracetamol: not as safe as we thought? A systematic literature review of observational studies. Ann. Rheum. Dis. 75 (3), 552–559. Available from: PM: 25732175.

Rollefstad, S., Ikdahl, E., Hisdal, J., Kvien, T.K., Pedersen, T.R., Holme, I., Semb, A.G., 2015. Systemic inflammation in patients with inflammatory joint diseases does not influence statin dose needed to obtain LDL cholesterol goal in cardiovascular prevention. Ann. Rheum. Dis. 74 (8), 1544–1550. Available from: PM: 24699940.

Ross, R., 1999. Atherosclerosis—an inflammatory disease. N. Engl. J. Med. 340 (2), 115–126. Available from: PM: 9887164.

Roubille, C., Richer, V., Starnino, T., McCourt, C., McFarlane, A., Fleming, P., Siu, S., Kraft, J., Lynde, C., Pope, J., Gulliver, W., Keeling, S., Dutz, J., Bessette, L., Bissonnette, R., Haraoui, B., 2015. The effects of tumour necrosis factor inhibitors, methotrexate, non-steroidal anti-inflammatory drugs and corticosteroids on cardiovascular events in rheumatoid arthritis, psoriasis and psoriatic arthritis: a systematic review and meta-analysis. Ann. Rheum. Dis. Available from: PM: 25561362.

Saag, K.G., Cerhan, J.R., Kolluri, S., Ohashi, K., Hunninghake, G.W., Schwartz, D.A., 1997. Cigarette smoking and rheumatoid arthritis severity. Ann. Rheum. Dis. 56 (8), 463–469. Available from: PM: 9306868.

Sandoo, A., Panoulas, V.F., Toms, T.E., Smith, J.P., Stavropoulos-Kalinoglou, A., Metsios, G.S., Gasparyan, A.Y., Carroll, D., Veldhuijzen van Zanten, J.J., Kitas, G.D., 2011a. Anti-TNFalpha therapy may lead to blood pressure reductions through improved endothelium-dependent microvascular function in patients with rheumatoid arthritis. J. Hum. Hypertens 25 (11), 699–702. Available from: PM: 21525886.

Sandoo, A., Veldhuijzen van Zanten, J.J., Metsios, G.S., Carroll, D., Kitas, G.D., 2011b. Vascular function and morphology in rheumatoid arthritis: a systematic review. Rheumatology (Oxford) 50 (11), 2125–2139. Available from: PM: 21926155.

Sattar, N., McCarey, D.W., Capell, H., McInnes, I.B., 2003. Explaining how "high-grade" systemic inflammation accelerates vascular risk in rheumatoid arthritis. Circulation 108 (24), 2957–2963. Available from: PM: 14676136.

Schoenfeld, S.R., Lu, L., Rai, S.K., Seeger, J.D., Zhang, Y., Choi, H.K., 2015. Statin use and mortality in rheumatoid arthritis: a general population-based cohort study. Ann. Rheum. Dis. Available from: PM: 26245753.

Semb, A.G., Rollefstad, S., Provan, S.A., Kvien, T.K., Stranden, E., Olsen, I.C., Hisdal, J., 2013. Carotid plaque characteristics and disease activity in rheumatoid arthritis. J. Rheumatol. 40 (4), 359–368. Available from: PM: 23322468.

Shah, N.H., LePendu, P., Bauer-Mehren, A., Ghebremariam, Y.T., Iyer, S.V., Marcus, J., Nead, K.T., Cooke, J.P., Leeper, N.J., 2015. Proton pump inhibitor usage and the risk of myocardial infarction in the general population. PLoS One 10 (6), e0124653. Available from: PM: 26061035.

Silman, A.J., 2002. The changing face of rheumatoid arthritis: why the decline in incidence? Arthritis Rheum. 46 (3), 579–581. Available from: PM: 11920391.

Skoldstam, L., Hagfors, L., Johansson, G., 2003. An experimental study of a Mediterranean diet intervention for patients with rheumatoid arthritis. Ann. Rheum. Dis. 62 (3), 208–214. Available from: PM: 12594104.

Smolen, J.S., Landewe, R., Breedveld, F.C., Buch, M., Burmester, G., Dougados, M., Emery, P., Gaujoux-Viala, C., Gossec, L., Nam, J., Ramiro, S., Winthrop, K., de, W.M., Aletaha, D., Betteridge, N., Bijlsma, J.W., Boers, M., Buttgereit, F., Combe, B., Cutolo, M., Damjanov, N., Hazes, J.M., Kouloumas, M., Kvien, T.K., Mariette, X., Pavelka, K., van Riel, P.L., Rubbert-Roth, A., Scholte-Voshaar, M., Scott, D.L., Sokka-Isler, T., Wong, J.B., van der Heijde, D., 2014. EULAR recommendations for the management of rheumatoid arthritis with synthetic and biological disease-modifying antirheumatic drugs: 2013 update. Ann. Rheum. Dis. 73 (3), 492–509. Available from: PM: 24161836.

Sokka, T., Mottonen, T., Hannonen, P., 1999. Mortality in early "sawtooth" treated rheumatoid arthritis patients during the first 8–14 years. Scand. J. Rheumatol. 28 (5), 282–287. Available from: PM: 10568424.

Solomon, D.H., Karlson, E.W., Rimm, E.B., Cannuscio, C.C., Mandl, L.A., Manson, J.E., Stampfer, M.J., Curhan, G.C., 2003. Cardiovascular morbidity and mortality in women diagnosed with rheumatoid arthritis. Circulation 107 (9), 1303–1307. Available from: PM: 12628952.

Solomon, D.H., Kremer, J., Curtis, J.R., Hochberg, M.C., Reed, G., Tsao, P., Farkouh, M.E., Setoguchi, S., Greenberg, J.D., 2010. Explaining the cardiovascular risk associated with rheumatoid arthritis: traditional risk factors versus markers of rheumatoid arthritis severity. Ann. Rheum. Dis. 69 (11), 1920–1925. Available from: PM: 20444756.

Souto, A., Salgado, E., Maneiro, J.R., Mera, A., Carmona, L., Gomez-Reino, J.J., 2015. Lipid profile changes in patients with chronic inflammatory arthritis treated with biologic agents and tofacitinib in randomized clinical trials: a systematic review and meta-analysis. Arthritis Rheumatol. 67 (1), 117–127. Available from: PM: 25303044.

Sparks, J.A., Chang, S.C., Liao, K.P., Lu, B., Fine, A.R., Solomon, D.H., Costenbader, K.H., Karlson, E.W., 2015. Rheumatoid arthritis and mortality among women during 36 years of prospective follow-up: results from the Nurses' Health Study. Arthritis Care Res. (Hoboken). Available from: PM: 26473946.

Stavropoulos-Kalinoglou, A., Metsios, G.S., Panoulas, V.F., Douglas, K.M., Nevill, A.M., Jamurtas, A.Z., Kita, M., Koutedakis, Y., Kitas, G.D., 2008. Cigarette smoking associates with body weight and muscle mass of patients with rheumatoid arthritis: a cross-sectional, observational study. Arthritis Res. Ther. 10 (3), R59. Available from: PM: 18492239.

Stavropoulos-Kalinoglou, A., Metsios, G.S., Veldhuijzen van Zanten, J.J., Nightingale, P., Kitas, G.D., Koutedakis, Y., 2013. Individualised aerobic and resistance exercise training improves cardiorespiratory fitness and reduces cardiovascular risk in patients with rheumatoid arthritis. Ann. Rheum. Dis. 72 (11), 1819–1825. Available from: PM: 23155222.

Stolt, P., Bengtsson, C., Nordmark, B., Lindblad, S., Lundberg, I., Klareskog, L., Alfredsson, L., 2003. Quantification of the influence of cigarette smoking on rheumatoid arthritis: results from a population based case-control study, using incident cases. Ann. Rheum. Dis. 62 (9), 835–841. Available from: PM: 12922955.

Sugiyama, D., Nishimura, K., Tamaki, K., Tsuji, G., Nakazawa, T., Morinobu, A., Kumagai, S., 2010. Impact of smoking as a risk factor for developing rheumatoid arthritis: a meta-analysis of observational studies. Ann. Rheum. Dis. 69 (1), 70—81. Available from: PM: 19174392.

Summers, G.D., Metsios, G.S., Stavropoulos-Kalinoglou, A., Kitas, G.D., 2010. Rheumatoid cachexia and cardiovascular disease. Nat. Rev. Rheumatol. 6 (8), 445—451. Available from: PM: 20647995.

Symmons, D.P., 2002. Epidemiology of rheumatoid arthritis: determinants of onset, persistence and outcome. Best Pract. Res. Clin. Rheumatol. 16 (5), 707—722. Available from: PM: 12473269.

Symmons, D.P., Jones, M.A., Scott, D.L., Prior, P., 1998. Longterm mortality outcome in patients with rheumatoid arthritis: early presenters continue to do well. J. Rheumatol. 25 (6), 1072—1077. Available from: PM: 9632066.

Thomas, E., Symmons, D.P., Brewster, D.H., Black, R.J., Macfarlane, G.J., 2003. National study of cause-specific mortality in rheumatoid arthritis, juvenile chronic arthritis, and other rheumatic conditions: a 20 year followup study. J. Rheumatol. 30 (5), 958—965. Available from: PM: 12734889.

Tlustochowicz, W., Cwetsch, A., Cholewa, M., Raczka, A., Nowak, J., 1997. Echocardiographic evaluation of cardiac structures in patients with rheumatoid arthritis. Pol. Arch. Med. Wewn. 97 (4), 352—358. Available from: PM: 9411412.

Toms, T.E., Panoulas, V.F., Douglas, K.M.J., Nightingale, P., Smith, J.P., Griffiths, H., Sattar, N., Symmons, D.P.M., Kitas, G.D., 2011. Are lipid ratios less susceptible to change with systemic inflammation than individual lipid components in patients with rheumatoid arthritis? Angiology 62 (2), 167—175. Available from: PM: 20682616.

Troughton, R.W., Asher, C.R., Klein, A.L., 2004. Pericarditis. Lancet 363 (9410), 717—727. Available from: PM: 15001332.

Turesson, C., Jarenros, A., Jacobsson, L., 2004. Increased incidence of cardiovascular disease in patients with rheumatoid arthritis: results from a community based study. Ann. Rheum. Dis. 63 (8), 952—955. Available from: PM: 15051620.

Turesson, C., O'Fallon, W.M., Crowson, C.S., Gabriel, S.E., Matteson, E.L. 2002. Occurrence of extraarticular disease manifestations is associated with excess mortality in a community based cohort of patients with rheumatoid arthritis. J. Rheumatol. 29 (1), 62—67. Available from: PM: 11824973.

Turesson, C., Eberhardt, K., Jacobsson, L.T., Lindqvist, E., 2007. Incidence and predictors of severe extra-articular disease manifestations in an early rheumatoid arthritis inception cohort. Ann. Rheum. Dis. 66 (11), 1543—1544. PMID: 17934083.

van den Berg, M.H., de Boer, I.G., le, C.S., Breedveld, F.C., Vliet Vlieland, T.P., 2007. Are patients with rheumatoid arthritis less physically active than the general population? J. Clin. Rheumatol. 13 (4), 181—186. Available from: PM: 17762450.

van Halm, V.P., Peters, M.J., Voskuyl, A.E., Boers, M., Lems, W.F., Visser, M., Stehouwer, C.D., Spijkerman, A.M., Dekker, J.M., Nijpels, G., Heine, R.J., Bouter, L.M., Smulders, Y.M., Dijkmans, B.A., Nurmohamed, M.T., 2009. Rheumatoid arthritis versus diabetes as a risk factor for cardiovascular disease: a cross-sectional study, the CARRE Investigation. Ann. Rheum. Dis. 68 (9), 1395—1400. Available from: PM: 18697775.

van Sijl, A.M., Van Den Hurk, K., Peters, M.J., van Halm, V.P., Nijpels, G., Stehouwer, C.D., Smulders, Y.V., Voskuyl, A.E., Dekker, J.M., Nurmohamed, M.T., 2012. Different type of carotid arterial wall remodeling in rheumatoid arthritis compared with healthy subjects: a case-control study. J. Rheumatol. 39 (12), 2261—2266. Available from PM: 23027891.

van Schaardenburg, D., Hazes, J.M., de, B.A., Zwinderman, A.H., Meijers, K.A., & Breedveld, F.C., 1993. Outcome of rheumatoid arthritis in relation to age and rheumatoid factor at diagnosis. J. Rheumatol. 20 (1), 45–52. Available from: PM: 8441165.

Vanderpump, M.P., Tunbridge, W.M., French, J.M., Appleton, D., Bates, D., Clark, F., Grimley, E.J., Hasan, D.M., Rodgers, H., Tunbridge, F., 1995. The incidence of thyroid disorders in the community: a twenty-year follow-up of the Whickham Survey. Clin. Endocrinol. (Oxf) 43 (1), 55–68. Available from: PM: 7641412.

Versteeg, H.H., Heemskerk, J.W., Levi, M., Reitsma, P.H., 2013. New fundamentals in hemostasis. Physiol. Rev. 93 (1), 327–358. Available from: PM: 23303912.

Voskuyl, A.E., 2006. The heart and cardiovascular manifestations in rheumatoid arthritis. Rheumatology (Oxford) 45 (Suppl. 4), iv4–iv7. Available from: PM: 16980723.

Voskuyl, A.E., Zwinderman, A.H., Westedt, M.L., Vandenbroucke, J.P., Breedveld, F.C., Hazes, J.M., 1996. Factors associated with the development of vasculitis in rheumatoid arthritis: results of a case-control study. Ann. Rheum. Dis. 55 (3), 190–192. Available from: PM: 8712883.

Wallberg-Jonsson, S., Ohman, M.L., Dahlqvist, S.R., 1997. Cardiovascular morbidity and mortality in patients with seropositive rheumatoid arthritis in Northern Sweden. J. Rheumatol. 24 (3), 445–451. Available from: PM: 9058647.

Widdifield, J., Bernatsky, S., Paterson, J.M., Tomlinson, G., Tu, K., Kuriya, B., Thorne, J.C., Pope, J.E., Hollands, S., Bombardier, C., 2015. Trends in excess mortality among patients with rheumatoid arthritis in Ontario, Canada. Arthritis Care Res. (Hoboken) 67 (8), 1047–1053. Available from: PM: 25623141.

Wislowska, M., Sypula, S., Kowalik, I., 1999. Echocardiographic findings and 24-h electrocardiographic Holter monitoring in patients with nodular and non-nodular rheumatoid arthritis. Rheumatol. Int. 18 (5–6), 163–169. Available from: PM: 10399790.

Wolfe, F., 2000. The effect of smoking on clinical, laboratory, and radiographic status in rheumatoid arthritis. J. Rheumatol. 27 (3), 630–637. Available from: PM: 10743800.

Wolfe, F., Freundlich, B., Straus, W.L., 2003. Increase in cardiovascular and cerebrovascular disease prevalence in rheumatoid arthritis. J. Rheumatol. 30 (1), 36–40. Available from: PM: 12508387.

Wolfe, F., Mitchell, D.M., Sibley, J.T., Fries, J.F., Bloch, D.A., Williams, C.A., Spitz, P.W., Haga, M., Kleinheksel, S.M., Cathey, M.A., 1994. The mortality of rheumatoid arthritis. Arthritis Rheum. 37 (4), 481–494. Available from: PM: 8147925.

Wong, M., Toh, L., Wilson, A., Rowley, K., Karschimkus, C., Prior, D., Romas, E., Clemens, L., Dragicevic, G., Harianto, H., Wicks, I., McColl, G., Best, J., Jenkins, A., 2003. Reduced arterial elasticity in rheumatoid arthritis and the relationship to vascular disease risk factors and inflammation. Arthritis Rheum. 48 (1), 81–89. Available from: PM: 12528107.

Young, A., Koduri, G., Batley, M., Kulinskaya, E., Gough, A., Norton, S., Dixey, J., 2007. Mortality in rheumatoid arthritis. Increased in the early course of disease, in ischaemic heart disease and in pulmonary fibrosis. Rheumatology (Oxford) 46 (2), 350–357. Available from: PM: 16908509.

Zhang, J., Chen, L., Delzell, E., Muntner, P., Hillegass, W.B., Safford, M.M., Millan, I.Y., Crowson, C.S., Curtis, J.R., 2014. The association between inflammatory markers, serum lipids and the risk of cardiovascular events in patients with rheumatoid arthritis. Ann. Rheum. Dis. 73 (7), 1301–1308. Available from: PM: 24796336.

Zoller, B., Li, X., Sundquist, J., Sundquist, K., 2012. Autoimmune diseases and venous thromboembolism: a review of the literature. Am. J. Cardiovasc. Dis. 2 (3), 171–183. Available from: PM: 22937487.

Chapter 11

Cardiac Involvement in Systemic Lupus Erythematosus

L. Iaccarino,* M. Gatto,* M. Zen* and A. Doria[§]
*Division of Rheumatology, University of Padova, Padova, Italy; [§]University of Padova Medical School, Padova, Italy

Key Points

- Cardiac abnormalities are common in systemic lupus erythematosus (SLE) patients. Nowadays they are usually mild or asymptomatic and are frequently recognized by noninvasive tests such as echocardiography and cardiac magnetic resonance imaging.
- Pericarditis is the most common manifestation, usually mild and rarely complicated by cardiac tamponade.
- Lupus myocarditis, although rare, is usually associated with high lupus disease activity and high-risk mortality; therefore a prompt and aggressive treatment is required.
- The most characteristic valvular lesion in SLE patients is atypical verrucous endocarditis (Libman-Sacks endocarditis), which rarely leads to hemodynamically significant valvular abnormalities requiring surgical treatment.
- Severe conduction tissue involvement is very rare in SLE patients. Congenital heart block can occur in 1–2% of newborns from anti-SSA and anti-SSB positive mothers.
- Atherosclerosis in SLE patients is premature and accelerated, being one of the most important cause of mortality in SLE patients. Chronic inflammation and the recruitment of several immunological cells promote formation and progression of atherosclerotic plaques as well as the development of complications.

1. INTRODUCTION

Systemic lupus erythematosus (SLE) is a chronic autoimmune disease of unknown etiology, characterized by the production of autoantibodies by autoreactive B cells. Autoantibodies are able, through several mechanisms, to induce inflammatory changes in various organs and systems including skin, musculoskeletal, hematopoietic and nervous systems, kidney, lung, blood vessels, and heart. In SLE, all the cardiac structures can be involved: pericardium, endocardium and valves, myocardium, coronary arteries, and conduction tissue (Doria et al., 2005a,b; Garcia et al., 2014; Miner and Kim, 2014).

In the past the diagnosis of SLE was frequently made in severe and life-threatening cases where cardiac abnormalities were rather frequent, serious, and often leading to death. Therefore, cardiac changes were frequently found in post-mortem examinations (Harvey et al., 1954; Estes and Christian, 1971). Nowadays, using more sensitive diagnostic tools, that is, antinuclear and other autoantibody tests, it is possible to diagnose SLE in earlier stages of the disease. Thus, cardiac manifestations are diagnosed earlier and more often are mild and asymptomatic, frequently (>50% of cases) recognized by echocardiography (D'Cruz et al., 2001; Kao and Manzi, 2002; Shazzad et al., 2013) and other noninvasive tests, including computer tomography (CT) and magnetic resonance imaging (MRI) (Mavrogeni et al., 2015).

2. PERICARDIAL INVOLVEMENT

Pericarditis is one of the most characteristic manifestations of the disease and is included in the ARA/ACR and SLICC classification criteria for SLE (Petri et al., 2012; Tan et al., 1982).

2.1 Prevalence

The prevalence of pericardial involvement varies between 11% and 83% (Tables 11.1 and 11.2). This variability depends on the type of the study: post-mortem, clinical, or echocardiographic. In post-mortem studies, the frequency of pericardial involvement varies between 47% and 83% (Gross, 1940; Kong et al., 1962; Ropes, 1976). Echocardiography finds pericardial abnormalities (effusion or thickening of the layers) in between 11% and 54% of SLE patients (Table 11.1).

2.2 Histopathologic Findings/Pathogenesis

In necropsy studies, the pericardium was involved by acute and chronic inflammatory changes. Acute pericarditis can be serofibrinous or fibrinous; the latter form is also found post-mortem, although less frequently than it was in the precorticosteroid era (Bulkley and Roberts, 1975). In chronic pericarditis, the fibrous or fibrofibrinous aspects prevail and the pericardial space may be obliterated by fibrous adhesions (Kong et al., 1962). Very large effusions, leading to cardiac tamponade and constrictive pericarditis (Jacobson and Reza, 1978) are very rare.

TABLE 11.1 Prevalence of Pericarditis in Systemic Lupus Erythematosus (SLE) Patients: Echocardiographic Studies

Reference	No. Patients	No. Positive (%)
Collins et al. (1978)	17	6 (35)
Ito et al. (1979)	48	22 (46)
Chia et al. (1981)	21	5 (23)
Klinkhoff et al. (1985)	47	10 (21)
Badui et al. (1985)	100	39 (39)
Doherty et al. (1988)	50	21 (42)
Crozier et al. (1990)	50	27 (54)
Leung et al. (1990a,b)	75	28 (37)
Kahl (1992)	395	75 (19)
Ramonda et al. (1992)	35	15 (43)
Cervera et al. (1992)	70	19 (27)
Sturfelt et al. (1992)	75	14 (19)
Rantapää-Dahlquist et al. (1997)	50	20 (40)
Castier et al. (2000)	325	107 (33)
Gentile et al. (2000)	91	19 (21)
Falcão et al. (2002)	70	8 (11)
Shahin et al. (2004)	62	12 (19)
Smiti et al. (2009)	97	38 (39)
Yu and Li (2011)	85	22 (26)
Shazzad et al. (2013)	50	20 (40)
Total	*1813*	*527 (29)*

The granular deposition of immunoglobulin and C3, demonstrated by direct immunofluorescence in surgical specimens of pericardial tissues from SLE patients (Jacobson and Reza, 1978; Bidani et al., 1980), supports the role of immune complexes in the development of pericarditis.

2.3 Clinical Features

The most frequent symptoms of pericarditis are tachycardia, dyspnea, precordial, or substernal chest pain that is emphasized by breathing, coughing, swallowing, and worsened when lying flat. At clinical examination, an increase

TABLE 11.2 Prevalence of Anatomical Valvular Abnormalities in Systemic Lupus Erythematosus (SLE): Echocardiographic Studies of Valvular Abnormalities

Reference	Patients No.	Verrucae No. (%)	Thickening No. (%)	Association with aPL
Klinkhoff et al. (1985)	47	0 (0)	10 (21)	–
Galve et al. (1988)	74	7 (9)	6 (8)	–
Crozier et al. (1990)	50	0 (0)	3 (6)	–
Khamashta et al. (1990)	132	9 (7)	5 (4)	Yes
Nihoyannoupoulos et al. (1990)	93	8 (9)	18 (19)	Yes
Leung et al. (1990a,b)	75	9 (12)	7 (9)	Yes
Cervera et al. (1992)	70	3 (4)	12 (17)	Yes
Sturfelt et al. (1992)	75	3 (4)	17 (23)	Yes
Ong et al. (1992)	40	1 (2.5)	15 (38)	No
Ramonda et al. (1992)	35	1 (3)	2 (6)	No
Giunta et al. (1993)	75	0 (0)	9 (12)	Yes
Metz et al. (1994)	52	3 (6)	4 (8)	No
Roldan et al. (1996) [a]	69	30 (43)	35 (51)	–
Rantapää-Dahlquist et al. (1997)	50	0 (0)	5 (10)	No
Omdal et al. (2001) [a]	35	12 (34)	10 (29)	No
Leszczyński et al. (2003)	52	1 (2)	11 (21)	Yes
Perez-Villa et al. (2005)	61	4 (7)	16 (26)	Yes
Moyssakis et al. (2007)	342	38 (11)	14 (4)	Yes
Yu and Li (2011)	85	0 (0)	15 (18)	–
Total	*1513*	*129 (8)*	*214 (14)*	

aPL, Antiphospholipid antibodies.
[a] *Transesophageal echocardiography.*

of the cardiac area and/or pericardial rub is the classical finding, but rarely found in the modern era (Ropes, 1976; Cervera et al., 1993; D'Cruz et al., 2001).

Pericardial involvement appears more frequently during SLE relapses (Ramonda et al., 1992), and it is often associated with the involvement of other serous layers, leading to polyserositis.

The complications of pericarditis are rare. If the effusion is very large, it can lead to cardiac tamponade. This occurs in 1−2.5% of patients with pericarditis, considering all cases including asymptomatic ones (Doherty and Siegel, 1985; Kahl, 1992; Castier et al., 2000) and in up to 16% of cases with overt clinical manifestations (Kahl, 1992; Buppajamrntham et al., 2014).

Constrictive pericarditis is even more rare (Lustig et al., 2014; Oh et al., 2012). Purulent pericarditis, with or without tamponade (Doherty and Siegel, 1985), is extremely rare too; it represents an infectious complication of immunosuppressive therapy and it is often due to Staphylococcus aureus.

2.4 Diagnostic Investigations

Large pericardial effusion can be recognized by standard chest X-ray, which documents the widening of the cardiac silhouette. Mild effusions and other abnormalities of the pericardial layers are demonstrated by echocardiography (Smiti et al., 2009; Yu and Li, 2011; Shazzad et al., 2013). Many patients with pericardial effusion and/or thickening of a moderate extent are asymptomatic (Doherty et al., 1988).

Pericardial effusion can be better defined using other investigations such as CT and MRI (Kruzliak et al., 2013).

Like pleural and synovial fluids, pericardial fluid in lupus patients is an inflammatory exudate and very seldom is hemorrhagic. Acidity is high, which allows its differentiation from the effusion due to renal insufficiency, traumas, or idiopathic effusion (Kindig and Goodman, 1983). In the pericardial exudate antinuclear antibodies, anti-double stranded (ds) DNA antibodies, low levels of complement, immune complexes, and rheumatoid factor may be detectable; glucose levels are normal (Moder et al., 1999).

2.5 Treatment

Nonsteroidal antiinflammatory drugs and/or corticosteroids (prednisone 0.5 mg/kg/day) are effective in mild pericarditis. In more severe cases or in tamponade a higher dose of corticosteroid is necessary, often given as an intravenous bolus (such as 1 g of methylprednisolone daily for 3 days).

In patients with recurring pericarditis chronic immunosuppression with azathioprine, methotrexate, mycophenolate mofetil, or, in refractory cases, belimumab or rituximab are recommended (Muangchan et al., 2015). High-dose intravenous immunoglobulins (IVIG) (Meissner et al., 2000) and colchicine (Morel et al., 2015) have also been suggested.

Invasive procedures such as pericardiocentesis, pericardial window, or pericardial stripping are rarely needed.

3. MYOCARDIAL INVOLVEMENT

The most characteristic feature of myocardial involvement in SLE is myocarditis. However, myocardial dysfunction may be the result of other noninflammatory features including ischemic heart disease, hypertension, renal failure, valvular disease, and toxicity from medications, especially cyclophosphamide and chloroquine (Moder et al., 1999; D'Cruz et al., 2001; Kao and Manzi, 2002). Myocardial dysfunction may progress to dilated cardiomyopathy, characterized by enlargement of all chambers, or hypertrophic cardiomyopathy involving the left ventricle (Kao and Manzi, 2002). This last feature typically develops in patients with long-standing hypertension.

3.1 Prevalence

The prevalence of lupus myocarditis has very much decreased since the introduction of steroid therapy (Kong et al., 1962; Bulkley and Roberts, 1975; Ropes, 1976) and nowadays clinically overt myocarditis is uncommon.

In post-mortem studies myocarditis prevalence varied from 7% to 50% (Badui et al., 1985; Doherty and Siegel, 1985; Bulkley and Roberts, 1975; Bidani et al., 1980; Roberts and High, 1999).

The prevalence of clinical manifestations due to myocarditis in the years 50s–80s was 10% (Harvey et al., 1954; Estes and Christian, 1971; Ropes, 1976; Badui et al., 1985; Dubois and Tuffanelli, 1964; Borestein et al., 1978). Recent epidemiologic data report a lower prevalence of clinically overt myocarditis: from 0.5% in an early lupus cohort (disease duration $\leq$2 years) (Garcia et al., 2014) to 6.1% in a more recent study (Du Toit et al., 2016).

3.2 Histopathologic Findings/Pathogenesis

Histological findings include small foci of fibrinoid necrosis with infiltrates of plasma cells and lymphocytes and, more rarely, diffuse interstitial inflammatory changes. Hematoxylin bodies, monocyte infiltrates, and foci of myocyte necrosis have also been found; however, this last feature is rare. In patients treated with corticosteroids, the finding of small foci of myocardial fibrosis is common (Bulkley and Roberts, 1975; Doherty and Siegel, 1985; Bidani et al., 1980; Fairfax et al., 1988).

Immunofluorescence studies demonstrate fine granular immune complexes and complement deposition in the walls and perivascular tissues of myocardial blood vessels (Bidani et al., 1980). Moreover, foci of immune deposits are observed along or within the myocyte bundles (Bidani et al., 1980). These observations support the hypothesis that lupus myocarditis is primarily an immune complex-mediated vascular phenomenon. However, the association between myocarditis and some circulating autoantibodies including anti-Ro/SSA (Logar et al., 1990), anti-U1RNP (Borenstein et al., 1978; Lash et al., 1986; Du Toit et al., 2016), and antiheart (Das and Cassidy, 1973) antibodies has been reported. Although there are evidences supporting the role of anti-Ro/SSA in the fetal development of myocarditis, the pathogenetic effects of these antibodies in adult myocarditis remain uncertain.

3.3 Clinical Features and Outcome

The signs and symptoms are similar to those of myocarditis due to other causes, that is, viral myocarditis (Wijetunga and Rockson, 2002): fever; dyspnea; palpitations; resting tachycardia, which is disproportionate to the patient's body temperature; cardiomegaly; gallop rhythms; rarely extrasystoles or other arrhythmias; increase of creatine phosphokinase (CPK), particularly CPK-MB; and troponin release (Feldman and McNamara, 2000). Myocarditis can progress to ventricular dysfunction, dilated cardiomyopathy, and heart failure. Heart failure can develop if other factors such as valvulitis, pericarditis, anemia, and hypertension concomitantly occur (Del Rio et al., 1978; Borenstein et al., 1978; Berg et al., 1985; Badui et al., 1985).

Lupus myocarditis is usually associated with high lupus disease activity, lupus nephritis, lymphopenia, and anti-U1RNP positivity. Mortality due to myocarditis remain high (43%) and it is associated with low ventricular function at diagnosis shown by echocardiography (Du Toit. et al., 2016).

3.4 Diagnostic Investigations

Diagnosis of myocarditis largely depends on clinical suspicion rather than on definitive diagnostic tests.

Nonspecific ST-T wave changes, conduction abnormalities, frequent premature complexes, and supraventricular and ventricular tachycardia may be noted on the electrocardiogram (ECG) (Estes and Christian, 1971; Borenstein et al., 1978; Badui et al., 1985).

Echocardiography is a useful and widely used procedure (Feldman and McNamara, 2000). It is able to show findings that, although unspecific, are indicative of myocardial inflammation and/or dysfunction. The most relevant findings are global, regional, or segmental wall motion abnormalities; decreased ejection fraction; increased chamber size; and diastolic dysfunction (Klinkhoff et al., 1985; Doherty et al., 1988; Crozier et al., 1990; Leung et al., 1990a,b; Nihoyannopoulos et al., 1990; Sturfelt et al., 1992; Giunta et al., 1993; Du Toit et al., 2016). MRI with T1-weighted early gadolinium enhancement, T1-weighted late gadolinium enhancement, and T2-weighted imaging is an emerging and very helpful tool in supporting a diagnosis of myocarditis (Yilmaz et al., 2013; Mavrogeni et al., 2016) because it offers a noninvasive detection of changes in myocardial tissue composition and well correlates with findings from endomyocardial biopsy (Mavrogeni et al., 2009; Yilmaz et al., 2013).

Endomyocardial biopsy represents the gold standard for the diagnosis of myocarditis. This invasive procedure is useful not only in confirming the diagnosis of lupus myocarditis, but also in ruling out other causes of cardiomyopathy (Feldman and McNamara, 2000; Lopez-Ruiz and Uribe, 2014; Mavrogeni et al., 2016). Moreover, it can give some information about the severity and the extent of cardiac involvement (Fairfax et al., 1988).

3.5 Treatment

Myocarditis, although mild, has to be treated immediately with high-dose corticosteroids (Moder et al., 1999; Wijetunga and Rockson, 2002). In the most severe forms it is necessary to use intravenous pulse corticosteroid (methylprednisolone 0.5–1 g/day for three consecutive days) followed by high doses of oral prednisone. The use of immunosuppressants, cyclophosphamide or azathioprine is particularly recommended for patients in whom active myocarditis has been histologically confirmed (Fairfax et al., 1988; Naarendorp et al., 1999; Du Toit et al., 2016). There are some report indicating a beneficial effect of intravenous IVIG (Disla et al., 1993; Sherer et al., 1999). Finally, in case of severe and/or refractory myocarditis, rituximab was successfully used as add on therapy (Aggarwal et al., 2012; Du Toit et al., 2016).

In patients with heart failure additional supportive pharmacologic therapy, such as inotropes, afterload-reducing agents, and diuretics are used; moreover, factors which can worsen heart failure such as anemia, hypertension, and infections have to be resolved.

4. VALVULAR INVOLVEMENT

Anatomical and functional valvular abnormalities have been described in SLE (Moder et al., 1999; D'Cruz et al., 2001; Kao and Manzi, 2002; Leszczyński et al., 2003; Perez-Villa et al., 2005,Yu and Li, 2011; Shazzad et al., 2013). Libman-Sacks endocarditis (Libman and Sacks, 1924), also termed "atypical verrucous endocarditis," is the most characteristic lesion.

4.1 Prevalence

In necroscopic studies the prevalence of valvular abnormalities ranges between 13% and 74% (Kong et al., 1962; Dubois and Tuffanelli, 1964; Estes and Christian, 1971; Bulkley and Roberts, 1975; Lehman et al., 1989). Some authors have suggested that the frequency of valvular abnormalities decreased after the introduction of corticosteroids in treatment. A study by Doherty and Siegel (1985) showed that the prevalence of these lesions was 59% before the use of corticosteroids and 35% after their introduction.

In Table 11.2 the prevalence of valvular verrucae and thickening observed in transthoracic and transesophageal echocardiography are reported.

4.2 Histopathologic Findings/Pathogenesis

Libman-Sacks endocarditis is characterized by ovoid verrucae, rather flat, smaller than those observed in rheumatic fever or in bacterial endocarditis, with a diameter ranging from 1 to 4 mm, consisting of fine granular material. The verrucae can be isolated, but they tend to gather together forming blackberry-shaped areas. These lesions can occur in any valve, but are observed more frequently in the mitral valve, on both surfaces of the valve. The simultaneous involvement of several valves is not uncommon.

In most post-mortem studies vegetations were observed in the recess between the posterior valvular leaflet and the ventricular wall (Doherty and Siegel, 1985), a location differing from that observed in infectious endocarditis, in which they are mostly found on the atrial aspect of the valve (Harvey et al., 1954; Bulkley and Roberts, 1975).

In a more recent study (Eiken et al., 2001), considering a surgical population, vegetations were found along the closing edges of the leaflets and along the atrial surfaces, without any involvement of the ventricular aspect—a pattern differing from that previously reported in post-mortem investigations.

Although rare, the vegetations can occur in chordae tendinae, papillary muscles, and the parietal endocardium.

Histologic studies have shown two types of lesions (Bulkley and Roberts, 1975): (1) active lesions which consist of fibrin clumps, focal necrosis, and mononuclear cell infiltrates and (2) healed lesions characterized by vascularized fibrous tissue sometimes associated with calcifications; calcification of the mitral ring has also been described (Bulkley and Roberts, 1975; Barzizza et al., 1987; Doherty et al., 1988). These lesions have different prognostic implications. The active lesions have been more frequently observed in young patients with recent disease onset (Galve et al., 1988). These lesions can induce mild valve regurgitation, but they generally do not lead to a hemodynamically significant valvular lesion.

The healed lesions are found in patients with long-standing disease and who have taken corticosteroids for a long time. Healed lesions are frequently associated with functional valve abnormalities, especially valvular insufficiency (Doherty and Siegel, 1985).

According to some authors (Galve et al., 1988; Carette, 1988) corticosteroid therapy can heal the valvular lesion with consequent retraction of the cusps and, in turn, valvular defect. Other authors (Doherty et al., 1988) did not observe any relationship between corticosteroid use and valvular abnormality.

The association between valvular abnormalities and antiphospholipid antibodies (aPL) has been reported (Ford et al., 1988; Chartash et al., 1989;

Nesher et al., 1997; Leszczyński et al., 2003; Perez-Villa et al., 2005) (Table 11.2). Indeed, it has been shown that valvular lesions were more frequently observed in SLE patients with aPL syndrome (APS) or positive aPL than in those without (Vianna et al., 1994; Leszczyński et al., 2003; Perez-Villa et al., 2005; Moyssakis et al., 2007).

Pathogenetic mechanism involved in the development of verrucous valvular abnormalities has not been fully elucidated. There are two major pathogenetic hypothesis. The *primum movens* could be represented by a thrombus. According to this hypothesis, aPL and antiendothelium antibodies could bind to endothelial cells, which lead to their activation and, in turn, platelet aggregation and thrombus formation (Simantov et al., 1995; Del Papa et al., 1999; Yazici et al., 2001; Kaplanski et al., 2000). Alternatively, the *primum movens* could be immune complex deposition between the endothelium and the basal membrane, followed by the infiltration of inflammatory cells (Shapiro et al., 1977; Bidani et al., 1980; Ziporen et al., 1996; Amital et al., 1999).

4.3 Clinical Features

Verrucous endocarditis is generally asymptomatic and only occasionally leads to a cardiac murmur (Ropes, 1976; Straaton et al., 1988). In fact, the verrucae are near the edge of the valves and therefore do not tend to deform the closing line, even when they are very large and protrude into the cardiac chambers.

It is rather common to find cardiac murmurs in SLE patients. It can be soft, holosystolic, and of low tone, but occasionally it can be strong and rough, perceptible at the left cardiac thrust and/or at the base. However, it is difficult to evaluate the cause of a "cardiac murmur" in SLE patients because of the coexistence of fever, tachycardia, and anemia.

The prevalence of complications due to verrucous endocarditis is low: lesions are hemodynamically significant in only 3–4% of cases, making surgical treatment necessary in 1–2%. The indication for valve replacement rises to 9% in the subset of patients with valvular abnormalities (Roldan et al., 1996). Anatomical abnormalities are generally found in the mitral and aortic valves. Mitral and/or aortic insufficiency are more frequent than stenosis of the same valves (Harvey et al., 1954; Ropes, 1976; Elkayam et al., 1977; Thandroyen et al., 1978; Kinney et al., 1980; Doherty and Siegel, 1985; Roldan et al., 1996; Perez-Villa et al., 2005,Yu and Li, 2011, Shazzad et al., 2013).

Among the complications of verrucous endocarditis, infectious endocarditis, embolism, and rupture of chordae tendinae have to be considered. The prevalence of infectious endocarditis is 4.9% in post-mortem surveys and 1.3% in clinical studies (Doherty and Siegel, 1985). It was observed in 3 (7%) out of 45 patients with valvular disease in the study of Roldan et al. (1996). It is facilitated by dental surgical treatments carried out without an appropriate antibiotic prophylaxis. In the setting of such surgical procedures, antibiotics should be taken by all SLE patients with valvular abnormalities (including mitral prolapse), especially if they are taking immunosuppressants (Klinkhoff et al., 1985; Doherty and Siegel, 1985; Comens et al., 1989; Luce et al., 1990). Fever, cardiac murmur, and splinter hemorrhages are common clinical manifestations in infectious endocarditis.

Stroke or peripheral embolism were observed in 13% of patients with valvular abnormalities (Roldan et al., 1996). It has also been suggested that positive aPL could increase the risk of cardioembolism (Fox et al., 1980). Finally, the rupture of chordae tendinae has occasionally observed (Kinney et al., 1980).

Jensen-Urstad et al. (2002) reported a close association between valvular abnormalities and cardiovascular disease (CVD) as well as raised levels of homocysteine and triglycerides in SLE patients. Therefore, patients with valvular disease should be screened for clinical and subclinical atherosclerotic features. Moreover, it has been suggested that the presence of Libman-Sacks endocarditis in patients with SLE is associated with a higher risk for embolic CVD indicating that Libman-Sacks endocarditis may be a source of cerebral emboli (Roldan et al., 2013).

4.4 Diagnostic Investigations

Echocardiography has been shown to be much more sensitive than clinical examination in the detection of Libman-Sacks endocarditis and/or its complications. This procedure allows the visualization of verrucae, thickening and calcification of valvular rings, and, when it is completed by Doppler investigation, can show valvular regurgitation (Table 11.2) (Kahan et al., 1985; Klinkhoff et al., 1985; Galve et al., 1988; Crozier et al., 1990; Leung et al., 1990a,b; Khamashta et al., 1990; Nihoyannopoulos et al., 1990; Sturfelt et al., 1992; Ramonda et al., 1992; Cervera et al., 1992; Ong et al., 1992; Giunta et al., 1993; Metz et al., 1994; Perez-Villa et al., 2005,Yu and Li, 2011, Shazzad et al., 2013; Roldan et al., 2015). The transesophageal technique is more sensitive than the transthoracic one in revealing these abnormalities (Roldan et al., 1996; Shively, 2000; Omdal et al., 2001; Roldan et al., 2008).

4.5 Treatment

Since Libman-Sacks endocarditis is clinically silent in the majority of cases, generally it is not treated. When it is found in an early active stage, corticosteroids (prednisone 1 mg/kg/day) are recommended, especially if aPL results are negative. It has been reported that valvular abnormalities frequently resolved over time (Roldan et al., 1996). Although no direct relationship between treatment and changes in valvular disease was demonstrated, these data support the hypothesis that active valvular lesions may be modifiable by therapy.

When endocarditis is detected at a later stage during the course of the disease, careful clinical surveillance is necessary and, if the lesion becomes hemodynamically significant, valve surgery is needed (Comens et al., 1989; Hakim et al., 2001). It is necessary to carefully evaluate the type of surgical treatment: valve repair, replacement with mechanical valve, or replacement with bioprosthetic porcine graft. Valve repair is a more conservative surgical treatment with no need for anticoagulation. It is a feasible and effective procedure in young patients with relatively stable SLE and/or APS and localized valve abnormalities caused by Libman-Sacks endocarditis (Bouma et al., 2010). However, valve repair often leads to repeated surgery and later valve replacement (Hakim et al., 2001).

Valve replacement in patients with SLE is generally uneventful and makes surgery a feasible option without posing a major risk to patients with compensated organ dysfunction (Morin et al., 1996; Foroughi et al., 2014). SLE patients who need valve surgery have, in the majority of cases, an associated APS, which itself requires anticoagulation. Bioprosthetic porcine valves have also been hindered by complications such as valvulitis relapse (Gordon et al., 1996). Therefore, mechanical valve replacement seems to be the best choice in lupus patients.

5. CORONARY ARTERY INVOLVEMENT

Angina pectoris and acute myocardial infarction (MI) were rare in SLE patients in 50s (Harvey et al., 1954). Following the improvement of the survival of SLE patients (Doria et al., 2006), they become the most frequently observed complications occurring in about 10% of patients with long-standing disease (Fernández-Nebro et al., 2015). Interestingly, in a cohort of patients with early SLE (within 15 months of diagnosis) the prevalence of MI is 1.6% (Urowitz et al., 2016).

5.1 Prevalence and Risk Estimation

In post-mortem studies, a significant narrowing of coronary arteries was observed in 25–45% of cases (Bulkley and Roberts, 1975; Haider and Roberts, 1981; Fukumoto et al., 1987).

The risk of developing CVD is eight-fold higher in women with SLE than controls; in addition, patients with SLE have an overall standardized incidence ratio of MI of 2.31 (Bengtsson et al., 2012). Manzi's study (Manzi et al., 1997) shows a 50-fold increased risk of MI in women aged between 35 and 44 years of age.

In carotid ultrasound studies coronary artery disease (CAD) is reported with a prevalence ranging from 16% to 40% (Manzi et al., 1999; Svenungsson et al., 2001; Roman et al., 2003; Doria et al., 2003; Thompson et al., 2008) and in coronary-CT studies the prevalence of coronary calcifications ranges from 7.2% to 28% (Romero-Díaz et al., 2012; Plazak et al., 2011; Manger et al., 2003).

Abnormalities of the coronary circulation have been reported in 40% of SLE patients using scintigraphy with Tallium-201 (Hosepund et al., 1984; Bruce et al., 2000a,b; Ishida et al., 2000) and even a higher percentage using single photon emission computed tomography dual isotope myocardial perfusion imaging (DIMPI) (Schillaci et al., 1999; Sun et al., 2001).

5.2 Histopathology/Pathogenesis

Different mechanisms can play a part in the development of CAD. These include atherosclerosis, coronary arteritis, thrombotic events with or without aPL, vasospasm, or embolization of valvular material, and hypertension (Bulkley and Roberts, 1975; Doherty and Siegel, 1985; Meller et al., 1975; Rosenthal et al., 1980; Pritzker et al., 1980; Lerman et al., 1982; Englund and Lucas, 1983; Matayoshi et al., 1999).

Histologically, two major findings occur: (1) large transmural infarctions: in this case a remarkable reduction of the lumen of at least one of the three major extramural coronary arteries has been reported, more frequently due to atherosclerotic plaque and more seldom to embolism; (2) small areas of necrosis, detectable only histologically, adjacent to small intramural coronary arteries, the lumen of which appear restricted, and walls infiltrated by inflammatory cells.

The lesions of the major coronary arteries are predominantly of an atherosclerotic nature and, histologically, are not different from those seen in non-SLE subjects. In patients with SLE it has been shown that chronic inflammation (cytokines) and several immune cells, including, T-lymphocytes and macrophages, promotes not only the initiation and progression of the atherosclerotic lesion, but also the development of complications. The most common is the complete rupture of the plaque's fibrous cap, which allows prothrombotic tissue factor to contact coagulation factors in the bloodstream. In addition, the activated cells into the plaque, including endothelial cells and smooth muscle cells, produce considerable amounts of plasminogen activator inhibitor-1, which is a powerful inhibitor of the endogenous fibrinolytic enzymes such as urokinase and tissue-type plasminogen activator (Libby and Ridker, 2006).

The minor coronary arteries can be affected by a vasculitic process. Histologically, a fibrinoid reaction of the intima and the media layers with partial interruption of the elastic layer, swelling and scaling of the endothelial cells (which can be followed by thrombosis), and perivascular inflammatory infiltrates of lymphocytes and plasma cells can be detected. The evolution is toward healing sclerosis of all the arterial layers and fibrous hyperplasia of the intima with remarkable reduction of the lumen.

Another mechanism that has been hypothesized to lead to coronary thrombus formation is a superficial erosion of the endothelial cells, possibly caused by endothelial apoptosis or desquamation (Libby and Ridker, 2006).

5.3 Clinical Features and Outcome

The clinical manifestations of CAD in SLE are angina pectoris and MI. The distinction between atherosclerosis and coronary vasculitis is difficult, but of key importance for therapeutic decisions. Ischemia due to vasculitis is more frequent in young people with active disease, often of short duration. Moreover, in these patients the detection of vasculitic abnormalities in other organs is not uncommon; however, the absence of these last features does not rule out coronary arteritis (Wilson et al., 1992). Ischemia due to atherosclerosis, although occurring earlier in SLE patients than in the normal population, affects more frequently older SLE patients, with long-standing disease, long period of corticosteroid intake, and, usually, quiescent disease at the time of the cardiovascular event.

Ischemic cardiopathy could be due to APS (Asherson et al., 1989; Murpy and Leach, 1989; Leung et al., 1990a,b; MacGregor et al., 1992; Kattwinkel et al., 1992), and in this case could develop at any age and in any stage of the disease course.

5.4 Outcome

Urowitz et al. (1976) described a bimodal distribution of the causes of death in SLE: an "early" peak due to SLE severity/activity or infections and a "late" peak due to atherosclerotic CAD; this trend has been confirmed in other studies too (Rubin et al., 1985; Abu-Shakra et al., 1995). Further studies found that acute MI was the cause of death in between 3% and 25% of SLE patients (Jonsson et al., 1989; Wallace et al., 1981; Rosner et al., 1982; Cervera et al., 1999; Bruce et al., 2000a,b).

5.5 Traditional and Nontraditional Risk Factors for Premature Atherosclerosis in SLE Patients

Early atherosclerotic lesions cannot be explained by Framingham risk factors alone, that is, age, male sex, arterial hypertension, hypercholesterolemia, diabetes, obesity, sedentary life, and smoke (Manzi et al., 1999; Esdaile et al., 2001; Rahman et al., 1999; Bruce et al., 1999). Thus, premature atherosclerosis observed in patients with SLE has been attributed to complex interactions between traditional risk factors and factors associated with the disease per se or its treatment (Ward, 1999; Bruce et al., 2000a,b; Roman et al., 2001; Svenungsson et al., 2001; Roman et al., 2003; Doria et al., 2003; Doria et al., 2005a,b; Thompson et al., 2008; Lòpez-Pedrera et al., 2010; Thacker et al., 2012).

5.5.1 Traditional Risk Factors

Many studies have shown abnormality of lipids in SLE patients with an increase of total cholesterol, very low-density lipoprotein, and triglycerides and a decrease of HDL and LDL cholesterol. These abnormalities seem to be influenced by disease activity (Ilowite et al., 1988; Borba and Bonfa, 1997; Borba et al., 1998), corticosteroid therapy (Ettinger et al., 1987; MacGregor et al., 1992; Petri et al., 1992b; Leong et al., 1994), nephrotic syndrome (Leong et al., 1994), and diabetes mellitus. The prevalence of diabetes in SLE patients is approximately 7% (Manzi et al., 1997; Petri et al., 1992a) and that of metabolic syndrome 16% (Parker et al., 2012). A beneficial effect of hydroxychloroquine on the lipid profile in SLE patients has also been reported (Wallace et al., 1990; Petri et al., 1994; Iaccarino et al., 2013), with a reduction of total cholesterol, LDL, and triglycerides.

Other studies (Clarke et al., 1991; Fermo et al., 1995; Petri et al., 1996; Manzi et al., 1999; Petri et al., 1992b; Petri, 2000a; Doria et al., 2003) have shown an important role of hypertension, sedentary life style, and hyperhomocysteinemia in the development of atherosclerosis. Hypertension can be secondary to renal involvement, corticosteroid therapy, and insulin resistance induced by corticosteroid therapy, and, therefore, it is a common feature in SLE patients. A study by Petri et al. (1996) has also shown that corticosteroids and nephropathy could lead to an increase of homocysteine, which is significantly associated with arterial thrombosis and vascular events such as TIA and stroke.

5.5.2 Nontraditional Risk Factors

Besides cumulative dosage and/or length of corticosteroid therapy, disease duration, high disease activity, and damage accrual (Gladman and Urowitz, 1987; Petri et al., 1992a; Petri et al., 1994; Manzi et al., 1997; Manzi et al., 1999; Petri, 2000a, 2000b; Doria et al., 2003), some other inflammatory and immunologic parameters have been recently proposed, which could contribute to the development of atherosclerotic plaque.

Some markers of acute phase response, especially high-sensitivity C-reactive protein, increased C3 serum levels, and high white blood cell count were found to be associated with clinical or subclinical atherosclerosis in SLE. Cytokines, including interferon (IFN)-α and INFγ, tumor necrosis factor (TNF)-α, interleukin (IL)-6, IL-17, and B-lymphocytes stimulator, which are involved in the pathogenesis of SLE are also considered pivotal factors in CAD development by various mechanisms: IFNα leads to endothelial dysfunction by decreasing the number of endothelial progenitor cells; TNFα enhances hypertriglyceridemia and promotes atherosclerosis-related inflammation leading to IL-6 and IFNγ overexpression (Lòpez-Pedrera et al., 2010; Iaccarino et al., 2013). On the other hand, Pentraxin 3 was significantly associated with SLE activity but not with carotid atherosclerosis (Shimada et al., 2014).

Among autoantibodies, aPL can contribute to the development of the atherosclerotic plaque. Some studies pointed out that aPL cross-react with oxidized LDL (Vaarala et al., 1993). LDL contains phospholipids and apolipoprotein B, which could become "antigenic" after lipoprotein oxidation.

According to another hypothesis, β2GPI could bind oxidized LDL turning them into a target for anti-β2GPI antibodies (Bruce et al., 2000a,b; Witztum, 1994; Matsuura et al., 1994). It has been suggested that β2GPI can prevent the uptake of oxLDL by macrophages via scavenger receptors and anti-β2GPI antibodies bind β2GPI facilitating the uptake of oxLDL by macrophages via Fcγ receptor (Bassi et al., 2007). Although controversial, other autoantibodies such as anti-HSP65 and anti-oxidized LDL (Shoenfeld et al., 2001; Bassi et al., 2007) have been suggested to be associated with the development of atherosclerotic plaque.

5.6 Diagnostic Investigations

Resting and exercise ECG represent standard noninvasive techniques that can be used to routinely investigate CAD in SLE.

Moreover, several advances in nuclear cardiac imaging have emerged in the last decades. Thallium-201 scintigraphy was the first technique used for detecting perfusion abnormalities in SLE patients (Hosepud et al., 1984; Bruce et al., 2000a,b; Ishida et al., 2000). More recently, the technique of DIMPI has been introduced, which employs two isotopes: thallium-201 and technetium 99m sestamibi (Schillaci et al., 1999; Sun et al., 2001). This technique has several advantages in comparison with thallium scintigraphy including a better image resolution. However, both thallium scintigraphy and DIMPI are more sensitive than specific; therefore their results have to be considered with caution.

Coronary scanning by electron beam CT detects coronary calcification, which is considered to be a marker of coronary atherosclerosis (Von Felt, 1999).

In some cases angiography can be useful in differentiating coronary vasculitis from atherosclerosis. In fact, aneurysms and/or rapidly progressive narrowing of coronary arteries, showed by serial angiographies, although not pathognomonic, support the diagnosis of coronary vasculitis (Homcy et al., 1982; Englund and Lucas, 1983; Wilson et al., 1992; Nobrega et al., 1996).

For the investigation of subclinical atherosclerosis, carotid color Doppler ultrasonography (US) has been widely used (Manzi et al., 1999; Roman et al., 2001; Svenungsson et al., 2001; Doria et al., 2003; Thompson et al., 2008). Although carotid US directly investigates only the carotid artery, this technique provides an accurate measurement of subclinical coronary atherosclerosis (Li et al., 1996).

5.7 Prevention and Treatment of CAD in SLE Patients

Physicians should implement prevention strategies for CAD in SLE patients. It should include tight management of traditional risk factors as in patients with diabetes mellitus, treatment with angiotensin-converting enzyme (ACE) inhibitors, low-dose aspirin, and hydroxychloroquine, and prompt control of the underlying disease by using corticosteroid at the lowest effective dosage as well as steroid-sparing agents (Iaccarino et al., 2013; Benvenuti et al., 2015).

The therapeutical approach to SLE patients with CAD depends on the nature of the underlining pathological process. If it is due to vasculitis, corticosteroid therapy at high dosage is recommended (prednisone 1−1.5 mg/kg/day); if it is due to aPL and/or atherosclerosis, the use of anticoagulation and/or platelet antiaggregation as well as vasodilator drugs is suggested (D'Cruz et al., 2001; Kao and Manzi, 2002).

6. CONDUCTION TISSUE INVOLVEMENT

6.1 Prevalence

Sinus tachycardia is the most frequent rhythm abnormality and is quite common in SLE patients. Atrioventricular block and bundle branch block are the most common conduction defects; however, they are rare in adult (Logar et al., 1990; Martinez-Costa et al., 1991; Fonseca et al., 1994; Comín-Colet et al., 2001; Gómez-Barrado et al., 2002, Vereckei et al., 2013). In a prospective study congenital heart block (CHB) occurred in 2% of children born from mothers with anti-Ro/SSA antibodies (Brucato et al., 2001, 2002).

6.2 Histopathology/Pathogenesis

In about 90% of cases an explaining factor for sinus tachycardia including fever, volume depletion, congestive failure, perciarditis, myocarditis, thyroid dysfunction, and others can be found. In case of "unexplained" tachycardia (10%), it has been hypothesized as an asymptomatic myopericarditis, which usually respond well to corticosteroid therapy used to treat other disease manifestations (Lazzerini et al., 2006). It has also been suggested that in some patients an autonomic dysfunction could account for heart rate variability in SLE (Hogarth et al., 2002; Shalimar Handa et al., 2006; Stojanovich et al., 2007; Aydemir et al., 2010; Alam et al., 2015). Conduction defects may result from different pathological processes leading to structural damage of the conduction system. Histopathologic studies showed inflammatory abnormalities caused by arteritis or degenerative and necrotic changes due to ischemia. In both cases small blood vessels and capillaries of nodal and conduction tissue were involved. Inflammatory and ischemic lesions resulted in fibrous tissue formation (James et al., 1965; Bulkley and Roberts, 1975; Bharati et al., 1975). However, conduction defects can also be the result of antimalarial use (Comín-Colet et al., 2001) or simply represent a coexisting idiopathic conduction system disease.

The evidence that maternal anti-Ro and anti-La antibodies are important in the etiopathogenesis of autoimmune CHB is supported by many epidemiological and clinical studies as well as by a number of in vitro and in vivo experimental studies (Ambrosi and Wahren-Herlenius, 2012; Costedoat-Chalumeau et al., 2013). In a systematic review of 39 retrospective or case-control studies, it has been found that anti-Ro and/or anti-La antibodies were detected in 1230 (87%) out of 1416 CHB-affected mothers (Brito-Zerón et al., 2015).

6.3 Clinical Findings

Signs and symptoms of rhythm and conduction abnormalities depend on the type of the defect and its severity. However, they are mostly asymptomatic or may lead to some mild complaints such as palpitation or fatigue. They are recognized during follow-up clinical examination and/or by routine ECG. In some cases syncope may occur.

6.4 Diagnostic Investigations

In the case of a patient with rhythm and conduction abnormalities, examinations including 24-h Holter monitoring, echocardiography, cardiac MRI, electrolyte balance, and thyroid hormonal status should be considered.

6.5 Treatment

Arrhythmia therapy depends on the type of rhythm or conduction abnormality. Common antiarrhythmic drugs can be used, but in the most severe cases the implant of a pacemaker is necessary. All potential causes of the rhythm or conduction abnormality (i.e., pericarditis, myocarditis, cardiac ischemia, thyroid dysfunction, fluid depletion, anemia, etc.) have to be identified and treated.

7. CONCLUSIONS

The heart is frequently affected in SLE and any cardiac tissues can be involved, including pericardium, myocardium, coronary arteries, valves, and the conduction system. Nowadays, noninvasive diagnostic tools, such as echocardiography, and, in selected cases, cardiac MRI are used in the diagnostic workup of cardiac involvement in patients with SLE, being sensitive and specific techniques in detecting almost all cardiac abnormalities.

CAD is common and remains an important cause of mortality in SLE patients, especially in those with long-standing SLE. Therefore, we should make any efforts in order to minimize the risk. Indeed, physicians should tightly manage traditional risk factors as in patients with diabetes mellitus, using ACE-inhibitors, low-dose aspirin, and hydroxychloroquine as well as they should control SLE activity by using corticosteroids at the lowest effective dosage and, if needed, steroid-sparing agents.

REFERENCES

Abu-Shakra, M., Urowitz, M.B., Gladman, D.D., et al., 1995. Mortality studies in systemic lupus erythematosus. Results from a single centre. I. Causes of death. J. Rheumatol. 22, 1259.

Aggarwal, P., Singh, S., Suri, D., Rawat, A., Narula, N., ManojKumar, R., 2012. Rituximab in childhood lupus myocarditis. Rheumatol. Int. 32, 1843.

Alam, M.M., Das, P., Ghosh, P., Zaman, M.S., Boro, M., Sadhu, M., Mazumdar, A., 2015. Cardiovascular autonomic neuropathy in systemic lupus erythematosus. Indian J. Physiol. Pharmacol. 59, 155.

Ambrosi, A., Wahren-Herlenius, M., 2012. Congenital heart block: evidence for a pathogenic role of maternal autoantibodies. Arthritis Res. Ther. 14, 208.

Amital, H., Langevitz, P., Levy, Y., et al., 1999. Valvular deposition of antiphospholipid antibodies in the antiphospholipid syndrome: a clue to the origin of the disease. Clin. Exp. Rheumatol. 17, 99.

Asherson, R.A., Khamashta, M.A., Baguley, E., et al., 1989. Myocardial infarction and antiphospholipid antibodies in SLE and related disorders. Q. J. Med. 73, 1100.

Aydemir, M., Yazisiz, V., Basarici, I., Avci, A.B., Erbasan, F., Belgi, A., Terzioglu, E., 2010. Cardiac autonomic profile in rheumatoid arthritis and systemic lupus erythematosus. Lupus 19, 255.

Badui, E., Garcia-Rubi, D., Robles, E., et al., 1985. Cardiovascular manifestations in systemic lupus erythematosus. Prospective study of 100 patients. Angiology 36, 452.

Barzizza, F., Venco, A., Grandi, A.M., et al., 1987. Mitral valve prolapse in systemic lupus erythematosus. Clin. Exp. Rheumatol. 5, 59.

Bassi, N., Ghiradello, A., Iaccarino, L., Zampieri, S., Rampudda, M.E., Atzeni, F., et al., 2007. OxLDL/β2-GPI – anti-OxLDL/β2-GPI complex and atherosclerosis in SLE patients. Autoimmun. Rev. 7, 52.

Bengtsson, C., Öhman, M.L., Nived, O., Rantapää Dahlqvist, S., 2012. Cardiovascular event in systemic lupus erythematosus in northern Sweden: incidence and predictors in a 7-year follow-up study. Lupus 21, 452.

Benvenuti, F., Gatto, M., Larosa, M., Iaccarino, L., Punzi, L., Doria, A., 2015. Cardiovascular risk factors, burden of disease and preventive strategies in patients with systemic lupus erythematosus: a literature review. Expert Opin. Drug Saf. 14, 1373.

Berg, G., Bodet, J., Webb, K., et al., 1985. Systemic lupus erythematosus presenting as isolated congestive heart failure. J. Rheumatol. 12, 1182.

Bharati, S., de la Fuente, D.J., Kallen, R.J., 1975. Conduction system in systemic lupus erythematosus with atrioventricular block. Am. J. Cardiol. 35, 299.

Bidani, A.K., Roberts, J.L., Schwartz, M.M., et al., 1980. Immunopathology of cardiac lesions in fatal systemic lupus erythematosus. Am. J. Med. 69, 849.

Borba, E.F., Bonfa, E., Vinagre, C.G., 1998. Impaired metabolism of artificial chylomicronis in systemic lupus erythematosus (abstract). Arthritis Rheum. 41 (Suppl.), S79.

Borba, E.F., Bonfa, E., 1997. Dyslipoproteinemias in systemic lupus erythematosus: influence of disease, activity and anticardiolipin antibodies. Lupus 6, 533.

Borenstein, D.G., Fye, W.B., Arnett, F.C., et al., 1978. The myocarditis of systemic lupus erythematosus: association with myositis. Ann. Intern. Med. 89, 619.

Bouma, W., Klinkenberg, T.J., van der Horst, I.C., Wijdh-den Hamer, I.J., Erasmus, M.E., Bijl, M., Suurmeijer, A.J., Zijlstra, F., Mariani, M.A., 2010. Mitral valve surgery for mitral regurgitation caused by Libman-Sacks endocarditis: a report of four cases and a systematic review of the literature. J. Cardiothorac. Surg. 5, 13.

Brito-Zerón, P., Izmirly, P.M., Ramos-Casals, M., Buyon, J.P., Khamashta, M.A., 2015. The clinical spectrum of autoimmune congenital heart block. Nat. Rev. Rheumatol. 11, 301.

Brucato, A., Frassi, M., Franceschini, F., et al., 2001. Risk of congenital complete heart block in newborns of mothers with anti-Ro/SSA antibodies detected by counterimmunoelectrophoresis: a prospective study of 100 women. Arthritis Rheum. 44, 1832.

Brucato, A., Doria, A., Frassi, M., et al., 2002. Pregnancy outcome in 100 women with autoimmune diseases and anti-Ro/SSA antibodies: a prospective controlled study. Lupus 11, 716.

Bruce, I.N., Burns, R.J., Gladman, D.D., et al., 2000a. Single photon emission computed tomograpy dual isotope myocardial perfusion imaging in women with systemic lupus erythematosus. I. Prevalence and distribution of abnormalities. J. Rheumatol. 27, 2372.

Bruce, I.N., Gladman, D.D., Urowitz, M.B., 2000b. Premature atherosclerosis in systemic lupus erythematosus. Rheum. Dis. Clin. N. Am. 26, 257.

Bruce, I.N., Urowitz, M.B., Galdman, D.D., et al., 1999. Natural history of hypercholesterolemia in systemic lupus erythematosus. J. Rheumatol. 26, 2137.

Bulkley, B.H., Roberts, W.C., 1975. The heart in systemic lupus erythematosus and the changes induced in it by corticosteroid therapy: a study of 36 necropsy patients Am. J. Med. 58, 243.

Buppajamrntham, T., Palavutitotai, N., Katchamart, W., 2014. Clinical manifestation, diagnosis, management, and treatment outcome of pericarditis in patients with systemic lupus erythematosus. J. Med. Assoc. Thai. 97, 1234.

Carette, S., 1988. Cardiopulmonary manifestations of systemic lupus erythematosus. Rheum. Dis. Clin. North. Am. 14, 135.

Castier, M.B., Albuquerque, E.M., Menezes, M.E., et al., 2000. Cardiac tamponade in systemic lupus erythematosus. Report of four cases. Arq. Bras. Cardiol. 75, 446.

Cervera, R., Font, J., Pare, C., et al., 1992. Cardiac disease in systemic lupus erythematosus: prospective study of 70 patients. Ann. Rheum. Dis. 51, 156.

Cervera, R., Khamashta, M.A., Font, J., et al., 1993. Systemic lupus erythematosus: clinical and immunonologic patterns of disease expression in a cohort of 1000 patients. The European working party on systemic lupus erythematosus. Medicine (Baltimore) 72, 113.

Cervera, R., Khamashta, M.A., Font, J., et al., 1999. Morbidity and mortality in systemic lupus erythematosus during a 5 year period. A multicenter prospective study of 1000 patients. European Working Party on Systemic lupus erythematosus. Medicine (Baltimore) 78, 167.

Chartash, E.K., Lans, D.M., Paget, S.A., et al., 1989. Aortic insufficiency and mitral regurgitation in patients with systemic lupus erythematosus and the antiphospholipid syndrome. Am. J. Med. 86, 407.

Chia, B.L., Mah, E.P., Feng, P.H., 1981. Cardiovascular abnormalities in systemic lupus erythematosus. J. Clin. Ultrasound 9, 237.

Clarke, R., Daly, L., Robinson, K., et al., 1991. Hyperhomocysteinemia. An independent risk factor for vascular disease. N. Engl. J. Med. 324, 1149.

Collins, R.L., Turner, R.A., Nomeir, A.M., et al., 1978. Cardiopulmonary manifestations of systemic lupus erythematosus. J. Rheumatol. 5, 299.

Comens, S.M., Alpert, M.A., Sharp, G.C., et al., 1989. Frequency of mitral valve prolapse in systemic lupus erythematosus, progressive systemic sclerosis and mixed connective tissue disease. Am. J. Cardiol. 63, 369.

Comín-Colet, J., Sánches-Corral, M.A., Alegre-Sancho, J.J., et al., 2001. Complete heart block in an adult with systemic lupus erythematosus and recent onset of hydroxychloroquine therapy. Lupus 10, 59.

Costedoat-Chalumeau, N., et al., 2013. Letter to the editor in response to the article "Preventing congenital neonatal heart block in offspring of mothers with anti-SSA/Ro and SSB/La antibodies: a review of published literature and registered clinical trials." by Gleicher N, Elkayam U, Autoimmun Rev. 2013 Sep; 12(11): 1039–1045. Autoimmun. Rev. 13, 70.

Crozier, I.G., Li, E., Miline, M.J., et al., 1990. Cardiac involvement in systemic lupus erythematosus detected by echocardiography. Am. J. Cardiol. 65, 1145.

Das, S.K., Cassidy, J.T., 1973. Anti-heart antibodies in patients with systemic lupus erythematosus. Am. J. Med. Sci. 265, 275.

D'Cruz, D., Khamashta, M., Huges, G., 2001. Cardiovascular manifestation of systemic lupus erythematosus. In: Wallace, D., Hahn, B.H. (Eds.), Dubois' Lupus Erythematosus. Lippincott Williams & Wilkins, Philadelphia, p. 645.

Del Papa, N., Raschi, E., Moroni, G., et al., 1999. Anti-endothelial cell IgG fractions from systemic lupus erythematosus patients bind to human endothelial cells induce a pro-adhesive and a pro-inflammatory phenotype in vitro. Lupus 8, 423.

Del Rio, A., Vazquez, J.J., Sobrino, J.A., et al., 1978. Myocardial involvement in systemic lupus erythematosus. A noninvasive study of left ventricular function. Chest 74, 414.

Disla, E., Rhim, H.R., Reddy, A., et al., 1993. Reversible cardiogenic shock in a patients with lupus myocarditis. J. Rheumatol. 20, 2174.

Doherty III, N.E., Feldman, G., Maurer, G., et al., 1988. Echocardiographic findings in systemic lupus erythematosus. Am. J. Cardiol. 61, 1144.

Doherty, N.E., Siegel, R.J., 1985. Cardiovascular manifestation of systemic lupus erythematosus. Am. Heart J. 110, 1257.

Doria, A., Iaccarino, L., Ghirardello, A., Zampieri, S., Arienti, S., Sarzi-Puttini, P., Atzeni, F., Piccoli, A., Todesco, S., 2006. Long-term prognosis and causes of death insystemic lupus erythematosus. Am. J. Med. 119 (8), 700–707.

Doria, A., Iaccarino, L., Sarzi-Puttini, P., Atzeni, F., Turriel, M., Petri, M., 2005a. Cardiac involvement in systemic lupus erythematosus. Lupus 14, 683.

Doria, A., Shoenfeld, Y., Wu, R., et al., 2003. Risk factors for subclinical atherosclerosis in a prospective cohort of patients with Systemic Lupus Erythematosus. Ann. Rheum. Dis. 62, 1071.

Doria, A., Sherer, Y., Meroni, P.L., Shoenfeld, Y., 2005b. Inflammation and accelerated atherosclerosis: basic mechanisms. Rheum. Dis. Clin. North. Am. 31, 355.

Du Toit, R., Herbst, P.G., van Rensburg, A., du Plessis, L.M., Reuter, H., Doubell, A.F., 2016. Clinical features and outcome of lupus myocarditis in the Western Cape, South Africa. Lupus [Epub ahead of print].

Dubois, E.L., Tuffanelli, D.L., 1964. Clinical manifestation of systemic lupus erythematosus. Computer analysis of 520 cases. JAMA 190, 104.

Eiken, P.W., Edwards, W.D., Tazelaar, H.D., et al., 2001. Surgical pathology of nonbacterial thrombotic endocarditis in 30 patients, 1985-2000. Mayo Clin. Proc. 76, 1204.

Elkayam, U., Weiss, S., Laniado, S., 1977. Pericardial effusion and mitral valve involvement in systemic lupus erythematosus: echocardiographic study. Ann. Rheum. Dis. 36, 349.

Englund, J.A., Lucas Jr., R.V., 1983. Cardiac complications in children with systemic lupus erythematosus. Pediatrics 72, 724.

Esdaile, J.M., Abrahamowicz, M., Grodzicky, T., Li, Y., et al., 2001. Traditional Framingham risk factors fail to fully account for accelerated atherosclerosis in systemic lupus erythematosus. Arthritis Rheum. 44, 2231.

Estes, D., Christian, C.L., 1971. The natural history of systemic lupus erythematosus by prospective analysis. Medicine (Baltimore) 50, 85.

Ettinger, W.H., Glodberg, A.P., Applebaum-Bowden, D., et al., 1987. Dyslipoproteinemia in systemic lupus erythematosus. Effect of corticosteroids. Am. J. Med. 83, 503.
Fairfax, M.J., Osborn, T.G., Williams, G.A., et al., 1988. Endomyocardial biopsy in patients with systemic lupus erythematosus. J. Rheumatol. 15, 593.
Falcão, C.A., Alves, I.C., Chahade, W.H., et al., 2002. Echocardiographic abnormalities and antiphospholipid antibodies in patients with systemic lupus erythematosus. Arq. Bras. Cardiol. 79, 285.
Feldman, A.M., McNamara, D., 2000. Myocarditis. N. Engl. J. Med. 343, 1388.
Fermo, I., D'Angelo, S.V., Paroni, R., et al., 1995. Prevalence of moderate hyperhomocysteinemia in patients with early onset venous and arterial occlusive disease. Ann. Intern. Med. 123, 747.
Fernández-Nebro, A., Rúa-Figueroa, Í., López-Longo, F.J., Galindo-Izquierdo, M., Calvo-Alén, J., Olivé-Marqués, A., et al., 2015. Cardiovascular events in systemic lupus erythematosus: a nationwide study in Spain from the RELESSER Registry. Medicine (Baltimore) 94, e1183.
Fonseca, E., Crespo, M., Sobrino, J.A., 1994. Complete heart block in an adult with systemic lupus erythematosus. Lupus 3, 129.
Foroughi, M., Hekmat, M., Ghorbani, M., Ghaderi, H., Majidi, M., Beheshti, M., 2014. Mitral valve surgery in patients with systemic lupus erythematosus. Sci. World J. 2014, 216291.
Ford, P.M., Ford, S.E., Lillicrap, D.P., 1988. Association of lupus anticoagulant with severe valvular heart disease in systemic lupus erythematosus. J. Rheumatol. 15, 597.
Fox, I.S., Spence, A.M., Wheelis, R.F., et al., 1980. Cerebral embolism in Libman-Sacks endocarditis. Neurology 30, 487.
Fukumoto, S., Tsumagari, T., Kinjo, M., et al., 1987. Coronary atherosclerosis in patients with systemic lupus erythematosus at autopsy. Acta Pathol. Jpn. 37, 1.
Galve, E., Candell-Riera, J., Pigrau, C., et al., 1988. Prevalence, morphologic types and evolution of cardiac valvular disease in systemic lupus erythematosus. N. Engl. J. Med. 319, 817.
Garcia, M.A., Alarcòn, G.S., Boggio, G., Hauchuel, L., Marcos, A.I., Marcos, J.C., Gentiletti, S., Caeiro, F., et al., 2014. Primary cardiac disease in sistemi lupus erythematosus patients: protective and risk factors — data from a multi-ethnic Latin American color. Rheumatology (oxford) 53, 1431.
Gentile, R., Laganaà, B., Tubani, M., et al., 2000. Assessment of echocardiographic abnormalities in patients with systemic lupus erythematosus: correlation with levels of antiphospholipid antibodies. Ital. Heart J. 1, 487.
Giunta, A., Picillo, U., Maione, S., et al., 1993. Spectrum of cardiac involvement in systemic lupus erythematosus: echocardiographic, echo-Doppler observations and immunologivcal investigation. Acta Cardiol. 48, 183.
Gladman, D.D., Urowitz, M.B., 1987. Morbidity in systemic lupus erythematosus. J. Rheumatol. 14 (Suppl.), 223.
Gómez-Barrado, J.J., García-Rubira, J.C., Polo Ostáriz, M.A., et al., 2002. Complete atrioventricular block in a woman with systemic lupus erythematosus. Int. J. Cardiol. 82, 289.
Gordon, R.J., Weilbaecher, D., Davy, S.M., et al., 1996. Valvulitis involving a bioprosthetic valve in a patients with systemic lupus erythematosus. J. Am. Soc. Echocardiogr. 9, 104.
Gross, L., 1940. The cardiac lesions in Libman-Sacks disease: with a consideration of its relationship to acute diffuse lupus erythematosus. Am. J. Pathol. 16, 375.
Haider, Y.S., Roberts, W.C., 1981. Coronary arterial disease in systemic lupus erythematosus: quantification of degrees of narrowing in 22 necropsy patients (21 women) ages 16 to 37 years. Am. J. Med. 70, 775.
Harvey, A.M., Shulman, L.E., Tumulty, P.A., et al., 1954. Systemic lupus erythematosus: review of the literature and clinical analysis of 138 cases. Medicine 33, 291.

Hakim, J.P., Mehta, A., Jain, A.C., et al., 2001. Mitral valve replacement and repair. Report of 5 patients with systemic lupus erythematosus. Tex. Heart Inst. J. 28, 47.

Hogarth, M.B., Judd, L., Mathias, C.J., et al., 2002. Cardiovascular autonomic function in systemic lupus erythematosus. Lupus 11, 308.

Homcy, C.J., Libertson, R.R., Fallon, J.T., et al., 1982. Ischemic heart coronary vasculitis in systemic lupus erythematosus in the young patient: report of six cases. Am. J. Cardiol. 49, 478.

Hosepund, J.D., Montanaro, A., Hart, M.V., et al., 1984. Myocardial perfusion abnormalities in asymptomatic patients with systemic lupus erythematosus. Am. J. Med. 77, 286.

Iaccarino, L., Bettio, S., Zen, M., Nalotto, L., Gatto, M., Ramonda, R., Punzi, L., Doria, A., 2013. Premature coronary heart disease in SLE: can we prevent progression? Lupus 22, 1232.

Ilowite, N.T., Samuel, P., Ginzler, E., et al., 1988. Dyslipoproteinemia in pediatric systemic lupus erythematosus. Arthritis Rheum. 31, 859.

Ishida, R., Murata, Y., Sawada, Y., et al., 2000. Thallium-201 myocardial SPECT in patients with collagen disease. Nucl. Med. Commun. 21, 729.

Ito, M., Kagiyama, Y., Omura, I., et al., 1979. Cardiovascular manifestation of systemic lupus erythematosus. Jpn. Circ. J. 43, 985.

Jacobson, E.J., Reza, M.J., 1978. Constrictive pericarditis in systemic lupus erythematosus: demonstration of immunoglobulins in the pericardium. Arthritis Rheum. 21, 972.

James, T.N., Rupe, C.E., Monto, R.W., 1965. Pathology of the cardiac conduction system in systemic lupus erythematosus. Ann. Intern. Med. 63, 402.

Jensen-Urstad, K., Svenungsson, E., de Faire, U., et al., 2002. Cardiac valvular abnormalities are frequent in systemic lupus erythematosus with manifest arterial disease. Lupus 11, 744.

Jonsson, H., Nived, O., Surfelt, G., 1989. Outcome in systemic lupus erythematosus: a prospective study of patients from a defined population. Medicine 68, 141.

Kahan, A., Amor, B., De Vernejoul, F., et al., 1985. Libman-Sacks endocarditis. The diagnostic importance of two-dimensional echocardiography. Br. J. Rheum. 24, 187.

Kahl, L.E., 1992. The spectrum of pericardial tamponade in systemic lupus erythematosus: report of ten patients. Arthritis Rheum. 35, 1343.

Kao, A.H., Manzi, S., 2002. How to manage patients with cardiopulmonary disease? Best Pract. Res. Clin. Rheumatol. 16, 211.

Kaplanski, G., Cacoub, B., Farnarier, C., et al., 2000. Increased soluble vascular cell adhesion molecule 1 concentration in patients with primary or lupus erythematosus related antiphospholipid syndrome: correlation with the severity of thrombosis. Arthritis Rheum. 43, 55.

Kattwinkel, N., Villanueva, A.G., Labib, S.B., et al., 1992. Myocardial infarction caused by cardiac microvasculopathy in a patient with the primary antiphospholipid syndrome. Ann. Intern. Med. 116, 974.

Khamashta, M.A., Cervera, R., Asherson, R.A., et al., 1990. Association of antibodies against phospholipid with heart valve disease in systemic lupus erythematosus. Lancet 335, 1541.

Kindig, J.R., Goodman, M.R., 1983. Clinical utility of pericardial fluid pH determination. Am. J. Med. 75, 1077.

Kinney, E.L., Wynn, J., Ward, S., et al., 1980. Ruptured chordae tendinae: its association with systemic lupus erythematosus. Arch. Pathol. Lab. Med. 104, 595.

Klinkhoff, A.V., Thompson, C.R., Reid, G.D., et al., 1985. M-mode and two-dimensional echocardiogrphic abnormalities in systemic lupus erythematusus. JAMA 253, 3273.

Kong, T.Q., Kellum, R.E., Haserich, J.R., 1962. Clinical diagnosis of cardiac involvement in systemic lupus erythematosus: a correlation of clinical and autopsy findings in thirty. Circulation 26, 7.

Kruzliak, P., Novak, M., Piler, P., Kovacova, G., 2013. Pericardial involvement in systemic lupus erythematosus: current diagnosis and therapy. Acta Cardiol. 68, 629.

Lash, A.D., Wittman, A.L., Quisimoro Jr., F.P., 1986. Myocarditis in mixed connective tissue disease: clinical and pathologic study of three cases and review of literature. Semin. Arthritis Rheum. 15, 288.

Lazzerini, P.E., Capecchi, P.L., Guideri, F., Acampa, M., Galeazzi, M., Laghi Pasini, F., 2006. Connective tissue diseases and cardiac rhythm disorders: an overview. Autoimmun. Rev. 5, 306.

Lehman, T.J.A., Mc Curdy, D.K., Bernstein, B.H., et al., 1989. Systemic lupus erythematosus in the first decade of life. Pediatrics 83, 235.

Leong, K.H., Koh, E.T., Feng, P.H., et al., 1994. Lipid profiles in patients with systemic lupus erythematosus. J. Rheumatol. 21, 1264.

Lerman, B.B., Thomas, L.C., Abrams, G.D., et al., 1982. Aortic stenosis associated with systemic lupus erythematosus. Am. J. Med. 72 (4), 707–710.

Leung, W.H., Wong, K.L., Lau, C.P., et al., 1990a. Cardiac abnormalities in systemic lupus erythematosus: a prospective M-mode, cross-sectional and Doppler echocardiographic study. Int. J. Cardiol. 27, 367.

Leung, W.H., Wong, K.L., Llau, C.P., et al., 1990b. Association between antiphospholipid antibodies and cardiac abnormalities in patients with systemic lupus erythematosus. Am. J. Med. 89, 411.

Leszczyński, P., Straburzyńska-Migaj, E., Korczowska, I., Łacki, J.K., Mackiewicz, S., 2003. Cardiac valvular disease in patients with systemic lupus erythematosus. Relationship with anticardiolipin antibodies. Clin. Rheumatol. 22, 405.

Li, R., Cai, J., Tegeler, C., Sorlie, P., et al., 1996. Reproducibility of extracranial carotid atherosclerotic lesion assessed by B-mode ultrasound: the artherosclerosis risk in communities study. Ultrasound Med. Biol. 22, 791.

Libby, P., Ridker, P.M., 2006. Inflammation and atherothrombosis: from population biology and bench research to clinical practice. J. Am. Coll. Cardiol. 48, A33.

Libman, E., Sacks, B., 1924. A hitherto undescribed form of valvular and mural endocarditis. Arch. Intern. Med. 33, 701.

Logar, D., Kveder, T., Rozman, B., et al., 1990. Possible association between anti-Ro antibodies and myocarditis or cardiac conduction defects in adults with systemic lupus erythematosus. Ann. Rheum. Dis. 49, 627.

Lòpez-Pedrera, C., Angeles Aguirre, M., Barbarroja, N., Cuadrado, M.J., 2010. Accelerated atherosclerosis in systemic lupus erythematosus: role of proinflammatory cytokines and therapeutic approaches. J. Biomed. Biotechnol. 2010 pii: 607084.

Lopez-Ruiz, N., Uribe, C.E., 2014. Chloroquine cardiomyopathy: beyond ocular adverse effects. BMJ Case Rep. 5, 2014.

Luce, E.B., Montgomery, M.T., Redding, S.W., 1990. The prevalence of cardiac valvular pathosis in patients with systemic lupus erythematosus. Oral Surg. Oral Med. Oral Pathol. 70, 590.

Lustig, N., Florenzano, P., Sanhueza, L.M., Cid, X., Ramos, G., Thone, N., Fullerton, D.A., 2014. Constrictive pericarditis as a serious and rare presentation of systemic lupus erythematosus: report of one case. Rev. Med. Chil. 142, 1065.

MacGregor, A.J., Dhillon, V.B., Binder, A., et al., 1992. Fastings lipids and antiacardiolipin antibodies as risk factors for vascular disease in systemic lupus erythematosus. Ann. Rheum. Dis. 51, 152.

Manger, K., Kusus, M., Forster, C., Ropers, D., Daniel, W.G., Kalden, J.R., Achenbach, S., Manger, B., 2003. Factors associated with coronary artery calcification in young female patients with SLE. Ann. Rheum. Dis. 62, 846.

Manzi, S., Meilahn, E.N., Rairie, J.E., et al., 1997. Age-specific incidence rates of myocardial infarction and angina in women with systemic lupus erythematosus: comparison with Framingham Study. Am. J. Epidemiol. 145, 408.

Manzi, S., Selzer, F., Sutton-Tyrrel, K., et al., 1999. Prevalence and risk factors of carotid plaque in women with systemic lupus erythematosus. Arthritis Rheum. 42, 51.

Martinez-Costa, X., Ordi, J., Barbera, J., et al., 1991. High grade atrioventricular heart block in 2 adults with systemic lupus erythematosus. J. Rheumatol. 18, 1926.

Matayoshi, A.H., Dhond, M.R., Laslett, L.J., 1999. Multiple coronary aneurysms in a case of systemic lupus erythematosus. Chest 116, 1116.

Matsuura, E., Igarashi, Y., Yasuda, T., et al., 1994. Anticardiolipin antibodies recognize β2-glycoprotein I structure altered by interacting with an oxigen modified solid phase surface. J. Exp. Med. 179, 457.

Mavrogeni, S., Spargias, K., Markussis, V., Kolovou, G., Demerouti, E., Papadopoulou, E., Stavridis, G., Kaklamanis, L., Douskou, M., Constantoulakis, P., Cokkinos, D.V., 2009. Myocardial inflammation in autoimmune diseases: investigation by cardiovascular magnetic resonance and endomyocardial biopsy. Inflamm. Allergy Drug Targets 8, 39.

Mavrogeni, S.I., Kitas, G.D., Dimitroulas, T., et al., 2016. Cardiovascular magnetic resonance in rheumatology: current status and recommendations for use. Int. J. Cardiol. 217, 135.

Meissner, M., Sherer, Y., Levy, Y., et al., 2000. Intravenous immunoglobulin therapy in a patient with lupus serositis and nephritis. Rheumatol. Int. 19, 199.

Meller, J., Conde, C.A., Deppisch, L.M., et al., 1975. Myocardial infarction due to coronary atherosclerosis in three young adults with systemic lupus erythematosus. Am. J. Cardiol. 35, 309.

Metz, D., Jolly, D., Graciet-Richard, J., et al., 1994. Prevalence of valvular involvement in systemic lupus erythematosus and association with antiphospholipid syndrome: a matched echocardiographic study. Cardiology 85, 129.

Miner, J.J., Kim, A.H., 2014. Cardiac manifestations of systemic lupus erythematosus. Rheum. Dis. Clin. North Am. 40, 51.

Moder, K.G., Miller, T.D., Tazelaar, H.D., 1999. Cardiac involvement in systemic lupus erythematosus. Mayo Clin. Proc. 74, 275.

Morel, N., Bonjour, M., Le Guern, V., Le Jeunne, C., Mouthon, L., Piette, J.C., Costedoat-Chalumeau, N., 2015. Colchicine: a simple and effective treatment for pericarditis in systemic lupus erythematosus? A report of 10 cases. Lupus 24, 1479.

Morin, A.M., Boyer, A.S., Nataf, P., et al., 1996. Mitral insufficiency caused by systemic lupus erythematosus requiring valve replacement: three case reports and a review of the literature. Torac. Cardiovasc. Surg. 44, 313.

Moyssakis, I., Tektonidou, M.G., Vasilliou, V.A., Samarkos, M., Votteas, V., Moutsopoulos, H.M., 2007. Libman-Sacks endocarditis in systemic lupus erythematosus: prevalence, associations, and evolution. Am. J. Med. 120, 636.

Muangchan, C., van Vollenhoven, R.F., Bernatsky, S.R., et al., 2015. Treatment algorithms in systemic lupus erythematosus. Arthritis Care Res. (Hoboken) 67, 1237.

Murpy, J.J., Leach, I.H., 1989. Findings at necropsy in the heart of patients with the primary antiphospholipid syndrome. Br. Heart J. 62, 61.

Naarendorp, M., Kerr, L.D., Khan, A.S., et al., 1999. Dramatic improvement of left ventricular function after cytotoxic therapy in lupus patients with acute cardiomyopathy: report of 6 cases. J. Rheumatol. 26, 2257.

Nesher, G., Ilany, J., Rosemann, D., et al., 1997. Valvular dysfunction in antiphospholipid syndrome: prevalence, clinical features, and treatment. Semin. Artthritis. Rheum. 27, 27.

Nihoyannopoulos, P., Gomez, P.M., Joshi, J., Loizou, S., Walport, M.J., Oakley, C.M., 1990. Cardiac abnormalities in systemic lupus erythematosus. Association with raised anti-cardiolipin antibodies. Circulation 82, 369.

Nobrega, T.P., Klodas, E., Breen, J.F., et al., 1996. Giant coronary artery aneurysm in systemic lupus erythematosus. Cathet. Cardiovasc. Diagn. 39, 75.
Oh, J.Y., Chang, S.A., Choe, Y.H., Kim, D.K., 2012. Transient constrictive pericarditis in systemic lupus erythematous. Eur. Heart J. Cardiovasc. Imaging 13, 793.
Omdal, R., Lunde, P., Rasmussen, K., et al., 2001. Transesophageal and trans thoracic echocardiography and Doppler-examination in systemic lupus erythematosus. Scand. J. Rheumatol. 30, 275.
Ong, M.L., Veerapen, K., Chambers, J.B., et al., 1992. Cardiac abnormalities in systemic lupus erythematosus: prevalence and relationship to disease activity. Int. J. Cardiol. 34, 69.
Parker, B., Urowitz, M.B., Gladman, D.D., Lunt, M., Bae, S.C., Sanchez-Guerrero, J., et al., 2012. Clinical associations of the metabolic syndrome in systemic lupus erythematosus: data from an international inception cohort. Ann. Rheum. Dis. 72, 1308.
Perez-Villa, F., Font, J., Azqueta, M., Espinosa, G., Pare, C., Cervera, R., Reverter, J.C., Ingelmo, M., Sanz, G., 2005. Severe valvular regurgitation and antiphospholipid antibodies in systemic lupus erythematosus: a prospective, long-term, followup study. Arthritis Rheum. 53, 460.
Petri, M., Perez-Gutthann, S., Spence, D., et al., 1992a. Risk factors for coronary artery disease in patients with systemic lupus erythematosus. Am. J. Med. 93, 513.
Petri, M., Spence, D., Bone, L.R., et al., 1992b. Coronary artery disease risk factors in the Johns Hopkins Lupus Cohort: prevalence, recognition by patients and preventing pratices. Medicine 71, 291.
Petri, M., Lakatta, C., Magder, L., et al., 1994. Effect of prednisone and hydroxychloroquine on coronary artery disease risk factors in systemic lupus erythematosus: a longitudinal data analysis. Am. J. Med. 96, 254.
Petri, M., Roubenoff, R., Dallal, G.E., et al., 1996. Plasma homocysteine as a risk factor for atherothrombotic events in systemic lupus erythematosus. Lancet 348, 1120.
Petri, M., 2000a. Detection of coronary artery disease and the role of traditional risk factors in the Hopkins Lupus Cohort. Lupus 9 (3), 170.
Petri, M., 2000b. Hopkins lupus cohort. 1999 update. Rheum. Dis. Clin. North. Am. 26, 199.
Petri, M., Am, O., Alarcòn, G.S., et al., 2012. Derivation and validation of the Systemic Lupus International Collaborating Clinics classification criteria for systemic lupus erythematosus. Arthritis Rheum. 64, 2677.
Plazak, W., Pasowicz, M., Kostkiewicz, M., Podolec, J., Tomkiewicz-Pajak, L., Musial, J., Podolec, P., 2011. Influence of chronic inflammation and autoimmunity on coronarycalcifications and myocardial perfusion defects in systemic lupus erythematosus patients. Inflamm. Res. 60, 973.
Pritzker, M.R., Ernst, J.D., Caudill, C., et al., 1980. Acquired aortic stenosis in systemic lupus erythematosus. Ann. Intern. Med. 93, 434.
Rahman, P., Urowitz, M.B., Galdman, D.D., et al., 1999. Contribution of traditional risk factors to coronary artery disease in patients with systemic lupus erythematosus. J Rheumatol. 26, 2363.
Ramonda, R., Doria, A., Villanova, C., et al., 1992. Évaluation de l'atteinte cardiaque au cours du lupus érythémateux disséminé: étude clinique et échocardiographique. Rev. Rhum. Mal. Ostéoartic. 59 (12), 790.
Rantapää-Dahlquist, S., Neumann-Andersen, G., Backman, C., et al., 1997. Echocardiographic findings, lipids and lipoprotein (a) in patients with systemic lupus erythematosus. Clin. Rheumatol. 16, 140.
Roberts, W.C., High, S.T., 1999. The heart in systemic lupus erythematosus. Curr. Probl. Cardiol. 24, 1.

Roldan, C.A., Qualls, C.R., Sopko, K.S., Sibbitt Jr., W.L., 2008. Transthoracic versus transesophageal echocardiography for detection of Libman-Sacks endocarditis: a randomized controlled study. J. Rheumatol. 35, 224.

Roldan, C.A., Shively, B.K., Crawford, M.H., 1996. An echocardiographic study of valvular heart disease associated with systemic lupus erythematosus. N. Engl. J. Med. 335, 1424.

Roldan, C.A., Sibbitt Jr., W.L., Qualls, C.R., Jung, R.E., Greene, E.R., Gasparovic, C.M., Hayek, R.A., Charlton, G.A., Crookston, K., 2013. Libman-Sacks endocarditis and embolic cerebrovascular disease. JACC Cardiovasc. Imaging 6, 973.

Roldan, C.A., Tolstrup, K., Macias, L., Qualls, C.R., Maynard, D., Charlton, G., Sibbitt Jr., W.L., 2015. Libman-sacks endocarditis: detection, characterization, and clinical correlates by three-dimensional transesophageal echocardiography. J. Am. Soc. Echocardiogr. 28, 770.

Roman, M.J., Salmon, J.E., Sobel, R., et al., 2001. Prevalence and relation to risk factors of carotid atherosclerosis and left ventricular hypertrophy in systemic lupus erythematosus and antiphospholipid antibody syndrome. Am. J. Cardiol. 87, 663.

Roman, M.J., Shanker, B.A., Davis, A., Lockshin, M.D., Sammaritano, L., Simantov, R., et al., 2003. Prevalence and correlates of accelerated atherosclerosis in systemic lupus erythematosus. N. Engl. J. Med. 349, 2399.

Romero-Díaz, J., Vargas-Vóracková, F., Kimura-Hayama, E., et al., 2012. Systemic lupus erythematosus risk factors for coronary artery calcifications. Rheumatology (Oxford) 51, 110.

Ropes, M.W. (Ed.), 1976. Systemic Lupus Erythematosus. Harvard University Press, Cambridge (MA).

Rosenthal, T., Neufeld, H., Kishon, Y., et al., 1980. Myocardial infarction in a young woman with systemic lupus erythematosus. Angiology 31, 573.

Rosner, S., Ginzler, E.M., Diamond, H.S., et al., 1982. A multicenter study of outcome in systemic lupus erythematosus. II. Causes of death. Arthritis Rheum. 25, 612.

Rubin, L.A., Urowitz, M.B., Gladman, D.D., 1985. Mortality in systemic lupus erythematosus: the bimodal pattern revisited. Q. J. M 55, 87.

Shalimar Handa, R., Deepak, K.K., Bhatia, M., Aggarwal, P., Pandey, R.M., 2006. Autonomic dysfunction in systemic lupus erythematosus. Rheumatol. Int. 26, 837.

Schillaci, O., Laganà, B., Danieli, R., et al., 1999. Technetium-99m sestamibi single-photon emission tomography detects subclinical myocardial perfusion abnormalities in patients with systemic lupus erythematosus. Eur. J. Nucl. Med. 26, 713.

Shahin, A.A., Shahin, H.A., Hamid, M.A., Amin, M.A., 2004. Cardiac involvement in patients with systemic lupus erythematosus and correlation of valvular lesions with anti-Ro/SS-A and anti-La/SS-B antibody levels. Mod. Rheumatol. 14, 117.

Shapiro, R.F., Gamble, C.N., Wiesner, K.B., et al., 1977. Immunopathogenesis of Libman Sacks endocarditis. Assessment by light and immunofluorescent microscopy in two cases. Ann. Rheum. Dis. 36, 508.

Shazzad, M.N., Islam, M.N., Ara, R., Ahmed, C.M., Fatema, N., Azad, A.K., et al., 2013. Echocardiographic assessment of cardiac involvement in systemic lupus erythematosus patients. Mymensingh Med. J. 22, 736.

Sherer, Y., Levy, Y., Shoenfeld, Y., 1999. Marked improvement of severe cardiac dysfunction after one course of intravenous immunoglobulin in a patient with systemic lupus erythematosus. Clin. Rheumatol. 18, 238.

Shimada, Y., Asanuma, Y.F., Yokota, K., Yoshida, Y., Kajiyama, H., Sato, K., et al., 2014. Pentraxin 3 is associated with disease activity but not atherosclerosis in patients with systemic lupus erythematosus. Mod. Rheumatol. 24, 78.

Shively, B.K., 2000. Transesophageal echocardiography (TEE) evaluation of the aortic valve, left ventricular outflow tract, and pulmonic valve. Cardiol. Clin. 18, 711.

Shoenfeld, Y., George, J., Sherer, Y., et al., 2001. Atherosclerosis: evidence for the role of autoimmunity. In: Shoenfeld, Y., Harats, D., Wick (Eds.), Atherosclerosis and Autoimmunity. Elsevier Science B.V. pp. 139–142

Smiti, M., Salem, T.B., Larbi, T., Sfaxi, A.B., Ghorbel, I.B., Lamloum, M., Houman, M.H., 2009. Pericarditis in systemic lupus erythematosus: prevalence and clinical and immunologic characteristics. Presse Med. 38, 362.

Simantov, R., LaSale, S.M., Lo, S.K., et al., 1995. Activation of cultured vascular endothelial cells by antiphospholipid antibodies. J. Clin. Invest. 96, 2211.

Straaton, K.V., Chatham, W.W., Reveille, J.D., et al., 1988. Clinically significant valvular heart disease in systemic lupus erythematosus. Am. J. Med. 85, 645.

Stojanovich, L., Milovanovich, B., de Luka, S.R., et al., 2007. Cardiovascular autonomic dysfunction in systemic lupus, rheumatoid arthritis, primary Sjögren syndrome and other autoimmune diseases. Lupus 16, 181.

Sturfelt, G., Eskilsson, J., Nived, O., et al., 1992. Cardiovascular disease in systemic lupus erythematosus: a study of 75 patients from a defined population. Medicine 71, 216.

Sun, S.S., Shiau, Y.C., Tsai, S.C., et al., 2001. The role of technetium-99m sestamibi myocardial perfusion single-photon emission tomography (SPECT) in the detection of cardiovascular involvement in systemic lupus erythematosus patients with non-specific chest complaints. Rheumatology 40, 1106.

Svenungsson, E., Jensen-Urstad, K., Heimbürger, M., et al., 2001. Risk factors for cardiovascular disease in systemic lupus erythematosus. Circulation 104, 1887.

Tan, E.M., Cohen, A.S., Fries, J.F., Masi, A.T., McShane, D.J., Rothfiled, N.F., et al., 1982. The 1982 revised criteria for the classification of systemic lupus erythematosus. Arthritis Rheum. 25, 1271.

Thacker, S.G., Zhao, W., Smith, C.K., Luo, W., Wang, H., Vivekanandan-Giri, A., et al., 2012. Type I interferons modulate vascular function, repair, thrombosis, and plaque progression in murine models of lupus and atherosclerosis. Arthritis Rheum. 64, 2975.

Thandroyen, F.T., Matisonn, R.E., Weir, E.K., 1978. Severe aortic incompetence caused by systemic lupus erythematosus: a case report. S. Afr. Med. J. 54, 166.

Thompson, T., Sutton-Tyrrell, K., Wildman, R.P., et al., 2008. Progression of carotid intima-media thickness and plaque in women with systemic lupus erythematosus. Arthritis Rheum. 58, 835.

Urowitz, M.B., Bookman, A.A.M., Koehler, B.E., et al., 1976. The bimodal mortality pattern of systemic lupus erythematosus. Am. J. Med. 60, 221.

Urowitz, M.B., Gladman, D.D., Anderson, N.M., Su, J., Romero-Diaz, J., Bae, S.C., et al., 2016. Cardiovascular events prior to or early after diagnosis of systemic lupus erythematosus in the systemic lupus international collaborating clinics cohort. Lupus Sci. Med. 3, e000143.

Vaarala, O., Alfthan, G., Jauhiainen, M., et al., 1993. Cross-reaction between antibodies to oxidized low-density lipoprotein and to cardiolipin in systemic lupus erythematosus. Lancet 341, 923.

Vianna, J.L., Khamashta, M.A., Ordi-Ros, J., et al., 1994. Comparison of the primary and secondary antiphospholipid syndrome: an European Multicenter Study of 114 patients. Am. J. Med. 96, 3.

Vereckei, A., Fazakas, A., Baló, T., Fekete, B., Molnár, M.J., Karádi, I., 2013. Chloroquine cardiotoxicity mimicking connective tissue disease heart involvement. Immunopharmacol. Immunotoxicol. 35, 304.

Von Felt, J.M., 1999. Coronary electron beam computed tomography (EBCT) in 13 patients with 2 or more cardiovascular risk factors. Arthritis Rheum. 41, S139.

Wallace, D.J., Metzger, A.L., Stecher, V.J., et al., 1990. Cholesterol-lowering effect of hydroxychloroquine in patients with rheumatic disease: effects on lipid metabolism. Am. J. Med. 89, 322.

Wallace, D.J., Podell, T., Weiner, J., et al., 1981. Systemic lupus erythematosus- survival patterns. Experience with 609 patients. JAMA 245, 934.

Ward, M.M., 1999. Premature morbidity from cardiovascular and cerebrovascular disease in women with systemic lupus erythematosus. Arthritis Rheum. 42, 338.

Wijetunga, M., Rockson, S., 2002. Myocarditis in systemic lupus erythematosus. Am. J. Med. 113, 419.

Wilson, V.E., Eck, S.L., Bates, E.R., 1992. Evaluation and treatment of acute myocardial infarction complicating systemic lupus erythematosus. Chest 101, 420.

Witztum, J.L., 1994. The oxidation hypothesis of atherosclerosis. Lancet 344, 793.

Yazici, Z.A., Raschi, E., Patel, A., et al., 2001. Human monoclonal anti-endothelial cell IgG--derived from a systemic lupus erythematosus patient bind and activates human endothelium in vitro. Int. Immunol. 13, 349.

Yilmaz, A., Ferreira, V., Klingel, K., Kandolf, R., Neubauer, S., Sechtem, U., 2013. Role of cardiovascular magnetic resonance imaging (CMR) in the diagnosis of acute and chronic myocarditis. Heart Fail. Rev. 18, 747.

Yu, X.H., Li, Y.N., 2011. Echocardiographic abnormalities in a cohort of Chinese patients with systemic lupus erythematosus—a retrospective analysis of eighty-five cases. J. Clin. Ultrasound 39, 519.

Ziporen, L., Goldberg, I., Arad, M., et al., 1996. Libman-Sacks endocarditis in the antiphospholipid syndrome. Immunopathologic findings in deformed heart valves. Lupus 5, 196.

Chapter 12

Cardiac Involvement in the Antiphospholipid Syndrome

I. Rodriguez-Pintó, G. Espinosa and R. Cervera
Department of Autoimmune Diseases, Hospital Clínic, Barcelona, Spain

1. INTRODUCTION

The heart is one of the main target organs in antiphospholipid syndrome (APS). Cardiac involvement has been found in up to 40% of patients with this syndrome, but significant morbidity appears in only 4–6% of these patients (Cervera, 2004). APS cardiac manifestations range from asymptomatic valvular lesions to life-threating diffuse myocardial microthrombosis involvement described in catastrophic APS (CAPS) setting (Table 12.1) (Levine et al., 2002; Cervera et al., 2014). However, the attribution of some of these clinical manifestations to the APS is still under debate. According to the largest series on APS published so far, heart valve diseases are the most common cardiac manifestations followed by myocardial infarcts (Cervera et al., 2002; Denas et al., 2015). Most of these manifestations could be explained on the basis of thrombotic lesions either in coronary circulation or

TABLE 12.1 Cardiac Manifestations of Antiphospholipid Syndrome

Valvular heart disease
Leaflet thickening
Valvular regurgitation
Valve stenosis
Vegetations
Ischemic cardiac disease
Nonischemic cardiac disease
Diastolic dysfunction
Systolic dysfunction
Intracardiac thrombosis

on the valves while other manifestations may be explained based on the deposition of immune complexes (Cervera, 2004).

Two different patterns of heart valve disease can be discerned: valve thickening and dysfunction and valve masses. Valve thickening and regurgitation is the most common abnormalities while one quarter presents valve masses (vegetations) (Cervera et al., 2011b). According to the international consensus published in 2006, heart valve disease in patients with antiphospholipid antibodies (aPL) is defined by the presence of valve lesions more than 3 mm thick or by localized thickening involving the proximal or middle portion of the leaflet, and irregular nodules on the atrial face of the mitral or vascular face of aortic valve in the absence of a history of rheumatic fever and infective endocarditis (Miyakis et al., 2006). Libman-Sacks endocarditis is a sterile mulberry-like cluster of fibro-fibrinous verrucae that develop anywhere in the endocardial surface but especially in the ventricular surface of the mitral valve (Libman and Sacks, 1924).

As mentioned before, ischemic cardiac disease has been found to be the second most prevalent cardiac manifestation of APS. While the exact pathophysiology of ischemic involvement in APS is not yet clear, systemic lupus erythematosus (SLE) patients' ischemic cardiac disease seem to be more often due to atherosclerosis than due to vasculitis. Additionally, other cardiac ventricle dysfunctions not clinically related to ischemic events have been found in several studies although their clinical significance is not yet clear. They have mainly been found in the diastolic phase of the cardiac cycle and, thus, the name preclinical diastolic dysfunction has been proposed. Finally, several reports have highlighted the risk for intracardiac thrombosis in patients with aPL.

This chapter will discuss each cardiac manifestation related to aPL separately.

2. EPIDEMIOLOGY

2.1 Valve Disease and Libman-Sacks

Several observational studies have described a higher prevalence of valve abnormalities in APS patients with respect to healthy controls (Brenner et al., 1991; Cervera et al., 1991; Galve et al., 1992; Badui et al., 1995). However, the prevalence of valvular abnormalities across different studies is very variable. Differences between transthoracic (TTE) and transesophagic echocardiography (TEE) have been pointed as one of the main reasons accounting for them (Table 12.2). TEE has showed to provide a higher sensitivity to detect valve abnormalities in primary APS patients than TTE (Cervera et al., 2011a). The prevalence of valve abnormalities in studies that used transthoracic echocardiography ranges from 20% to 65% while those that used TTE found a higher prevalence from 61% to 84% (Espínola-Zavaleta et al., 1999; Zavaleta et al., 2004; Turiel et al., 2000; Erdogan et al., 2005; Turiel et al., 2005) (see Table 12.2). Additionally, although not all of them were able to find statistically significant

TABLE 12.2 Prevalence of Valvular Abnormalities in Patients With Primary Antiphospholipid Syndrome (APS)

Study	Study Type	Technique	Primary APS	Controls	*p*
Brenner et al. (1991)	CC	TTE	11/34 (32%)	1/22 (5%)	0.038
Cervera et al. (1991)	CC	TTE	21/55 (38%)	2/55 (4%)	<0.001
Galve et al. (1992)	CC	TTE	10/28 (36%)	0/28 (0%)	0.002
Badui et al. (1995)	CC	TTE	13/20 (65%)	0/20 (0%)	<0.0001
García-Torres et al.	T	TTE	6/20 (30%)		
Espinola-Zavaleta et al. (1999)	T	TEE	22/29 (76%)		
Turiel et al. (2000)	T	TEE	33/40 (82%)		
Espinola-Zavaleta et al. (2006)	T	TEE	17/24 (71%)		
Erdogan et al. (2005)	T	TEE	26/31 (84%)		
Turiel et al. (2005)	Ch	TEE	34/56 (61%)		

CC, case-control study; *Ch*, cohort study; *T*, transversal.

differences, most studies have shown the higher frequency of valve abnormalities in SLE patients with circulating aPL with respect to those SLE patients without aPL (Khamashta et al., 1990; Nihoyannopoulos et al., 1990; Leung et al., 1990; Cervera et al., 1992; Roldan et al., 1992; Jouhikainen et al., 1994; Gabrielli et al., 1995; Leszczyński et al., 2003; Perez-Villa et al., 2005; Roldan et al., 2005, 2007; Amoroso et al., 2006) (see Table 12.3). Moreover, almost 90% of patients with SLE and valvular disease have been found to have aPL with respect to 44% of patients without valvular involvement (Table 12.4).

Fewer studies have addressed directly the prevalence of Libman-Sacks valve lesions. Verrucous endocarditis was detected in 9% and up to 16% of SLE patients (Khamashta et al., 1990; Moyssakis et al., 2007; Nihoyannopoulos et al., 1990). Further the detection of lupus anticoagulant (LA) in SLE patients has been found to account for a 5.9 relative risk of developing Libman-Sacks endocarditis in SLE patients (Zuily et al., 2011).

TABLE 12.3 Prevalence of Valvular Abnormalities in Systemic Lupus Erythematosus (SLE) Patients According to the Presence of Antiphospholipid Antibodies (aPL)

			SLE			
Author (Year)	Study Type	Tech.	aPL +ve	aPL −ve	Controls	*p*
Khamashta et al. (1990)	CC/Ch	TTE	30/132 (22.7%)		2/68 (2.9%)	<0.001
			1/50 (1.2%)	10/82 (12%)		<0.001
Nihoyannopoulos et al. (1990)	T	TTE	26/93 (28%)		4/40	
			20/50 (40%)	6/43 (14%)		<0.0001
Leung et al. (1990)	CC	TTE	NS		NS	<0.001
			(70%)	(8%)		<0.005
Cervera et al. (1992)	CC	TTE	31/70 (44%)		2/40 (5%)	<0.001
			15/23 (65%)	16/47 (34%)		<0.03
Roldan et al. (1992)	CC	TTE	40/54 (74%)		8/35 (23%)	<0.001
			17/22 (77%)	23/32 (72%)		0.92
Jouhikainen et al. (1994)	Ch	TTE	5/74 (7%)			
			5/37 (14%)	0/37 (0%)		<0.057
Gabrielli et al. (1995)	CC	TTE	15/39 (38%)		0/20 (0%)	0.001
			11/27 (41%)	4/12 (33%)		0.91

Leszczyński et al. (2003)	CC	TTE	18/52 (34.6%)		2/34 (5.9%	<0.05
			14/28 (50%)	4/24 (17%)		<0.05
Perez-Villa et al. (2005) [a]	CC/Ch	TTE	24/61 (39%)		2/40 (5%)	<0.01
			6/7 (86%)	17/52 (33%)		0.01
Roldan et al. (2005)	T	TEE	28/37 (76%)			
			13/16 (81%)	15/21 (71%)		0.68
Amoroso et al. (2006)	CC	TTE	19/34 (56%)		1/34 (3%)	<0.001
			69.6%	27.3%		NS
Farzaneh-Far et al. (2006) [b]	T	TTE	13/200			
			6/42 (14%)	7/158 (4%)		0.02
Roldan et al. (2007)	T	TEE	38/69 (55%)			
			31/46 (67%)	7/23 (30%)		0.008
All studies using TTE			131/300 (44%)	120/488 (25%)		<0.0005
All studies using TEE			30/50 (60%)	26/41 (63%)		0.9

aPL, antiphospholipid antibodies; *aPL +ve*, patients with aPL; *aPL −ve*, patients without aPL; *CC*, case-control; *Ch*, cohort; *NS*, not specified; *NSig*, not significant; *T*, transversal; *Tech.*, technique.
[a]*Data are referred as severe valvular regurgitation.*
[b]*Data are referred as moderate to severe mitral regurgitation.*

TABLE 12.4 **Prevalence of Valve Abnormalities in Systemic Lupus Erythematosus (SLE), SLE Associated to Antiphospholipid Syndrome (APS), SLE With Antiphospholipid Antibodies (aPL), SLE Without aPL, and Primary Antiphospholipid Syndrome (PAPS) Patients**

			SLE					
	Study	**Tech.**	**APS**	**aPL +ve**	**aPL −ve**	**PAPS**	**Healthy**	***P***
Roldan et al. (1992)	CC	TEE	**17/40 (77%)**			3/10 (30%)	8/35 (23%)	<0.001
			-	17/22 (77%)	23/32 (72%)			NS
Gleason et al. (1993)	CC	NS	**8/20 (40%)**			6/10 (60%)	/20	NS
			-	-	-			
Vianna et al. (1994)		NS	**-/56**			-/58	-	<0.001
			-	-	-			
Gabrielli et al. (1995)	CC	NS	**15/39 (38%)0**			0/20	0/20	0.001
			-	11/27 (41%)	4/12 (33%)			NS
Krause et al. (2005)	T	NS	-			29/159 (18%)	-	0.009
			27/97 (28%)	-				
Pardos-Gea et al. (2010)	Ch	TTE				19/34 (56)	-	0.82
			10/19 (52)	-	-			
Kampolis et al. (2014)	Ch	TEE	**23/65 (35%)**			9/17 (53%)	-	NS
			7/23 (30%)	8/19 (42%)	8/23 (35%)			NS

CC, case-control study; *Ch*, cohort study; *NS*, not specified; *NSig*, not significant; *S*, series.

2.2 Ischemic Cardiomyopathy

According to the Euro-phospholipid cohort, myocardial infarction is diagnosed in 5.5% of APS patients and is the presenting manifestation in up to 2.8% of patients (Cervera et al., 2002). Ten-year follow-up of the Euro-phospholipid cohort found an incidence of 180–190 patients/100,000 patients/year (Cervera et al., 2015; Cervera et al., 2009b). Most authors recognize a higher incidence of ischemic cardiomyopathy in APS patients despite the same cardiovascular risk when assessed by traditional Framingham risk factors (Sacré et al., 2010). However, others argue that the association of aPL and myocardial infarct is controversial since, although anticardiolipin antibodies (aCL) are found in 5–15% of patients with myocardial infarction and increases up to 21% of patients under 45 years old (Cuadrado and Hughes, 2001; Hamsten et al., 1986), not all studies were able to find an association between aCL and myocardial infarction (Sletnes et al., 1992). Further, aCL were not found to be predictors of mortality nor recurrent infarcts in survivors of myocardial infarcts (Sletnes et al., 1992). Nevertheless, the lack of association in this case might be attributed to an incomplete assessment of aPL profile since other authors did report an increased risk of myocardial infarct in patients with lupus anticoagulant (Petri, 2004). Anyhow, considering the low sensitivity of clinical symptoms and Q waves on electrocardiography for diagnosis of myocardial infarction, the true frequency might be higher because when myocardial ischemia is assessed with very sensitive techniques as high as 30% can be proved (Sacré et al., 2010). Moreover, cardiac involvement is described in up to 50% of cases with CAPS where several organs are affected at the same time due to widespread microthrombosis (Cervera, unpublished data) (Rodríguez-Pintó et al., 2015).

Additionally, some studies indicate a relation between a faster atherosclerosis evolution and the presence of aPL (Ames et al., 2009a,b).

2.3 Nonischemic Ventricular Dysfunction

Limited data have been published regarding ventricular dysfunction not attributable to valvular disease in APS patients. The few case-control and cohort studies published agree that systolic left ventricular function remains preserved in APS patients without ischemic cardiomyopathy; however, a higher prevalence of left ventricular diastolic dysfunction was found in some studies (Pardos-Gea et al., 2013; Kampolis et al., 2014; Hasnie et al., 1995). Diastolic dysfunction is reported in up to 22.6% of patients while left ventricle hypertrophy was shown in up to 18% (Pardos-Gea et al., 2013).

Some studies reported a higher prevalence of right ventricular diastolic dysfunction although its relation to pulmonary hypertension secondary to previous thromboembolic disease is not yet clear because routine catheterization was not undertaken (Pardos-Gea et al., 2013; Coudray et al., 1995). No difference has been found in right ventricular systolic function in APS patients (Kampolis et al., 2014).

2.4 Intracardiac Thrombus

Intracardiac thrombosis is a very rare event. There is very scarce data regarding the epidemiology of intracardiac thrombosis in APS. Only 0.4% of cases with APS from the 1000 patients with APS reported intracardiac thrombosis (Cervera et al., 2002). Pardos-Gea et al. (2013) were able to find a single case of intracardiac thrombosis in a cohort of 53 cases of APS patients observed during 10 years corresponding to a 1.8%; however, the low number of cases precludes the study to find any statistical difference from the controls. Further, this patient developed a cancer and died. The rarity of this presentation makes difficult to understand the relationship between intracardiac thrombosis and APS. However, APS was the only explanation for 2.2% of cases with an intracardiac thrombosis found in a series of autopsies (Vaideeswar et al., 2012).

3. PATHOPHYSIOLOGY

3.1 Valve Disease and Libman-Sacks Endocarditis

The pathophysiology and the role of aPL in APS valvular heart diseases is not yet clear. Some authors support that valve thickening and vegetation reflect the same pathological process while other suggest to differentiate between noninflammatory and inflammatory valvulopathy (Amigo and García-Torres, 2000). Indeed, nonbacterial vegetations may be found combined with valve thickening (Turiel et al., 2000; Espínola-Zavaleta et al., 1999). Some authors agree that a continuous progression takes place in APS valvular heart disease. In this sense, vegetations may eventually heal with a fibrous plaque, sometimes with focal calcification, scarring, and deformity leading to valve dysfunction. Valve thickening might represent an early stage of valve disease that sometimes might evolve into severe inflammation.

Macroscopic evaluation of valves shows thickened valves with a rough surface, verrucous thrombosis, and commissural fusions while microscopic evaluation shows recent and old lesions (García-Torres et al., 1996). Histologic evaluation of recent lesion shows intravalvular capillary thrombosis with hemorrhages and necrosis with laminar and verrucous thrombosis while old lesions show nodular and laminar fibrosis with vascular hyperplasia and proliferation with focal calcifications (Ford et al., 1989; Ziporen et al., 1996; García-Torres et al., 1996). Inmunohistological evaluation observed aCL deposits along the leaflets or cusps surface together with granular complement deposition suggesting immune complex deposition (Ziporen et al., 1996;

Shapiro et al., 1977; García-Torres et al., 1996). Inflammatory infiltrate is scanty on microscopical examination (Afek et al., 1999). These observations support the hypothesis reported by Amigo et al., which proposes that valve endocardial interaction with circulating aPL leads to valvular endocardial damage resulting in thrombosis and subendocardial fibroblastic infiltration. Otherwise, intravalvular immune complex deposition would lead to intracapillary thrombosis, edema and hemorrhages with necrosis, and fibroblast infiltration and valvular retraction. Both pathways would lead to fibrosis, scarring, focal calcification, deformities, and finally to subsequent valve dysfunction (Amigo and García-Torres, 2000).

3.2 Ischemic Cardiomyopathy

An increased thrombotic risk is well known in patients with APS. aPL are both diagnostic markers and pathogenic drivers of the syndrome (Meroni et al., 2011). However, no more than 15% of general population patients with aPL develop thrombosis (Ortega-Hernandez et al., 2009). This observation led to propose the requirement of a "second hit" to explain the only occasionally clinical observation of thrombotic events in patients with circulating aPL (Shoenfeld et al., 2009). In this hypothesis, a "first hit" would induce a thrombophilic state but clotting would only take place in the presence of a second event. This "second event" (or "second hit") would be another thrombophilic condition that increases the risk of a clot formation. In these sense, the presence of an environmental trigger as a "second hit" has been reported in more than half of cases of CAPS (Cervera et al., 2009a,b). Several authors showed the binding of aPL to toll-like and annexin V receptors in the cell membrane (Pierangeli et al., 2007; Raschi et al., 2008; Xie et al., 2014). This interaction engages intracellular mediators as nuclear factor kappa B and mTORC, the mammalian target of rapamycin, leading to prothrombotic endothelial changes that might involve a disturbance in the redox balance (Eikelboom and Weitz, 2014; Giannakopoulos and Krilis, 2013; Poulton et al., 2012). The second hit that led to a thrombotic event has been less clearly identified; however, up to 50% of cases with CAPS event and an identified trigger, it is an infectious microrganism (Cervera et al., 2009a,b).

Furthermore, some studies suggested that APS may result in early atherosclerosis (Petri, 2000; Barón et al., 2005). However, although a clear relationship between SLE and preclinical and clinical atherosclerosis is accepted, the association of aPL with atherosclerosis is not yet that clear (Petri, 2004; Roman et al., 2003; Asanuma et al., 2003; Ames et al., 2009a,b). An increase in traditional risk factors and risk factors associated to the disease have been proposed to account of an increase of atherosclerotic risk in APS patients (Ames et al., 2009a,b). Nevertheless, some evidence point in this direction. Ames et al. found a direct relation between IgG aCL titter and carotid intimal-medial thickness (IMT) suggesting an early accelerated atherosclerosis in APS patients (Ames et al., 2009a,b; Ambrosino et al., 2014). Further, anti-β2 glycoprotein I (anti-β2 GPI) antibodies have been found to block the reduction of oxidized LDL (oxLDL) intake by macrophages in the vessel wall drove by β2- gycoprotein I (Matsuura and Koike, 2000). Thus, aPL seem to increase macrophages oxLDL uptake leading to accelerated atherosclerosis. Further, anti-β2 GPI have been found in atheroma plaques from endarterectomy samples, and an increase of homocysteine in APS patients has been correlated with an accelerated atherosclerosis as assessed by the IMT (George et al., 1999; Ames et al., 2002).

3.3 Nonischemic Ventricular Dysfunction

The pathogenesis of nonischemic ventricular dysfunction is unclear. Some authors have related circulating antibodies to the development of left ventricular myocardial hypertrophy and dysfunction (Leung et al., 1990). In these sense, some authors proposed ischemic myocardial injury and myocardial fibrosis to be responsible for a left ventricular compliance decrease leading to an impaired left ventricular relaxation and filling (Hasnie et al., 1995; Tektonidou et al., 2001). However, Pardos-gea et al., in a study where they found a higher prevalence of left ventricle hypertrophy, rose the hypothesis of an impairment in left ventricle filling related to hypertension secondary to an accelerated atherosclerosis (Pardos-Gea et al., 2013). Indeed, accelerate atherosclerosis is a known phenomenon in inflammatory and specially in autoimmune disease although its relation to APS is not that clear (Hollan et al., 2013). In this sense, diastolic dysfunction has been linked to the association of APS to SLE and specially to SLE activity (Roman et al., 2001; Paran et al., 2007). However, other studies found no association between left ventricular diastolic dysfunction and hypertension (Hasnie et al., 1995; Kampolis et al., 2014; Coudray et al., 1995). Others found even worst diastolic function in patients with primary APS with respect to those with APS associated to SLE; yet, differences in age and hypertension prevalence might have acted as confounders in this study (Hasnie et al., 1995). Anyhow, the physiological hallmarks of left ventricle diastolic dysfunction are impaired relaxation, loss of restoring forces, reduced diastolic compliance and an elevated left ventricle filling pressure.

Although rare, left ventricle systolic dysfunction due to myocardial thrombotic microangiopathy in cases of catastrophic APS has been reported (Cervera et al., 2014). Nevertheless, more frequently, a complete workup in patients with left ventricle systolic dysfunction leads to valvulopathy or atherosclerotic coronary artery disease as the main reason that leads to left ventricular dilated myocardiopathy and systolic dysfunction (Pardos-Gea et al., 2013) (see below the discussion on the differential diagnosis of ischemic cardiomyopathy).

Finally, other authors have attributed right ventricular dysfunction to pulmonary artery hypertension secondary to chronic thromboembolic disease or to myocardial ischemia (Tektonidou et al., 2001).

3.4 Intracardiac Thrombus

The pathophysiology of intracardiac thrombosis is unknown. Partially because the infrequency of intracardiac thrombosis in APS patients precludes any mechanistic study on this clinical manifestation. However, an intravascular thrombophilic environment related to the contact of circulating aPL antibodies with the endothelial surface has been proposed as the probable trigger.

4. CLINICAL MANIFESTATIONS

4.1 Valve Disease

Valve heart disease in APS vary from minimal thickening and regurgitation to severe deformity and valvular dysfunction. Left-sided valves, and specially the mitral valve, are the most frequently involved (Cervera et al., 2011b). Regurgitation is more commonly found than stenosis (Zuily et al., 2011). Generally, mitral affection leads to regurgitation with minor hemodynamic significance (Brenner et al., 1991; Espínola-Zavaleta et al., 1999). However, Turiel et al. showed progression or new valves involvement in up to 36% of patients with primary APS and found high IgG aCL to be an independent risk factor for new and progressive valve abnormalities (Turiel et al., 2005). Perez-Villa et al. (2005) demonstrated an increase in frequency of mitral regurgitation in up to 20% of patients with SLE after an 8-year follow-up and an increase of 19% of cases with mitral valve thickening. Conversely, Pardos-Gea et al. (2010) found that up to 93% of patients with APS and thrombosis with valvulopathy remained stable after 10-year follow-up and only 8%, from those without valvulopathy at the initial evaluation, developed valve defects. Thus, it seems that there is no way to predict which lesions will continue stable over time and which will worsen or improve to disappear (Cervera et al., 1992). Severe valve disease worsening might lead to heart failure with dyspnea, orthopnea and nocturnal cough, or paroxysmal nocturnal dyspnea episodes requiring valve replacement (Espínola-Zavaleta et al., 1999; Zavaleta et al., 2004; Turiel et al., 2000, 2005).

However, heart valve disease is important not only because of valve dysfunction and its hemodynamic consequences but also because it is related to other clinical manifestations like stroke, epilepsy, migraine, or livedo reticularis (Cervera et al., 1991; Pardos-Gea et al., 2010). An increased risk of arterial thrombosis and specially of cerebrovascular ischemic events has been found in APS patients with heart valve disease (Pardos-Gea et al., 2010; Krause et al., 2005). Other authors described uncommon complications including infective endocarditis and pseudoinfective endocarditis (Asherson and Cervera, 1991).

4.2 Libman-Sacks Endocarditis

Usually, Libman-Sacks endocarditis has no hemodynamic significance initially, but hemodynamic instability might develop over time requiring valve replacement (Moyssakis et al., 2007). Libman-Sacks endocarditis might progress to mitral regurgitation or stenosis with regurgitation leading to hear failure. Some patients present aortic involvement with aortic regurgitation, stenosis, or both while tricuspid involvement is rare, although it has been reported (Moyssakis et al., 2007). A significant association was found between Libman-Sacks endocarditis and disease duration, the presence of aCL, and thrombocytopenia in SLE patients (Moyssakis et al., 2007).

Thromboembolic events remain the major fear for patients with Libman-Sacks endocarditis. The brain is the most frequent embolic target. Some patients with Libman-Sacks endocarditis might present like an infective endocarditis, the so-called pseudoendocarditis, with fever, splinter hemorrhages, cardiac murmurs with echocardiographic evidence of valve vegetations, moderate to high levels of aPL, and repeated negative blood cultures (Font et al., 1991).

4.3 Ischemic Cardiomyopathy

Cardiac ischemic disease might present with a wide spectrum of clinical manifestations from asymptomatic myocardial lesions to sudden death. Chest pain is the most frequent clinical presentation of patients with coronary insufficiency while others might present other more unspecific complaints like dyspnea or palpitations.

Acute large cardiac infarcts or small diffuse coronary occlusions and those affecting valvular function might lead to left ventricular systolic dysfunction or right heart failure. Patients might present with edema, orthopnea or severe dyspnea, and respiratory insufficiency requiring immediate ventilation support. Other patients present with ventricular arrhythmias and require pharmacologic or electric cardioversion. Acute cardiac collapse (often together with respiratory decompensation) is frequent in patients with the catastrophic APS and is one of the most common causes of death in this group of patients (Bucciarelli et al., 2006).

Chronic small vascular occlusion might be responsible for diffuse myocardial systolic dysfunction finally leading to a dilated myocardiopathy (Lauwerys et al., 2001). Dilated myocardiopathy might evolve to a chronic cardiac inefficiency with dyspnea or chronic cough specially when lying down.

4.4 Nonischemic Ventricular Dysfunction

Left ventricular hypertrophy as left ventricular diastolic dysfunction are cardiac manifestations usually not related to symptomatic manifestations (Paran et al., 2007). However, ventricular dysfunction associated or not associated to left ventricular hypertrophy might progress to clinical chronic heart failure in some patients. Right ventricular function seems to become worse over time; however, most patients remain asymptomatic. Rarely, some patients might evolve and develop limbs edema, pleural effusion, and liver congestion, or even ascites.

4.5 Intracardiac Thrombus

Although intracardiac thrombosis is often an unexpected finding during an echocardiography requested due to other reasons, sometimes it is the only finding to explain systemic or pulmonary embolic disease (Abanador-Kamper et al., 2012; Mottram and Gelman, 2002). Rarely, some patients might present with fever or chest pain. Unfortunately, most published cases account for tragic situations where patients presented with systemic emboli to their physician or to the emergency room. In these cases, intracardiac thrombosis are found when looking for an embolic source. Usually, embolic clinical manifestations take place as ischemic stroke. However, although thrombus might form in any heart cavity some authors reported that they are most usually found on the right side. However, this finding could be explained by an underdetection of lung embolisms or lower embolic risk of the right side thrombosis possibly due to lower shear hemodynamic forces on the right heart side (Weiss et al., 2008).

5. DIAGNOSTIC PROCEDURES

5.1 Valve Disease and Libman-Sacks Endocarditis

Echocardiography is the main tool for cardiac valve evaluation in APS patients. It gives valuable information on heat function and valvular involvement. Additionally, echocardiography is inexpensive and widely available. However, its operator-dependent nature limits its reproducibility and transthoracic echocardiography might not be appropriate for some obese or emphysematous patients with a poor acoustic window. TTE is more specific but more sensible than transthoracic echocardiography, especially when evaluating the left side valves. However, TTE might result in higher frequency of nonspecific valvular thickenings detection (Roldan et al., 2008; Cervera et al., 2011a). An initial echocardiography in all APS patients is recommended at the time of diagnosis, especially after an arterial thrombosis has been diagnosed (Cervera et al., 2011a). Generally, a double step process is implemented. Transthoracic evaluation is first used due to its noninvasive nature as a first screening tool. When a clinically significant valve dysfunction is found in transthoracic echocardiography, transesophagic evaluation is then undertaken. If valves are normal, serial echocardiographic controls are not recommended while periodic echocardiographic evaluation are warranted in patients with valvular abnormalities to follow functional changes that may require surgery (Perez-Villa et al., 2005).

Recently, valvular heart disease evaluation by cardiac magnetic resonance (CMR) has been proposed, especially when echocardiography imaging is not possible particularly for surgical decision making (Reddy et al., 2013). However, to the best of our knowledge, this technique has not yet been validated in APS patients.

5.2 Ischemic Cardiomyopathy

Coronary insufficiency is generally diagnosed by electrocardiography performed during chest pain while elevation of circulating serum troponin levels reveals myocardial injury. Unstable angina is usually studied by coronarography. Angiographic studies provide a morphologic evaluation of coronary arteries and permits the differential diagnosis between coronary disease related to atherosclerosis and thrombosis triggered directly by aPL. Stable angina may be diagnosed by stress tests either by conventional exercise testing or stress echocardiography or SPECT when there is a left bundle branch block or a limitation to perform enough effort. However, stable angina does not seem to be more frequent in APS patients than in the general population. A high degree of agreement was found between contrast echocardiography and nuclear imaging for assessment of myocardial perfusion defects in patients with APS (Espinola-Zavaleta et al., 2006). Some studies point to the availability of PET scan to detect myocardial perfusion defects in patients with APS, although its role in APS assessment is still a matter of debate (Alexánderson et al., 2008). Additionally, CMR has been found to provide a high sensitivity to detect asymptomatic myocardial infarcts in patients with APS that are detected neither by electrocardiography nor by echocardiography, as characterized by late gadolinium enhancement, although their clinical significances are not yet clear (Sacré et al., 2010).

Routine testing for aPL in myocardial infarct patients is not recommended; however, testing should be considered in young patients with coronary artery disease and no other risk factors, family history, or recreational drug abuse.

5.3 Nonischemic Ventricular Dysfunction

Left and right ventricle systolic function are usually assessed by direct echographie observation of cardiac contraction. However, left ventricular is then objectivized by one of the several different echocardiographic techniques to assess the left ventricular ejection fraction (usually by volume or short axis dimensions change) (Lang et al., 2015). The tricuspid annular plane systolic excursion as assessed by M-mode is generally measured to evaluate right ventricle function although other measures are sometimes used. Whereas left ventricle systolic function is routinely quantified by measuring ejection fraction there is not a single clinical measure that quantifies left ventricle diastolic function. Instead a high number of indexes based on cardiac imaging have been used to determine if diastolic function is normal or impaired. Transmitral velocity curves reflect the relative pressure gradients between the left atrium and the ventricle throughout the diastole. They are influenced by ventricular relaxation, ventricle compliance, and their driving forces. Early (E) and late or atrial (A) peak filling velocities and their relation reflect ventricular diastolic function. A decrease in peak early filling velocity with a prolonged deceleration time and a compensatory increase in flow during atrial contraction (A wave) is best explained by an impairment in left ventricle relaxation in its early phase. Compensatory left atrial pressure increase in order to maintain left ventricle filling results in a higher early trasmitral velocity (E wave) leading to a normal E/A ratio typical of a progressed diastolic disease (pseudonormal pattern) (Maragiannis and Nagueh, 2015). In summary, impairment of diastolic function can be detected noninvasively in clinical routine practice by measuring transmitral filling pattern. Tissue Doppler echocardiography provides further information on the heart diastolic function by measuring the velocity of myocardial motion (Boyd et al., 2015). Recently, some studies point to the possible utility of stress echocardiography to unmask hidden diastolic dysfunction although they have not been used in APS patients and their clinical utility has not been established.

5.4 Intracardiac Thrombus

Intracardiac masses can be visualized on 2D echocardiography, provided that image quality is adequate. Intracardiac thrombosis is often first found by transthoracic echocardiography performed for other reasons. Thrombus mobility is predictive of embolic vents. Often, a TTE is then performed specially in myocardial masses under 1 cm in diameter in order to obtain further details regarding the anatomy and nature of intracardiac mass. A sensitivity as high as 86–95% has been found for transthoracic echocardiography for left ventricular thrombosis although a higher sensitivity is attributed tranesophagic echocardiography when thrombus is placed in the atrium or the left appendage where transthoracic echocardiography has a low sensitivity (39–63%) (Shrestha et al., 1983; Manning, 1995). However, when doubts still persist about the nature of an intracardiac mass, cardiac computed tomography or CMR scan can be undertaken providing a high predictive value for the detection of auricular thrombi (Hur et al., 2013). Indeed, contrast-enhanced cardiac resonance is now known to provide the highest sensitivity and specificity for left ventricle thrombi detection (Srichai et al., 2006). Additionally, CMR may predict the risk of embolism based on the thrombi organization (Barkhausen et al., 2012). Unfortunately, CMR is expensive and not widely available. Further, CMR cannot be performed in patients with metallic devices and might be not possible in patients with arrhythmias or with a limited respiratory reserve.

6. DIFFERENTIAL DIAGNOSIS

6.1 Valve Disease and Libman-Sacks Endocarditis

Valvular morphological pattern and clinical picture should base the differential diagnosis approach. In these sense two distinct scenarios of valve abnormalities can be distinguished: valve thickening and valve vegetations.

6.2 Valve Heart Disease

The differential diagnosis of valve heart disease in APS should include rheumatic heart disease, valvular aging as so as other less frequent valvular heat diseases like drug-induced valve disease, and collagen or glycogen storage diseases. Notable morphologic differences have been noted between rheumatic and APS-related valve heart disease by echocardiography. In these sense, subvalvular apparatus chordal structures thickening is typically seen in rheumatic valvular disease and is rare in APS. Rheumatic disease characteristically progresses from the free margins toward the leaflet bases. Leaflet tips and chordal thickening and calcification are prominent and often seen in these cases while APS valve disease is generally diffuse starting from the mid-portion or base to spread out (Roldan et al., 1992). Additionally, chordae tendineae involvement is rare in APS. Rarely, some drugs like ergot-derived dopamine agonists used to treat prolactin-secreting tumors and pergolide, formerly used to treat Parkinson disease, as so as recreational amphetaminic drugs, might induce valve thickening although in that case usually tendinous chords are involved and shortened but without valvular calcifications or commissural fusion (Cosyns et al., 2013; Bhattacharyya et al., 2009). Additionally, when mitral valve involvement is hemodynamically linked to mitral stenosis nonrheumatic mitral annular calcification should be included in the differential diagnosis especially in patients above 50 years old Bicuspid aortic valve, aortic root dilatation, ankylosing spondylitis, and systemic hypertension should be included in the differential diagnosis when aortic valve is the main valve affected, although most anamnesis and echocardiographic findings can rule out most cases (Reményi et al., 2012).

6.3 Libman-Sacks Endocarditis

The differential diagnosis of verrucous endocarditis in the setting of APS classically includes infective endocarditis and rheumatic disease although probably other clinical situations like marantic endocarditis (or cancer-related nonbacterial endocarditis), intracardiac thrombosis, chordae tendineae rupture, valvular sclerosis, mixoide valve degeneration, cardiac tumors, and rheumatoid nodules as so as Lambl's excrescences (small filiform images at the free edge of aortic cusps) should be taken into account (Gonzalez and Evangelista, 2011). Additionally, hypermobile Chiari net or a prominent Eustachian valve might cause some confusion when assessing the right side valves (Asherson et al., 1988; Gonzalez and Evangelista, 2011). However, several important features might help in the differential diagnosis.

The differential diagnosis with infectious endocarditis typically arises when patients present fever while infectious endocarditis without fever is rare. Further, in infectious endocarditis generally a bacteria growth can be proved in blood cultures sometimes; however, no microorganism can be demonstrated from blood cultures especially in patients to whom antibiotics have been prescribed (Gonzalez and Evangelista, 2011). Anyhow, patients with negative blood cultures who fulfill the Dukes criteria for a probable infectious endocarditis should undergo an accurate workup with serology tests and molecular biology techniques to rule out infective endocarditis as detailed elsewhere, because infectious endocarditis still is the most probable diagnosis (Fournier et al., 2010; Gonzalez and Evangelista, 2011). Infectious endocarditis often evolves rapidly to valve perforation or dysfunction leading to heart failure or acute pulmonary edema. Further, infectious endocarditis tends to form abscess resulting in rhythm abnormalities while Libman-Sacks endocarditis do not do so. Vegetations in the setting of Libman-Sacks are morphologically sessile, oval or tubular or coalescent in shape, nodular or protuberant, heterogeneously or homogeneously echoreflectant, and are predominantly located on the leaflets coaptation point but frequently extending through the leaflets into the opposite. Contrariwise, infectious vegetations are highly mobile and are attached to the valve through a narrow base (Roldan et al., 2015).

Rarely, Libman-Sacks endocarditis, especially in the setting of SLE, might present with clinical features of pseudoinfective endocarditis (fever, cardiac murmur, vegetations, splinter hemorrhages, and serological evidence of lupus activity). However, several clinical and serological features might distinguish both clinical pictures (Asherson and Cervera, 1991). To start with, white cell count is usually high in infective endocarditis while a low white cell count points to lupus activity. Additionally, autoimmune disease activity does not usually increase C-reactive protein or procalcitonin levels and, thus, elevated levels of these serum markers should point to the infectious origin of the clinical picture. To end with, although aPL might be found positive in up to 14% of patients with infective endocarditis their titters are usually low (Asherson et al., 1990; Kupferwasser et al., 1999).

Additionally, when there are doubts between Libman-Sacks endocarditis and morphologic normality variants or intracardiac tumors, CMR might provide a complementary view of the lesions and might distinguish between them (Dursun et al., 2015; Gaudio et al., 2004; Patel et al., 2016).

Up to 19% of patients with known malignancy might develop nonbacterial thrombotic endocarditis from whom 24% develop thrombotic phenomena (Edoute et al., 1997). The most frequent malignancies are adenocarcinomas (pulmonary or pancreatic) or hematologic neoplasia while carcinoid tumors tend to affect the right side valves (Edoute et al., 1997). Although the presence of circulating aPL might be detected in oncologic patients they are usually found in low titters (Font et al., 2011). A difficult unsolved situation might appear when patents with APS develop a malignancy and a vegetation is found in an echocardiography performed for other reason.

Finally, a cut-off of more than 3 mm in diameter is generally adopted to prevent misinterpretation of Lambl's excrescences as vegetations because they are usually thin (less $\leq$ 2 mm) and elongated (>5 mm in length).

6.4 Ischemic Cardiomyopathy

Conditions that should always be considered in the differential diagnosis of patients with acute chest pain include life-threatening conditions like aortic dissection, pulmonary embolism, and pneumothorax notwithstanding pericardic and musculoskeletal problems. Chest X-ray is recommended in patients to detect pneumonia, pneumothorax, rib fracture, or other thoracic disorders (Roffi et al., 2015). For patients with established ischemic cardiac disease angiographic studies usually provide information on the nature of coronary disease distinguishing patient with atherosclerotic coronary disease and those patients without. When no atherosclerotic disease is detected, sometimes ECG may be able to capture ST-shifts during and after chest pain indicating Prinzmetal angina (Task Force Members et al., 2013). Sometimes stress test result indicative of myocardial ischemia by coronary angiography do not show any abnormality, then primary microvascular disease such as that seen in aortic stenosis and hypertrophic cardiomyopathy should be suspected. Finally, the differential diagnosis workup should include other inherited thrombophilic disease specially activated protein C resistance or factor V Leiden, protein C or S deficiency, and factor XII deficiency (Pasupathy et al., 2015). Additionally, some authors have reported some cases of coronary arteritis although this is a rare event.

6.5 Nonischemic Ventricular Dysfunction

Although, ventricular dysfunction has been described in APS patients, other reasons should be ruled out. In these instances ventricular dysfunction related to other primary causes should be suspected. Initially by basic anamnesis and exploratory workup but even when this reason is not apparent some further studies are warranted. Diastolic dysfunction related to aging is the first differential diagnosis. Later, unapparent hypertension might be found sometimes related to an undiagnosed obstructive sleep apnea-hypopnea syndrome.

Obstructive heart disease is usually apparent by echocardiography. Asymmetric myocardial hypertrophy should lead to suspect inborn myocardial disease.

6.6 Intracardiac Thrombus

Suspected cardiac masses may be benign, malign, or ultimately found to be artifacts. In patients with APS an echo-dense mass attached to the valve leaftlets caution should be taken not to mistake a verrucous endocarditis. Often a transesophageal is performed in order to best assess intracardiac abnormality. Solid masses appear as echo-dense structures inside the cardiac chambers or infiltrating the myocardium while atrial myxoma are well-circumscribed mobile not calcified masses attached to the atrial septum (Gertner and Leatherman, 1992). When echocardiography is inconclusive CMR might assist in the differential diagnosis between thrombosis and tumoral masses because while tumors enhance when gadolinium is administered, intracardiac thrombosis does not (Erkan et al., 2002). Further, on CMR evaluation, fresh thrombus show high intensity whereas old clot has low signal intensity. These differences allow thrombus aging that has important consequences in order to determinate the more appropriate therapeutic approach. Anyhow, detection of intracardiac thrombi without apparent explanation warrants aPL testing (Miyakis et al., 2006).

7. TREATMENT

7.1 Valve Disease and Libman-Sacks Endocarditis

Unfortunately, no therapeutic randomized trials have been undertaken to evaluate the role of treatment in heart valve disease. Although different pathophysiology pathways are suspected to lead to valve heart disease or valve vegetation respectively, treatment results are not distinguished in most publications. Observational studies could find neither anticoagulants nor antiaggregation to be able to reverse established valvular lesions or prevent their appearance (Espínola-Zavaleta et al., 1999; Zavaleta et al., 2004; Kampolis et al., 2014). However, a consensus international committee on occasion of the 10th International Congress on aPL recommended anticoagulation with warfarin/heparin for patients with vavulopathy who have had evidence of thromboembolic diseases based on the premise that valve lesion might serve as a substrate for embolism (Lockshin et al., 2003). Prophylactic antiplatelet treatment was suggested by the committee members for asymptomatic APS patients with valvular lesions (Lockshin et al., 2003). Finally, although case reports pointed to a possible efficacy of corticosteroid therapy in APS patients with heart valvular disease (Nesher et al., 1997), follow-up studies show clinical effects of neither corticosteroids nor immunosuppression treatment and, thus, no consensus was achieved by the international committee. Nowadays, the role of steroids in the treatment of APS valve disease is uncertain (Kampolis et al., 2014; Erkan et al., 2012). Therefore, distinguishing among reversible valve deformity, irreversible cicatricial valve deformity, and vegetations is suggested when considering treatment in heart valve disease in APS (Lockshin et al., 2003). Patients with APS and valve lesions do not require infective endocarditis prophylaxis (Habib et al., 2009).

Although, only 4–6% of patients with valvular disease develop severe dysfunction, valve replacement surgery should be considered in patients with severe valvulopathy. Data on long-term outcome after surgery are scarce. Heart valve surgery in patients with APS carries a considerable morbidity and mortality specially due to thromboembolic complications. Thus, a careful anticoagulation monitoring is warranted to avoid frequent hemorrhagic and thrombotic complications after surgery.

7.2 Ischemic Cardiomyopathy

Aggressive treatment of all traditional risk factors for atherosclerosis (hypertension, hypercholesterolemia, smoking) is recommended. Additionally, folic acid, vitamin B, and statins should be considered. Statins therapy is beneficial not only because of its effect on lipid profile but also because statins enhance atherosclerosis plaques stability, decrease oxidative stress, block the thrombogenic properties of aPL and upregulate endothelial nitric oxide synthesis (Ferrara et al., 2003; Laufs et al., 1998). An international committee on the treatment of cardiac APS manifestations recommended warfarin anticoagulation for those who suffered thrombosis in the absence of atherosclerosis. Aspirin prophylaxis did not show to provide additional effect over warfarin alone. Moreover, hydroxychloroquine might be considered, specially in patients with clinical features of SLE, due to its possible antithrombotic effects.

7.3 Nonischemic Ventricular Dysfunction

No study has been published regarding the treatment of nonischemic ventricular manifestations in APS and thus it is difficult to be established if these patients would benefit from any specific treatment (Lockshin et al., 2003). According to international consensus, meanwhile, standard therapeutic approach to hypertension and heart failure due to other etiologies is recommended.

7.4 Intracardiac Thrombus

No data exist regarding the best approach to patients with intracardiac thrombosis in APS. International guidelines recommended long-term anticoagulation for intracardiac thrombosis not related to APS and most authors would suggest this approach in patients with APS (O'Neill, 1995; Albers et al., 2004). However, some authors, and especially those who reported cases with systemic emboli proposed cardiac surgery in order to remove the intracardiac thrombus (Abanador-Kamper et al., 2012). An international committee on cardiac disease in APS recommended intensive warfarin anticoagulation and consultation with cardiac surgery when appropriated (Lockshin et al., 2003).

8. FINAL REMARKS

Cardiac involvement is very common in patients with APS. Whether the aPL are the cause of all the heart complications that have been described or simply accompany more basic underlying immunological disturbances cannot be assessed for most of them. However, serial screening of aPL in patients who develop these complications will help to assess the prevalence and usefulness of these antibodies in cardiac diseases. Until these studies become available, clinicians should consider a search for aPL in those patients with the previously reported cardiac complications in whom no other etiology could be found.

Take Home Messages

- Cardiac involvement is frequent in APS.
- Cardiac manifestations of APS include heart valve disease, ischemic cardiomyopathy, nonischemic myocardial involvement, and intracardiac thrombosis.
- The most frequent cardiac manifestation of APS is heart valve disease.
- Left side valves are more usually affected.
- Valve heart disease is most frequently characterized by mitral valve regurgitation and valve thickening while some patients develop noninfectious vegetations called Libman-Sacks endocarditis.
- Ischemic cardiac disease due to aPL-driven thrombosis or due to accelerated atherosclerosis is the next most frequent cardiac manifestation.
- Nonischemic cardiac disease has been suggested in some studies, although its exact prevalence and clinical significance is not yet clear.
- Several publications have reported cases of intracardiac thrombosis in patients with APS, although their real incidence in these patients is not yet known.

REFERENCES

Abanador-Kamper, N., et al., 2012. Disseminated intracardiac thrombosis: a rare manifestation of antiphospholipid syndrome. Eur. Heart J. Cardiovasc. Imaging 13 (6), 537.

Afek, A., et al., 1999. Increased endothelial cell expression of alpha3beta1 integrin in cardiac valvulopathy in the primary (Hughes) and secondary antiphospholipid syndrome. Lupus 8 (7), 502–507.

Albers, G.W., et al., 2004. Antithrombotic and thrombolytic therapy for ischemic stroke: the Seventh ACCP Conference on Antithrombotic and Thrombolytic Therapy. Chest 126 (3 Suppl.), 483S–512S.

Alexánderson, E., et al., 2008. Myocardial ischaemia in patients with primary APS: a 13N-ammonia PET assessment. Rheumatology (Oxford, England) 47 (6), 894–896.

Ambrosino, P., et al., 2014. Markers of cardiovascular risk in patients with antiphospholipid syndrome: a meta-analysis of literature studies. Ann. Med. 46 (8), 693–702.

Ames, P.R., et al., 2002. Anticardiolipin antibody titre and plasma homocysteine level independently predict intima media thickness of carotid arteries in subjects with idiopathic antiphospholipid antibodies. Lupus 11 (4), 208–214.

Ames, P.R.J., et al., 2009a. Atherosclerosis in thrombotic primary antiphospholipid syndrome. J. Thromb. Haemost. 7 (4), 537–542.

Ames, P.R.J., Margarita, A., Alves, J.D., 2009b. Antiphospholipid antibodies and atherosclerosis: insights from systemic lupus erythematosus and primary antiphospholipid syndrome. Clin. Rev. Allergy Immunol. 37 (1), 29–35.

Amigo, M.C., García-Torres, R., 2000. Morphology of vascular, renal, and heart lesions in the antiphospholipid syndrome: relationship to pathogenesis. Curr. Rheumatol. Rep. 2 (3), 262–270.

Amoroso, A., et al., 2006. The adjunctive role of antiphospholipid antibodies in systemic lupus erythematosus cardiac involvement. Clin. Exp. Rheumatol. 24 (3), 287–294.

Asanuma, Y., et al., 2003. Premature coronary-artery atherosclerosis in systemic lupus erythematosus. N. Engl. J. Med. 349 (25), 2407–2415.

Asherson, R.A., et al., 1988. Diagnostic and therapeutic problems in two patients with antiphospholipid antibodies, heart valve lesions, and transient ischaemic attacks. Ann. Rheum. Dis. 47 (11), 947–953.

Asherson, R.A., et al., 1990. Infective endocarditis, rheumatoid factor, and anticardiolipin antibodies. Ann. Rheum. Dis. 49 (2), 107–108.

Asherson, R.A., Cervera, R., 1991. Antiphospholipid antibodies and the heart. Lessons and pitfalls for the cardiologist. Circulation 84 (2), 920–923.

Badui, E., et al., 1995. The heart in the primary antiphospholipid syndrome. Arch. Med. Res. 26 (2), 115–120.

Barkhausen, J., et al., 2012. Detection and characterization of intracardiac thrombi on MR imaging. Am. J. Roentgenol. 179 (6), 1539–1544.

Barón, M. a, et al., 2005. Prevalence of an abnormal ankle-brachial index in patients with primary antiphospholipid syndrome: preliminary data. Ann. Rheum. Dis. 64 (1), 144–146.

Bhattacharyya, S., et al., 2009. Drug-induced fibrotic valvular heart disease. Lancet (London, England) 374 (9689), 577–585.

Boyd, A.C., Schiller, N.B., Thomas, L., 2015. Principles of transthoracic echocardiographic evaluation. Nat. Rev. Cardiol. 12 (7), 426–440.

Brenner, B., et al., 1991. Cardiac involvement in patients with primary antiphospholipid syndrome. J. Am. Coll. Cardiol. 18 (4), 931–936.

Bucciarelli, S., et al., 2006. Mortality in the catastrophic antiphospholipid syndrome: causes of death and prognostic factors in a series of 250 patients. Arthritis Rheum. 54 (8), 2268–2576.

Cervera, R., et al., 2014. 14th international congress on antiphospholipid antibodies task force report on catastrophic antiphospholipid syndrome. Autoimmun. Rev. 13 (7), 699–707.

Cervera, R., et al., 2002. Antiphospholipid syndrome: clinical and immunologic manifestations and patterns of disease expression in a cohort of 1,000 patients. Arthritis Rheum. 46 (4), 1019–1027.

Cervera, R., et al., 1992. Cardiac disease in systemic lupus erythematosus: prospective study of 70 patients. Ann. Rheum. Dis. 51 (2), 156–159.

Cervera, R., et al., 2009a. Catastrophic antiphospholipid syndrome (CAPS): descriptive analysis of a series of 280 patients from the "CAPS Registry". J. Autoimmun. 32 (3–4), 240–245.

Cervera, R., 2004. Coronary and valvular syndromes and antiphospholipid antibodies. Thromb. Res. 114 (5–6), 501–507.

Cervera, R., et al., 1991. High prevalence of significant heart valve lesions in patients with the "primary" antiphospholipid syndrome. Lupus 1 (1), 43–47.

Cervera, R., et al., 2015. Morbidity and mortality in the antiphospholipid syndrome during a 10-year period: a multicentre prospective study of 1000 patients. Ann. Rheum. Dis. 74 (6), 1011–1018.

Cervera, R., et al., 2009b. Morbidity and mortality in the antiphospholipid syndrome during a 5-year period: a multicentre prospective study of 1000 patients. Ann. Rheum. Dis. 68 (9), 1428–1432.

Cervera, R., et al., 2011a. Task force on catastrophic antiphospholipid syndrome (APS) and non-criteria APS manifestations (I): catastrophic APS, APS nephropathy and heart valve lesions. Lupus 20 (2), 165–173.

Cervera, R., et al., 2011b. Task force on catastrophic antiphospholipid syndrome (APS) and non-criteria APS manifestations (II): thrombocytopenia and skin manifestations. Lupus 20 (2), 174–181.

Cosyns, B., et al., 2013. Drug-induced valvular heart disease. Heart (British Cardiac Society) 99 (1), 7–12.

Coudray, N., et al., 1995. M mode and Doppler echocardiographic assessment of left ventricular diastolic function in primary antiphospholipid syndrome. Br. Heart J. 74 (5), 531–535.

Cuadrado, M.J., Hughes, G.R., 2001. Hughes (antiphospholipid) syndrome. Clinical features. Rheum. Dis. Clin. North Am. 27 (3), 507–524 (v).

Denas, G., et al., 2015. Antiphospholipid syndrome and the heart: a case series and literature review. Autoimmun. Rev. 14 (3), 214–222.

Dursun, M., et al., 2015. The utility of cardiac MRI in diagnosis of infective endocarditis: preliminary results. Diagn. Interv. Radiol. 21, 28–33 (August 2014).

Edoute, Y., et al., 1997. Cardiac valvular vegetations in cancer patients: a prospective echocardiographic study of 200 patients. Am. J. Med. 102 (3), 252–258.

Eikelboom, J.W., Weitz, J.I., 2014. The mTORC pathway in the antiphospholipid syndrome. N. Engl. J. Med. 371 (4), 369–371.

Erdogan, D., et al., 2005. Assessment of cardiac structure and left atrial appendage functions in primary antiphospholipid syndrome: a transesophageal echocardiographic study. Stroke 36 (3), 592–596.

Erkan, D., et al., 2012. A pilot open label phase II trial of rituximab for non-criteria manifestations of antiphospholipid syndrome. Arthritis Rheum. 1–26.

Erkan, D., et al., 2002. The role of cardiac magnetic resonance imaging in antiphospholipid syndrome. J. Rheumatol. 29 (12), 2658–2659.

Espinola-Zavaleta, N., et al., 2006. Myocardial perfusion defects in patients with autoimmune diseases: a prospective study. Analysis of two diagnostic tests. Lupus 15 (1), 38–43.

Espínola-Zavaleta, N., et al., 1999. Echocardiographic evaluation of patients with primary antiphospholipid syndrome. Am. Heart J. 137 (5), 973–978.

Farzaneh-Far, A., et al., 2006. Relationship of antiphospholipid antibodies to cardiovascular manifestations of systemic lupus erythematosus. Arthritis Rheum. 54 (12), 3918–3925.

Ferrara, D.E., et al., 2003. Inhibition of the thrombogenic and inflammatory properties of antiphospholipid antibodies by fluvastatin in an in vivo animal model. Arthritis Rheum. 48 (11), 3272–3279.

Font, C., et al., 2011. Solid cancer, antiphospholipid antibodies, and venous thromboembolism. Autoimmun. Rev. 10 (4), 222–227.

Font, J., et al., 1991. Non-infective verrucous endocarditis in a patient with "primary" antiphospholipid syndrome. Br. J. Rheumatol. 30 (4), 305–307.

Ford, S.E., et al., 1989. Thrombotic endocarditis and lupus anticoagulant. A pathogenetic possibility for idiopathic "rheumatic type" valvular heart disease. Arch. Pathol. Lab. Med. 113 (4), 350–353.

Fournier, P.-E., et al., 2010. Comprehensive diagnostic strategy for blood culture-negative endocarditis: a prospective study of 819 new cases. Clin. Infect. Dis. 51 (2) 131–140.

Gabrielli, F., et al., 1995. Cardiac valve involvement in systemic lupus erythematosus and primary antiphospholipid syndrome: lack of correlation with antiphospholipid antibodies. Int. J. Cardiol. 51 (2), 117–126.

Galve, E., et al., 1992. Valvular heart disease in the primary antiphospholipid syndrome. Ann. Intern. Med. 116 (4), 293–298.

García-Torres, R., et al., 1996. Valvular heart disease in primary antiphospholipid syndrome (PAPS): clinical and morphological findings. Lupus 5 (1), 56–61.

Gaudio, C., et al., 2004. Prominent crista terminalis mimicking a right atrial mixoma: cardiac magnetic resonance aspects. Eur. Rev. Med. Pharmacol. Sci. 8 (4), 165–168.

George, J., et al., 1999. Immunolocalization of beta2-glycoprotein I (apolipoprotein H) to human atherosclerotic plaques: potential implications for lesion progression. Circulation 99 (17), 2227–2230.

Gertner, E., Leatherman, J.W., 1992. Intracardiac mural throm-bus mimicking atrial myxoma in the antiphos- phollpid syndrome. J. Rheumatol. 19 (8), 1293–1298.

Giannakopoulos, B., Krilis, S. a, 2013. The pathogenesis of the antiphospholipid syndrome. N. Engl. J. Med. 368 (11), 1033–1044.

Gleason, C.B., et al., 1993. A comparison of cardiac valvular involvement in the primary antiphospholipid syndrome versus anticardiolipin-negative systemic lupus erythematosus. Am. Heart J. 125 (4), 1123–1129.

Gonzalez, M., Evangelista, A., 2011. Diagnóstico de la endocarditis infecciosa. In: Almirante, B., Tornos, P. (Eds.), Actualizacion en la endocarditis infecciosa. Marge Medica Books, Barcelona, pp. 31–50.

Habib, G., et al., 2009. Guidelines on the prevention, diagnosis, and treatment of infective endocarditis (new version 2009): the task force on the prevention, diagnosis, and treatment of infective endocarditis of the european society of cardiology (ESC). Endorsed by the European. Eur. Heart J. 30 (19), 2369–2413.

Hamsten, A., et al., 1986. Antibodies to cardiolipin in young survivors of myocardial infarction: an association with recurrent cardiovascular events. Lancet (London, England) 1 (8473), 113–116.

Hasnie, A.M.A., et al., 1995. Diastolic dysfunction is a feature of the antiphospholipid syndrome. Am. Heart J. 129 (5), 1009–1013.

Hollan, I., et al., 2013. Cardiovascular disease in autoimmune rheumatic diseases. Autoimmun. Rev. 12 (10), 1004–1015.

Hur, J., et al., 2013. Dual-enhancement cardiac computed tomography for assessing left atrial thrombus and pulmonary veins before radiofrequency catheter ablation for atrial fibrillation. Am. J. Cardiol. 112 (2), 238–244.

Jouhikainen, T., Pohjola-Sintonen, S., Stephansson, E., 1994. Lupus anticoagulant and cardiac manifestations in systemic lupus erythematosus. Lupus 3 (3), 167–172.

Kampolis, C., et al., 2014. Evolution of cardiac dysfunction in patients with antiphospholipid antibodies and/or antiphospholipid syndrome: a 10-year follow-up study. Semin. Arthritis Rheum. 43 (4), 558–565.

Khamashta, M.A., et al., 1990. Association of antibodies against phospholipids with heart valve disease in systemic lupus erythematosus. Lancet 335 (8705), 1541–1544.

Krause, I., et al., 2005. Close association between valvar heart disease and central nervous system manifestations in the antiphospholipid syndrome. Ann. Rheum. Dis. 64 (10), 1490–1493.

Kupferwasser, L.I., et al., 1999. The presence of infection-related antiphospholipid antibodies in infective endocarditis determines a major risk factor for embolic events. J. Am. Coll. Cardiol. 33 (5), 1365–1371.

Lang, R.M., et al., 2015. Recommendations for cardiac chamber quantification by echocardiography in adults: an update from the American Society of Echocardiography and the European Association of Cardiovascular Imaging. Eur. Heart J. Cardiovasc. Imaging 16 (3), 233–270.

Laufs, U., et al., 1998. Upregulation of endothelial nitric oxide synthase by HMG CoA reductase inhibitors. Circulation 97 (12), 1129–1135.

Lauwerys, B.R., et al., 2001. Myocardial microangiopathy associated with antiphospholipid antibodies. Lupus 10 (2), 123–125.

Leszczyński, P., et al., 2003. Cardiac valvular disease in patients with systemic lupus erythematosus. Relationship with anticardiolipin antibodies. Clin. Rheumatol. 22 (6), 405–408.

Leung, W.H., et al., 1990. Association between antiphospholipid antibodies and cardiac abnormalities in patients with systemic lupus erythematosus. Am. J. Med. 89 (4), 411–419.

Levine, J.S., Branch, D.W., Rauch, J., 2002. The antiphospholipid syndrome. N. Engl. J. Med. 346 (10), 752–763.

Libman, E., Sacks, B., 1924. A hitherto undescribed form of valvular and mural endocarditis. Arch. Intern. Med. 33 (6), 701.

Lockshin, M., et al., 2003. Cardiac disease in the antiphospholipid syndrome: recommendations for treatment. Committee consensus report. Lupus 12 (7), 518–523.

Manning, W.J., 1995. Accuracy of transesophageal echocardiography for identifying left atrial thrombi: a prospective, intraoperative study. Ann. Intern. Med. 123 (11), 817.

Maragiannis, D., Nagueh, S.F., 2015. Echocardiographic evaluation of left ventricular diastolic function: an update. Curr. Cardiol. Rep. 17 (2), 3.

Matsuura, E., Koike, T., 2000. Accelerated atheroma and anti-beta2-glycoprotein I antibodies. Lupus 9, 210–216.

Meroni, P.L., et al., 2011. Pathogenesis of antiphospholipid syndrome: understanding the antibodies. Nat. Rev. Rheumatol. 7 (6), 330–339.

Miyakis, S., et al., 2006. International consensus statement on an update of the classification criteria for definite antiphospholipid syndrome (APS). J. Thromb. Haemost. 4 (2), 295–306.

Mottram, P.M., Gelman, J.S., 2002. Mitral valve thrombus mimicking a primary tumor in the antiphospholipid syndrome. J. Am. Soc. Echocardiogr. 15 (7), 746–748.

Moyssakis, I., et al., 2007. Libman-Sacks endocarditis in systemic lupus erythematosus: prevalence, associations, and evolution. Am. J. Med. 120 (7), 636–642.

Nesher, G., et al., 1997. Valvular dysfunction in antiphospholipid syndrome: prevalence, clinical features, and treatment. Semin. Arthritis Rheum. 27 (1), 27–35.

Nihoyannopoulos, P., et al., 1990. Cardiac abnormalities in systemic lupus erythematosus. Association with raised anticardiolipin antibodies. Circulation 82 (2), 369–375.

O'Neill, D., 1995. Dissolution of intracardiac mass lesions in the primary antiphospholipid antibody syndrome. Arch. Intern. Med. 155 (3), 325.

Ortega-Hernandez, O.-D., et al., 2009. The physiopathology of the catastrophic antiphospholipid (Asherson's) syndrome: compelling evidence. J. Autoimmun. 32 (1), 1–6.

Paran, D., et al., 2007. Cardiac dysfunction in patients with systemic lupus erythematosus and antiphospholipid syndrome. Ann. Rheum. Dis. 66 (4), 506–510.
Pardos-Gea, J., et al., 2013. Cardiac manifestations other than valvulopathy in antiphospholipid syndrome: long-time echocardiography follow-up study. Int. J. Rheum. Dis. 76–83.
Pardos-Gea, J., et al., 2010. Echocardiography at diagnosis of antiphospholipid syndrome provides prognostic information on valvular disease evolution and identifies two subtypes of patients. Lupus 19 (5), 575–582.
Pasupathy, S., et al., 2015. Systematic review of patients presenting with suspected myocardial infarction and nonobstructive coronary arteries. Circulation 131 (10), 861–870.
Patel, R., et al., 2016. Diagnostic performance of cardiac magnetic resonance imaging and echocardiography in evaluation of cardiac and paracardiac masses. Am. J. Cardiol. 117 (1), 135–140.
Perez-Villa, F., et al., 2005. Severe valvular regurgitation and antiphospholipid antibodies in systemic lupus erythematosus: a prospective, long-term, followup study. Arthritis Rheum. 53 (3), 460–467.
Petri, M., 2000. Detection of coronary artery disease and the role of traditional risk factors in the Hopkins Lupus Cohort. Lupus 9 (3), 170–175.
Petri, M., 2004. The lupus anticoagulant is a risk factor for myocardial infarction (but not atherosclerosis): Hopkins Lupus Cohort. Thromb. Res. 114 (5–6), 593–595.
Pierangeli, S.S., et al., 2007. Toll-like receptor and antiphospholipid mediated thrombosis: in vivo studies. Ann. Rheum. Dis. 66 (10), 1327–1333.
Poulton, K., Rahman, A., Giles, I., 2012. Examining how antiphospholipid antibodies activate intracellular signaling pathways: a systematic review. Semin. Arthritis Rheum. 41 (5), 720–736.
Raschi, E., et al., 2008. Toll-like receptors: another player in the pathogenesis of the anti-phospholipid syndrome. Lupus 17 (10), 937–942.
Reddy, S.T., et al., 2013. Evaluation of cardiac valvular regurgitant lesions by cardiac MRI sequences: comparison of a four-valve semi-quantitative versus quantitative approach. J. Heart Valve Dis. 22 (4), 491–499.
Reményi, B., et al., 2012. World Heart Federation criteria for echocardiographic diagnosis of rheumatic heart disease—an evidence-based guideline. Nat. Rev. Cardiol. 9 (5), 297–309.
Rodríguez-Pintó, I., Espinosa, G., Cervera, R., 2015. Catastrophic APS in the context of other thrombotic microangiopathies. Curr. Rheumatol. Rep. 17 (1), 482.
Roffi, M., et al., 2015. 2015 Esc guidelines for the management of acute coronary syndromes in patients presenting without persistent ST-segment elevation. Revista española de cardiologia (English ed.) 68 (12), 1125.
Roldan, C. A, et al., 2008. Transthoracic versus transesophageal echocardiography for detection of Libman-Sacks endocarditis: a randomized controlled study. J. Rheumatol. 35 (2), 224–229.
Roldan, C.A., et al., 2015. Libman-sacks endocarditis: detection, characterization, and clinical correlates by three-dimensional transesophageal echocardiography. J. Am. Soc. Echocardiogr. 28 (7), 770–779.
Roldan, C.A., et al., 1992. Systemic lupus erythematosus valve disease by transesophageal echocardiography and the role of antiphospholipid antibodies. J. Am. Coll. Cardiol. 20 (5), 1127–1134.
Roldan, C.A., et al., 2005. Valvular heart disease as a cause of cerebrovascular disease in patients with systemic lupus erythematosus. Am. J. Cardiol. 95 (12), 1441–1447.
Roldan, C.A., et al., 2007. Valvular heart disease by transthoracic echocardiography is associated with focal brain injury and central neuropsychiatric systemic lupus erythematosus. Cardiology 108 (4), 331–337.

Roman, M.J., et al., 2003. Prevalence and correlates of accelerated atherosclerosis in systemic lupus erythematosus. N. Engl. J. Med. 349 (25), 2399–2406.

Roman, M.J., et al., 2001. Prevalence and relation to risk factors of carotid atherosclerosis and left ventricular hypertrophy in systemic lupus erythematosus and antiphospholipid antibody syndrome. Am. J. Cardiol. 87 (5), 663–666.

Sacré, K., et al., 2010. Asymptomatic myocardial ischemic disease in antiphospholipid syndrome: a controlled cardiac magnetic resonance imaging study. Arthritis Rheum. 62 (7), 2093–2100.

Shapiro, R.F., et al., 1977. Immunopathogenesis of Libman-Sacks endocarditis. Assessment by light and immunofluorescent microscopy in two patients. Ann. Rheum. Dis. 36 (6), 508–516.

Shoenfeld, Y., Meroni, P.L., Toubi, E., 2009. Antiphospholipid syndrome and systemic lupus erythematosus: are they separate entities or just clinical presentations on the same scale? Curr. Opin. Rheumatol. 21 (5), 495–500.

Shrestha, N.K., et al., 1983. Two-dimensional echocardiographic diagnosis of left-atrial thrombus in rheumatic heart disease. A clinicopathologic study. Circulation 67 (2), 341–347.

Sletnes, K.E.E., et al., 1992. Antiphospholipid antibodies after myocardial infarction and their relation to mortality, reinfarction, and non-haemorrhagic stroke. Lancet (London, England) 339 (8791), 451–453.

Srichai, M.B., et al., 2006. Clinical, imaging, and pathological characteristics of left ventricular thrombus: a comparison of contrast-enhanced magnetic resonance imaging, transthoracic echocardiography, and transesophageal echocardiography with surgical or pathological validation. Am. Heart J. 152 (1), 75–84.

Task Force Members, et al., 2013. 2013 ESC guidelines on the management of stable coronary artery disease: the Task Force on the management of stable coronary artery disease of the European Society of Cardiology. Eur. Heart J. 34 (38), 2949–3003.

Tektonidou, M.G., et al., 2001. Right ventricular diastolic dysfunction in patients with anticardiolipin antibodies and antiphospholipid syndrome. Ann. Rheum. Dis. 60 (1), 43–48.

Turiel, M., et al., 2000. Evaluation of cardiac abnormalities and embolic sources in primary antiphospholipid syndrome by transesophageal echocardiography. Lupus 9 (6), 406–412.

Turiel, M., et al., 2005. Five-year follow-up by transesophageal echocardiographic studies in primary antiphospholipid syndrome. Am. J. Cardiol. 96 (4), 574–579.

Vaideeswar, P., Divate, S., Harke, M., 2012. Intracardiac thrombi in extracardiac disorders: an autopsy study. Cardiovasc. Pathol. 21 (2), e1–9.

Vianna, J.L., et al., 1994. Comparison of the primary and secondary antiphospholipid syndrome: a European Multicenter Study of 114 patients. Am. J. Med. 96 (1), 3–9.

Weiss, S., et al., 2008. Antiphospholipid syndrome: intraoperative and postoperative anticoagulation in cardiac surgery. J. Cardiothorac. Vasc. Anesth. 22 (5), 735–739.

Xie, H., et al., 2014. The role of TLR4 in pathophysiology of antiphospholipid syndrome-associated thrombosis and pregnancy morbidity. Br. J. Haematol. 164 (2), 165–176.

Zavaleta, N.E., et al., 2004. Primary antiphospholipid syndrome: a 5-year transesophageal echocardiographic followup study. J. Rheumatol. 31 (12), 2402–2407.

Ziporen, L., et al., 1996. Libman-Sacks endocarditis in the antiphospholipid syndrome: immunopathologic findings in deformed heart valves. Lupus 5 (3), 196–205.

Zuily, S., et al., 2011. Increased risk for heart valve disease associated with antiphospholipid antibodies in patients with systemic lupus erythematosus: meta-analysis of echocardiographic studies. Circulation 124 (2), 215–224.

Chapter 13

Cardiac Involvement in Scleroderma

J.G. Coghlan* and C.P. Denton[§]
*Royal Free Hospital, London, United Kingdom; [§]Royal Free and University College Medical School, London, United Kingdom

1. INTRODUCTION

Cardiac involvement in scleroderma (systemic sclerosis; SSc) may present as primary cardiac involvement (small vessel ischemia, inflammation, or replacement fibrosis) or secondary involvement (due to pulmonary hypertension, coronary disease, or systemic hypertension). Primary cardiac involvement may lead to systolic dysfunction, and/or diastolic dysfunction, pericardial disease, conduction abnormalities (including brady- and tachyarrhythmias), and less commonly valvular disease. Autopsy studies and cardiac MRI studies have shown that subclinical cardiac involvement is extremely common.

Modalities such as tissue Doppler echocardiography and cardiac MRI have proven more sensitive in detecting cardiac involvement than standard Doppler echocardiography. Screening for Cardiac disease is often undertaken as part of the pulmonary hypertension screening package that includes a yearly echocardiography, B-type natriuretic peptide (BNP) or N-terminal proBNP, serum urate, and an ECG.

In this updated chapter we focus on some areas where new data have emerged. We have clearer data on the prevalence and contribution to outcome of cardiac involvement, and a somewhat better understanding of the role of coronary disease. Initial CMR data showing that diffuse patchy fibrosis is common, though conflicting data on the cause of this. Data are also accumulating to suggest that ventricular tachyarrhythmia may be an important treatable cause of mortality in patients with primary cardiac involvement.

The absence of a disease-specific evidence base for the management of cardiac involvement remains an issue, thus management should be in accordance with standard cardiology guideline recommendations, for example, ACE inhibitors and cautious use of beta blockers for systolic dysfunction.

2. EVIDENCE FOR AND PROGNOSTIC IMPACT OF CLINICAL CARDIAC INVOLVEMENT

Large older registry studies provided clear evidence of the poor prognosis associated with scleroderma and identified cardiac abnormalities as a major adverse factor (Ruangjutipopan et al., 2002; Steen and Medsger, 2000; Abbott et al., 2002; Bulpitt et al., 1993; Follansbee et al., 1993; Lee et al., 1992). More recent registries suggest that the prognosis associated with scleroderma may be much more benign (Vlachoyiannopoulos et al., 2000; Nishioka et al., 1996) and not predicted by cardiac abnormalities noted at study entry. This suggests that either the initial registries were excessively pessimistic or that the outcome has improved. In any event it led to some confusion as to the role of cardiac disease in predicting outcome. However, more recent data with more contemporary methodology have confirmed a significant prognostic impact of clinical cardiac involvement, though the prevalence may be lower than previously thought.

A recent all-comer incident case registry (Nihtyanova et al., 2014) included 398 consecutives that were followed-up for up to 15 years. Cardiac involvement was defined as pericardial effusion, hemodynamically significant cardiac arrhythmias, or heart failure requiring specific treatment. In this study the incidence of clinically important cardiac complications was found to be higher in patients with diffuse cutaneous SSc (dcSSc) than those with limited cutaneous SSc (lcSSc) especially early in the disease course (prevalence at 5 years: 7% dSSc versus 1% lSSc). No new cases of cardiac SSc among dcSSc patients were observed after 5 years of follow-up; however, new cardiac involvement continued to emerge during follow-up in the lSSc cohort. Importantly, in that study cardiac SSc was associated with a five-fold increase in hazard ratio for mortality (HR = 5.436; CI: 2.396−12.332; $p < 0.001$) compared to SSc patients without cardiac involvement. These findings are supported by a previous meta-analysis of 578 deaths from registry data (Ioannidis et al., 2005) involving seven different centers that showed a significant increase in cardiovascular mortality in patients with clinically evident cardiac involvement (HR = 2.8; 95% CI: 2.1−3.8).

3. PREVALENCE OF SUBCLINICAL CARDIAC INVOLVEMENT

Autopsy data (D'Angelo et al., 1969; Buckley et al., 1976; Murata et al., 1998; Follansbee et al., 1990; Fernandes et al., 2003) have consistently shown widespread patchy myocardial fibrosis in patients with SSc with or without clear prior known cardiac involvement. These data are now supported by the frequent finding of fibrosis on cardiac biopsy, late gadolinium enhancement on CMR, and recent data on expansion of extracellular myocardial volume using tissue phase CMR mapping (Ntusi et al., 2014).

Diastolic dysfunction has historically been found in 50–80% of patients in association with scleroderma, whether studied using echocardiography (Plazak et al., 2002; Candell-Riera et al., 1996; Di Bello et al., 1999; Armstrong et al., 1996) or nuclear medicine (Nakajima et al., 2001). More recent studies using more reliable parameters such as EE′ suggest a lower rate of diastolic dysfunction (de Groote et al., 2008) or abnormal trends (Cadeddu et al., 2015; D'Alto et al., 2014) that worsen over time (Faludi et al., 2014). No clear association with outcome has been defined, though it has been suggested that the observed diastolic abnormalities are likely a result of intermittent vasospastic ischemia, and therapy directed at relieving ischemia may improve parameters of diastolic dysfunction in patients with scleroderma.

Nuclear studies using older techniques suggest a high prevalence of perfusion defects (Alexander et al., 1986; Morelli et al., 1997; Lekakis et al., 1998); abnormalities whether fixed or reversible perfusion defects have been found in 50–100% of patients with scleroderma. Other studies fail to confirm these findings (Nakajima et al., 2001) or suggest that only minor abnormalities can be found (Ishida et al., 2000).

Troponin is markedly sensitive in active myocarditis and in advanced heart failure. Combined elevation of BNP and troponin has been reported to be highly specific for cardiac involvement as indicated by an elevated E/E′ ratio, but with a low prevalence (Avouac et al., 2015).

4. ISCHEMIC HEART DISEASE

One of the most widely accepted hypotheses is that ischemic damage underlies much of the cardiac pathology found in scleroderma. Recent systematic reviews appear to confirm a significant increase in the prevalence of coronary atherosclerotic disease based on autopsy, CT coronary angiography, and coronary angiography (Ali et al., 2015) or clinical diagnosis (Ali et al., 2015; Ungprasert et al., 2014).

However, most data in the literature focus on possible microvascular ischemia. Histology shows replacement fibrosis and contraction band necrosis (Follansbee et al., 1993; Bulkley et al., 1978, 1976), which in other situations is associated with ischemic injury (Follansbee et al., 1985). The histological evidence for myocardial ischemia are much more problematic showing either normal intramyocardial vessels (Bulkley et al., 1976) or occasional mild intimal or medial thickening (Follansbee et al., 1985). The presence of an excess of focal fibrosis has nevertheless been proposed as evidence of an ischemic pathogenesis (Follansbee et al., 1990) even though in this study the hallmark abnormality of contraction band necrosis was not found to be more prevalent in the hearts of patients with scleroderma when compared to controls. More recent methodology including cell typing raises the possibility that a low-grade inflammation is the actual driver (Liangos et al., 2000). Histological features which are not readily explained by ischemic injury are also frequent—fibrinous pericarditis, subvalvular thickening (Bulkley et al., 1976; Follansbee et al., 1990).

ECG abnormalities, in particular septal q waves, are advanced as further evidence of ischemic damage (Follansbee et al., 1985). ECG abnormalities in scleroderma range from loss of R waves particularly in the septal leads to right or left ventricular hypertrophy, nonspecific ST-T changes, and p-wave notching (Lubitz et al., 2008). Increased QT dispersion and decreased heart rate variability have also been reported (Wozniak et al., 2009). Conduction disturbances in SSc are often caused by conduction tissue fibrosis (Femenía et al., 2010). Septal "r" waves require functioning septal conduction tissue and are thus absent in left bundle branch block without infarction (Josephson, 1993); a possible alternate explanation thus is conducting tissue fibrosis rather than infarction. However, one then has the issue of whether microvascular ischemia is responsible for the conducting tissue fibrosis.

Several publications using thallium scintigraphy have found an increased prevalence of resting (Morelli et al., 1997), exercise-induced (Steen et al., 1996) or cold pressor–induced (Alexander et al., 1986; Lekakis et al., 1998) perfusion defects in patients with scleroderma, and these have in some cases been associated with an adverse prognosis (Candell-Riera et al., 1996). Further, with the development of more specific techniques such as technetium scanning, stress echocardiography, and stress MUGA scanning, these inducible perfusion defects have not been persistent (Nakajima et al., 2001; Ishida et al., 2000).

The results of the studies examining coronary sinus blood flow invasively are contradictory with one showing impaired vasodilator reserve (Nitenberg et al., 1986) and another showing the absence of vasospasm in response to cold pressor testing (Colfer et al., 1993). However, using a noninvasive technique, Vacca et al. (2013) recently documented impaired vasodilator reserve in 46% of 41 patients with SSc, further the presence of abnormal coronary reserve was associated with a worse prognosis.

Three potential mechanisms of ischemic damage have been proposed: coronary arterial vasospasm, small vessel disease, and occlusive coronary disease. The theoretical basis for assuming an excess of macrovascular coronary disease is derived from the observed endothelial dysfunction and fibroproliferative tendency, which have been proposed as the pathobiological model of scleroderma (Kissin and Korn, 2002), and reports of an excess of lower limb macrovascular disease in the scleroderma population. Recent studies have also identified altered large blood vessel elasticity as a general feature of scleroderma (Cheng et al., 2003a,b). Vascular lesions in the skin, kidney, and lungs of patients with scleroderma show consistent features, with medial hypertrophy followed by luminal occlusion (Taylor et al., 2002). TGFB1 overexpression has been found, with evidence of upregulation of CTGF and PDGF (Schachna and Wigley, 2002). Downstream endothelin levels and adrenaline levels have also been shown to increase. These changes are thought to drive the smooth muscle and fibromuscular hypertrophy observed. Histology of the coronaries have not shown any excess of fibromuscular hypertrophy to date (Follansbee et al., 1993, 1990; Bulkley et al., 1976, 1978).

There is evidence of abnormal thickening of the large vessels in the leg (Veale et al., 1995; Youssef et al., 1993) and carotid (Cheng et al., 2003b; Ho et al., 2000), yet to date there have been no publications showing an excess of large vessel coronary disease either angiographically or on post-mortem studies. Whether or not macrovascular coronary disease is more common in patients with scleroderma is clinically significant, as this may provide a treatable cause of cardiac dysfunction. In the absence of evidence for macrovascular disease or significant pathology of the small vessels of the myocardium, vasospasm has been promoted as the cause of the observed myocardial damage (Steen et al., 1996). Unfortunately, 30 years after cardiac Raynaud was first proposed (Gupta et al., 1975) as the unifying cause of myocardial ischemia in scleroderma, clear confirmation that this exists as a clinically important entity is lacking.

5. MYOCARDITIS

Myositis is well known to occur in scleroderma evidenced by histological findings and electromyography. Follansbee et al. (1993) have shown an association between cardiac mortality and myositis raising the possibility that associated myocarditis is occurring in these patients. Myocarditis may well explain the frequent occurrence of exudative pericardial effusions, and could explain the endocardial lesions found on histology. The ECG evidence of conducting tissue damage could readily be the consequence of an autoimmune inflammatory process. At present, there are few published data suggesting that widespread low-grade myocarditis occurs in this population leading to diastolic dysfunction and the other cardiac abnormalities seen. We have observed an excess of troponin T release from patients with scleroderma (Mukerjee et al., 2003), and noted a weak association with outcome at 5 years. A recent CMR study supports the concept of widespread low-grade myocardial inflammation with abnormalities of tissue phase mapping likely to represent a response to a diffuse inflammatory process found in 53% of 19 patients with scleroderma and none of the controls (Ntusi et al., 2014). Mavrogeni et al. (2015) by contrast found that tissue phase mapping abnormalities were uncommon but that reduced perfusion during stress was present in almost all patients, with most patients that underwent follow up scanning developing subendocardial scar. Thus the precise picture remains confused.

6. HYPERTENSION

Surprisingly little has been published about the impact of systemic and pulmonary hypertension on the heart given the prevalence of these conditions. Renal impairment is one of the acknowledged predictors of poor prognosis in patients with scleroderma, and this effect is aggravated by evidence of cardiac involvement, unsurprisingly therefore a recent analysis by Al-Dhaher et al. (2010) has identified the presence of systemic hypertension as an independent predictor of mortality in a cohort of patients with SSc.

Pulmonary hypertension has been suggested as occurring in up to 50% of patients with scleroderma, though a prevalence of 12% is probably closer to the mark (Mukerjee et al., 2003). Recent registry data have suggested a prevalence closer to 5%; however, this must be balanced against the finding of pulmonary hypertension in 30% of patients enrolled in a screening study where the definitive diagnostic test of cardiac catheterization was performed in over 400 patients (Coghlan et al., 2014).

In patients with scleroderma, pulmonary hypertension carries a particularly adverse prognosis; however, death is still primarily cardiac (Mukerjee et al., 2003). The fact that an adverse outcome relative to primary pulmonary hypertension is seen at relatively low pressures suggests that there is, in patients with scleroderma, an additional cardiac impairment, which compromises cardiac adaptation to afterload. This has been recently confirmed (Hsu et al., 2016) in a study comparing the response of the right ventricle to low-intensity exercise in nine patients with idiopathic pulmonary hypertension to 15 patients with scleroderma-associated pulmonary arterial hypertension (PAH). Though afterload rose similarly in both populations right ventricular contractility only increased in those with idiopathic PAH, whereas in those with scleroderma the right ventricle simply dilated to maintain cardiac output. These data strongly suggest an intrinsic abnormality of cardiac function in patients with scleroderma leading to poorer tolerance of increased workload.

7. ARRHYTHMIAS

A number of recent case series have raised the prospect that malignant ventricular arrhythmias may be much more common in SSc than previously recognized. The first series related to implantable cardioverter defibrillator (ICD) implantation in 10 patients who had a high burden of ventricular ectopics (>1000/24 h) or nonsustained ventricular tachycardia (Bernardo et al., 2011). During three years of follow-up, three individuals had appropriate device discharge.

In a second series of 25 patients who had undergone cardiac biopsy to evaluate noninvasively determined cardiac involvement, 12 received ICD for primary prevention. Four of the 25 died of cardiovascular causes, including three with sudden death (one of whom had VT documented immediately prior to death). The fourth had an ICD in place and died with VT/VF unresponsive to device therapy. Three others had appropriate successful device therapy for VT/VF. Thus in total seven patients had probable or proven ventricular arrhythmias (Mueller et al., 2015).

The third report concerns six patients with device implantation as primary prevention prior to autologous stem cell transplantation (aSCT) of whom half (three) had appropriate device therapy during or after aSCT (Chung et al., 2012). Only two of these patients are reported as having an abnormal echo (either an ejection fraction of <50% or pericardial effusion).

A fourth case series (De Luca et al., 2016) describes 100 patients with cardiac involvement as evidenced by symptoms or raised cardiac enzymes.

Evaluation included 24-h monitoring, echocardiography, and catheterization where recommended by the DETECT protocol. More than 1000 ventricular ectopics (VE)/24 h was identified in 24 patients. The number of VEs correlated positively with troponin levels and inversely with left ventricular ejection fraction. Seven patients either died suddenly (5) or required ICD (2); the presence of >1190 VE/24 h had a sensitivity of 100% and specificity of 82% for these events.

8. THE FUTURE

After more than half a century of contradictory information, we now have the tools to adequately characterize the subtler forms of cardiac involvement present in SSc. With widespread use of troponin testing, CMR scanning, CT coronary angiography, and implantable monitors it should be possible to determine the precise prevalence and prognostic significance of the various manifestations of cardiac involvement and we have reasonable therapeutic options available. Standardized and widespread use of such techniques will shed light on the natural history associated with these cardiac abnormalities, however, will not immediately uncover the pathobiological mechanisms underlying such abnormalities. If one accepts that this is an autoimmune condition, then it is unlikely that a purely vascular explanation will suffice; we shall need to explore the nature of the process in a more sophisticated manner. We need to identify patients with active cardiac involvement, analyze vasoreactivity invasively, and obtain myocardial biopsies for study using modern immunofluorescent techniques. Only through studying such patients invasively can the basic disease mechanisms underlying cardiac scleroderma be unequivocally elucidated.

REFERENCES

Abbott, K.C., Trespalacios, F.C., Welch, P.G., Agodoa, L.Y., 2002. Scleroderma at end stage renal disease in the United States: patient characteristics and survival. J. Nephrol. 15, 236.

Al-Dhaher, F.F., Pope, J.E., Ouimet, J.M., 2010. Determinants of morbidity and mortality in systemic sclerosis in Canada. Semin. Arthritis Rheum. 39, 269.

Alexander, E.L., Firestein, G.S., Weiss, J.L., Heuser, R.R., Leitl, G. Wagner Jr., H.N., Brinker, J.A., Ciuffo, A.A., Becker, L.C., 1986. Reversible cold-induced abnormalities in myocardial perfusion and function in systemic sclerosis. Ann. Intern. Med. 105, 661.

Ali, H., Kiat, R., Low, A., 2015. A qualitative systematic review of the prevalence of coronary artery disease in systemic sclerosis. Int. J. Rheum. Dis. 18, 276.

Armstrong, G.P., Whalley, G.A., Doughty, R.N., Gamble, G.D., Flett, S.M., Tan, P.L., Sharpe, D.N., 1996. Left ventricular function in scleroderma. Br. J. Rheumatol. 35, 983.

Avouac, J., Meune, C., Chenevier-Gobeaux, C., Borderie, D., Lefevre, G., Kahan, A., Allanore, Y., 2015. Cardiac biomarkers in systemic sclerosis: contribution of high-sensitivity cardiac troponin in addition to N-terminal pro-brain natriuretic peptide. Arthritis Care Res. (Hoboken) 67, 1022.

Bernardo, P., Conforti, M.L., Bellando-Randone, S., Pieragnoli, P., Blagojevic, J., Kaloudi, O., et al., 2011. Implantable cardioverter defibrillator prevents sudden cardiac death in systemic sclerosis. J. Rheumatol. 38, 1617.

Bulkley, B.H., Ridolfi, R.L., Salyer, W.R., Hutchins, G.M., 1976. Myocardial lesions of progressive systemic sclerosis. A cause of cardiac dysfunction. Circulation 53, 483.

Bulkley, B.H., Klacsmann, P.G., Hutchins, G.M., 1978. Angina pectoris, myocardial infarction and sudden cardiac death with normal coronary arteries: a clinicopathologic study of 9 patients with progressive systemic sclerosis. Am. Heart J. 95, 563. An Early Series Recognizing That Cardiac Involvement Was an Important Cause of Death in Systemic Sclerosis but Was not Always Associated With Structural Pathology.

Bulpitt, K.J., Clements, P.J., Lachenbruch, P.A., Paulus, H.E., Peter, J.B., Agopian, M.S., Singer, J.Z., Steen, V.D., Clegg, D.O., Ziminski, C.M., 1993. Early undifferentiated connective tissue disease: III. Outcome and prognostic indicators in early scleroderma (systemic sclerosis). Ann. Intern. Med. 118, 602.

Cadeddu, C., Deidda, M., Giau, G., Lilliu, M., Cadeddu, F., Binaghi, G., Mura, M.N., Farci, M., Del Giacco, S., Manconi, P.E., Mercuro, G., 2015. Contractile reserve in systemic sclerosis patients as a major predictor of global cardiac impairment and exercise tolerance. Int. J. Cardiovasc. Imaging 31, 529.

Candell-Riera, J., Armadans-Gil, L., Simeon, C.P., Castell-Conesa, J., Fonollosa-Pla, V., Garcia-del-Castillo, H., Vaque-Rafart, J., Vilardell, M., Soler-Soler, J., 1996. Comprehensive noninvasive assessment of cardiac involvement in limited systemic sclerosis. Arthritis Rheum. 39, 1138.

Cheng, K.S., Tiwari, A., Boutin, A., Denton, C.P., Black, C.M., Morris, R., Seifalian, A.M., Hamilton, G., 2003a. Differentiation of primary and secondary Raynaud's disease by carotid arterial stiffness. Eur. J. Vasc. Endovasc. Surg. 25, 336.

Cheng, K.S., Tiwari, A., Boutin, A., Denton, C.P., Black, C.M., Morris, R., Hamilton, G., Seifalian, A.M., 2003b. Carotid and femoral arterial wall mechanics in scleroderma. Rheumatology 42, 1299.

Chung, H.H., Kim, J.B., Hong, S.H., Lee, H.J., Joung, B., Lee, M.H., 2012. Radiofrequency catheter ablation of hemodynamically unstable ventricular tachycardia associated with systemic sclerosis. J. Korean Med. Sci. 27, 215.

Coghlan, J.G., Denton, C.P., Grünig, E., et al., 2014. Evidence-based detection of pulmonary arterial hypertension in systemic sclerosis: the DETECT study. Ann. Rheum. Dis. 73, 1340.

Colfer, H.T., Das, S.K., Dabich, L., Randall, O.S., Pitt, B., 1993. Effect of cold stress on coronary sinus blood flow in patients with scleroderma. J. Assoc. Acad. Minor. Phys. 4, 62.

D'Alto, M., Cuomo, G., Romeo, E., Argiento, P., Iudici, M., Vettori, S., Giovanna Russo, M., Calabrò, R., Valentini, G., 2014. Tissue Doppler imaging in systemic sclerosis: a 3-year longitudinal study. Semin. Arthritis Rheum. 43, 673.

D'Angelo, W.A., Fries, J.F., Masi, A.T., Shulman, L.E., 1969. Pathologic observations in systemic sclerosis (scleroderma). A study of fifty-eight autopsy cases and fifty-eight matched controls. Am J. Med. 46, pp 428.

Di Bello, V., Ferri, C., Giorgi, D., Bianchi, M., Bertini, A., Martini, A., Storino, F.A., Paterni, M., Pasero, G., Giusti, C., 1999. Ultrasonic videodensitometric analysis in scleroderma heart disease. Coron. Artery Dis. 10, 103.

de Groote, P., Gressin, V., Hachulla, E., Carpentier, P., Guillevin, L., Kahan, A., Cabane, J., Francès, C., Lamblin, N., Diot, E., Patat, F., Sibilia, J., Petit, H., Cracowski, J.L., Clerson, P., Humbert, M., 2008. ItinerAIR-Scleroderma Investigators. Evaluation of cardiac abnormalities by Doppler echocardiography in a large nationwide multicentric cohort of patients with systemic sclerosis. Ann. Rheum. Dis. 31.

De Luca, G., Bosello, S., Leone, A.M., Gabrielli, F., Pelargonio, G., Inzani, F., Crea, F., Ferraccioli, G., 2016. Life-threatening arrhythmias in a scleroderma patient: the role of myocardial inflammation in arrhythmic outburst. Scand. J. Rheumatol. 21, 1.

Faludi, R., Költő, G., Bartos, B., Csima, G., Czirják, L., Komócsi, A., 2014. Five-year follow-up of left ventricular diastolic function in systemic sclerosis patients: determinants of mortality and disease progression. Semin. Arthritis Rheum. 44, 220.

Femenía, F., Arce, M., Arrieta, M., 2010. [Systemic sclerosis complicated with syncope and complete AV block]. Medicina (B Aires) 70, 442.

Fernandes, F., Ramires, F.J., Arteaga, E., Ianni, B.M., Bonfá, E.S., Mady, C., 2003. Cardiac remodeling in patients with systemic sclerosis with no signs or symptoms of heart failure: an endomyocardial biopsy study. J. Card Fail. 9, 311.

Follansbee, W.P., Curtiss, E.I., Rahko, P.S., Medsger Jr., T.A., Lavine, S.J., Owens, G.R., Steen, V.D., 1985. The electrocardiogram in systemic sclerosis (scleroderma). Study of 102 consecutive cases with functional correlations and review of the literature. Am. J. Med. 79, 183.

Follansbee, W.P., Miller, T.R., Curtiss, E.I., Orie, J.E., Bernstein, R.L., Kiernan, J.M., Medsger Jr., T.A., 1990. A controlled clinicopathologic study of myocardial fibrosis in systemic sclerosis (scleroderma). J. Rheumatol. 17, 656. Seminal Paper Describing Cardiac Involvement With Fibrosis in Systemic Sclerosis That Establishes a Substantial Prevalence of Subclinical Disease.

Follansbee, W., Zerbe, T., Medsger, T., 1993. Cardiac and skeletal muscle disease in systemic sclerosis (scleroderma): a high risk association. Am. Heart J. 125, 194.

Gupta, M.P., Zoneraich, S., Zeitlin, W., Zoneraich, O., D'Angelo, W., 1975. Scleroderma heart disease with slow flow velocity in coronary arteries. Chest 67, 116.

Ho, M., Veale, D., Eastmond, C., Eastmond, C., Nuki, G., Belch, J., 2000. Macrovascular disease and systemic sclerosis. Ann. Rheum. Dis. 59, 39.

Hsu, S., Houston, B.A., Tampakakis, E., et al., 2016. Right ventricular functional reserve in pulmonary arterial hypertension. Circulation 133, 2413.

Ioannidis, J.P., Vlachoyiannopoulos, P.G., Haidich, A.B., Medsger Jr., T.A., Lucas, M., Michet, C.J., Kuwana, M., Yasuoka, H., van den Hoogen, F., Te Boome, L., van Laar, J.M., Verbeet, N.L., Matucci-Cerinic, M., Georgountzos, A., Moutsopoulos, H.M., 2005. Mortality in systemic sclerosis: an international meta-analysis of individual patient data. Am. J. Med. 118, 2.

Ishida, R., Murata, Y., Sawada, Y., Nishioka, K., Shibuya, H., 2000. Thallium-201 myocardial SPECT in patients with collagen disease. Nucl. Med. Commun. 21, 729.

Josephson, M., 1993. Intraventricular Conduction Disturbances. Clinical Cardiac Electrophysiology, second ed. Lea and Febiger, Philadelphia, PA, p. 117.

Kissin, E., Korn, J.H., 2002. Poptosis and myofibroblasts in the pathogenesis of systemic sclerosis. Curr. Rheumatol. Rep. 4, 129.

Lee, P., Langevitz, P., Alderdice, C.A., Aubrey, M., Baer, P.A., Baron, M., Buskila, D., Dutz, J.P., Khostanteen, I., Piper, S., 1992. Mortality in systemic sclerosis (scleroderma). Q. J. Med. 82, 139.

Lekakis, J., Mavrikakis, M., Emmanuel, M., Prassopoulos, V., Papazoglou, S., Papamichael, C., Moulopoulou, D., Kostamis, P., Stamatelopoulos, S., Moulopoulos, S., 1998. Cold-induced coronary Raynaud's phenomenon in patients with systemic sclerosis. Clin. Exp. Rheumatol. 16, 135.

Liangos, O., Neure, L., Kuhl, U., Pauschinger, M., Sieper, J., Distler, A., Schwimmbeck, P.L., Braun, J., 2000. The possible role of myocardial biopsy in systemic sclerosis. Rheumatology (Oxford) 39, 674.

Lubitz, S.A., Goldbarg, S.H., Mehta, D., 2008. Sudden cardiac death in infiltrative cardiomyopathies: sarcoidosis, scleroderma, amyloidosis, hemachromatosis. Prog. Cardiovasc. Dis. 51, 58.

Mavrogeni, S.I., Bratis, K., Karabela, G., et al., 2015. Cardiovascular Magnetic resonance imaging clarifies cardiac pathophysiology in early asymptomatic diffuse systemic sclerosis. Inflamm. Allergy Drug Targets 14, 29.

Morelli, S., Sgreccia, A., De Marzio, P., Perrone, C., Ferrante, L., Gurgo, A.M., Gurgo diCastelmenardo, A.M., Aguglia, G., De Vincentiis, G., Scopinaro, F., Calvieri, S., 1997. Noninvasive assessment of myocardial involvement in patients with systemic sclerosis: role of signal averaged electrocardiography. J. Rheumatol. 24, 2358.

Mueller, K.A.L., Mueller II, Eppler, D., Zuern, C.S., Seizer, P., Kramer, U., et al., 2015. Clinical and histopathological features of patients with systemic sclerosis undergoing endomyocardial biopsy. PLoS One 10 (5), e0126707. http://dx.doi.org/10.1371/journal.pone.0126707.

Mukerjee, D., St George, D., Coleiro, B., Denton, C.P., Devar, J., Black, C.M., Coghlan, J.G., 2003. Prevalence and outcome in systemic sclerosis associated pulmonary arterial hypertension (SScPAH): application of a registry approach. Ann. Rheum. Dis. 62, 1088–1093.

Murata, I., Takenaka, K., Shinohara, S., Suzuki, T., Sasaki, T., Yamamoto, K., 1998. Diversity of myocardial involvement in systemic sclerosis: an 8-year study of 95 Japanese patients. Am. Heart J. 135, 960.

Nakajima, K., Taki, J., Kawano, M., Higuchi, T., Sato, S., Nishijima, C., Takehara, K., Tonami, N., 2001. Diastolic dysfunction in patients with systemic sclerosis detected by gated myocardial perfusion SPECT: an early sign of cardiac involvement. J. Nucl. Med. 42, 183.

Nishioka, K., Katayama, I., Kondo, H., Shinkai, H., Ueki, H., Tamaki, K., Takehara, K., Tajima, S., Maeda, M., Hayashi, S., Kodama, H., Miyachi, Y., Mizutani, H., Fujisaku, A., Sasaki, T., Shimizu, M., Kaburagi, J., 1996. Epidemiological analysis of prognosis of 496 Japanese patients with progressive systemic sclerosis (SSc). Scleroderma Research Committee Japan. J. Dermatol. 23, 677.

Nihtyanova, S.I., Schreiber, B.E., Ong, V.H., Rosenberg, D., Moinzadeh, P., Coghlan, J.G., Wells, A.U., Denton, C.P., 2014. Prediction of pulmonary complications and long term survival in systemic sclerosis. Arthritis Rheumatol. 66, 1625.

Nitenberg, A., Foult, J.M., Kahan, A., Perennec, J., Devaux, J.Y., Menkes, C.J., Amor, B., 1986. Reduced coronary flow and resistance reserve in primary scleroderma myocardial disease. Am. Heart J. 112, 309.

Ntusi, N.A., Piechnik, S.K., Francis, J.M., Ferreira, V.M., Rai, A.B., Matthews, P.M., Robson, M.D., Moon, J., Wordsworth, P.B., Neubauer, S., Karamitsos, T.D., 2014. Subclinical myocardial inflammation and diffuse fibrosis are common in systemic sclerosis—a clinical study using myocardial T1-mapping and extracellular volume quantification. J. Cardiovasc. Magn. Reson. 16, 21.

Plazak, W., Zabinska-Plazak, E., Wojas-Pelc, A., Podolec, P., Olszowska, M., Tracz, W., Bogdaszewska-Czabanowska, J., 2002. Heart structure and function in systemic sclerosis. Eur. J. Dermatol. 12, 257.

Ruangjutipopan, S., Kasitanon, N., Louthrenoo, W., Sukitawut, W., Wichainun, R., 2002. Causes of death and poor survival prognostic factors in Thai patients with systemic sclerosis. J. Med. Assoc. Thai. 85, 1204.

Schachna, L., Wigley, F.M., 2002. Targeting mediators of vascular injury in scleroderma. Curr. Opin. Rheumatol. 14, 686.

Steen, V.D., Medsger Jr., T.A., 2000. Severe organ involvement in systemic sclerosis with diffuse scleroderma. Arthritis Rheum. 43, 2437.

Steen, V.D., Follansbee, W.P., Conte, C.G., Medsger Jr., T.A., 1996. Thallium perfusion defects predict subsequent cardiac dysfunction in patients with systemic sclerosis. Arthritis Rheum. 39, 677.

Taylor, M.H., McFadden, J.A., Bolster, M.B., Silver, R.M., 2002. Ulnar artery involvement in systemic sclerosis (scleroderma). J. Rheumatol. 29, 102.

Ungprasert, P., Charoenpong, P., Ratanasrimetha, P., Thongprayoon, C., Cheungpasitporn, W., Suksaranjit, P., 2014. Risk of coronary artery disease in patients with systemic sclerosis: a systematic review and meta-analysis. Clin. Rheumatol. 33, 1099.

Vacca, A., Montisci, R., Garau, P., Siotto, P., Piga, M., Cauli, A., Ruscazio, L., Iliceto, S., Mathieu, A., 2013. Prognostic impact of coronary microcirculation abnormalities in systemic sclerosis: a prospective study to evaluate the role of non invasive tests. Arthitis Res. Ther. 15, R8.

Veale, D.J., Collidge, T.A., Belch, J.J., 1995. Increased prevalence of symptomatic macrovascular disease in systemic sclerosis. Ann. Rheum. Dis. 54, 853.

Vlachoyiannopoulos, P.G., Dafni, U.G., Pakas, I., Spyropoulou-Vlachou, M., Stavropoulos-Giokas, C., Moutsopoulos, H.M., 2000. Systemic scleroderma in Greece: low mortality and strong linkage with HLA-DRB1*1104 allele. Ann. Rheum. Dis. 59, 359.

Wozniak, J., Dabrowski, R., Luczak, D., et al., 2009. Evaluation of heart rhythm variability and arrhythmia in children with systemic and localized scleroderma. J. Rheumatol. 36, 191.

Youssef, P., Englert, H., Bertouch, J., 1993. Large vessel occlusive disease associated with CREST syndrome and scleroderma. Ann. Rheum. Dis. 52, 464.

FURTHER READING

Geirsson, A., Danielsen, R., Petursson, E., 1996. Left ventricular myocardial perfusion and function in systemic sclerosis before and after diltiazem treatment. Scand. J. Rheumatol. 25, 317.

Morelli, S., Piccirillo, G., Fimognari, F., Sgreccia, A., Ferrante, L., Morabito, G., DeMarzio, P., Valesini, G., Marigliano, V., 1996. Twenty-four hour heart period variability in systemic sclerosis. J. Rheumatol. 23, 643.

Chapter 14

Cardiac Involvement in Systemic Vasculitis

M. Sebastiani, A. Manfredi and C. Ferri
Rheumatology Unit, Azienda Policlinico of Modena, Department of Medical and Surgical Sciences, University of Modena and Reggio Emilia, Modena, Italy

Key Points

- Despite cardiac involvement can be observed in all primary vasculitides, it is frequently unrecognized.
- Subclinical involvement is frequently observed in pathology and heart imaging studies, but its impact on prognosis and survival is unclear.
- Takayasu's arteritis, polyarteritis nodosa, and Behçet disease are the vasculitides with more frequent heart involvement.
- Pericarditis, myocarditis, coronary arteritis, and valvular heart disease can be observed with different incidence in all primary vasculitides.
- A correct treatment of cardiac involvement in patients with vasculitis requires a multidisciplinary approach, including rheumatologist, cardiologist, and radiologist.

1. INTRODUCTION

Systemic vasculitides are a heterogeneous group of diseases characterized by inflammation of vessels, which can result in their obstruction and/or aneurysm formation. The evidence of the inflammation of blood vessel walls in at least one occasion during the course is a shared defining feature of all categories of vasculitis. Their classification varies according to etiology, pathogenesis, type of vessel affected, type of inflammation, and favored organ distribution (Fig. 14.1).

Almost all primary vasculitides can target the heart; even if cardiac manifestations are rarely predominant, they can be life threatening and, therefore, require specific diagnostic and therapeutic strategies.

Although cardiac involvement occurs in less than 10% of all patients affected by systemic vasculitides, certain entities, such as eosinophilic

The Heart in Systemic Autoimmune Diseases.

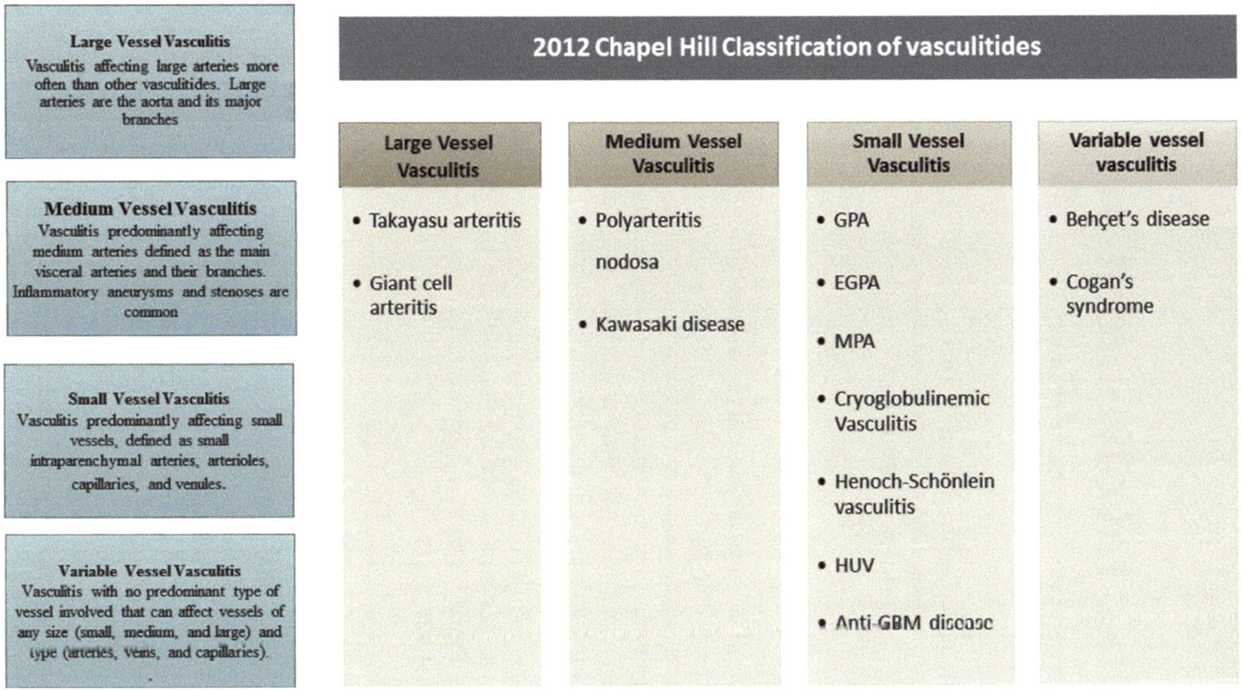

FIGURE 14.1 **2012 Chapel Hill classification of vasculitides.** *EGPA*, eosinophilic granulomatosis with polyangiitis; *GBM*, glomerular basal membrane; *GPA*, granulomatosis with polyangiitis; *HUV*, hypocomplementemic urticarial vasculitis; *MPA*, microscopic polyangiitis.

granulomatosis with polyangiitis (EGPA) and Takayasu's arteritis (TAK) can cause heart complications in up to 60% of patients.

After briefly reviewing the definitions, classification, and pathogenic mechanisms of vasculitides, we describe the cardiac manifestations that can occur in each vasculitis and their corresponding therapies.

2. PATHOGENESIS OF VASCULITIDES

Pathogenesis of vasculitides differs according to the type of vasculitis. Despite several pathogenic pathways have been implicated in the development of these diseases, the exact mechanisms are only partly understood and some are probably still unknown. Small vessel vasculitides (granulomatosis with polyangiitis, EGPA, microscopic polyangiitis) are strongly associated with the presence of antineutrophil cytoplasmic antibodies (ANCA), whereas immune complexes may be responsible for Henoch-Schönlein purpura (HSP), cryoglobulinemic vasculitis, and polyarteritis nodosa (PAN).

2.1 Immune Complexes

Immune complex small vessel vasculitis is defined as vasculitis with moderate to marked vessel wall deposits of immunoglobulin and complement components, predominantly affecting small vessels. These deposits differ from the few or no immune deposits in vessel walls, which is characteristic for ANCA-associated vasculitides. The precipitation of immune complexes in the vessel walls causes the complement fixation, leading to an intense immune reaction, with the recruitment of neutrophils, which attempt to engulf the immune complexes. During this process the neutrophils degranulate, releasing lysosomal enzymes and oxygen free radicals, responsible for tissue necrosis. Immune complexes seem to be relevant in some vasculitides, like PAN, cryoglobulinemia, and necrotizing vasculitis occurring in rheumatoid arthritis.

2.2 Antineutrophil Cytoplasmic Antibodies

First detected in a small cohort of patients with pauci-immune glomerulonephritis (Davies et al., 1982), antibodies specific to antigens in the cytoplasm of ethanol-fixed neutrophils have been shown to be strongly associated with three major small vessel vasculitides: granulomatosis with polyangiitis (GPA), microscopic polyangiitis (MPA), and EGPA (Falk and Jennette, 1988; Van der Woude et al., 1985). Despite ANCA are considered a useful immunological marker of disease, in particular c-ANCA, in vitro data and animal models have not so far been able to support a clear pathogenic role of these autoantibodies.

Witko-Sarsat identified proteinase 3 (PR3), a major target antigen, in plasma membrane secretory vesicles (Witko-Sarsat et al., 1999). By indirect immunofluorescence (IIF), ANCA are identified as cytoplasmic (c-ANCA), with coarse granular stain of cytoplasm; perinuclear (p-ANCA), with staining of the nucleus and perinuclear area; and atypical ANCA. The antigen responsible for homogeneous cytoplasmic fluorescence is usually PR3, while myeloperoxidase (MPO) showed more frequently a perinuclear IIF. Antibodies to other neutrophil constituents such as elastase, cathepsin G, and lactoferrin produce perinuclear or atypical pattern (Ledford, 1997; Specks et al., 1993).

Pathogenetic activity of MPO-ANCA has been demonstrated in MPO-knockout mice immunized with murine MPO. The recipient mice developed necrotizing glomerulonephritis and systemic necrotizing vasculitis (Xiao et al., 2002). Another murine model for anti-MPO–mediated glomerulonephritis and vasculitis has been performed using MPO-knockout mice ($MPO^{-/-}$) (Schreiber et al., 2006). Chimeric $MPO^{-/-}$ mice with circulating MPO-positive neutrophils developed pauci-immune necrotizing and crescentic glomerulonephritis, whereas chimeric $MPO^{+/+}$ mice with circulating MPO-negative neutrophils did not.

c-ANCA are detected in 60–90% of cases of systemic GPA, and in 50–75% of those with localized forms of GPA (Kallenberg et al., 1992). ANCA titer changes according to the disease activity, but this relationship is not constant; therefore, the therapy should not be modified using ANCA titer (Girard et al., 2001; Tervaert et al., 1990). p-ANCA are more often associated with pauci-immune glomerulonephritis (80% of the patients), MPA (50–75%), or EGPA (47%) (Ewert et al., 1991; Guillevin et al., 1999a; Hagen et al., 1998). However, ANCA have also been detected in some nonvasculitic pathologies, such as inflammatory bowel and autoimmune liver diseases, rheumatoid arthritis, tuberculosis (Flores-Suarez et al., 2003), and drug reactions (Guillevin et al., 1995a; Halbwachs-Mecarelli et al., 1992; Specks et al., 1993).

2.3 Cytokines and Adhesion Molecules

Many cytokines and adhesion molecules are present at sites of inflammation and their circulating levels are high in patients with vasculitis (Sundy and Haynes 2000; Tesar et al., 1998). Recently, high levels of different chemokins have also been detected in patients with vasculitis (Millet et al., 2015), and potentially correlated with clinical symptoms (fever and weight loss induced by interleukin-1, tumor necrosis factor α, and interleukin 6). Some of them may favor fibrosis and thrombosis (transforming growth factor β), while others may act as chemoattractants for polymorphonuclear leukocytes, or have inflammatory capacities [interferon-γ (IFNγ)]. Adhesion molecules are involved in the interactions between endothelial cells and activated neutrophils (Sundy and Haynes, 2000). In patients with active GPA, MPA, TKA, and HSP, high levels of soluble endothelial receptors for neutrophils, E-selectin, and vascular cell adhesion molecule-1 have been detected. Moreover, expression of chemokines, such as CXCL9, CXCL10, CXCL11, and CCL2, was higher in vascular smooth muscle cells isolated from giant cells arteritis-involved arteries (Corbera-Bellalta et al., 2016).

2.4 Other Pathogenic Factors

Other immunopathogenic factors and mechanisms may play a role in vasculitides. For example, dysfunction of T and B regulatory (reg) cells is implicated in pathogenesis of ANCA-associated vasculitis. Normally, Treg cells control the production of pathogenic ANCA by B cells; in patients with active disease, there is a decrease in the FOXP3 positive Treg cell, which normalizes during remission. Infiltration by T lymphocytes secreting Th1 proinflammatory cytokines, essentially IFNγ, has been observed in granulomatous lesions of the nasal mucosa in GPA patients. Thus, in GPA, Th1 lymphocytes would play a major role in localized and granulomatous upper respiratory tract involvement, whereas a shift toward Th2 lymphocytes would tend to be more predominant in systemic forms (Balding et al., 2001; Csernok et al., 1999).

Also eosinophils are a part of inflammatory infiltrate in necrotizing small and medium vessel vasculitis. Tissue and circulating eosinophils are characteristic of EGPA. Eosinophilic cationic proteins, CCL-11, CCL-26, and IL-25, secreted by eosinophils are associated with disease activity in EGPA.

A role for antiendothelial cell antibodies (AECA) has been supposed from their presence in GPA, MPA, as well as in vasculitis secondary to rheumatoid arthritis and systemic lupus erythematosus. It still remains unclear whether AECA are involved in the pathogenesis of vasculitis or if they are the result of vasculitis-associated inflammation (Chan and Cheng, 1996; Falcini et al., 1997; Gobel et al., 1996). Viral etiologies for vasculitides have been clearly demonstrated in hepatitis B virus (HBV)-related PAN (Guillevin et al., 1995b), hepatitis C virus (HCV)-related mixed cryoglobulinemia (Ferri et al., 1991a,b), and in HIV vasculitides (Gisselbrecht et al., 1997).

Finally, environmental, genetic, and infectious factors have been proposed to explain the different geographic distribution observed for many vasculitides (Fig. 14.2).

3. CARDIOVASCULAR CLINICAL MANIFESTATIONS IN VASCULITIDES

3.1 Main Cardiovascular Manifestations

Frequency, characteristics, and severity of heart involvement vary according to the type of vasculitis. Each cardiac tissue may be affected, from myocardium to epicardium, endocardium, conductive nodal tissue, and coronary arteries. Cardiovascular manifestations (Table 14.1) may thus be categorized as detailed below.

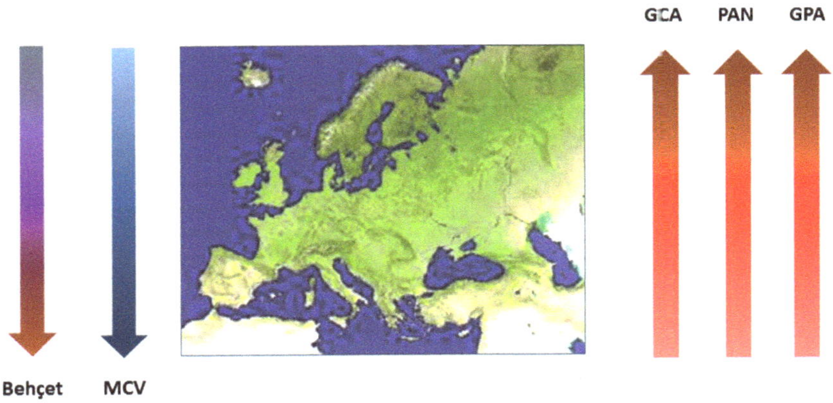

FIGURE 14.2 **Different geographic distribution of vasculitides.** Many vasculitides show differences in geographical distribution. For Behçet disease and mixed cryoglobulinemic vasculitis a North-South gradient is described; on the contrary giant cell arteritis (GCA), polyarteritis nodosa (PAN), and granulomatosis with polyangiitis (GPA) are more frequently observed in North-European than Mediterranean countries. Environmental, genetic, and infectious factors have been proposed to explain this different distribution.

3.1.1 Cardiomyopathy

Cardiomyopathy consists of a group of diseases involving the heart muscle itself in absence of ischemic, hypertensive, congenital, valvular or pericardial diseases. A functional classification includes dilated or congestive cardiomyopathy, hypertrophic cardiomyopathy, and restrictive cardiomyopathy. These distinctions are not absolute and overlaps can occur.

Cardiovascular manifestations in systemic vasculitis include initially silent cardiomyopathy due to either ischemic or inflammatory causes. The combination of vasculitis and cardiomyopathy is usually associated with a poor prognosis.

The reported frequencies of specific myocarditis vary widely from not-even-mentioned (Chumbley et al., 1977; Savage et al., 1985) up to 78% in an anatomical study (Holsinger et al., 1962), depending on the examinations used to diagnose small- and medium-sized vessel vasculitides with a mean of 25–30% (Forstot et al., 1980; Lanham et al., 1985). In the context of vasculitis, specific cardiomyopathy is reported in ANCA-associated vasculitides, and also in TAK and giant cell arteritis (GCA). However, cardiomyopathy leading to heart failure may reflect either specific myocardial involvement or myocardial ischemia in most patients or may be the consequence of associated conditions (e.g., hypertensive cardiomyopathy, steroid-induced coronary arteries atheromatosis). Specific cardiomyopathy could result from necrotizing vasculitis of the arterioles and venules supplying cardiac muscle, with inflammatory infiltration and/or granulomas and/or fibrosis formation within cardiac tissue. Endoventricular biopsies are technically possible, but rarely

TABLE 14.1 Heart Involvement in Primary Vasculitides

	Pericarditis	Myocarditis	Valvulopathy	Coronary Arteritis	Intracavitary Thrombus	Aortitis
Takayasu's arteritis	+	+	+	+	+	+
Giant cell arteritis	+	+	+	+	−	+
Polyarteritis nodosa	+	+	−	+	−	−
Kawasaki disease	+	+	+	+	−	−
Granulomatosis with polyangiitis	+	+	+	+	+	+
Eosinophilic granulomatosis with polyangiitis	+	+	+	+	+	−
Microscopic polyangiitis	+	+	+	+	+	−
Henoch-Schönlein purpura	−	−	−	+	−	−
Crioglobulinemic vasculitis	+	−	−	+	−	−
Behçet disease	+	+	+	+	+	−
Buerger disease	−	−	−	+	−	−
Cogan syndrome	+	−	−	+	−	+

obtained (Lanham et al., 1985; Leung et al., 1989) and may be helpful in understanding the causal process. However, vasculitis is rarely diagnosed based on the detection of granulomatous or necrotizing vasculitis in biopsy samples.

3.1.2 Coronary Arteritis

Coronary arteritis may manifest as aneurysms, thromboses, dissections, and/or stenoses, all of which can lead to myocardial infarction. Although coronary angiography may show some abnormalities, it is only occasionally performed. Therefore, diagnosis of coronary arteritis is rare in clinical practice, even if autopsy studies have found coronary involvement in 50% of PAN (Schrader et al., 1985), and specific abnormalities have been also reported in GPA, EPGA, and Behçet disease patients. Nonetheless, in clinical practice, Kawasaki disease remains the vasculitis with the highest frequency of coronary arteritis, with up to 25% of untreated children developing coronary lesions.

3.1.3 Pericarditis

Pericardial effusion is a frequent cardiac manifestation during vasculitis and may be associated with cardiomyopathy, mainly in EGPA, occurring in about 15–30% (Dennert et al., 2010), but also in up to 19% of GPA (Fig. 14.3A) (Oliveira et al., 2005) and in 5–10% of PAN (Fig. 14.3B) (Pagnoux et al., 2010). Manifestations may range from acute pericarditis and pericardial effusions to chronic constrictive pericarditis. Less life threatening than myocardial involvement, pericardial disease typically responds to immunosuppressive therapy, but pericardiocentesis may be required in cases of cardiac

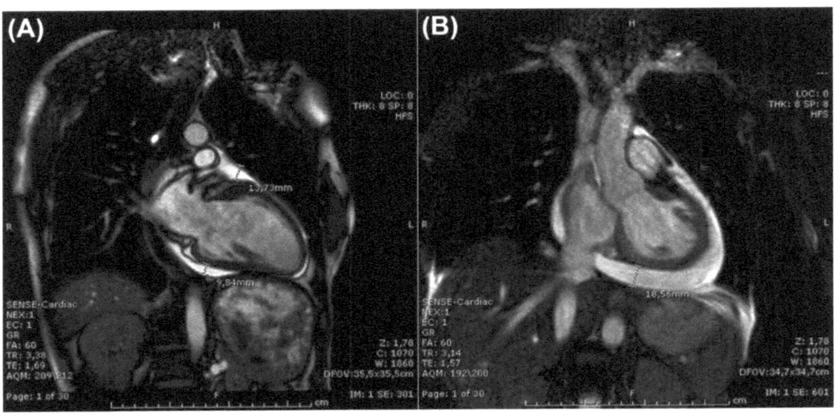

FIGURE 14.3 **Pericarditis.** Pericardial effusion: (A) Patient with granulomatosis with polyangiitis: thickening of pericardial layer. Fibrotic nodule in the context of pericardial fluid. (B) Large pericardial effusion in a patient with polyarteritis nodosa.

tamponade. An epicardial biopsy may provide the diagnosis of vasculitis, particularly of EGPA (Sharma et al., 1993).

3.1.4 Endocarditis and Valvular Disease

Endocardium involvement is thought to be rare in vasculitides. Functional inorganic murmurs or valvular pathologies that are not related to vasculitis comprise most of the reported cases. However, especially in EGPA, myocardial vasculitis, in addition to predisposing to arterial thromboembolus, endocardial thickening, and thrombus may extend down the myocardial surface to engulf the valvular apparatus or leaflets, classically affecting the atrioventricular valves, leading to significant valve dysfunction (Ramakrishna et al., 2000). Also in GPA, significant valvular stenosis or regurgitation is frequently detected by echocardiography (about 15% of patients), with the mitral and tricuspid valves most commonly affected (Oliveira et al., 2005).

Moreover, specific valve damage may sometimes occur during the acute phase of the vasculitis and progress to valve distortion during lesion repair and cicatrization (Davenport et al., 1994).

3.1.5 Conduction Tissue Involvement

Vasculitic or ischemic cardiomyopathy may involve nodal tissue, more frequently the sinus node than atrioventricular branches, leading to secondary heart block. Vasculitic or granulomatous involvement of the atrioventricular node or bundle of His has also been reported (Eisen et al., 2009). Hence, patients with vasculitis may develop a variety of conduction system disorders and potentially require permanent pace-maker implantation (Sumitomo et al., 2008). Complete atrioventricular heart blocks and bundle-branch blocks have been mentioned particularly in medium- to small-sized vasculitides, as GPA (Handa et al., 1997), EGPA (Rabusin et al., 1998), or PAN (Blétry et al., 1980).

3.1.6 Arrhythmia

Supraventricular, but also ventricular tachyarrhythmias may occur in the setting of myopathic-induced elevations in left ventricular filling pressures or ischemia or both. They mainly resolve within a few days of treatment for vasculitis (Hu et al., 1997; Schiavone et al., 1985).

3.1.7 Aortic Dissections and Aneurysms

The aorta and its proximal branches are frequently involved in large vessel vasculitis, that is, TAK and GCA (Fig. 14.4). Nevertheless, arteritis of the aorta may occur in the setting of small vessel vasculitis such as Kawasaki disease (Cormier et al., 2000; Kerr et al., 2000). Subclinical inflammation of the aorta can be detected by transesophageal echocardiography and magnetic resonance angiography. Rarely, aortitis resulting by a vasculitis of the vasa vasorum of the aorta can be observed in ANCA-associated vasculitides (Schildhaus et al., 2002).

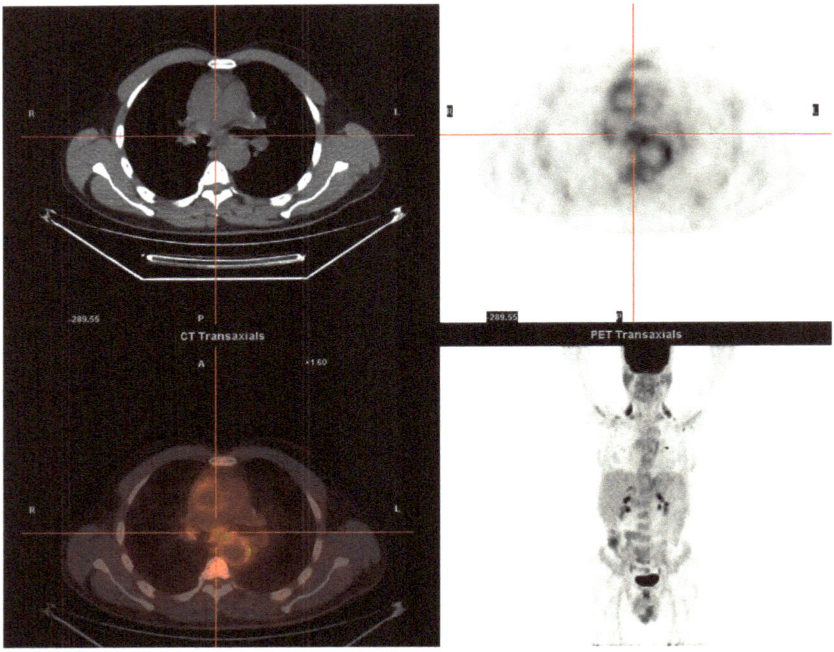

FIGURE 14.4 **Aortitis in patients with Takayasu's arteritis.** Positron emission tomography—computed tomography: hypermetabolic activity and enlargement of the thoracic aorta in a patient with Takayasu's arteritis.

3.1.8 Pulmonary Hypertension

Pulmonary hypertension is infrequent, but can be secondary to concomitant lung disease or recurrent lung embolism or by direct involvement of pulmonary arteries. Pulmonary arteries are affected in 15—70% of patients with TAK (Endo et al., 2003). In some instances, it can be the consequence of constrictive pericarditis and/or restrictive cardiomyopathy (Grant et al., 1994).

3.1.9 Thromboembolic and Proximal Vascular Complications

Intracardiac thrombosis has been documented in EGPA and GPA, and patients with active small vessel vasculitis have also been found to be at an increased risk for venous thromboembolic disease (Merkel et al., 2005). Moreover, thromboembolic events can commonly complicate necrotizing vasculitis, that is, Kawasaki disease, Behçet disease, Buerger disease, PAN, and the vasculitis of rheumatoid arthritis. Intracardiac thrombus with or without endomyocardial fibrosis or endomyocarditis can represent the onset manifestation of Behçet disease (Ng et al., 2015).

3.1.10 Secondary Cardiovascular Manifestations and Differential Diagnoses

A careful differential diagnosis should be performed in all cardiovascular manifestations occurring in vasculitides. In fact, primary cardiovascular diseases should be distinguished by the involvement consequent to vasculitis. Moreover, heart involvement can be secondary to other vasculitic organ involvement or to treatment side effects.

3.2 Large Vessel Vasculitides

3.2.1 Giant Cell Arteritis

GCA, also called temporal or granulomatous arteritis, is the most common vasculitis in populations with Northern European ancestry. This large vessel vasculitis seldom presents below the age of 50 years (Salvarani et al., 2002). The incidence increases with age and is higher in populations of northern European origin than in Mediterranean countries (Fig. 14.2; Salvarani et al., 1995).

It rarely causes cardiac problems but the considerably increased relative risk, up to 17 times, to develop thoracic aortic aneurysm and aortic dissection is poorly known. This was initially reported in a population-based cohort study of 96 patients of whom 11 had thoracic aortic aneurysm. At least 20% of patients with GCA develop aortitis. Many of these develop an aortic aneurysm as a consequence. Although there is a risk of spontaneous aortic rupture without aneurysmal dilatation secondary to vessel wall weakening and necrosis, this event is exceedingly rare, with only rare cases reported in the literature (Klein et al., 1975; Salvarani et al., 2002). Bruits may be heard on auscultation over the carotid, subclavian, axillary, and brachial arteries. Absent or decreased pulses are present in the neck or arms. Such patients may have few of the usual symptoms of GCA, so the diagnosis may be initially overlooked.

Data from surgical case series and autopsy studies suggested a high rate of aortic involvement in GCA. In retrospective studies of patients treated surgically for aneurysms of the thoracic aorta, routine histological examination of the operative specimen indicated noninfectious aortitis in 4–12% of cases. GCA was the second most common cause after idiopathic aortitis, with 8–30% of case.

Thoracic aortic aneurysms are 17 times more likely to develop in patients with GCA than in persons without this disease (Evans et al., 1995). This complication occurs as a late event, usually several years after the diagnosis and often after the patient's other symptoms have subsided. The aneurysm may rupture and cause the patient's death. However, the mortality rate in patients with GCA is similar to that expected in general populations of similar age and sex (Salvarani et al., 2002).

In the clinical suspicion of large vessel GCA, arteriography, computerized tomography (CT) scanning, and magnetic resonance (MR) angiography are the diagnostic modalities required. Contrast-enhanced CT and MR angiography are largely replacing conventional angiography in delineating extent of disease. In large vessel arteritis, these will show thickening of the arterial wall with crescents and indistinct vascular borders. They may also show alternating stenotic segments or occlusion. Additionally, these studies are excellent at detecting aneurysms or dissections secondary to vasculitis (Stanson, 2000).

Ultrasound can be useful in determining flow patterns and stenosis in vessels. It may also show a "halo sign" (hypoechoic halo around the vessel lumen on color duplex ultrasound of the involved artery), which has been shown to be associated with active inflammation on temporal artery biopsy.

Coronary arteritis is a rare but potentially fatal complication of GCA. Patients may present with chest pain, dyspnea, chronic heart failure, arrhythmia, and sudden cardiac death (Karger and Fechner, 2006). Concomitant cardiovascular risk factors, commonly present in this elderly population, make the differentiation between vasculitis- and atherosclerosis-induced coronary artery disease challenging. Pericarditis has been described in several case reports (Guillaume et al., 1991).

3.2.2 Takayasu's Arteritis

TAK is a systemic granulomatous large vessel vasculitis with a phenotype that overlaps with GCA. In the Chapel Hill Consensus Conference 2012, these two syndromes were the only categories within the LVV classification without a change in definition from the first, 1993, consensus statement (Jennette et al., 2013). Similarities in the pathology and distribution of vascular lesions have led to claims that TAK and GCA are one disease (Grayson et al., 2012), but genotypic, phenotypic, and racial differences have been described (Furuta et al., 2015).

TAK affects the aortic arch and its proximal branches (see Fig. 14.4). Ethnic differences in the pattern of involvement of the aorta are reported both in adult and in child. Japanese adults have been shown to have predominant aortic arch involvement, while Asian Indian patients seem to have preponderance of thoracic and abdominal aorta involvement. North American patients with childhood TAK also tend to have aortic involvement similar to that seen in adult patients from the Asian Indian population.

The disease characteristically evolves in three phases (Kerr, 1994). Systemic symptoms develop and then resolve over several weeks, while arteritis takes root. This arteritis also resolves, with an ensuing asymptomatic period (mean duration of 8 years) before vasoocclusive signs and symptoms develop. During the initial phase, systemic symptoms are noted only in less than half of the cases, especially European patients, whereas they are rare in Japanese patients. The disease is monophasic and self-limited for 20% of the patients.

Cardiac and vascular features include blood pressure difference of extremities (45–69%), claudication (38–81%), carotidynia or vessel tenderness (13–32%), hypertension (28–53%), aortic regurgitation (20–24%), pericarditis (<8%), and congestive heart failure (<7%).

Severe cardiovascular complications of TAK are caused by fibrotic thickening of the aortic arch and its branches and, more rarely, complicated by thromboembolic events. Histological findings are granulomatous inflammation and adventitial sclerosis, predominantly at the adventitia-media junction. Occasionally, vascular inflammation spreads from the aorta to the proximal epicardial coronary arteries and may cause coronary insufficiency and myocardial infarctions (Park et al., 2005).

3.3 Medium-Sized Vessel Vasculitides

3.3.1 Polyarteritis Nodosa

PAN is a primary systemic necrotizing vasculitis predominantly targeting medium-sized arteries defined as the main visceral arteries and their branches. Small arteries may also be involved but small vessels, including arterioles, capillaries, and venules, are characteristically spared. The diagnosis is made by biopsy of affected tissue(s) and/or by angiography revealing characteristic microaneurysms and/or stenoses. In the past, systemic necrotizing vasculitis was generally considered as PAN or related variants. The annual incidence of PAN currently ranges from 0 to 1.6 cases/million inhabitants in European countries and its prevalence is about 31 cases/million. PAN affects patients of any gender, age, or ethnic background (Fig. 14.2). The peak incidence occurs in the fifth to sixth decades of life. Before vaccination against HBV was available, more than one-third of adults with PAN were infected by HBV. Currently, less than 5% of patients with PAN are HBV-infected in developed countries.

Cardiac involvement in PAN was already mentioned in the first publication (Küssmaul and Maier, 1866), which described a case of "nodular coronaritis," and it was subsequently reported with frequencies ranging from 10% in clinical studies of PAN patients (Frohnert and Sheps, 1967) to 78% in histopathological study (Holsinger et al., 1962).

In clinical and necropsy series including 283 patients, congestive heart failure (27%) and hypertension (37%) were found to be common cardiac presentations of PAN, whereas myocardial infarction was rare (2%). PAN presenting with acute myocardial infarction and complicated by multiple coronary aneurysms is also very rare.

Several reports describe PAN in patients with coronary artery disease. Most of these patients had myocardial infarctions due to angiographically or pathologically diagnosed narrowing or occlusion of the coronary arteries. Multiple vascular aneurysms are the most typical angiographic finding of PAN and is also one of the criteria for the disease. Some case reports have demonstrated aneurysms and stenotic changes in the coronary arteries (2–4). A few case reports have described acute myocardial infarctions with coronary dissection.

Congestive heart failure occurs in 6–57% in PAN. It is specific and/or can result from other vasculitis-related organ involvement or disorders, mainly hypertension and/or renal involvement (Blétry et al., 1980). Congestive heart failure may thus also be attributed to coronary artery or myocardial arteriolar infarcts, caused by immune complex deposition, resulting in disseminated necrotic foci, mostly in the left ventricle. The right ventricle may also be involved (Blétry et al., 1980).

Pericardial involvement occurs in 5 to 30% of PAN patients (Fig. 14.3B; Hu et al., 1997; Schrader et al., 1985). About half of the first reported cases of pericardial effusion were indeed secondary to uremia, which is much less frequent nowadays since diagnosis and therapeutic management of PAN patients has been improved.

Sinus tachycardia is usual and nonspecific. Arrhythmias and conduction disorders, mainly supraventricular, can occur in 2–19% of patients because of arteritis of the sinus node or neighboring nerve fibers.

Aortic dissection is a rare complication, resulting from diffuse vasculitis of the vasa vasorum, but was reported in one patient with HBV-related PAN, which evolved to fatal tamponade (Iino et al., 1992). Dissections of proximal aortic branches have also been reported, but some were attributed to other causes, such as atherosclerotic aneurysms (Hachulla et al., 1993; Hautekeete et al., 1990; Lomeo et al., 1989), syphilis, cystic media necrosis, trauma, sepsis, or hypertension.

3.3.2 Kawasaki Disease

Kawasaki disease, or mucocutaneous lymph-node syndrome, was first reported in Japanese with clinical observation of 50 cases by Dr. Kawasaki in 1967 (Kawasaki, 1967). The disease affects children mostly those aged 8–24 months in North America and 6–11 months in Asia and is associated with arterial vasculitis. Although inflammation is present in medium-sized and small arteries throughout the body, coronary arteries are the main target.

After myocardial infarction in Kawasaki disease was reported in 1974, many reports showed that cardiac lesions, such as coronary dilatation, coronary aneurysms, coronary narrowing, myocardial infarction, and valvular lesions, often occur in patients with Kawasaki disease, which is now recognized as the leading cause of acquired heart disease in children in the developed world.

Up to 25% of untreated children develop coronary lesions, with a peak 3–4 weeks into the illness, but treatment with intravenous immunoglobulin improves clinical outcomes and reduces the proportion of coronary lesions to less than 5%. Patients with cardiac lesions are more likely to be older, male, and to have higher white blood cells count, C-reactive protein levels, and platelet count, as well as lower albumin levels.

In 2014 the Japanese Circulation Society (JCS) published a consensus guideline, where patients are risk stratified based on the severity of the coronary artery lesions and likelihood of complications, including myocardial ischemia and congestive heart failure. In patients with coronary artery aneurysms (CAA) or with early, transient coronary artery dilatations, the JCS advises an ECG and echocardiogram at 1, 2, 6, and 12 months, and a final evaluation at 5 years with an exercise ECG. For patients diagnosed with persisting CAA after the acute phase, the guideline advises a more intensive and prolonged follow-up with additional imaging modalities.

The JCS recommends follow-up for patients with small aneurysms at 30 days after the acute illness with an echocardiogram and ECG every 3 months until the dilatation has disappeared. Patients with medium-sized aneurysms should be more intensely evaluated, that is, every 1–3 months with (exercise) ECG, echocardiography, and chest X-ray until dilatation is no longer observed and should undergo MR Coronary Angiography every 5 years.

Patients with persistent large coronary artery aneurysms may, however, develop acute coronary syndromes in adulthood (Takahashi, 1993). Fewer than 1–2% of the patients succumb to sudden death due to coronary artery thrombosis or aneurysm rupture with subsequent acute myocardial infarctions (responsible for 80% of the deaths), myopericarditis, congestive heart failure, and/or arrhythmia.

Half the patients may have electrocardiographic abnormalities (first-degree atrioventricular block, or sinus tachycardia, but rarely ventricular arrhythmia). Myocarditis and pericarditis are rare, occurring in half and 25% of the patients with cardiac complications during the initial phase of the disease, respectively.

Mitral insufficiency has been observed in less than 1% of the cases and aortic regurgitation even less frequently.

3.4 Small Vessel Vasculitides

3.4.1 Granulomatosis With Polyangiitis

GPA, formerly Wegener granulomatosis, is a necrotizing vasculitis of medium and small size vessels with granulomatous lesions classically involving the upper and lower respiratory tract and the kidneys. Evidence of C-ANCA detected in the sera of more than 80% of WG patients with systemic forms (Kallenberg et al., 1992), is useful in making the diagnosis.

Symptomatic heart involvement is seen in a small percentage of patients with GPA. Pericarditis and arrhythmias are the most commonly reported abnormalities, occurring in 1–6% of patients (Fig. 14.3A). Coronary arteritis, aortic regurgitation, and aortic valvular lesions simulating endocarditis have also been reported. Arrhythmias tend to be supraventricular and are hypothesized to occur as a result of sinus node dysfunction, which may be secondary to pericardial inflammation (Forstot et al., 1980). Involvement of the conduction system structures is uncommon, although atrioventricular block has been reported (Eisen et al., 2009).

Myocarditis, coronary arteritis, and cardiac thrombus are less frequent manifestations, each occurring in less than 1–2% of patients. Valvular lesions (mainly aortic) are rare, but histological examination can demonstrate specific lesions, with polymorphous microabscesses with minute and remarkable geographic necrosis and granulomatous inflammation. Subclinical cardiac involvement, however, may be much more frequent. In an echocardiographic study of patients with GPA, 31% were found to have abnormalities attributable to vasculitis or granulomatosis. Of these, wall motion defects were seen in 65% of patients, decreased left ventricular ejection fraction in 50%, pericardial effusions in 19%, and valvular lesions in 15% (Oliveira et al., 2005).

Coronary arteritis, as in PAN, is clinically silent in most GPA patients, but can nonetheless be responsible for foci of myocardial infarcts and eventually lead to congestive heart failure, with left ventricular systolic dysfunction detected echocardiographically in 22% of the patients (Morelli et al., 2000).

GPA is a vasculitis of small- and medium-sized and vessels and therefore involvement of the aorta and its proximal branches is not expected. However, they, as well as the more distal branches such as iliac or popliteal arteries (Allen et al., 1984) can sometimes be involved, causing proximal dilatation (Grant et al., 1994), dissection (Blockmans et al., 2000), or thickening (Fink et al., 1994; Goodfield et al., 1995).

3.4.2 Eosinophilic Granulomatosis With Polyangiitis

EGPA, formerly Churg-Strauss syndrome, is an eosinophil-rich necrotizing vasculitis of small-to-medium blood vessels (Jennette et al., 2013), with an incidence of 2–4 cases per million patients per year in the UK (Watts et al., 2000). Diagnostic criteria require the presence of any four or more of the following: asthma, eosinophilia greater than 10%, neuropathy, pulmonary infiltrates, paranasal sinus abnormality, or extravascular eosinophils (Masi et al., 1990). Prognosis is usually good, with 91% of patients achieving remission, 25% relapsing, and 11% dying from complications of vasculitis, although Guillevin et al. (1999b) showed that the strongest predictors of poor outcome are cardiac involvement, severe gastrointestinal disease, and proteinuria greater than 1 g/day (Hemmett et al., 2015).

Cardiac involvement is well documented in EGPA with a widely varying incidence of 17–92% depending on the diagnostic modality used for diagnosis, including postmortem examination. Recent reviews showed a prevalence of 60% after detailed cardiac evaluation using cardiac MRI (Dennert et al., 2010; Marmursztejn et al., 2009).

Recently, a distinction between ANCA-positive and ANCA-negative EGPA has been emphasized, the first being significantly associated with renal involvement, peripheral neuropathy, and biopsy-proven vasculitis, whereas the latter is associated with cardiac involvement.

Histologically, myocardial damage is rarely caused by small-vessel vasculitis but rather by the in situ production of toxic mediators, thus supporting the phenotypic differences between ANCA-positive and ANCA-negative EGPA.

Any cardiac structure can be involved, and patients present with myocarditis, heart failure, pericarditis, arrhythmia, coronary arteritis, valvulopathy, and intracavitary cardiac thrombosis. Although cardiovascular involvement is usually an early manifestation, it can also occur later in the course of the disease.

A significant proportion of patients with cardiac involvement are asymptomatic. In the absence of symptoms and major ECG abnormalities, cardiac involvement may be detected in nearly 40% of the patients. All patients with EGPA should be studied not only with a detailed history of cardiac symptoms and ECG, but also with echocardiography; if abnormalities are detected, a cardiac magnetic resonance study should be performed. Coronary angiography and endomyocardial biopsy should be reserved to selected cases.

Pulmonary hypertension secondary to concomitant pulmonary involvement may also induce right ventricular dysfunction. Moreover, heart failure associated with dilatative cardiomyopathy is possible but uncommon, and only few cases have been described.

Cardiomyopathy may result from vasculitis-related ischemia affecting small myocardial vessels and coronary arteries (Hellemans et al., 1997), from myocardial eosinophilic infiltration sometimes followed by fibrotic scar tissue or, more rarely, from granulomatous infiltration of the myocardium (Cohen et al., 1995).

Many features of EGPA cardiomyopathy are shared with eosinophilic endomyocardiopathy, which includes different pathologies: idiopathic hypereosinophilic syndrome, hypersensitivity myocarditis, Loeffler disease and endomyocardial fibrosis, transplant rejection, giant cell myocarditis, toxic myocarditis, parasitic infections, eosinophilic leukemias, T-cell lymphomas, and carcinomas (Pearce et al., 1999). During the first stage of these eosinophilic cardiomyopathies, eosinophils infiltrate the tissue and the proteins (major basic protein, cationic protein, eosinophil-derived neurotoxin) they release induce local toxic reactions (Tai et al., 1984; Terasaki et al., 1997) that potentially evolve to scarring and fibrosis. However, EGPA is distinguished from idiopathic hypersensitivity syndrome by its less intense eosinophilic infiltration, less frequent fibrosis, and the presence of myocardial foci of necrosis and angiitis.

Acute and chronic constrictive pericarditis, valvular disease, and sudden cardiac arrest are other known features of heart involvement in EGPA (Azzopardi et al., 1999).

Pericardial effusion occurs in up to 22% of EGPA patients. Tamponade has been reported and is usually easily controlled with corticosteroids, but may have a relapsing course (Hasley et al., 1990). Pericardial biopsy or pericardiectomy may show granulomatous nodules in the epicardium and can serve as the basis for a histological diagnosis of EGPA (Sharma et al., 1993).

Echocardiography may show wall-motion abnormalities, signs of pericarditis, or intraventricular thrombus. Coronary abnormalities can be ruled out by left-heart catheterization. Cardiac MRI provides a detailed anatomic description of the lesions; both first-pass deficits and late gadolinium enhancements are suitable to detect myocarditis and myocardial fibrosis. Therefore, active inflammation and fibrous changes are difficult to differentiate. Cardiac MRI anomalies were also described in patients with no clinical symptoms and otherwise normal cardiac work-up, but the clinical and therapeutic implications of such findings are not clear.

In 32 patients with EGPA Dennert observed no relationship between the duration of EGPA, prior corticosteroid or immunosuppressive therapy, and cardiac manifestations. Seventy-four percent of ANCA-negative patients showed cardiac involvement, and wall motion disturbances were the most frequent finding in up to 64% of the patients. In contrast, cardiac abnormalities could be detected in only 23% of ANCA-positive patients (Dennert et al., 2010).

Pathology findings suggest that myocardial fibrosis develops rapidly during the course of EGPA; consequently, immediate and aggressive immunosuppressant treatment might be indicated to prevent chronic heart failure. Whereas there are reports of partial and complete recovery of left ventricular function in patients treated with corticosteroid monotherapy or combination of corticosteroid with cytotoxic agents, it appears that patients treated with cytotoxic agents have better responses as compared with those treated with corticosteroid alone.

Although steroids and immunosuppressants may be effective during the early stages of EGPA myocarditis, fibrosis or residual cardiac insufficiency may thereafter progress on their own and require heart transplantation. The results of heart engraftments in EGPA have been mitigated: in two transplanted patients, one recipient had no EGPA recurrence, but died of infectious complications 3 years post-transplant (Yeatman et al., 1996) and EGPA reappeared either in the transplanted heart (Henderson et al., 1993) or at extracardiac sites (Thomson et al., 1989) despite potent immunosuppression in the other patients.

3.4.3 Microscopic Polyangiitis

MPA was classified by the Chapel Hill Consensus Conference as an ANCA-associated necrotizing small-sized vessel vasculitis, with little or no immune-complex deposition, that primarily affects the kidneys and lungs.

Medium-sized arteries might be concerned, even though the disease is predominantly considered to involve small-sized arteries, arterioles, capillaries, and venules.

Involvement of small vessels of the heart is quite rare. MPA-associated cardiac insufficiency is found in approximately 10% of the patients. Pericarditis is equally rare. Among 85 French MPA patients, respective heart failure and/or pericarditis rates were 17.6% and 10%. Severe, acute, congestive heart failure was reported, but rarely with documented myocardial infarction due to myocardial or coronary small vessel arteritis. However, subclinical myocardial infarctions may be more frequent, as in PAN and other small vessel vasculitides (Villiger and Guillevin, 2010).

MPA with lung and kidney involvement appears to be associated with P-ANCA whereas heart involvement may be more frequent in ANCA-negative patients (Wang et al., 2002) as in EGPA.

3.4.4 Henoch-Schönlein Purpura

HSP is the most common of the systemic vasculitides and affects people of all ages, but is mainly a disease of children under 10 years. It is characterized by leukocytoclastic vasculitis, affecting the skin, kidney, joints, and gastrointestinal tract.

Cardiac involvement is not recognized as a feature of HSP, with only isolated cases described, but can be severe, even if it generally responds to immunosuppressive therapy.

Subclinical cardiac involvement can be hypothesized by the observation of deposits of IgA and C3 in intramyocardial vessel walls, resolving after immunosuppressive therapy (Kereiakes et al., 1984). Myocardial infarction (Agraharkar et al., 2000), conduction abnormalities, and/or congestive heart failure (Polizzotto et al., 2006) have also been described.

3.4.5 Cryoglobulinemic Vasculitis

Cryoglobulinemic vasculitis is one of the most important extrahepatic manifestations of HCV chronic infection. Vasculitis and other extrahepatic HCV-related manifestations are recently included in so-called HCV syndrome (Fig. 14.5). More than 80% of the cases of mixed cryoglobulinemia are now attributed to HCV infection (Ferri et al., 1991b; Rieu et al., 2002). Cardiac manifestations are reported in 4–8% of patients with cryoglobulinemic vasculitis. Pericarditis, myocardial ischemia, and acute heart failure, the usual presenting syndromes, are caused by immune complex–mediated vasculitis (Terrier et al., 2013).

Congestive heart failure may be seen in up to 30% of the patients, even though myocardial infarction is often clinically silent, concerning less than 8.5% of the patients, and rarely diagnosed during the patients' lifetime (Rieu et al., 2002). Other cardiovascular manifestations, such as hypertrophic

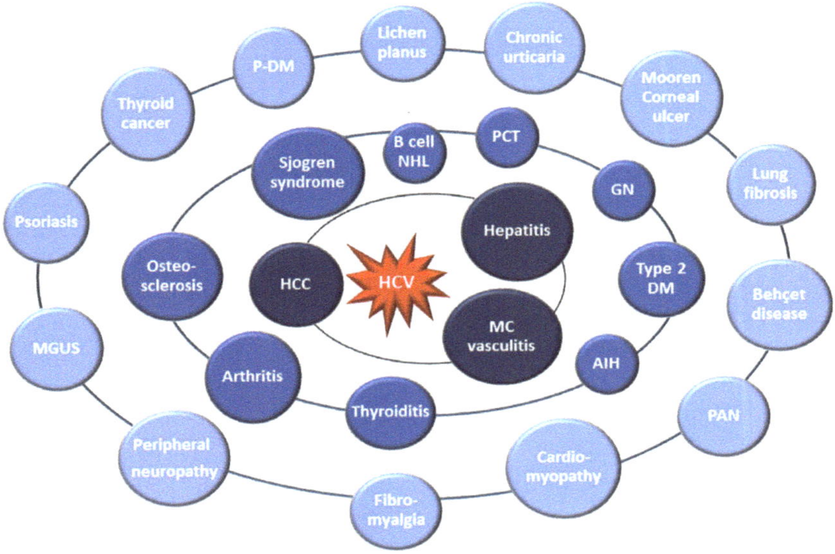

FIGURE 14.5 **Clinical manifestations of HCV.** The spectrum of different HCV-associated immunological and neoplastic disorders may be classified on the basis of clinicoepidemiological, histopathological, and molecular biology studies, into three different levels: (1) high: the association with HCV infection has been largely demonstrated and HCV infection is one of the major triggering agents of the disease; (2) medium: the disease shows a significantly higher prevalence of HCV infection compared to controls; (3) low: the possible association is suggested by limited clinicoepidemiological observations. *AIH*, autoimmune hepatitis; *B cell NHL*, B cell non-Hodgkin lymphoma; *GN*, glomerulonephritis; *HCC*, hepatocellular carcinoma; *HCV*, hepatitis C virus, MC *vasculitis*, mixed cryoglobulinemia vasculitis; *MGUS*, monoclonal gammopathy of undetermined significance; *PAN*, polyarteritis nodosa; *PCT*, porphyria cutanea tarda; *P-DM*, poly- and dermatomyositis; *Type 2 DM*, type 2 diabetes mellitus.

myocardiopathy, have been reported in HCV-infected patients, mainly in series from countries of eastern Asia (Matsumori, 2005).

3.5 Other Vasculitic Diseases

3.5.1 Behçet Disease

Behçet disease involves widespread vasculitis with recurrent oral and genital ulcers and ocular symptoms as well as musculoskeletal, neurological, cardiac, pulmonary, and gastrointestinal system involvement. The disease is generally seen in the third and fourth decades; it is rare for the disease to occur during adolescence or after the age of 40 years. The prevalence in males and females differs according to the region. In countries of the Middle East, the disease is seen more among males, whereas it is more frequent among females in the countries of North Europe and the United States (Saadoun and Wechsler, 2012).

Cardiovascular involvement in Behçet disease ranges from 7% to 46%, with vasculitis lesions affecting both veins and arteries of all sizes. Cardiac involvement may occur in the form of intracardiac thrombus, endocarditis, myocarditis, pericarditis, endomyocardial fibrosis, coronary arteritis, myocardial infarction, and valvular disease. Recently, some studies have demonstrated subclinical left ventricular dysfunction in the early stage of disease.

Cardiovascular manifestations occur within the first year after diagnosis in one-quarter of the cases and can even reveal the disease. Venous lesions (30% of the patients) are more common than arterial disease. Most arterial involvement is clinically silent (Lakhanpal et al., 1985; Wechsler et al., 1999). The main localizations are the abdominal aorta and the pulmonary arteries. Pulmonary artery aneurysms and/or thrombosis, with subsequent caval syndrome (Hughes-Stovin syndrome), may occur in 1.1% of the patients and carries a poor prognosis (Hamuryudan et al., 1994; Stricker and Malinverni, 1989).

Pericardial involvement has been reported as the most common manifestation of cardiac involvement in some series (Bletry et al., 1988). The clinical presentation may be acute pericarditis, hemorrhagic pericardial tamponade, constrictive pericarditis, recurrent pericarditis, or asymptomatic pericardial effusion (Okcun et al., 2003). Endomyocardial involvement typically manifests as endomyocardial fibrosis on the right and/or left side of the heart.

Intracardiac thrombus is a frequently reported serious complication of Behçet disease and it is especially common in Middle Eastern and Mediterranean countries. Intracardiac thrombosis is more commonly seen in young adults, and sometimes is the first manifestation of disease (Mendes et al., 1994).

Coronary arteries are involved in 33% of patients with cardiac manifestations (Bletry et al., 1988), including occlusions, stenoses, aneurysms, or spasms. Coronary thrombosis arteritis has been also histologically documented (Lakhanpal et al., 1985).

The prognosis of cardiac lesions is poorer than that of lesions in others organs involved in Behçet disease, but anticoagulation, immunosuppressant agents, and colchicine seem to improve the prognosis of these patients (Hatemi et al., 2008).

3.5.2 Buerger Disease

Thromboangiitis obliterans, or Buerger disease, was found in 0.5–5% of hospitalized patients with arterial occlusive disease in Europe and up to 16% of patients in Japan. It can affect all races (Horton, 1988).

Since 1966 less than 20 patients with coronary arteries or myocardium involvement have been described. Coronary angiography revealed predominant involvement of the left anterior descending and right coronary arteries;

one patient presented a normal arteriography. Coronary involvement may be seen only as another clinical consequence of tobacco toxicity, known to be the leading causative factor of this disease (Joyce, 1990; Shionoya, 1993; Somer, 1993).

3.5.3 Cogan Syndrome

Cogan syndrome is a rare idiopathic chronic inflammatory disease of the eye and the inner ear in young adults. There is no predisposition for race or gender. The characteristics of Cogan syndrome are nonsyphilitic interstitial keratitis and audiovestibular dysfunction resembling Ménière disease. Systemic nonspecific features (fever, fatigue, weight loss, lymphadenopathy, arthritis, and urticarial) are frequent, while in 15–20% of patients with Cogan syndrome, there are overt signs of systemic vasculitis. The vasculitis mainly involves small, medium-sized, and/or large vessels (Vollertsen et al., 1986). Aortitis is described in 10% of patients and can lead to proximal aorta dilation, aortic valvular regurgitation, ostial coronary artery involvement, and thoracoabdominal aneurysms. Aortitis is usually associated with ostium coronary artery stenosis.

Distal coronary artery stenoses and aneurysms, pericarditis, and conductive heart tissue involvement have also been reported (Cochrane and Tatoulis, 1991).

3.6 Hypersensitivity Myocarditis

Hypersensitivity myocarditis is relatively rare. Its clinical signs are nonspecific, occur in the setting of generalized drug reactions with eosinophilia, and can mimic vasculitis. Among many drugs that have been linked to the development of hypersensitivity myocarditis, the main ones include: sulfonamides, methyldopa, and penicillins, which are incriminated in 75% of cases (Kounis et al., 1989). Prior uneventful exposure to the suspected medication is one of the criteria for diagnosing hypersensitivity myocarditis. Clinical and in vivo recognition of eosinophilic myocarditis is infrequent, whereas it accounts for up to 0.5% of unselected myocarditis autopsy series (Ginsberg and Parrillo, 2005; Kendell et al., 1995; Kounis et al., 1989). No vasculitis is seen and myocardial damage is usually less extensive than in EGPA.

The diagnosis of hypersensitivity myocarditis is suggested by the presence of signs and symptoms of drug hypersensitivity (rash, fever, eosinophilia) associated with nonspecific cardiac findings. These may include ECG changes, unexplained tachycardia, or serum cardiac enzyme elevations. Clinically the patient may present with symptoms of heart failure, ECG abnormalities such as nonspecific ST-T changes or sinus tachycardia, arrhythmias, or even sudden death. An endomyocardial biopsy remains the gold standard for diagnosis of myocarditis. However, this is a highly invasive procedure that is not routinely performed. Other noninvasive strategies include scintigraphy, contrast-enhanced MRI, and echocardiography. However, the diagnosis of myocarditis is still largely dependent on clinical suspicion rather than definitive diagnostic tests.

After withdrawal of the responsible medication, the majority of the patients recover in a few days without sequelae. Immunosuppressive treatment may, however, be required when cardiac involvement is severe and/or because of late diagnosis.

4. EVOLUTION AND PROGNOSTIC FACTORS

Outcome of vasculitides largely varies among different diseases; the relapse rate also varies, from 5% for HBV-related PAN (Guillevin et al., 1995b) to 23.4% for EGPA (Guillevin et al., 1999b), 34.1% for MPA (Guillevin et al., 1999b), and more than 50% for GPA (Hoffman et al., 1992). However, the introduction of more recent drugs, such as rituximab, could bring significant change in the prognosis of these diseases. Cardiac involvement may dramatically worsen the prognosis, particularly for EGPA patients. Death due to acute heart failure, arrhythmia, or massive myocardial infarction can occur during the initial acute phase, or later during the course of the disease, from refractory residual cardiac failure.

Cardiac, renal, gastrointestinal, and/or central nervous system involvements have been shown to be associated with poor outcome in 342 patients with PAN or EGPA (Guillevin et al., 1996). The five-factor score (FFS) is a prognostic score including all these parameters. Five-year mortality is 12% when FFS is null, 26% when FFS is 1, and 46% when FFS is 2 or more ($p < .001$). Application of the FFS to MPA patients has also been validated (Gayraud et al., 2001).

Birmingham vasculitis activity score (BVAS) (Luqmani et al., 1994; Stone et al., 2001), another scale aiming to assess the activity of systemic necrotizing vasculitis, also includes the cardiac involvement. Cardiac manifestations included in the BVAS are new loss of pulse(s) with/without threatened loss of limb, aortic incompetence, myocardial infarction/angina, cardiomyopathy, bruits, and pericarditis. However, because this score was designed only to reflect the severity and current extent of active disease in patients, its use should be restricted to the evaluation of therapeutic efficacy, primarily in trials.

Finally, the vasculitis damage index (VDI) (Exley et al., 1997) has been developed to assess organ damage in systemic necrotizing vasculitides. It includes some cardiovascular manifestations, namely angina/coronary bypass, myocardial infarction, second myocardial infarction, cardiomyopathy, valvular disease, pericarditis, and hypertension.

5. TREATMENT

In combination with symptomatic therapies (e.g., angiotensin inhibitors, angiotensin II-receptor blockers, antiarrhythmic drugs, anticoagulants) or cardiac surgery (valve replacement, pericardiectomy) when needed, specific treatments for these vasculitides have to be used in patients with vasculitis and cardiovascular involvement. Before the introduction of corticosteroids (CS) in the 1970s, survival was 10% for untreated PAN patients (Frohnert and Sheps, 1967). Since then, it has increased to 55% with the use of CS alone, and to 82% at 5 years with combined CS and immunosuppressive therapy (Guillevin et al., 1988; Leib et al., 1979). Therapeutic decisions to treat and with which agents should rely on the presence or not of a poor prognosis at FFS.

5.1 Large Vessel Vasculitides

5.1.1 Giant Cell Arteritis

Treatment of GCA, with or without large vessel disease, is principally based upon high-dose corticosteroids with the dose titrated according to symptoms and inflammatory indices. A dose of 40–60 mg/day is usually accepted for the first 2 weeks before a slow taper (maximum of 10% reduction every one to 2 weeks) according to response with a total treatment time of 2 years. Initial intravenous pulse methylprednisolone (1000 mg every day for 3 days) can be tried in patients with recent or impending visual loss. CS may prevent, but usually do not reverse fixed visual loss.

The response to CS is rapid, with resolution of many symptoms after a few days of therapy. A gradual tapering of 10% of the total every 4 weeks should be evaluated after 2–4 weeks from the beginning of the treatment. A relapse can occur when the CS dose is reduced or withdrawn too quickly. However, in about 30–50% of the patients, spontaneous disease exacerbations occur, more frequently in the first 2 years, independent of the CS reduction schedule (Salvarani et al., 1987). No consistently reliable predictors of duration of CS therapy have been found.

Even despite apparently effective steroid therapy, there is some evidence that a high risk of thoracic aortic complication persists in the GCA patient. Among 5 of 13 patients previously requiring ascending aortic surgery developed, or showed progression of, aneurysmal change in the remaining aorta during follow-up despite medical therapy (Zehr et al., 2005).

CS-sparing agents have been tried, such as methotrexate, azathioprine, dapsone, hydroxychloroquine, or tumor necrosis factor alpha (TNFα) blockers, with inconstant results (De Silva and Hazleman, 1986; Jover et al., 2001; Mahr et al., 2007).

The only immunosuppressant with proven benefits in this situation is methotrexate, which has been reported to diminish both the cumulative corticosteroid dosage and the relapse risk (Salvarani et al., 2002). However, this drug may be added in patients who need high CS doses to control active disease and have developed major side effects or when a relapse occurs.

A recent pilot study found that infliximab was efficacious in patients with CS-resistant GCA (Cantini et al., 2001).

Cyclophosphamide (CYC) has been proposed in CS-dependent GCA or for patients suffering from the iatrogenic effects of CS. Several case reports also highlight that CYC has been successfully used in life-threatening or severe GCA, for example, with central nervous system or digestive involvement (de Boysson et al., 2013).

Three randomized clinical trials investigated the efficacy of anti-TNFα drugs in GCA, two enrolling patients with newly diagnosed GCA (Hoffman et al., 2007; Seror et al., 2014), the third one enrolling patients with long-standing GCA (Martínez-Taboada et al., 2008). These studies globally showed a marginal role for anti-TNFα in patients with recent onset disease, while anti-TNF biologic agents could have a role in relapsing, long-standing GCA.

Balloon angioplasty has been widely described for treatment of stenoses and occlusions owing to TA and GCA. The balloon sizing should be conservative to avoid vessel dissection or rupture. Stents are rarely needed and should only be employed for the management of a flow-limiting dissection or significant vessel recoil and should be avoided in younger patients. Stents may be needed in older patients with GCA who may have concomitant atherosclerotic disease.

No clear evidences are available for the timing of elective surgical repair of GCA-related disease; therefore, current criteria for elective intervention are based on the strategies applied to other noninfective disease processes, such as arteriosclerotic disease (Isselbacher, 2005). The same principles should be applied for aortic valvular disease and any combination of potentially affected structures.

5.1.2 Takayasu's Arteritis

Treatment of TAK arteritis aims to contrast the ischemic manifestations, reducing vascular surgery and bypass procedures. CS are still the mainstay of treatment for TAK arteritis.

However, despite a frequent initial disease remission, relapses and CS dependence are observed in more than 60% of patients (Kötter et al., 2012). More than half of the patients need a combination therapy to achieve a sustained remission with low-dose CS.

In these cases, immunosuppression may also be required, and might include cyclophosphamide or methotrexate (Hoffman et al., 1994). Recently, some retrospective studies have showed that anti-TNFα drugs are able to induce remission in the majority (70–90%) of TAK patients unable to achieve or maintain remission with CS and synthetic immunosuppressants alone (Comarmond et al., 2012). However, about half of the patients who achieve remission will have further relapse(s), thereby implying the need for long-term therapy in some patients.

5.2 Medium-Sized and Small Vessel Vasculitides

5.2.1 Kawasaki Disease

Intravenous immunoglobulin and aspirin remain the first-line standard initial therapy. Although the mechanism of action of intravenous immunoglobulins is unknown, a single dose of 2 g/kg, given over 10–12 h, together with high-dose oral aspirin (80–100 mg/kg/day) within 10 days of fever onset results in rapid resolution of clinical symptoms in 80–90% of patients and has been shown to reduce the risk of coronary disease from 20–25% to about 2–4% (Newburger et al., 1991). Aspirin should be decreased to 3–5 mg/kg/day with long-term maintenance therapy in patients who have developed coronary aneurysms (Leung et al., 1998). Two recent important Japanese studies evaluated the utility of adjunctive steroids as initial therapy in "high-risk" patients (Ogata et al., 2012; Kobayashi et al., 2012). In selected, nonresponder patients, infliximab, methotrexate, or cyclosporine could be proposed (Burns et al., 2008; Suzuki et al., 2011; Lee et al., 2008). Coronary angioplasty, endoarterial procedures, or coronary bypass surgery may be needed in severe progressing forms (Sugimura et al., 1997).

5.2.2 Primary Systemic Necrotizing Vasculitides

The introduction of CS and cyclophosphamide transformed more necrotizing vasculitides from a fatal to a largely treatable condition. Over the past 40 years, considerable progress has been made in optimize immunosuppressive regimens with a significant increase of safety.

Recently, anti-CD20 antibody rituximab has been approved for the treatment of ANCA-associated vasculitis, increasing the therapeutic options. Rituximab is also superior to cyclophosphamide for maintaining remission. Blocking the C5a-receptor seems promising as well as an alternative for high-dose corticosteroids during induction of remission.

5.2.3 Corticosteroids

Despite there are no randomized controlled trials to support their use, CS remain the first choice for all necrotizing vasculitides with cardiac manifestations. Evidence is also lacking to guide dosage and overall duration of therapy, but usually initial therapy includes 1–3 days of methylprednisolone pulse (15 mg/kg/day), followed by high-dose oral prednisone (at least 1 mg/kg/day). This full oral dose should be maintained until clinical and biological improvement is achieved, generally within 1 month, and then gradually tapered over 12–18 months.

5.2.4 Cyclophosphamide

CYC was introduced empirically for induction treatment of ANCA associated vasculitis over 40 years ago, and remains one of the two recommended induction strategies (alongside rituximab) for patients with severe disease. Fauci et al. (1979) demonstrated the efficacy of adjunctive CYC in patients whose vasculitides were not controlled with CS alone. Pulse intravenous CYC should be combined with CS for patients with PAN, MPA, or EGPA and a high FFS, like those with cardiomyopathy and every patient with systemic GPA.

Pulse therapy acts more rapidly and engenders fewer side effects (hemorrhagic cystitis, leukopenia) than oral administration. However, oral CYC is also effective as first-line therapy for GPA, and may nonetheless achieve remission in patients who did not respond to the pulse CYC regimen (Gayraud et al., 1997; Reinhold-Keller et al., 1993). Doses, intervals between pulses, and duration of CYC treatment have to be adjusted for each patient. Briefly, each CYC pulse (0.5–0.7 mg/m^2) is administered every 15 days for the first three boluses, then every 3 weeks (for GPA and MPA), or monthly (for PAN and EGPA). When preferred (in GPA) or needed (e.g., after failure of pulse CYC), oral CYC (2 mg/kg/day) should be prescribed.

To reduce exposure and cumulative toxicity of CYC, sequential therapy with azathioprine, mycophenolate mofetil, or methotrexate is frequently prescribed (Walsh et al., 2014; Faurschou et al., 2012; Hiemstra et al., 2010). Moreover, methotrexate was also proposed as induction therapy (De Groot et al., 2005).

Anyway, in long-term follow-up, less cyclophosphamide was associated with a higher risk of relapse, and methotrexate was associated with less-effective disease control, although ultimately there was no increase in mortality or long-term morbidity.

In patients with cardiac dysfunction, hydration during pulse CYC administration has to be carefully monitored. However, the potential but rarely reported cardiac side effects of CYC (Gharib and Burnett, 2002; Hochster et al., 1995) must definitely not prevent its use in patients with specific cardiomyopathy, because CYC is clearly the most effective drug used to date. It has been shown that delaying treatment can favor the progression to myocardial infarction, intractable cardiac failure, and eventual myocardial fibrosis in EGPA patients with heart involvement. Conversely, the rare cases of valvulitis occurring in the context of GPA have been reported to respond to therapy (Gerbracht et al., 1987), as conductive heart blocks, even though a pacemaker might be needed temporarily (Forstot et al., 1980; Handa et al., 1997; Schiavone et al., 1985; Suleymenlar et al., 2002).

5.2.5 Rituximab

Rituximab is an unconjugated chimeric monoclonal IgG1κ antibody against CD20, a transmembrane protein exclusively expressed by B cells. CD20 is expressed by mature B cells, but not by stem cells, early B-cell precursors, or plasma cells. Rituximab has become a valuable alternative treatment for necrotizing vasculitides and it has been approved for the treatment of MPA or GPA by several international regulatory agencies. Two randomized controlled trials have independently shown its noninferiority to CYC in severe newly diagnosed or relapsing MPA or GPA (Jones et al., 2010; Stone et al., 2010). There is also growing evidence of efficacy in eosinophilic GPA patients (Muñoz et al., 2015).

CYC and rituximab showed similar efficacy in patients with renal involvement, irrespective of diagnosis or antibody specificity (Geetha et al., 2015). In PR3-ANCA patients, rituximab was superior to cyclophosphamide and noninferior in MPO-ANCA patients (Sanders et al., 2006). Whereas vasculitic manifestations responded well to rituximab treatment, significantly lower response rates were seen in granulomatous manifestations, in particular in cases with orbital masses.

The available evidence provides some guidance for the choice of treatment in the individual patient. It may be reasonable to treat young patients with fertility concerns, relapsing patients, and PR3-positive GPA patients with rituximab rather than with cyclophosphamide. Rituximab demonstrated also to be able to reverse myocarditis with atrioventricular block in a GPA patient (Brihaye et al., 2008).

However, the long-term efficacy of rituximab remains to be further characterized, and the established long-standing experience with cyclophosphamide as an effective remission-inducing drug justifies its further use, in particular in areas of uncertainty, such as life-threatening disease, ANCA-negative disease, or severe granulomatous disease.

5.2.6 Other Therapies

Plasma exchanges may be useful as second-line therapy for refractory PAN or MPA with rapidly progressive glomerulonephritis (Guillevin and Bussel, 2000; Pusey et al., 1991), but are contraindicated for patients with unstable cardiac conditions. Other immunosuppressants (methotrexate, azathioprine, mycophenolate mofetil) should preferentially be kept for maintenance therapy, when indicated, that is, for GPA and MPA, or PAN and EPGA with multiple relapses (De Groot et al., 1996; Nowack et al., 1999).

Other biologic drugs than rituximab have been evaluated useful for patients with intractable vasculitides, in particular anti-TNFα antibodies (Bartolucci et al., 2002), but they should be carefully monitored since these antibodies are theoretically contraindicated in patients with coronary artery disease and/or heart failure (Weisman, 2002). Abatacept, in addition to CS and azathioprine, methotrexate, or mycophenolate mofetil, was safe and effective in a small number of patients and allowed to discontinued CS in 11/15 patients (Langford et al., 2014). Because they can prevent aneurysms formation in Kawasaki disease, it may be expected that parenteral immunoglobulins would also be effective in ANCA-associated vasculitides. First reports of their use in patients with refractory vasculitides have yielded encouraging but mixed results (Jayne et al., 1991, 2000).

5.2.7 Virus-Related Vasculitides

When vasculitides are related to viral infection, a specific approach is needed, combining antiviral treatments and plasma exchanges.

5.2.7.1 Hepatitis B Virus-Related Polyarteritis Nodosa

Current therapeutic approaches consider treating mild forms of primary PAN (with FFS = 0) with prednisone at doses of 1 mg/kg/day and subsequent tapering when remission is achieved (Ribi et al., 2010) and in life-threatening situations or rapidly progressive disease, therapy with intravenous CS pulses. When prednisone cannot be tapered below 15−20 mg/day without recurrence or in presence of critical organ involvement indicated by an FFS $\geq$ 1, immunosuppressants are given in addition to CS; usually orally or intravenous CYC (1000 mg/day of 6-methylprednisolone for 3 days) may be tried (Guillevin et al., 2003). After the induction of the remission with CYC, azathioprine or methotrexate are advised to maintain remission. Surgery may be required only for some disease complications, such as perforation/rupture, ischemia, or hemorrhage of the gastrointestinal organs or kidneys (Pagnoux et al., 2005).

In patients with HBV-associated vasculitis, combination of short corticosteroid treatment with plasma exchanges and antiviral therapy, such as lamivudine or entecavir, may be effective in controlling disease activity and in facilitating viral seroconversion. Contrarily to idiopathic or primary PAN, relapses are rare in HBV-related PAN and never occur when viral replication has ceased and seroconversion has been achieved (Pagnoux et al., 2010). Although the existing experience is more limited, the same approach (short glucocorticoid treatment followed by specific antiviral therapy) may be suitable for other virus-associated PAN.

5.2.7.2 Hepatitis C Virus-Related Mixed Cryoglobulinemic Vasculitis

A correct strategy should deal with two concomitant factors: HCV infection and autoimmune disorder. Considering the HCV as triggering and possibly perpetuating agent of the cryoglobulinemic vasculitis through a chronic trigger on the immune system, HCV eradication treatment should be attempted in all patients with HCV infection. The long-term effects of HCV eradication need to be deeply investigated, particularly the outcome of HCV-related immunological alterations, including cryoglobulinemia and its clinical manifestations. Immunosuppression with rituximab or CYC represents the pathogenetic treatment of patients with vasculitis (Ferri et al., 2011). These treatments also include steroids, low antigen content diet, and plasma exchange (Durand et al., 1998; Pietrogrande et al., 2011; Guillevin and Bussel, 2000). Immunosuppressants are typically reserved for patients with severe disease features, such as MPGN, sensory-motor neuropathy, and life-threatening complications.

5.2.8 Henoch-Schönlein Purpura

Patients with HSP and cardiac involvement must receive at least CS. Anecdotal data show that cytotoxic immunosuppressive therapy may prevent infarction and a deleterious outcome (Osman and McCreery, 2000). In a case report, treatment with steroids/cyclophosphamide has proved effective in severe HSP with multiple organ involvement (Lutz et al., 2009).

5.3 Other Vasculitides

5.3.1 Behçet Disease

Pharmacological agents used for the treatment of Behçet disease include CS, colchicine, azathioprine, and anti-TNFα drugs. Pericarditis has always been treated with aspirin and immunosuppressive agents (Godeau et al., 1980). Because of the high frequency of thromboses, anticoagulants are widely prescribed, sometimes associated to CS and immunosuppressants. CS, colchicine, or immunosuppressive drugs have been proposed for the treatment of myocardial involvement, almost always associated with endomyocarditis (Geri et al., 2012). High-dose prednisolone and azathioprine can be used, along with the routine treatment of cardiac failure. Prognosis in these patients becomes better with early diagnosis and intense immunosuppressive treatment. Coronary artery aneurysms seem to carry a poorer prognosis than stenoses and may therefore warrant immunosuppression. Valve disease and myocardial dysfunction(s) may resolve with CS alone.

5.3.2 Buerger Disease

The only definitive therapy for Buerger disease is smoking cessation. In one study, 94% of patients who quit smoking avoided limb amputation. Of the patients who continued to smoke, 43% had at least one amputation (Olin, 2000). Vasodilators may be used to treat peripheral disease, with anti-platelet-aggregating agents, such as aspirin, or anticoagulants. When cardiac ischemic manifestations occur, patients should be managed as for common coronary artery disease (Shionoya, 1993). There are no indications for CS or immunosuppressants used to treat this entity.

5.3.3 Cogan Syndrome

While ocular manifestations may sometimes be treated with topical CS alone, audiovestibular and systemic features of Cogan syndrome require systemic therapy. The first choices in immunosuppressive therapy are glucocorticoids (prednisolone 1 mg/kg). In case of treatment failure or corticosteroid-sparing therapy, other immunosuppressive drugs can be used such as cyclophosphamide, azathioprine, methotrexate, cyclosporine, mycophenolate mofetil, and TNFα blockers. Bypass surgery or aortic valve replacement may be necessary where there are severe ischemic symptoms or heart failure (Raza et al., 1998; Vollertsen et al., 1986).

6. CONCLUSIONS

Cardiac involvement can be observed in all primary vasculitides, but often it is unrecognized. Therefore, cardiovascular risk should be evaluated in all patients with vasculitis and a careful follow-up should be reserved to the patients at risk; since differential diagnosis with ischemic cardiomyopathies can be difficult, a multidisciplinary approach with cardiologist and radiologist should be taken in account in these patients.

Finally, since inflammatory and ischemic damage are not easily distinguishable, management of cardiac involvement should always consider immunosuppressant, heart failure, ischemia-targeted drugs, and surgery; the appropriated therapeutic approach should be evaluated in the single patient by rheumatologist and cardiologist.

REFERENCES

Agraharkar, M., Gokhale, S., Le, L., Rajaraman, S., Campbell, G.A., 2000. Cardiopulmonary manifestations of Henoch-Schönlein purpura. Am. J. Kidney Dis. 35, 319.

Allen, D.C., Doherty, C.C., O'Reilly, D.P., 1984. Pathology of the heart and the cardiac conduction system in Wegener's granulomatosis. Br. Heart J. 52, 674.

Azzopardi, C., Montefort, S., Mallia, C., 1999. Cardiac involvement and left ventricular failure in a patient with the Churg-Strauss syndrome. Adv. Exp. Med. Biol. 455, 547.

Balding, C.E., Howie, A.J., Drake-Lee, A.B., Savage, C.O., 2001. Th2 dominance in nasal mucosa in patients with Wegener's granulomatosis. Clin. Exp. Immunol. 125, 332.

Bartolucci, P., Ramanoelina, J., Cohen, P., Mahr, A., Godmer, P., Le Hello, C., Guillevin, L., 2002. Efficacy of the anti-TNF-alpha antibody infliximab against refractory systemic vasculitides: an open pilot study on 10 patients. Rheumatology (Oxford) 41, 1126.

Blétry, O., Godeau, P., Charpentier, G., Guillevin, L., Herreman, G., 1980. Cardiac manifestations of periarteritis nodosa. Incidence of non-hypertensive cardiomyopathy. Arch. Mal. Coeur. Vaiss. 73, 1027.

Bletry, O., Mohattane, A., Wechsler, B., Beaufils, P., Valère, P., Petit, J., Gourgon, R., Grosgogeat, Y., Godeau, P., 1988. Cardiac manifestations of Behcet's disease 12 cases. Presse Med. 17, 2388.

Blockmans, D., Baeyens, H., Van Loon, R., Lauwers, G., Bobbaers, H., 2000. Periaortitis and aortic dissection due to Wegener's granulomatosis. Clin. Rheumatol. 19, 161.

Brihaye, B., Aouba, A., Pagnoux, C., Vignaux, O., Le Hello, C., Guillevin, L., 2008. Rituximab reversed cardiac involvement of Wegener's granulomatosis: magnetic resonance imaging assessment. Presse Med. 37, 412–415.

Burns, J.C., Best, B.M., Mejias, A., Mahony, L., Fixler, D.E., Jafri, H.S., Melish, M.E., Jackson, M.A., Asmar, B.I., Lang, D.J., Connor, J.D., Capparelli, E.V., Keen, M.L.,

Mamun, K., Keenan, G.F., Ramilo, O., 2008. Infliximab treatment of intravenous immunoglobulin-resistant Kawasaki disease. J. Pediatr. 153, 833.
Cantini, F., Niccoli, L., Salvarani, C., Padula, A., Olivieri, I., 2001. Treatment of longstanding active giant cell arteritis with iniximab: report of four cases. Arthritis Rheum. 44, pp.2933.
Chan, T.M., Cheng, I.K., 1996. A prospective study on anti-endothelial cell antibodies in patients with systemic lupus erythematosus. Clin. Immunol. Immunopathol. 78, 41.
Chumbley, L.C., Harrison Jr., E.G., DeRemee, R.A., 1977. Allergic granulomatosis and angiitis (Churg-Strauss syndrome). Report and analysis of 30 cases. Mayo Clin. Proc. 52, 477.
Cochrane, A.D., Tatoulis, J., 1991. Cogan's syndrome with aortitis, aortic regurgitation, and aortic arch vessel stenosis. Ann. Thorac. Surg. 52, 1166.
Cohen, A., Johnson, N., Prier, A., Zerbib, E., Chauvel, C., Kaplan, G., Valty J., 1995. Segmental myocarditis in Churg-Strauss syndrome. Review of the literature apropos of a case. Rev. Med. Interne 16, 58 (in French).
Comarmond, C., Plaisier, E., Dahan, K., Mirault, T., Emmerich, J., Amoura, Z., Cacoub, P., Saadoun, D., 2012. Anti TNF-α in refractory Takayasu's arteritis: cases series and review of the literature. Autoimmun. Rev. 11, 678.
Corbera-Bellalta, M., Planas-Rigol, E., Lozano, E., Terrades-García, N., Alba, M.A., Prieto-González, S., García-Martínez, A., Albero, R., Enjuanes, A., Espígol-Frigolé, G., Hernández-Rodríguez, J., Roux-Lombard, P., Ferlin, W.G., Dayer, J.M., Kosco-Vilbois, M.H., Cid, M.C., 2016. Blocking interferon γ reduces expression of chemokines CXCL9, CXCL10 and CXCL11 and decreases macrophage infiltration in ex vivo cultured arteries from patients with giant cell arteritis. Ann. Rheum. Dis. 75, 1177.
Cormier, J.M., Cormier, F., Laridon, D., Vuong, P.N., 2000. Horton's disease and aortic aneurysm: coincidence or causality? 5 cases. J. Mal. Vasc. 25, 92 (in French).
Csernok, E., Trabandt, A., Muller, A., Wang, G.C., Moosig, F., Paulsen, J., Schnabel, A., Gross, W.L., 1999. Cytokine profiles in Wegener's granulomatosis: predominance of type 1 (Th1) in the granulomatous inflammation. Arthritis Rheum. 42, 742.
Davenport, A., Goodfellow, J., Goel, S., Maciver, A.G., Walker, P., 1994. Aortic valve disease in patients with Wegener's granulomatosis. Am. J. Kidney Dis. 24, 205.
Davies, D.J., Moran, J.E., Niall, J.F., Ryan, G.B., 1982. Segmental necrotising glomerulonephritis with antineutrophil antibody: possible arbovirus aetiology? Br. Med. J. (Clin. Res. Ed.) 285, 606.
de Boysson, H., Boutemy, J., Creveuil, C., Ollivier, Y., Letellier, P., Pagnoux, C., Bienvenu, B., 2013. Is there a place for cyclophosphamide in the treatment of giant-cell arteritis? A case series and systematic review. Semin. Arthritis Rheum. 43, pp.105.
De Groot, K., Rasmussen, N., Bacon, P.A., Tervaert, J.W., Feighery, C., Gregorini, G., et al., 2005. Randomized trial of cyclophosphamide versus methotrexate for induction of remission in early systemic antineutrophil cytoplasmic antibody-associated vasculitis. Arthritis Rheum. 52, 2461.
De Groot, K., Reinhold-Keller, E., Tatsis, E., Paulsen, J., Heller, M., Nolle, B., Gross, W.L., 1996. Therapy for the maintenance of remission in sixty-five patients with generalized Wegener's granulomatosis. Methotrexate versus trimethoprim/sulfamethoxazole. Arthritis Rheum. 39, 2052.
De Silva, M., Hazleman, B.L., 1986. Azathioprine in giant cell arteritis/polymyalgia. rheumatica: a double-blind study. Ann. Rheum. Dis. 45, 136.
Dennert, R.M., van Paassen, P., Schalla, S., Kuznetsova, T., Alzand, B.S., Staessen, J.A., Velthuis, S., Crijns, H.J., Tervaert, J.W., Heymans, S., 2010. Cardiac involvement in Churg-Strauss syndrome. Arthritis Rheum. 62, 627.
Durand, J.M., Cacoub, P., Lunel-Fabiani, F., Cosserat, J., Cretel, E., Kaplanski, G., Frances, C., Bletry, O., Soubeyrand, J., Godeau, P., 1998. Ribavirin in hepatitis C related cryoglobulinemia. J. Rheumatol. 25, 1115.

Eisen, A., Arnson, Y., Dovrish, Z., Hadary, R., Amital, H., 2009. Arrhythmias and conduction defects in rheumatological diseases—a comprehensive review. Semin. Arthritis Rheum. 39, 145.

Endo, M., Tomizawa, Y., Nishida, H., Aomi, S., Nakazawa, M., Tsurumi, Y., Kawana, M., Kasanuki, H., 2003. Angiographic findings and surgical treatments of coronary artery involvement in Takayasu arteritis. J. Thorac. Cardiovasc. Surg. 125, 570.

Evans, J.M., O'Fallon, W.M., Hunder, G.G., 1995. Increased incidence of aortic aneurysm and dissection in giant cell (temporal) arteritis. A population-based study. Ann. Intern. Med. 122, 502.

Ewert, B.H., Jennette, J.C., Falk, R.J., 1991. The pathogenic role of antineutrophil cytoplasmic autoantibodies. Am. J. Kidney Dis. 18, 188.

Exley, A.R., Bacon, P.A., Luqmani, R.A., Kitas, G.D., Gordon, C., Savage, C.O., Adu, D., 1997. Development and initial validation of the vasculitis damage index for the standardized clinical assessment of damage in the systemic vasculitides. Arthritis Rheum. 40, 371.

Falcini, F., Trapani, S., Turchini, S., Farsi, A., Ermini, M., Keser, G., Khamashta, M.A., Hughes, G.R., 1997. Immunological findings in Kawasaki disease: an evaluation in a cohort of Italian children. Clin. Exp. Rheumatol. 15, 685.

Falk, R.J., Jennette, J.C., 1988. Anti-neutrophil cytoplasmic autoantibodies with specificity for myeloperoxidase in patients with systemic vasculitis and idiopathic necrotizing and crescentic glomerulonephritis. N. Engl. J. Med. 318, 1651.

Fauci, A., Katz, P., Haynes, B., Wolff, S., 1979. Cyclophosphamide therapy of severe necrotizing vasculitis. N. Engl. J. Med. 301, 235—238.

Faurschou, M., Westman, K., Rasmussen, N., de Groot, K., Flossmann, O., Hoglund, P., et al., 2012. Brief report: long-term outcome of a randomized clinical trial comparing methotrexate to cyclophosphamide for remission induction in early systemic antineutrophil cytoplasmic antibody-associated vasculitis. Arthritis Rheum. 64, 3472.

Ferri, C., Marzo, E., Longombardo, G., Lombardini, F., Greco, F., Bombardieri, S., 1991a. Alpha-interferon in the treatment of mixed cryoglobulinemia patients. International Cancer Update. Focus on Interferon Alfa 2b. Cannes, France. November 1—4, 1990. Eur. J. Cancer 27, S81.

Ferri, C., Greco, F., Longombardo, G., Palla, P., Moretti, A., Marzo, E., Mazzoni, A., Pasero, G., Bombardieri, S., Highfield, P., 1991b. Association between hepatitis C virus and mixed cryoglobulinemia. Clin. Exp. Rheumatol. 9, 621.

Ferri, C., Cacoub, P., Mazzaro, C., Roccatello, D., Scaini, P., Sebastiani, M., Tavoni, A., Zignego, A.L., De Vita, S., 2011. Treatment with rituximab in patients with mixed cryoglobulinemia syndrome: results of multicenter cohort study and review of the literature. Autoimmun. Rev. 11, 48.

Fink, A.M., Miles, K.A., Wraight, E.P., 1994. Indium-111 labelled leucocyte uptake in aortitis. Clin. Radiol. 49, 863.

Flores-Suarez, L.F., Cabiedes, J., Villa, A.R., van der Woude, F.J., Alcocer-Varela, J., 2003. Prevalence of antineutrophil cytoplasmic autoantibodies in patients with tuberculosis. Rheumatology (Oxford) 42, 223.

Forstot, J.Z., Overlie, P.A., Neufeld, G.K., Harmon, C.E., Forstot, S.L., 1980. Cardiac complications of Wegener granulomatosis: a case report of complete heart block and review of the literature. Semin. Arthritis Rheum. 10, 148.

Frohnert, P., Sheps, S., 1967. Long term follow-up study of periarteritis nodosa. Am. J. Med. 43, 8.

Furuta, S., Cousins, C., Chaudhry, A., Jayne, D., 2015. Clinical features and radiological findings in large vessel vasculitis: are Takayasu arteritis and giant cell arteritis 2 different diseases or a single entity? J. Rheumatol. 42, 300.

Gayraud, M., Guillevin, L., Cohen, P., Lhote, F., Cacoub, P., Deblois, P., Godeau, B., Ruel, M., Vidal, E., Piontud, M., Ducroix, J.P., Lassoued, S., Christoforov, B., Babinet, P., 1997. Treatment of good-prognosis polyarteritis nodosa and Churg-Strauss syndrome: comparison of steroids and oral or pulse cyclophosphamide in 25 patients. French Cooperative Study Group for Vasculitides. Br. J. Rheumatol. 36, 1290.

Gayraud, M., Guillevin, L., Le Toumelin, P., Cohen, P., Lhote, F., Casassus, P., Jarousse, B., 2001. Long-term followup of polyarteritis nodosa, microscopic polyangiitis, and Churg-Strauss syndrome: analysis of four prospective trials including 278 patients. Arthritis Rheum. 44, 666.

Geetha, D., Specks, U., Stone, J.H., Merkel, P.A., Seo, P., Spiera, R., Langford, C.A., Hoffman, G.S., Kallenberg, C.G., St Clair, E.W., Fessler, B.J., Ding, L., Tchao, N.K., Ikle, D., Jepson, B., Brunetta, P., Fervenza, F.C., 2015. Rituximab versus cyclophosphamide for ANCA-associated vasculitis with renal involvement. J. Am. Soc. Nephrol. 26, 976.

Gerbracht, D.D., Savage, R.W., Scharff, N., 1987. Reversible valvulitis in Wegener's granulomatosis. Chest 92, 182.

Geri, G., Wechsler, B., Thi Huong du, L., Isnard, R., Piette, J.C., Amoura, Z., Resche-Rigon, M., Cacoub, P., Saadoun, D., 2012. Spectrum of cardiac lesions in Behcet disease: a series of 52 patients and review of the literature. Medicine 91, 25.

Gharib, M.I., Burnett, A.K., 2002. Chemotherapy-induced cardiotoxicity: current practice and prospects of prophylaxis. Eur. J. Heart Fail. 4, 235.

Ginsberg, F., Parrillo, J.E., 2005. Eosinophilic myocarditis. Heart Fail. Clin 1, 419.

Girard, T., Mahr, A., Noël, L.H., Cordier, J.F., Lesavre, P., André, M.H., Guillevin, L., 2001. Are antineutrophil cytoplasmic antibodies a marker predictive of relapse in Wegener's granulomatosis? A prospective study. Rheumatology (Oxford) 40, 147.

Gisselbrecht, M., Cohen, P., Lortholary, O., Jarrousse, B., Gayraud, M., Gherardi, R., Baudrimont, M., Guillevin, L., 1997. HIV-related vasculitis: clinical presentation and therapeutic approach on six patients. AIDS 11, 121.

Gobel, U., Eichhorn, J., Kettritz, R., Briedigkeit, L., Sima, D., Lindschau, C., Haller, H., Luft, F.C., 1996. Disease activity and autoantibodies to endothelial cells in patients with Wegener's granulomatosis. Am. J. Kidney Dis. 28, 186.

Godeau, P., Wechsler, B., Maaouni, A., Fagard, M., Herreman, G., 1980. Cardiovascular involvement in Behcet's disease. Ann. Dermatol. Venereol. 107, 741.

Goodfield, N.E., Bhandari, S., Plant, W.D., Morley-Davies, A., Sutherland, G.R., 1995. Cardiac involvement in Wegener's granulomatosis. Br. Heart J. 73, 110.

Grant, S.C., Levy, R.D., Venning, M.C., Ward, C., Brooks, N.H., 1994. Wegener's granulomatosis and the heart. Br. Heart J. 71, 82.

Grayson, P.C., Maksimowicz-McKinnon, K., Clark, T.M., Tomasson, G., Cuthbertson, D., Carette, S., Khalidi, N.A., Langford, C.A., Monach, P.A., Seo, P., Warrington, K.J., Ytterberg, S.R., Hoffman, G.S., Merkel, P.A., 2012. Distribution of arterial lesions in Takayasu's arteritis and giant cell arteritis. Ann. Rheum. Dis. 71, 1329

Guillaume, M., Vachiery, F., Cogan, E., 1991. Pericarditis: an unusual manifestation of giant cell arteritis. Am. J. Med. 91, 662.

Guillevin, L., Bussel, A., 2000. Indications of plasma exchanges in 2000. Ann. Méd. Interne (Paris) 151, 123.

Guillevin, L., Le Thi Huong, D., Godeau, P., Jais, P., Wechsler, B., 1988. Clinical findings and prognosis of polyarteritis nodosa and Churg-Strauss angiitis: a study in 165 patients. Br. J. Rheumatol. 27, 258.

Guillevin, L., Lhote, F., Brauner, M., Casassus, P., 1995a. Antineutrophil cytoplasmic antibodies (ANCA) and abnormal angiograms in polyarteritis nodosa and Churg-Strauss syndrome: indications for the diagnosis of microscopic polyangiitis. Ann. Méd. Interne (Paris) 146, 548.

Guillevin, L., Lhote, F., Cohen, P., Sauvaget, F., Jarrousse, B., Lortholary, O., Noel, L.H., Trep, C., 1995b. Polyarteritis nodosa related to hepatitis B virus. A prospective study with long-term observation of 41 patients. Medicine (Baltimore) 74, 238.

Guillevin, L., Lhote, F., Gayraud, M., Cohen, P., Jarrousse, B., Lortholary, O., Thibult, N., Casassus, P., 1996. Prognostic factors in polyarteritis nodosa and Churg-Strauss syndrome. A prospective study in 342 patients. Medicine (Baltimore) 75, 17.

Guillevin, L., Durand Gasselin, B., Cevallos, R., Gayraud, M., Lhote, F., Callard, P., Amouroux, J., Casassus, P., Jarrousse, B., 1999a. Microscopic polyangiitis: clinical and laboratory findings in eighty-five patients. Arthritis Rheum. 42, 421.

Guillevin, L., Cohen, P., Gayraud, M., Lhote, F., Jarrousse, B., Casassus, P., 1999b. Churg-Strauss syndrome. Clinical study and long-term follow-up of 96 patients. Medicine (Baltimore) 78, 26.

Guillevin, L., Cohen, P., Mahr, A., Arène, J.P., Mouthon, L., Puéchal, X., Pertuiset, E., Gilson, B., Hamidou, M., Lanoux, P., Bruet, A., Ruivard, M., Vanhille, P., Cordier, J.F., 2003. Treatment of polyarteritis nodosa and microscopic polyangiitis with poor prognosis factors: a prospective trial comparing glucocorticoids and six or twelve cyclophosphamide pulses in sixty-five patients. Arthritis Rheum. 49, 93.

Hachulla, E., Bourdon, F., Taieb, S., Robert, Y., Amrouni, N., Steckolorom, T., Jabinet, J.L., Hatron, P.Y., Devulder, B., 1993. Embolization of two bleeding aneurysms with platinum coils in a patient with polyarteritis nodosa. J. Rheumatol. 20, 158.

Hagen, E.C., Daha, M.R., Hermans, J., Andrassy, K., Csernok, E., Gaskin, G., Lesavre, P., Ludemann, J., Rasmussen, N., Sinico, R.A., Wiik, A., Woude, F.J., 1998. Diagnostic value of standardized assays for anti-neutrophil cytoplasmic antibodies in idiopathic systemic vasculitis. EC/BCR Project for ANCA assay standardization. Kidney Int. 53, 743.

Halbwachs-Mecarelli, L., Nusbaum, P., Noël, L.H., Reumaux, D., Erlinger, S., Grunfeld, J.P., Lesavre, P., 1992. Antineutrophil cytoplasmic antibodies (ANCA) directed against cathepsin G in ulcerative colitis. Crohn's disease and primary sclerosing cholangitis. Clin. Exp. Immunol. 90, 79.

Hamuryudan, V., Yurdakul, S., Moral, F., Numan, F., Tuzun, H., Tuzuner, N., Mat, C., Tuzun, Y., Ozyazgan, Y., Yazici, H., 1994. Pulmonary arterial aneurysms in Behçet's syndrome: a report of 24 cases. Br. J. Rheumatol. 33, 48.

Handa, R., Wali, J.P., Aggarwal, P., Wig, N., Biswas, A., Kumar, A.K., 1997. Wegener's granulomatosis with complete heart block. Clin. Exp. Rheumatol. 15, 97.

Hasley, P.B., Follansbee, W.P., Coulehan, J.L., 1990. Cardiac manifestations of Churg-Strauss syndrome: report of a case and review of the literature. Am. Heart J. 120, 996.

Hatemi, G., Silman, A., Bang, D., Bodaghi, B., Chamberlain, A.M., Gul, A., Houman, M.H., Kötter, I., Olivieri, I., Salvarani, C., Sfikakis, P.P., Siva, A., Stanford, M.R., Stübiger, N., Yurdakul, S., Yazici, H., 2008. EULAR recommendations for the management of Behçet disease. Ann. Rheum. Dis. 68, 1656.

Hautekeete, M.L., Babany, G., Marcellin, P., Gayno, S., Palazzo, E., Erlinger, S., Benhamou, J.P., 1990. Retroperitoneal fibrosis after surgery for aortic aneurysm in a patient with periarteritis nodosa: successful treatment with corticosteroids. J. Intern. Med. 228, 533.

Hellemans, S., Dens, J., Knockaert, D., 1997. Coronary involvement in the Churg-Strauss syndrome. Heart 77, 576.

Hemmett, J., Qirjazi, E., Weir, M.A., Moussa, M., Landry, Y.D., Gunaratnam, L., 2015. Cardiac, renal, and central nervous system dysfunction with eosinophilia: eosinophilic granulomatosis with polyangiitis. Lancet 385, 480.

Henderson, R.A., Hasleton, P., Hamid, B.N., 1993. Recurrence of Churg Strauss vasculitis in a transplanted heart. Br. Heart J. 70, 553.

Hiemstra, T.F., Walsh, M., Mahr, A., Savage, C.O., de Groot, K., Harper, L., Hauser, T., Neumann, I., Tesar, V., Wissing, K.M., Pagnoux, C., Schmitt, W., Jayne, D.R., 2010. Mycophenolate mofetil vs azathioprine for remission maintenance in antineutrophil cytoplasmic antibody-associated vasculitis: a randomized controlled trial. JAMA 304, 2381.

Hochster, H., Wasserheit, C., Speyer, J., 1995. Cardiotoxicity and cardioprotection during chemotherapy. Curr. Opin. Oncol. 7, 304.

Hoffman, G.S., Kerr, G.S., Leavitt, R.Y., Hallahan, C.W., Lebovics, R.S., Travis, W.D., Rottem, M., Fauci, A.S., 1992. Wegener granulomatosis: an analysis of 158 patients. Ann. Intern. Med. 116, 488.

Hoffman, G.S., Leavitt, R.Y., Kerr, G.S., Rottem, M., Sneller, M.C., Fauci, A.S., 1994. Treatment of glucocorticoid-resistant or relapsing Takayasu arteritis with methotrexate. Arthritis Rheum. 37, 578.

Hoffman, G.S., Cid, M.C., Rendt-Zagar, K.E., Merkel, P.A., Weyand, C.M., Stone, J.H., Salvarani, C., Xu, W., Visvanathan, S., Rahman, M.U., 2007. Infliximab for maintenance of glucocorticosteroid-induced remission of giant cell arteritis: a randomized trial. Ann. Intern. Med. 146, 621.

Holsinger, D.R., Osmundson, P.J., Edwards, J.E., 1962. The heart in periarteritis nodosa. Circulation 25, 610.

Horton, B.T., 1988. The outlook in thromboangiitis obliterans. JAMA 111, 2184.

Hu, P.J., Shih, I.M., Hutchins, G.M., Hellmann, D.B., 1997. Polyarteritis nodosa of the pericardium: antemortem diagnosis in a pericardiectomy specimen. J. Rheumatol. 24, 2042.

Isselbacher, E.M., 2005. Thoracic and abdominal aortic aneurysms. Circulation 111, 816.

Iino, T., Eguchi, K., Sakai, M., Nagataki, S., Ishijima, M., Toriyama, K., 1992 Polyarteritis nodosa with aortic dissection: necrotizing vasculitis of the vasa vasorum. J. Rheumatol. 19, 1632.

Jayne, D.R., Davies, M.J., Fox, C.J., Black, C.M., Lockwood, C.M., 1991. Treatment of systemic vasculitis with pooled intravenous immunoglobulin. Lancet 337, 1137.

Jayne, D.R., Chapel, H., Adu, D., Misbah, S., O'Donoghue, D., Scott, D., 2000. Intravenous immunoglobulin for ANCA-associated systemic vasculitis with persistent disease activity. QJM 93, 433.

Jennette, J.C., Falk, R.J., Bacon, P.A., Basu, N., Cid, M.C., Ferrario, F., Flores-Suarez, L.F., Gross, W.L., Guillevin, L., Hagen, E.C., Hoffman, G.S., Jayne, D.R., Kallenberg, C.G., Lamprecht, P., Langford, C.A., Luqmani, R.A., Mahr, A.D., Matteson, E.L., Merkel, P.A., Ozen, S., Pusey, C.D., Rasmussen, N., Rees, A.J., Scott, D.G., Specks, U., Stone, J.H., Takahashi, K., Watts, R.A., 2013. 2012 revised international Chapel Hill consensus conference nomenclature of vasculitides. Arthritis Rheum. 65, 1.

Jones, R.B., Tervaert, J.W., Hauser, T., Luqmani, R., Morgan, M.D., Peh, C.A., Savage, C.O., Segelmark, M., Tesar, V., van Paassen, P., Walsh, D., Walsh, M., Westman, K., Jayne, D.R., 2010. Rituximab versus cyclophosphamide in ANCA-associated renal vasculitis. N. Engl. J. Med. 363, 211.

Jover, J.A., Hernandez-Garcia, C., Morado, I.C., Vargas, E., Banares, A., Fernandez-Gutierrez, B., 2001. Combined treatment of giant-cell arteritis with methotrexate and prednisone. a randomized, double-blind, placebo-controlled trial. Ann. Intern. Med. 134, 106.

Joyce, J.W., 1990. Buerger's disease (thromboangiitis obliterans). Rheum. Dis. Clin. North Am. 16, 463.

Kallenberg, C.G., Mulder, A.H., Tervaert, J.W., 1992. Antineutrophil cytoplasmic antibodies: a still-growing class of autoantibodies in inflammatory disorders. Am. J. Med. 93, 675.

Karger, B., Fechner, G., 2006. Sudden death due to giant cell coronary arteritis. Int. J. Legal Med. 120, 377.

Kawasaki, T., 1967. Acute febrile mucocutaneous syndrome with lymphoid involvement with specific desquamation of the fingers and toes in children. Arerugi 16, 178.

Kendell, K.R., Day, J.D., Hruban, R.H., Olson, J.L., Rosenblum, W.D., Kasper, E.K., Baughman, K.L., Hutchins, G.M., 1995. Intimate association of eosinophils to collagen bundles in eosinophilic myocarditis and ranitidine-induced hypersensitivity myocarditis. Arch. Pathol. Lab. Med. 119, 1154.

Kereiakes, D.J., Ports, T.A., Finkbeiner, W., 1984. Endomyocardial biopsy in Henoch-Schönlein purpura. Am. Heart J. 107, 382.

Kerr, G., 1994. Takayasu's arteritis. Curr. Opin. Rheumatol. 6, 32.

Kerr, L.D., Chang, Y.J., Spiera, H., Fallon, J.T., 2000. Occult active giant cell aortitis necessitating surgical repair. J. Thorac. Cardiovasc. Surg. 120, 813.

Klein, R.G., Hunder, G.G., Stanson, A.W., Sheps, S.G., 1975. Large artery involvement in giant cell (temporal) arteritis. Ann. Intern. Med. 83, 806.

Kobayashi, T., Saji, T., Otani, T., Takeuchi, K., Nakamura, T., Arakawa, H., Kato, T., Hara, T., Hamaoka, K., Ogawa, S., Miura, M., Nomura, Y., Fuse, S., Ichida, F., Seki, M., Fukazawa, R., Ogawa, C., Furuno, K., Tokunaga, H., Takatsuki, S., Hara, S., Morikawa, A., 2012. Efficacy of immunoglobulin plus prednisolone for prevention of coronary artery abnormalities in severe Kawasaki disease (RAISE study): a randomized. open-label. blinded-endpoints trial. Lancet 379, 571.

Kötter, I., Henes, J.C., Wagner, A.D., Loock, J., Gross, W.L., 2012. Does glucocorticosteroid-resistant large-vessel vasculitis (giant cell arteritis and Takayasu arteritis) exist and how can remission be achieved? A critical review of the literature. Clin. Exp. Rheumatol. 30, S114.

Kounis, N.G., Zavras, G.M., Soufras, G.D., Kitrou, M.P., 1989. Hypersensitivity myocarditis. Ann. Allergy 62, 71.

Küssmaul, A., Maier, K., 1866. Uber eine bischer nicht beschreibene eigenthumliche Arterienerkrankung (Periarteritis Nodosa), die mit Morbus Brightii und rapid fortschreitender allgemeiner Muskellähmung einhergeht. Dtsch. Arch. Klein. Med. 1, 484.

Lakhanpal, S., Tani, K., Lie, J.T., Katoh, K., Ishigatsubo, Y., Ohokubo, T., 1985. Pathologic features of Behçet's syndrome: a review of Japanese autopsy registry data. Hum. Pathol. 16, 790.

Langford, C.A., Monach, P.A., Specks, U., Seo, P., Cuthbertson, D., McAlear, C.A., Ytterberg, S.R., Hoffman, G.S., Krischer, J.P., Merkel, P.A., 2014. An open-label trial of abatacept (CTLA4-IG) in non-severe relapsing granulomatosis with polyangiitis (Wegener's). Ann. Rheum. Dis. 73, 1376.

Lanham, J.G., Cooke, S., Davies, J., Hughes, G.R., 1985. Endomyocardial complications of the Churg-Strauss syndrome. Postgrad. Med. J. 61, 341.

Ledford, D.K., 1997. Immunologic aspects of vasculitis and cardiovascular disease. JAMA 278, 1962.

Lee, T.J., Kim, K.H., Chun, J.K., Kim, D.S., 2008. Low dose methotrexate therapy for intravenous immunoglobulin-resistant Kawasaki disease. Yonsei Med. J. 49, 714.

Leib, E.S., Restivo, C., Paulus, H.E., 1979. Immunosuppressive and corticosteroid therapy of polyarteritis nodosa. Am. J. Med. 67, 941.

Leung, W.H., Wong, K.K., Lau, C.P., Wong, C.K., Cheng, C.H., So, K.F., 1989. Myocardial involvement in Churg-Strauss syndrome: the role of endomyocardial biopsy. J. Rheumatol. 16, 828.

Leung, D.Y., Schlievert, P.M., Meissner, H.C., 1998. The immunopathogenesis and management of Kawasaki syndrome. Arthritis Rheum. 41, 1538.

Lomeo, R.M., Silver, R.M., Brothers, M., 1989. Spontaneous dissection of the internal carotid artery in a patient with polyarteritis nodosa. Arthritis Rheum. 32, 1625.

Luqmani, R.A., Bacon, P.A., Moots, R.J., Janssen, B.A., Pall, A., Emery, P., Savage, C., Adu, D., 1994. Birmingham vasculitis activity score (BVAS) in systemic necrotizing vasculitis. QJM 87, 671.

Mahr, A.D., Jover, J.A., Spiera, R.F., Hernández-García, C., Fernández-Gutiérrez, B., Lavalley, M.P., Merkel, P.A., 2007. Adjunctive methotrexate for treatment of giant cell arteritis: an individual patient data meta-analysis. Arthritis Rheum. 56, 2789.

Marmursztejn, J., Vignaux, O., Cohen, P., et al., 2009. Impact of cardiac magnetic resonance imaging for assessment of Churg-Strauss syndrome: a cross-sectional study in 20 patients. Clin. Exp. Rheumatol. 27 (Suppl. 52), S70.

Martínez-Taboada, V.M., Rodríguez-Valverde, V., Carreño, L., López-Longo, J., Figueroa, M., Belzunegui, J., Mola, E.M., Bonilla, G., 2008. A double-blind placebo controlled trial of etanercept in patients with giant cell arteritis and corticosteroid side effects. Ann. Rheum. Dis. 67, 625.

Masi, A.T., Hunder, G.G., Lie, J.T., Michel, B.A., Bloch, D.A., Arend, W.P., Calabrese, L.H., Edworthy, S.M., Fauci, A.S., Leavitt, R.Y., 1990. The American College of Rheumatology 1990 criteria for the classification of Churg-Strauss syndrome (allergic granulomatosis and angiitis). Arthritis Rheum. 33, 1094.

Matsumori, A., 2005. Hepatitis C virus infection and cardiomyopathies. Circ. Res. 96, 144.

Mendes, L.A., Magraw, L.L., Aldea, G.S., Davidoff, R., 1994. Right ventricular thrombus: an unusual manifestation of Behçet's disease. J. Am. Soc. Echocardiogr. 7 438.

Merkel, P.A., Lo, G.H., Holbrook, J.T., Tibbs, A.K., Allen, N.B., Davis Jr., J.C., Hoffman, G.S., McCune, W.J., St Clair, E.W., Specks, U., Spiera, R., Petri, M., Stone, J.H., 2005. Brief communication: high incidence of venous thrombotic events among patients with Wegener granulomatosis: the Wegener's Clinical Occurrence of Thrombosis (WeCLOT) study. Ann. Intern. Med. 142, 620.

Millet, A., Martin, K.R., Bonnefoy, F., Saas, P., Mocek, J., Alkan, M., Terrier, B., Kerstein, A., Tamassia, N., Satyanarayanan, S.K., Ariel, A., Ribeil, J.A., Guillevin, L., Cassatella, M.A., Mueller, A., Thieblemont, N., Lamprecht, P., Mouthon, L., Perruche, S., Witko-Sarsat, V., 2015. Proteinase 3 on apoptotic cells disrupts immune silencing in autoimmune vasculitis. J. Clin. Invest. 125, 4107.

Morelli, S., Gurgo Di Castelmenardo, A.M., Conti, F., Sgreccia, A., Alessandri, C., Bernardo, M.L., 2000. Cardiac involvement in patients with Wegener's granulomatosis. Rheumatol. Int. 19, 209.

Muñoz, S.A., Gandino, I.J., Orden, A.O., Allievi, A., 2015. Rituximab in the treatment of eosinophilic granulomatosis with polyangiitis. Reumatol Clin. 11, 165.

Newburger, J.W., Takahashi, M., Beiser, A.S., Burns, J.C., Bastian, J., Chung, K.J., Colan, S.D., Duffy, C.E., Fulton, D.R., Glode, M.P., 1991. A single intravenous infusion of gamma globulin as compared with four infusions in the treatment of acute Kawasaki syndrome. N. Engl. J. Med. 324, 1633.

Ng, M.Y., Boutet, A., Carette, S., de Perrot, M., Cusimano, R.J., Nguyen, E.T., 2015. Behcet disease presenting with cardiac and pulmonary masses. Can. J. Cardiol. 31, 1204.

Nowack, R., Gobel, U., Klooker, P., Hergesell, O., Andrassy, K., Woude, F.J., 1999. Mycophenolate mofetil for maintenance therapy of Wegener's granulomatosis and microscopic polyangiitis: a pilot study in 11 patients with renal involvement. J. Am. Soc. Nephrol. 10, 1965.

Ogata, S., Ogihara, Y., Honda, T., Kon, S., Akiyama, K., Ishii, M., 2012. Corticosteroid pulse combination therapy for refractory Kawasaki disease: a randomized trial. Pediatrics 129, e17.

Okcun, B., Baran, T., Babalik, E., Kücükoglu, S., 2003. Multichamber masses and constrictive pericarditis in Behcet's disease. Clin. Exp. Rheumatol. 21, 55.
Olin, J.W., 2000. Thromboangiitis obliterans (Buerger's disease). N. Engl. J. Med. 343, 864.
Oliveira, G.H., Seward, J.B., Tsang, T.S., Specks, U., 2005. Echocardiographic findings in patients with Wegener granulomatosis. Mayo Clin. Proc. 80, 1435.
Osman, A., McCreery, C.J., 2000. Cardiac vasculitis in Henoch-Schönlein purpura. Circulation 101, E69.
Pagnoux, C., Mahr, A., Cohen, P., Guillevin, L., 2005. Presentation and outcome of gastrointestinal involvement in systemic necrotizing vasculitides: analysis of 62 patients with polyarteritis nodosa, microscopic polyangiitis, Wegener granulomatosis, Churg-Strauss syndrome, or rheumatoid arthritis-associated vasculitis. Medicine 84, 115.
Pagnoux, C., Seror, R., Henegar, C., Mahr, A., Cohen, P., Le Guern, V., Bienvenu, B., Mouthon, L., Guillevin, L., 2010. French Vasculitis Study Group. Clinical features and outcomes in 348 patients with polyarteritis nodosa: a systematic retrospective study of patients diagnosed between 1963 and 2005 and entered into the French Vasculitis Study GroupDatabase. Arthritis Rheum. 62, 616.
Park, M.C., Lee, S.W., Park, Y.B., Chung, N.S., Lee, S.K., 2005. Clinical characteristics and outcomes of Takayasu's arteritis: analysis of 108 patients using standardized criteria for diagnosis. activity assessment. and angiographic classification. Scand. J. Rheumatol. 34, 284.
Pearce, C.B., McMeekin, J.D., Moyana, T.N., Sibley, J., 1999. A case of peripartum eosinophilic myocarditis. Can. J. Cardiol. 15, 465.
Pietrogrande, M., De Vita, S., Zignego, A.L., Pioltelli, P., Sansonno, D., Sollima, S., Atzeni, F., Saccardo, F., Quartuccio, L., Bruno, S., Bruno, R., Campanini, M., Candela, M., Castelnovo, L., Gabrielli, A., Gaeta, G.B., Marson, P., Mascia, M.T., Mazzaro, C., Mazzotta, F., Meroni, P., Montecucco, C., Ossi, E., Piccinino, F., Prati, D., Puoti, M., Riboldi, P., Riva, A., Roccatello, D., Sagnelli, E., Scaini, P., Scarpato, S., Sinico, R., Taliani, G., Tavoni, A., Bonacci, E., Renoldi, P., Filippini, D., Sarzi-Puttini, P., Ferri, C., Monti, G., Galli, M., 2011. Recommendations for the management of mixed cryoglobulinemia syndrome in hepatitis C virus-infected patients. Autoimmun. Rev. 10, 444.
Polizzotto, M.N., Gibbs, S.D., Beswick, W., Seymour, J.F., 2006. Cardiac involvement in Henoch-Schönlein purpura. Intern. Med. J. 36, 328.
Pusey, C.D., Rees, A.J., Evans, D.J., Peters, D.K., Lockwood, C.M., 1991. Plasma exchange in focal necrotizing glomerulonephritis without anti-GBM antibodies. Kidney Int. 40, 757.
Rabusin, M., Lepore, L., Costantinides, F., Bussani, R., 1998. A child with severe asthma. Lancet 351, 32.
Ramakrishna, G., Connolly, H.M., Tazelaar, H.D., Mullany, C.J., Midthun, D.E., 2000. Churg-Strauss syndrome complicated by eosinophilic endomyocarditis. Mayo Clin. Proc. 75, 631.
Raza, K., Karokis, D., Kitas, G.D., 1998. Cogan's syndrome with Takayasu's arteritis. Br. J. Rheumatol. 37, 369.
Reinhold-Keller, E., Kekow, J., Schnabel, A., Schwarz-Eywill, M., Schmitt, W.H., Gross, W.L., 1993. Effectiveness of cyclophosphamide pulse treatment in Wegener's granulomatosis. Adv. Exp. Med. Biol. 336, 483.
Ribi, C., Cohen, P., Pagnoux, C., Mahr, A., Arène, J.P., Puéchal, X., Carli, P., Kyndt, X., Le Hello, C., Letellier, P., Cordier, J.F., Guillevin, L., 2010. French Vasculitis Study Group. Treatment of polyarteritis nodosa and microscopic polyangiitis without poor-prognosis factors: a prospective randomized study of one hundred twenty-four patients. Arthritis Rheum. 62, 1186.
Rieu, V., Cohen, P., Andre, M.H., Mouthon, L., Godmer, P., Jarrousse, B., Lhote, F., Ferriere, F., Dény, P., Buchet, P., Guillevin, L., 2002. Characteristics and outcome of 49 patients with symptomatic cryoglobulinaemia. Rheumatology (Oxford) 41, 290.

Saadoun, D., Wechsler, B., 2012. Behçet's disease. Orphanet J. Rare Dis. 7.
Salvarani, C., Macchioni, P.L., Tartoni, P.L., Rossi, F., Baricchi, R., Castri, C., Chiaravalloti, F., Portioli, I., 1987. Polymyalgia rheumatica and giant cell arteritis: a 5-year epidemiologic and clinical study in Reggio Emilia. Italy Clin. Exp. Rheumatol. 5, 205.
Salvarani, C., Gabriel, S.E., O'Fallon, W.M., Hunder, G.G., 1995. The incidence of giant cell arteritis in Olmsted County, Minnesota: apparent fluctuations in a cyclic pattern. Ann. Intern. Med. 123, 192.
Salvarani, C., Cantini, F., Boiardi, L., Hunder, G.G., 2002. Polymyalgia rheumatica and giant-cell arteritis. N. Engl. J. Med. 347, 261.
Sanders, J.S., Huitma, M.G., Kallenberg, C.G., Stegeman, C.A., 2006. Prediction of relapses in PR3-ANCA-associated. vasculitis by assessing responses of ANCA titres to treatment. Rheumatology (Oxford) 45, 724.
Savage, C.O., Winearls, C.G., Evans, D.J., Rees, A.J., Lockwood, C.M.. 1985. Microscopic polyarteritis: presentation. pathology and prognosisv. QJM 56, 467.
Schiavone, W.A., Ahmad, M., Ockner, S.A., 1985. Unusual cardiac complications of Wegener's granulomatosis. Chest 88, 745.
Schildhaus, H.U., Von Netzer, B., Dombrowski, F., Pfeifer, U., 2002. Atypical manifestation of a cytoplasmic antineutrophil cytoplasmic antibody (PR3-ANCA)-associated vasculitis with involvement of aortic intima and parietal endocardium. Hum. Pathol. 33, 441.
Schrader, M.L., Hochman, J.S., Bulkley, B.H., 1985. The heart in polyarteritis nodosa: a clinicopathologic study. Am. Heart J. 109, 1353.
Schreiber, A., Xiao, H., Falk, R.J., Jennette, J.C., 2006. Bone marrow-derived cells are sufficient and necessary targets to mediate glomerulonephritis and vasculitis induced by anti-myeloperoxidase antibodies. J. Am. Soc. Nephrol. 17, 3355.
Seror, R., Baron, G., Hachulla, E., Debandt, M., Larroche, C., Puéchal, X., Maurier, F., de Wazieres, B., Quéméneur, T., Ravaud, P., Mariette, X., 2014. Adalimumab for steroid sparing in patients with giant-cell arteritis: results of a multicentre randomized controlled trial. Ann. Rheum. Dis. 73, 2074.
Sharma, A., De Varennes, B., Sniderman, A.D., 1993. Churg-Strauss syndrome presenting with marked eosinophilia and pericardial effusion. Can. J. Cardiol. 9, 329.
Shionoya, S., 1993. Buerger's disease: diagnosis and management. Cardiovasc. Surg. 1, 207.
Somer, T., 1993. Thrombo-embolic and vascular complications in vasculitis syndromes. Eur. Heart J. 14, 24.
Specks, U., Homburger, H.A., DeRemee, R.A., 1993. Implications of c-ANCA testing for the classification of Wegener's granulomatosis: performance of different detection systems. Adv. Exp. Med. Biol. 336, 65.
Stanson, A.W., 2000. Imaging findings in extracranial (giant cell) temporal arteritis. Clin. Exp. Rheumatol. 18, S43.
Stone, J.H., Hoffman, G.S., Merkel, P.A., Min, Y.I., Uhlfelder, M.L., Hellmann, D.B., Allen, N.B., Davis, J.C., Spiera, R.R., Calabrese, L.H., Wigley, F.M., Maiden, N., Valente, R.M., Niles, J.L., Fye, K.H., McCune, J.W., Clair, E.W., Luqmani, R.A., 2001. A disease-specific activity index for Wegener's granulomatosis: modification of the Birmingham vasculitis activity score. International network for the study of the systemic vasculitides (INSSYS). Arthritis Rheum. 44, 912.
Stone, J.H., Merkel, P.A., Spiera, R., Seo, P., Langford, C.A., Hoffman, G.S., Kallenberg, C.G., St Clair, E.W., Turkiewicz, A., Tchao, N.K., Webber, L., Ding, L., Sejismundo, L.P., Mieras, K., Weitzenkamp, D., Ikle, D., Seyfert-Margolis, V., Mueller, M., Brunetta, P., Allen, N.B., Fervenza, F.C., Geetha, D., Keogh, K.A., Kissin, E.Y., Monach P.A., Peikert, T.,

Stegeman, C., Ytterberg, S.R., Specks, U., 2010. Rituximab versus cyclophosphamide for ANCA-associated vasculitis. N. Engl. J. Med. 363, 221.

Stricker, H., Malinverni, R., 1989. Multiple. large aneurysms of pulmonary arteries in Behçet's disease. Clinical remission and radiologic resolution after corticosteroid therapy. Arch. Intern. Med. 149, 925.

Sugimura, T., Yokoi, H., Sato, N., Akagi, T., Kimura, T., Iemura, M., 1997. Interventional treatment for children with severe coronary artery stenosis with calcification after long-term Kawasaki disease. Circulation 96, 3928.

Suleymenlar, G., Sarikaya, M., Sari, R., Tuncer, M., Sevinc, A., 2002. Complete heart block in a patient with Wegener's granulomatosis in remission—a case report. Angiology 53, 337.

Sumitomo, N., Karasawa, K., Taniguchi, K., Ichikawa, R., et al., 2008. Association of sinus node dysfunction. atrioventricular node conduction abnormality and ventricular arrhythmia in patients with Kawasaki disease and coronary involvement. Circ. J. 72, 274—280.

Sundy, J.S., Haynes, B.F., 2000. Cytokines and adhesion molecules in the pathogenesis of vasculitis. Curr. Rheumatol. Rep. 2, 402.

Suzuki, H., Terai, M., Hamada, H., Honda, T., Suenaga, T., Takeuchi, T., Yoshikawa, N., Shibuta, S., Miyawaki, M., Oishi, K., Yamaga, H., Aoyagi, N., Iwahashi, S., Miyashita, R., Onouchi, Y., Sasago, K., Suzuki, Y., Hata, A., 2011. Cyclosporin A treatment of Kawasaki disease refractory to initial and additional intravenous immunoglobulin. Pediatr. Infect. Dis. J. 30, 871.

Tai, P.C., Holt, M.E., Denny, P., Gibbs, A.R., Williams, B.D., Spry, C.J., 1984. Deposition of eosinophil cationic protein in granulomas in allergic granulomatosis and vasculitis: the Churg-Strauss syndrome. Br. Med. J. (Clin. Res. Ed.) 289, 400.

Takahashi, M., 1993. Inflammatory diseases of the coronary artery in children. Coron. Artery Dis. 4, 133—138.

Terasaki, F., Hayashi, T., Hirota, Y., Okabe, M., Suwa, M., Deguchi, H., Kitaura, Y., Kawamura, K., 1997. Evolution to dilated cardiomyopathy from acute eosinophilic pancarditis in Churg-Strauss syndrome. Heart Vessels 12, 43.

Terrier, B., Karras, A., Cluzel, P., Collet, J.P., Sène, D., Saadoun, D., Cacoub, P., 2013. Presentation and prognosis of cardiac involvement in hepatitis C virus-related vasculitis. Am. J. Cardiol. 111, 265.

Tervaert, J.W., Huitema, M.G., Hene, R.J., Sluiter, W.J., The, T.H., Hem, G.K., Kallenberg, C.G., 1990. Prevention of relapses in Wegener's granulomatosis by treatment based on anti-neutrophil cytoplasmic antibody titre. Lancet 336, 709.

Tesar, V., Jelinkova, E., Masek, Z., Jirsa, M., Zabka, J., Bartunkova, J., Stejskalova, A., Janatkova, I., Zima, T., 1998. Influence of plasma exchange on serum levels of cytokines and adhesion molecules in ANCA-positive renal vasculitis. Blood Purif. 16, 72.

Thomson, D., Chamsi-Pasha, H., Hasleton, P., 1989. Heart transplantation for Churg-Strauss syndrome. Br. Heart J. 62, 409.

Van der Woude, F.J., Rasmussen, N., Lobatto, S., Wiik, A., Permin, H., Giessen, M., Hem, G.K., The, T.H., 1985. Autoantibodies against neutrophils and monocytes: tool for diagnosis and marker of disease activity in Wegener's granulomatosis. Lancet 1, 425.

Villiger, P.M., Guillevin, L., 2010. Microscopic polyangiitis: clinical presentation. Autoimmun. Rev. 9, 812.

Vollertsen, R.S., McDonald, T.J., Younge, B.R., Banks, P.M., Stanson, A.W., Ilstrup, D.M., 1986. Cogan's syndrome: 18 cases and a review of the literature. Mayo Clin. Proc. 61, 344.

Walsh, M., Faurschou, M., Berden, A., Flossmann, O., Bajema, I., Hoglund, P., Smith, R., Szpirt, W., Westman, K., Pusey, C.D., Jayne, D.R., 2014. Long-term follow-up of cyclophosphamide compared with azathioprine for initial maintenance therapy in ANCA-associated vasculitis. Clin. J. Am. Soc. Nephrol. 9, 1571.

Wang, L., Thelmo, W.L., Axiotis, C.A., 2002. Microscopic polyangiitis with massive myocardial necrosis and diffuse pulmonary hemorrhage. Virchows Arch. 441, 202.

Watts, R.A., Lane, S.E., Bentham, G., Scott, D.G., 2000. Epidemiology of systemic vasculitis: a ten year study in the United Kingdom. Arthritis Rheum. 43, 414.

Wechsler, B., Du, L.T., Kieffer, E., 1999. Cardiovascular manifestations of Behcet's disease. Ann. Méd. Interne (Paris) 150, 542 (in French).

Weisman, M.H., 2002. What are the risks of biologic therapy in rheumatoid arthritis? An update on safety. J. Rheumatol. Suppl. 65, 33.

Witko-Sarsat, V., Cramer, E.M., Hieblot, C., Guichard, J., Nusbaum, P., Lopez, S., Lesavre, P., Halbwachs-Mecarelli, L., 1999. Presence of proteinase 3 in secretory vesicles: evidence of a novel. highly mobilizable intracellular pool distinct from azurophil granules. Blood 94, 2487.

Xiao, H., Heeringa, P., Hu, P., Liu, Z., Zhao, M., Aratani, Y., Maeda, N., Falk, R.J., Jennette, J.C., 2002. Antineutrophil cytoplasmic autoantibodies specific for myeloperoxidase cause glomerulonephritis and vasculitis in mice. J. Clin. Invest. 110, 955.

Yeatman, M., McNeil, K., Smith, J.A., Stewart, S., Sharples, L.D., Higenbottam, T., Wells, F.C., Wallwork, J., 1996. Lung transplantation in patients with systemic diseases: an eleven-year experience at Papworth Hospital. J. Heart Lung Transpl. 15, 144.

Zehr, K.J., Mathur, A., Orszulak, T.A., Mullany, C.J., Schaff, H.V., 2005. Surgical treatment of ascending aortic aneurysms in patients with giant cell aortitis. Ann. Thorac. Surg. 79, 1512.

FURTHER READING

Anderson, G., Coles, E.T., Crane, M., Douglas, A.C., Gibbs, A.R., Geddes, D.M., Gibbs, Peel, E.T., Wood, J.B., 1992. Wegener's granuloma. A series of 265 British cases seen between 1975 and 1985. A report by a sub-committee of the British Thoracic Society Research Committee. QJM 83, 427.

Andersson, R., Malmvall, B.E., Bengtsson, B.A., 1986a. Long-term corticosteroid treatment in giant cell arteritis. Acta Med. Scand. 220, 465.

Andersson, R., Malmvall, B.E., Bengtsson, B.A., 1986b. Long-term survival in giant cell arteritis including temporal arteritis and polymyalgia rheumatica. A follow-up study of 90 patients treated with corticosteroids. Acta Med. Scand. 220, 361.

Anthony, D.D., Askari, A.D., Wolpaw, T., McComsey, G., 1999. Wegener granulomatosis simulating bacterial endocarditis. Arch. Intern. Med. 159, 1807.

Ara, J., Mirapeix, E., Arrizabalaga, P., Rodriguez, R., Ascaso, C., Abellana, R., Font, J., Darnell, A., 2001. Circulating soluble adhesion molecules in ANCA-associated vasculitis. Nephrol. Dial. Transpl. 16, 276.

Balestrieri, G.P., Valentini, U., Cerudelli, B., Spandrio, S., Renaldini, E., 1992. Reversible myocardial impairment in the Churg-Strauss syndrome: report of a case. Clin. Exp. Rheumatol. 10, 75.

Berbis, P., Carena, M.C., Auffranc, J.C., Privat, Y., 1986. Cutaneo-systemic necrotizing vasculitis occurring during desensitization. Ann. Dermatol. Venereol. 113, 805.

Bligny, D., Mahr, A., Toumelin, P.L., Mouthon, L., Guillevin, L., 2004. Predicting mortality in systemic Wegener's granulomatosis: a survival analysis based on 93 patients. Arthritis Rheum. 51, 83.

Bloch, D.A., Michel, B.A., Hunder, G.G., McShane, D.J., Arend, W.P., Calabrese, L.H., 1990. The American College of Rheumatology 1990 criteria for the classification of vasculitis. Patients and methods. Arthritis Rheum. 33, 1068.

Blockmans, D., Maes, A., Stroobants, S., Nuyts, J., Bormans, G., Knockaert, D., Bobbaers, H., Mortelmans, L., 1999. New arguments for a vasculitic nature of polymyalgia rheumatica using positron emission tomography. Rheumatology (Oxford) 38, 444.

Bookman, A.A., Goode, E., McLoughlin, M.J., Cohen, Z., 1983. Polyarteritis nodosa complicated by a ruptured intrahepatic aneurysm. Arthritis Rheum. 26, 106.

Brouet, J.C., Clauvel, J.P., Danon, F., Klein, M., Seligmann, M., 1974. Biologic and clinical significance of cryoglobulins. A report of 86 cases. Am. J. Med. 57, 775.

Calabrese, L.H., Michel, B.A., Bloch, D.A., Arend, W.P., Edworthy, S.M., Fauci, A.S., Fries, J.F., Hunder, G.G., Leavitt, R.Y., Lie, J.T., 1990. The American College of Rheumatology 1990 criteria for the classification of hypersensitivity vasculitis. Arthritis Rheum. 33, 1108.

Carlson, J.A., 2010. The histological assessment of cutaneous vasculitis. Histopathology 56, p3.

Chikamori, T., Doi, Y.L., Yonezawa, Y., Takata, J., Kawamura, M., Ozawa, T., 1990. Aortic regurgitation secondary to Behçet's disease. A case report and review of the literature. Eur. Heart J. 11, 572.

Churg, J., Strauss, L., 1951. Allergic granulomatosis, allergic angiitis and periarteritis nodosa. Am. J. Pathol. 27, 277.

Cohen, P., Nguyen, Q.T., Dény, P., Ferriere, F., Roulot, D., Lortholary, O., Jarrousse, B., Danon, F., Barrier, J.H., Ceccaldi, J., Constans, J., Crickx, B., Fiessinger, J.N., Hachulla, E., Jaccard, A., Seligmann, M., Kazatchkine, M., Laroche, L., Subra, J.F., Turlure, P., Guillevin, L., 1996. Treatment of mixed cryoglobulinemia with recombinant interferon alpha and adjuvant therapies. A prospective study on 20 patients. Ann. Méd. Interne (Paris) 147, 81.

Comparato, E., Toso, M., 1977. A case of polyarteritis nodosa associated with pulmonary hypertension. Minerva Med. 68, 2963 (in Italian).

D'Cruz, D., 1998. Vasculitis in systemic lupus erythematosus. Lupus 7, 270.

Demaziere, A., 1989. Dapsone in the long-term treatment of temporal arteritis. Am. J. Med. 87, 3.

D'Izarn, J.J., Boulet, C.P., Convard, J.P., Bonnin, A., Ledoux-Lebard, G., 1976. Arteriography in polyarteritis nodosa. 15 cases. J. Radiol. Electrol. Med. Nucl. 57, 505 (in French).

Drenkard, C., Villa, A.R., Reyes, E., Abello, M., Alarcon-Segovia, D., 1997. Vasculitis in systemic lupus erythematosus. Lupus 6, 235.

Durieux, P., Blétry, O., Huchon, G., Wechsler, B., Chrétien, J., Godeau, P., 1981. Multiple pulmonary arterial aneurysms in Behcet's disease and Hughes-Stovin syndrome. Am. J. Med. 71, 736.

Erkan, F., Kiyan, E., Tunaci, A., 2002. Pulmonary complications of Behçet's disease. Clin. Chest Med. 23, 493.

Fauci, A.S., Haynes, B.F., Katz, P., Wolff, S.M., 1983. Wegener's granulomatosis: prospective clinical and therapeutic experience with 85 patients for 21 years. Ann. Intern. Med. 98, 76.

Fong, C., Schmidt, G., Cain, N., Cranswick, P., Tonkin, A.M., 1992. Churg-Strauss syndrome, cardiac involvement and life threatening ventricular arrhythmias. Aust. N. Z. J. Med. 22, 167.

Fortin, P.R., Larson, M.G., Watters, A.K., Yeadon, C.A., Choquette, D., Esdaile, J.M., 1995. Prognostic factors in systemic necrotizing vasculitis of the polyarteritis nodosa group—a review of 45 cases. J. Rheumatol. 22, 78—84.

Fox, A.D., Robbins, S.E., 1994. Aortic valvulitis complicating Wegener's granulomatosis. Thorax 49, 1176.

Fries, J.F., Hunder, G.G., Bloch, D.A., Michel, B.A., Arend, W.P., Calabrese, L.H., 1990. The American College of Rheumatology 1990 criteria for the classification of vasculitis. Arthritis Rheum. 33, 1135 (Summary).

Frustaci, A., Chimenti, C., Pieroni, M., 1997. Idiopathic myocardial vasculitis presenting as restrictive cardiomyopathy. Chest 111, 1462.

Garcia-Porrua, C., Llorca, J., Gonzalez-Louzao, C., Gonzalez-Gay, M.A., 2001. Hypersensitivity vasculitis in adults: a benign disease usually limited to skin. Clin. Exp. Rheumatol. 19, 85.

Généreau, T., Lortholary, O., Leclerq, P., Grenet, D., Tubery, M., Sicard, D., Caubarrére, I., Guillevin, L., 1994. Treatment of systemic vasculitis with cyclophosphamide and steroids: daily oral low-dose cyclophosphamide administration after failure of a pulse intravenous high-dose regimen in four patients. Br. J. Rheumatol. 33, 959.

Généreau, T., Lortholary, O., Pottier, M.A., Michon-Pasturel, U., Ponge, T., de Wazières, B., Liozon, E., Pinède, L., Hachulla, E., Roblot, P., Barrier, J.H., Herson, S., Guillevin, L., 1999. Temporal artery biopsy: a diagnostic tool for systemic necrotizing vasculitis. French Vasculitis Study Group. Arthritis Rheum. 42, 2674.

Godeau, P., Blétry, O., Guillevin, L., Herson, S., Piette, J.C., 1985. Le coeur des collagénoses. Ann. Méd. Interne (Paris) 136, 496.

Golan, T.D., 2002. Lupus vasculitis: differential diagnosis with antiphospholipid syndrome. Curr. Rheumatol. Rep. 4, 18.

Gonzalez-Gay, M.A., Garcia-Porrua, C., Pujol, R.M., 2005. Clinical approach to cutaneous vasculitis. Curr. Opin. Rheumatol. 17, 56.

Gorevic, P.D., Kassab, H.J., Levo, Y., Kohn, R., Meltzer, M., Prose, P., 1980. Mixed cryoglobulinemia: clinical aspects and long-term follow-up of 40 patients. Am. J. Med. 69, 287.

Goronzy, J.J., Weyand, C.M., 1994. Vasculitis in rheumatoid arthritis. Curr. Opin. Rheumatol. 6, 290.

Gower, R.G., Sausker, W.F., Kohler, P.F., Thorne, G.E., McIntos, R.M., 1978. Small vessel vasculitis caused by hepatitis B virus immune complexes. Small vessel vasculitis and HBsAg. J. Allergy Clin. Immunol. 62, 222.

Greidinger, E.L., Lemes, V., Hellmann, D.B., 1996. Cardiac valve disease in Wegener's granulomatosis. J. Rheumatol. 23, 1485.

Guillevin, L., Lhote, F., Léon, A., Fauvelle, F., Vivitski, L., Trepo, C., 1993. Treatment of polyarteritis nodosa related to hepatitis B virus with short term steroid therapy associated with antiviral agents and plasma exchanges. A prospective trial in 33 patients. J. Rheumatol. 20, 289.

Guillevin, L., Lhote, F., Jarrousse, B., Cohen, P., Jacquot, C., Lesavre, P., 1995. Treatment of Wegener's granulomatosis: a prospective trial in 50 patients comparing prednisone, pulse cyclophosphamide versus prednisone and oral cyclophosphamide. Clin. Exp. Rheumatol. 101, 43 (Abstract).

Gunal, N., Kara, N., Cakar, N., Kocak, H., Kahramanyol, O., Cetinkaya, E., 1997. Cardiac involvement in childhood polyarteritis nodosa. Int. J. Cardiol. 60, 257.

Gupta, S., Piraka, C., Jaffe, M., 2001. Lamivudine in the treatment of polyarteritis nodosa associated with acute hepatitis B. N. Engl. J. Med. 344, 1645.

Ha, H.K., Lee, S.H., Rha, S.E., Kim, J.H., Byun, J.Y., Lim, H.K., Chung, J.W., Kim, J.G., Kim, P.N., Lee, M.G., Auh, Y.H., 2000. Radiologic features of vasculitis involving the gastrointestinal tract. Radiographics 20, 779.

Hamza, M., 1987. Large artery involvement in Behçet's disease. J. Rheumatol. 14, 554.

Heeringa, P., Brouwer, E., Tervaert, J.W., Weening, J.J., Kallenberg, C.G., 1998. Animal models of anti-neutrophil cytoplasmic antibody associated vasculitis. Kidney Int. 53, 253.

Hunder, G.G., Bloch, D.A., Michel, B.A., Stevens, M.B., Arend, W.P., Calabrese, L.H., Leavitt, R.Y., Lie, J.T., Lightfoot, R.W., Masi, A.T., 1990. The American College of Rheumatology 1990 criteria for the classification of giant cell arteritis. Arthritis Rheum. 33, 1122.

Huong, D.L., Wechsler, B., Papo, T., de Zuttere, D., Blétry, O., Hernigou, A., Delcourt, A., Godeau, P., Piette, J.C., 1997. Endomyocardial fibrosis in Behçet's disease. Ann. Rheum. Dis. 56, 205.

Imai, T., Matsumoto, S., 1970. Anaphylactoid purpura with cardiac involvement. Arch. Dis. Child. 45, 727.

Islim, I.F., Gill, M.D., Situnayake, D., Watson, R.D., 1994. Successful treatment of right atrial thrombus in a patient with Behçet's disease. Ann. Rheum. Dis. 53, 550.

Israel, H.L., 1988. Sulfamethoxazole-trimethoprim therapy for Wegener's granulomatosis. Arch. Intern. Med. 148, 2293.

Jee, K.N., Ha, H.K., Lee, I.J., Klim, J.K., Sung, K.B., Cho, K.S., Kim, P.N., Lee, M.G., Lim, H.K., Choi, C.S., Auh, Y.H., 2000. Radiologic findings of abdominal polyarteritis nodosa. Am. J. Roentgenol. 174, 1675.

Jennette, J.C., Falk, R.J., 2007. The role of pathology in the diagnosis of systemic vasculitis. Clin. Exp. Rheumatol. 25, S52.

Jennette, J.C., Falk, R.J., Andrassy, K., Bacan, P.A., Churg, J., Gross, W.L., Hagen, E.C., Hoffman, G.S., Hunder, G.G., Kallenberg, C.G., 1994. Nomenclature of systemic vasculitides. Proposal of an international consensus conference. Arthritis Rheum. 37, 187.

Jones, R.B., Furuta, S., Tervaert, J.W., Hauser, T., Luqmani, R., Morgan, M.D., Peh, C.A., Savage, C.O., Segelmark, M., Tesar, V., van Paassen, P., Walsh, M., Westman, K., Jayne, D.R., 2015. Rituximab versus cyclophosphamide in ANCA-associated renal vasculitis: 2-year results of a randomised trial. Ann. Rheum. Dis. 74, 1178.

Kato, H., Sugimura, T., Akagi, T., Sato, N., Hashino, K., Maeno, Y., Kazue, T., Eto, G., Yamakawa, R., 1996. Long-term consequences of Kawasaki disease. A 10- to 21-year follow-up study of 594 patients. Circulation 94, 1379.

Katsuyama, T., Sada, K.E., Makino, H., 2014. Current concept and epidemiology of systemic vasculitides. Allergol. Int. 63, 505.

Klinger, H., 1931. Grenzformen der Periarteritis Nodosa. Frankf. Z. Pathol. 42, 455.

Koldingsnes, W., Nossent, J.C., 2003. Baseline features and initial treatment as predictors of remission and relapse in Wegener's granulomatosis. J. Rheumatol. 30, 80.

Kosovsky, P.A., Ehlers, K.H., Rafal, R.B., Williams, W.M., O'Loughlin, J.E., Markisz, J.A., 1991. MR imaging of cardiac mass in Wegener granulomatosis. J. Comput. Assist. Tomogr. 15, 1028.

Kumar, S., Subramanyan, R., Mandalam, K.R., Rao, V.R., Gupta, A.K., Joseph, S., Unni, N.M., Rao, A.S., 1990. Aneurysmal form of aortoarteritis (Takayasu's disease): analysis of thirty cases. Clin. Radiol. 42, 342.

Lane, S.E., Watts, R.A., Bentham, G., Innes, N.J., Scott, D.G., 2003. Are environmental factors important in primary systemic vasculitis? A case-control study. Arthritis Rheum. 48, 814.

Lanham, J.G., Elkon, K.B., Pusey, C.D., Hughes, G.R., 1984. Systemic vasculitis with asthma and eosinophilia: a clinical approach to the Churg-Strauss syndrome. Medicine (Baltimore) 63, 65.

Le Thi Huong, D., Wechsler, B., De Gennes, C., Raguin, G., Piette, J.C., Blétry, O., Godeau, P., 1990. Treatment of Wegener's granulomatosis with cotrimoxazole (7 cases). Rev. Méd. Interne 11, 87 (in French).

Leavitt, R.Y., Fauci, A.S., Bloch, D.A., Michel, B.A., Hunder, G.G., Arend, W.P., Calabrese, L.H., Fries, J.F., Lie, J.T., Lightfoot, R.W., 1990. The American College of Rheumatology 1990 criteria for the classification of Wegener's granulomatosis. Arthritis Rheum. 33, 1101.

Lie, J.T., 1997. Wegener's granulomatosis: histological documentation of common and uncommon manifestations in 216 patients. Vasa 26, 261.

Lightfoot Jr., R.W., Michel, B.A., Bloch, D.A., Hunder, G.G., Zvaifler, N.J., McShane, D.J., 1990. The American College of Rheumatology 1990 criteria for the classification of polyarteritis nodosa. Arthritis Rheum. 33, 1088.

Lockwood, C.M., 1998. Refractory Wegener's granulomatosis: a model for shorter immunotherapy of autoimmune diseases. J. R. Coll. Phys. Lond. 32, 473–478.

Lockwood, C.M., Thiru, S., Stewart, S., Hale, G., Isaacs, J., Wraight, P., Elliott, J., Waldmann, H., 1996. Treatment of refractory Wegener's granulomatosis with humanized monoclonal antibodies. QJM 89, 903.

Lortholary, O., Généreau, T., Guillevin, I., 1999. Viral vasculitis not related to HBV, HCV and HIV. Pathol. Biol. (Paris) 47, 248 (in French).

Lunel, F., Cacoub, P., 2000. Treatment of autoimmune and extra-hepatic manifestations of HCV infection. Ann. Méd. Interne (Paris) 151, 58.

Lutz, H.H., Ackermann, T., Krombach, G.A., Gröne, H.J., Rauen, T., Floege, J., Mertens, P.R., 2009. Henoch-Schönlein purpura complicated by cardiac involvement: case report and review of the literature. Am. J. Kidney Dis. 54, e9–15.

Mahr, A., de Menthon, M., 2015. Classification and classification criteria for vasculitis: achievements. limitations and prospects. Curr. Opin. Rheumatol. 27, 1.

Mahr, A.D., Jover, J.A., Spiera, R.F., Hernandez-Garcia, C., Fernandez-Gutierrez, B., Maksimowicz-McKinnon, K., Clark, T.M., Hoffman, G.S., 2009. Takayasu arteritis and giant cell arteritis: a spectrum within the same disease? Medicine 88, 221.

Marette, P., Molle, B., Mas, J.L., Kahan, A., Devaux, J.Y., Toussaint, M., Volkringer, P., Fouchard, J., 1989. Angina without involvement of large coronary trunks and precapillary pulmonary hypertension in a patient with periarteritis nodosa. Ann. Cardiol. Angeiol. (Paris) 38, 305 (in French).

McLaren, J.S., McRorie, E.R., Luqmani, R.A., 2002. Diagnosis and assessment of systemic vasculitis. Clin. Exp. Rheumatol. 20, 854.

Miller, D.L., 2000. Angiography in polyarteritis nodosa. Am. J. Roentgenol. 175, 1747.

Mills, J.A., Michel, B.A., Bloch, D.A., Calabrese, L.H., Hunder, G.G., Arend, W.P., 1990. The American College of Rheumatology 1990 criteria for the classification of Henoch-Schönlein purpura. Arthritis Rheum. 33, 1114.

Mohan, N., Kerr, G., 2000. Spectrum of giant cell vasculitis. Curr. Rheumatol. Rep. 2, 390.

Morgan, J.M., Raposo, L., Gibson, D.G., 1989. Cardiac involvement in Churg-Strauss syndrome shown by echocardiography. Br. Heart J. 62, 462.

Mrowka, C., Sieberth, H.G., 1994. Circulating adhesion molecules ICAM-1, VCAM-1 and E-selectin in systemic vasculitis: marked differences between Wegener's granulomatosis and systemic lupus erythematosus. Clin. Investig. 72, 762.

Mrowka, C., Sieberth, H.G., 1995. Detection of circulating adhesion molecules ICAM-1, VCAM-1 and E-selectin in Wegener's granulomatosis, systemic lupus erythematosus and chronic renal failure. Clin. Nephrol. 43, 288.

Mrowka, C., Heintz, B., Sieberth, H.G., 1999. VCAM-1, ICAM-1, and E-selectin in IgA nephropathy and Schonlein-Henoch syndrome: differences between tissue expression and serum concentration. Nephrology 81, 256.

Murphy, D.J., Huhta, J.C., 1987. Treatment of Kawasaki syndrome with intravenous gamma globulin. N. Engl. J. Med. 316, 881.

Naarendorp, M., Kallemuchikkal, U., Nuovo, G.J., Gorevic, P.D., 2001. Longterm efficacy of interferon-alpha for extrahepatic disease associated with hepatitis C virus infection. J. Rheumatol. 28, 2466.

Nesher, G., Sonnenblick, M., Friedlander, Y., 1994. Analysis of steroid related complications and mortality in temporal arteritis: a 15-year survey of 43 patients. J. Rheumatol. 21, 1283.

Noguchi, S., Numano, F., Gravanis, M.B., Wilcox, J.N., 1998. Increased levels of soluble forms of adhesion molecules in Takayasu arteritis. Int. J. Cardiol. 66, S23.

Nuyts, G.D., Van Vlem, E., De Vos, A., Daelemans, R.A., Rorive, G., Elseviers, M.M., Schurgers, M., Segaert, M., D'Haese, P.C., Broe, M.E., 1995. Wegener granulomatosis is associated to exposure to silicon compounds: a case-control study. Nephrol. Dial. Transpl. 10, 1162.

Ohta, N., Fukase, S., Aoyagi, M., 2001. Serum levels of soluble adhesion molecules ICAM-1. VCAM-1 and E-selectin in patients with Wegener's granulomatosis. Auris Nasus Larynx 28, 311.

Pall, A.A., Adu, D., Drayson, M., Taylor, C.M., Richards, N.T., Michael, J., 1994. Circulating soluble adhesion molecules in systemic vasculitis. Nephrol. Dial. Transpl. 9, 770.

Paulley, J.W., 1980a. Coronary ischaemia and occlusion in giant cell (temporal) arteritis. Acta Med. Scand. 208, 257.

Paulley, J.W., 1980b. Ischaemic heart disease in giant cell arteritis. Lancet 1, 421.

Pinching, A.J., Lockwood, C.M., Pussell, B.A., Rees, A.J., Sweny, P., Evans, D.J., Bowley, N., Peters, D.K., 1983. Wegener's granulomatosis: observations on 18 patients with severe renal disease. QJM 52, 435.

Praprotnik, S., Rozman, B., Blank, M., Shoenfeld, Y., 2000. Pathogenic role of anti-endothelial cell antibodies in systemic vasculitis. Wien Klin. Wochenschr. 112, 660.

Rajani, R.M., Dalvi, B.V., D'Silva, S.A., Lokhandwala, Y.Y., Kale, P.A., 1991. Acute myocardial infarction with normal coronary arteries in a case of polyarteritis nodosa: possible role of coronary artery spasm. Postgrad. Med. J. 67, 78.

Rapezzi, C., Ortolani, P., Binetti, G., Picchio, F.M., Magnani, B., 1990. Idiopathic restrictive cardiomyopathy in the young: report of two cases. Int. J. Cardiol. 29, 121.

Reinhold-Keller, E., de Groot, K., Rudert, H., Nolle, B., Heller, M., Gross, W.L., 1996. Response to trimethoprim/sulfamethoxazole in Wegener's granulomatosis depends on the phase of disease. QJM 89, 15.

Reinhold-Keller, E., Beuge, N., Latza, U., de Groot, K., Rudert, H., Nolle, B., Heller, M., Gross, W.L., 2000. An interdisciplinary approach to the care of patients with Wegener's granulomatosis: long-term outcome in 155 patients. Arthritis Rheum. 43, 1021.

Rosen, N., Gaton, E., 1972. Takayasu's arteritis of coronary arteries. Arch. Pathol. 94, 225.

Salojin, K.V., Le Tonqueze, M., Saraux, A., Nassonov, E.L., Dueymes, M., Piette, J.C., Youinou, P.Y., 1997. Antiendothelial cell antibodies: useful markers of systemic sclerosis. Am. J. Med. 102, 178.

Salvarani, C., Macchioni, P., Zizzi, F., Mantovani, W., Rossi, F., Castri, C., Chiravalloti, F., Portioli, I., 1991. Epidemiologic and immunogenetic aspects of polymyalgia rheumatica and giant cell arteritis in northern Italy. Arthritis Rheum. 34, 351.

Sangle, S., Karim, M.Y., Hughes, G.R., D'Cruz, D.P., 2002. Sulphamethoxazole-trimethoprim in the treatment of limited paranasal Wegener's granulomatosis. Rheumatology (Oxford) 41, 589.

Saveuse, H., Dorra, M., Dechy, H., Baglin, C., Rouveix, E., Betourne, C., 1988. Temporal arteritis: a syndrome. From Horton's disease to periarteritis nodosa. Presse Méd. 17, 517 (in French).

Schiff, S., Moffatt, R., Mandel, W.J., Rubin, S.A., 1982. Acute myocardial infarction and recurrent ventricular arrhythmias in Behcet's syndrome. Am. Heart J. 103, 438.

Scolyer, R.A., 1999. Test and teach. Number ninety-four: Part 1. Churg-Strauss syndrome. Pathology 31, 217.

Shimizu, T., Ehrlich, G.E., Inaba, G., Hayashi, K., 1979. Behçet disease (Behçet syndrome). Semin. Arthritis Rheum. 8, 223.

Small, P., Brisson, M.L., 1991. Wegener's granulomatosis presenting as temporal arteritis. Arthritis Rheum. 34, 220.

Specks, U., Fervenza, F.C., McDonald, T.J., Hogan, M.C., 2001. Response of Wegener's granulomatosis to anti-CD20 chimeric monoclonal antibody therapy. Arthritis Rheum. 44, 2836.

Stanson, A.W., Klein, R.G., Hunder, G.G., 1976. Extracranial angiographic findings in giant cell (temporal) arteritis. Am. J. Roentgenol. 127, 957.

Stegeman, C.A., Tervaert, J.W., Huitema, M.G., de Jong, P.E., Kallenberg, C.G., 1994. Serum levels of soluble adhesion molecules intercellular adhesion molecule 1, vascular cell adhesion molecule 1, and E-selectin in patients with Wegener's granulomatosis. Relationship to disease activity and relevance during followup. Arthritis Rheum. 37, 1228.

Thomas-Golbanov, C., Sridharan, S., 2001. Novel therapies in vasculitis. Exp. Opin. Investig. Drugs 10, 1279.

Vollertsen, R.S., Conn, D.L., 1990. Vasculitis associated with rheumatoid arthritis. Rheum. Dis. Clin. North Am. 16, 445.

Wagner, J., Andrassy, K., Ritz, E., 1991. Is vasculitis in subacute bacterial endocarditis associated with ANCA? Lancet 337, 799.

Walton, E.W., 1958. Giant-cell granuloma of the respiratory tract (Wegener's granulomatosis). Br. Med. J. 2, 265.

Wegener, F., 1936. Uber generalisierte. septische Gefasserkrankungen. Verh. Dtsch. Ges. Pathol. 29, 202.

Woywodt, A., Streiber, F., de Groot, K., Regelsberger, H., Haller, H., Haubitz, M., 2003. Circulating endothelial cells as markers for ANCA-associated small-vessel vasculitis. Lancet 361, 206.

Yamashita, Y., Yorioka, N., Taniguchi, Y., Yamakido, M., Watanabe, C., Kitamura, T., Nakamura, S., 1998. Nonasthmatic case of Churg-Strauss syndrome with rapidly progressive glomerulonephritis. Intern. Med. 37, 561.

Yazici, H., Barnes, C.G., 1991. Practical treatment recommendations for pharmacotherapy of Behcet's syndrome. Drugs 42, 796.

Chapter 15

Cardiovascular Involvement in Ankylosing Spondylitis

I. Sari[*,§,¶] **and N. Haroon**[*,¶,||]
[*]*Division of Rheumatology, University Health Network, Toronto, ON, Canada;* [§]*Division of Rheumatology, Department of Internal Medicine, Dokuz Eylul University, Izmir, Turkey;* [¶]*University of Toronto, Toronto, ON, Canada;* [||]*Krembil Research Institute, Toronto, ON, Canada*

Key Points

- The available data on mortality in AS suggest that there is an increased overall mortality and reduced life expectancy, which is independent from radiation therapy. The increase in mortality is largely due to CV reasons.
- CV morbidity is also increased in AS. Current data suggest that the rate of IHD, MI, and stroke seem to be more prevalent in AS than healthy subjects.
- Men with AS face higher risk of CV morbidity and mortality.
- There is no clear association between traditional CV risk factors and increased CV mortality and morbidity in AS. This may be explained by complex multifactorial interactions between CV risk factors, inflammation, structural cardiac abnormalities (i.e., AI), genetic predisposition, and environmental agents.
- The prevalence of heart pathologies in patients with AS varies. Well-defined structural abnormalities are aortic valve and myocardial involvements. There is also an increased frequency of conduction system disturbances. Majority of the patients who have these abnormalities remain clinically asymptomatic.
- There is an increased prevalence of subclinical vascular involvement such as impaired endothelial function and increased aortic stiffness in AS. The further consequences of these findings in the development of macrovascular disease is currently unknown.
- Although there is a considerable gap in the literature, treatment modalities (both pharmacological and nonpharmacological) possibly have a beneficial effect on morbidity and mortality in AS. These may show their effects via reducing pain and stiffness and therefore improving mobility and

functional performance. Additionally, treatment may decrease inflammation, which is possibly an offending factor for vascular injury.
- Considering the increased CV morbidity and mortality, there is a need for developing prevention, treatment, and follow-up strategies in AS.

1. INTRODUCTION

Ankylosing spondylitis (AS) is a chronic inflammatory disease predominantly involving the axial skeleton. Presenting symptoms generally occur before the age of 30 and men are affected more commonly compared to women. The chronic and progressive nature of the disease may cause spinal restriction and can adversely affect quality of life, as well as the psychological and economic status of the patients (Poddubnyy and Sieper, 2012). The prevalence of AS has been reported to be as high as that of rheumatoid arthritis with estimates ranging from 0.03% to 1.4% (Haroon et al., 2014). There are several extraspinal manifestations that may complicate the clinical course such as arthritis, acute anterior uveitis, inflammatory bowel disease, and psoriasis. Involvement of the cardiovascular (CV) system and increased CV mortality and morbidity has been reported in AS (Braun and Pincus, 2002; Zochling and Braun, 2009; Nurmohamed et al., 2012; Haroon et al., 2015). This chapter focuses on various aspects of CV involvement in AS.

2. CARDIOVASCULAR MORTALITY IN ANKYLOSING SPONDYLITIS

Several studies reported an increased overall mortality in AS. In the initial reports, performed during 1950s, there was an excess mortality rate because of leukemia and cancer (Smith et al., 1977; Kaprove et al., 1980). This was mainly due to the radiation therapy, which was one of the treatment options for AS during that period. However, later studies in nonradiated patients have confirmed the decreased overall life expectancy in AS (Radford et al., 1977; Khan et al., 1981; Bakland et al., 2011; Mok et al., 2011; Exarchou et al., 2015) with CV disease being the leading cause of death in most studies (Khan et al., 1981; Bakland et al., 2011; Exarchou et al., 2015; Haroon et al., 2015).

In 1977, Radford et al. (1977) reported that AS patients (n = 836) with no history of radiation therapy had a relative risk (RR) of 1.3 for CV and 1.7 for cerebrovascular death. In this study total mortality from circulatory diseases was increased in both men and women with AS. In 1993, Lehtinen et al. reported increased overall mortality rates in AS (n = 398). The observed/expected deaths from circulatory disease were 1.2 in which coronary and cerebrovascular diseases were responsible for 60% and 25% of deaths, respectively (Lehtinen, 1993). In a small retrospective study by Khan et al. a life table analysis of survival was conducted in 56 white AS patients. The majority of patients (88%) in this study was male. There was a decrease in survival among AS patients that was significant after 20 years of diagnosis. Death was attributed to CV and cerebrovascular reasons in about half of the deceased patients (Khan et al., 1981). In a Canadian study, Kaprove et al. studied 62 male AS patients who did not receive radiation therapy and revealed an observed/expected ratio of 1.3 for total mortality. This number was not significant when compared to the general population (Kaprove et al., 1980). An observational study including 677 AS patients followed in a hospital in Norway reported that overall mortality was significantly increased in AS compared to age- and sex-matched controls [standardized mortality ratio (SMR): 1.61 [95% confidence interval (CI): 1.29−1.93]] (Bakland et al., 2011). The increased risk was only present in the male patients (SMR: 1.63 [95% CI: 1.29−1.97]). Circulatory diseases were the most common cause (40%) of death in that group (Bakland et al., 2011). In a Hong Kong study, among 2154 AS patients, overall age- and sex-adjusted SMR was significantly higher in the patients compared to the general population (SMR: 1.87 [95% CI: 1.61−2.13]) (Mok et al., 2011). The age-adjusted SMR was significantly higher in men (SMR: 1.94 [95% CI: 1.65−2.22]) but not in women (Table 15.1). The leading causes of death among AS patients were infection (29%), cancer (17%), respiratory diseases (14%), and CV diseases (12%) (Mok et al., 2011). A population-based cohort study in Sweden (8600 AS and 40,460 controls) also confirmed the results of previous studies indicating that all-cause mortality was significantly higher in patients with AS compared to the general population with an age- and sex-adjusted hazard ratio (HR) of 1.60 (95% CI: 1.44−1.77) (Exarchou et al., 2015). In the Swedish study, both men (HR: 1.83, 95% CI: 1.50−2.22) and women (HR: 1.53, 95% CI: 1.36−1.72) had increased overall mortality. The major cause of death in the AS cohort was CV disease (34.7% vs. 30.6% compared to controls) (Exarchou et al., 2015). In a recent, large population-based study (21473 AS and 86,606 controls) among Ontario residents in Canada, Haroon et al. (2015) showed that vascular mortality was significantly higher in AS patients compared to the general population. In the Canadian study, there was a 36% higher risk for vascular mortality when adjusted for baseline CV risk factors (HR: 1.36 [95% CI: 1.13−1.65]). When stratified according to sex, this risk was particularly significant among the male subjects (HR: 1.46 [95% CI: 1.13−1.87]). Compared to non-AS comparators, patients with AS had 60% higher risk for cerebrovascular mortality (HR: 1.60 [CI: 1.17−2.20]) and 35% higher risk for CV mortality (HR: 1.35 [CI: 1.07−1.70]) (Haroon et al., 2015) (Table 15.1).

In summary, there is convincing evidence that overall mortality is increased in AS compared to the general population. The enhanced mortality is largely due to the CV reasons and both sexes, particularly men, are at risk.

TABLE 15.1 Summary of Mortality Studies Focusing on Circulatory Diseases in Patients With Ankylosing Spondylitis (AS)

	AS (n)	Male (%)	Cardiovascular Mortality		Total Circulatory Mortality	Total Mortality
Radford[a,b], UK (Radford et al., 1977)	836	62	Male	1.4 (NA)	1.5 (NA)	1.8
			Female	1.1 (NA)	1.3 (NA)	1.2 (NS)
			Total	1.3 (NA)	1.4 (NA)	1.6
Lehtinen[a,b], Finland (Lehtinen, 1993)	398	87			1.2 (NA)	1.5 (NA)
Kaprove[a], Canada (Kaprove et al., 1980)	62	100	1.22 (NS)			1.3 (NS)
Bakland[c], Norway (Bakland et al., 2011)	611	76	Male			1.63
			Female			1.38 (NS)
			Total			1.61
Mok[c], Hong Kong (Mok et al., 2011)	2,154	83	Male			1.94
			Female			1.38 (NS)
			Total			1.87
Exarchou[d], Sweden (Exarchou et al., 2015)	8,600	66	Male			1.53
			Female			1.83
			Total			1.60
Haroon[b,d], Canada (Haroon et al., 2015)	21,473	53	Male		1.46	
			Female		1.24 (NS)	
			Total	1.35	1.36	

Note that patients in those studies did not expose to radiation therapy. Numbers indicate significant values unless NA (data not available) or NS (not significant) present.
[a]*Observed/expected ratio.*
[b]*Studies reporting cerebrovascular mortality in AS.*
[c]*Standardized mortality ratio.*
[d]*Hazard ratio.*

3. VASCULAR MORBIDITY IN ANKYLOSING SPONDYLITIS

Despite the association of AS with increased CV death, the underlying etiology of this enhanced mortality is still unknown. The occurrence of CV events, that is, myocardial infarction (MI) and stroke was evaluated in several studies. Han et al. (2006) studied 1843 AS patients and 7372 controls in PharMetrics Patient-Centric Database, a database that contains fully adjudicated medical service and prescription drug claims from health plans across the US, and revealed that age- and sex-adjusted prevalence ratio of ischemic heart disease (IHD; 1.2 [95% CI: 1−1.5]), peripheral vascular disease (PVD; 2.4 [95% CI: 1.2−2.2]), congestive heart failure (1.8 [95% CI: 1.2−2.6]), and cerebrovascular disease (1.7 [95% CI: 1.3−2.3]) were higher in patients than controls. Peters et al. (2010) performed a survey using a standardized questionnaire to estimate the prevalence of MI in patients with AS, aged between 50 and 75 years. Only 65% of the patients (n = 383) responded to the questionnaire. There was an increased prevalence of MI even taking into account the nonresponder patients (considered as non-MI) in the total group with an age- and gender-adjusted odds ratio (OR) of 1.9 (95% CI: 1.2−3.2). Interestingly, the sex-stratified analysis was significant only for women in this analysis (OR: 5.7 [95% CI: 2.1−15.8]) (Peters et al., 2010). Kang et al. (2010) studied 11,701 AS patients and documented an increased frequency of IHD both in male (OR: 2.32 [95% CI: 1.74−3.09]) and female (OR: 4.49 [95% CI: 2.78−7.26]) AS patients. In contrast, there was no increased risk for stroke among patients with AS (OR: 1.01 [95% CI: 0.87−1.17]) (Kang et al., 2010). A registry study from Southern Sweden evaluated the common comorbidities in AS (n = 935) (Bremander et al., 2011). They revealed higher prevalence of IHD both in male (SMR: 2.18 [95% CI: 1.71−2.74]) and female (SMR: 2.27 [95% CI: 1.32−3.64]) patients. However, the prevalence of MI specifically was not different from the general population (Bremander et al., 2011). A population-based study in Canada showed that age- and sex-standardized prevalence ratios with respect to IHD (1.37 [95% CI: 1.31−1.44]), cerebrovascular disease (1.25 [95% CI: 1.15−1.35]), and any hospitalization for a CV or cerebrovascular disease (1.31 [95% CI: 1.22−1.41]) was significantly increased in the AS group compared to the general population of Quebec (Szabo et al., 2011). A Taiwanese study in younger AS patients (n = 4794) showed a significant increase in IHD compared to age- and sex-matched controls, with an adjusted HR of 1.47 (95% CI: 1.13−1.92) (Huang et al., 2013). In a retrospective cohort study of 1686 AS patients recruited from primary care/general practitioner records, Brophy et al. (2012) found no significant differences in terms of age- and gender-adjusted HRs for MI 1.28 (95% CI: 0.93−1.74) and for cerebrovascular disease/stroke 1.0 (95% CI: 0.73−1.39) compared to the controls in the same registry. In another Taiwanese study, Chou et al. (2014) studied 6262 AS patients and found an increased risk of acute coronary syndrome in the AS cohort compared to the control population registered in the National Health Insurance Research Database in Taiwan (adjusted HR: 1.36 [1.16–1.59]). This risk was significant in both males (aHR: 1.34 [1.08–1.66]) and females (aHR: 1.33 [1.06–1.66]) (Chou et al., 2014). In a recent meta-analysis Mathieu et al. (2015) showed a higher frequency of MI (OR: 1.60 [95% CI: 1.32–1.93]) and stroke (OR: 1.50 [95% CI: 1.39–1.62]) in AS. Ungprasert et al. conducted a systematic review and meta-analysis of observational studies that compared the risk of coronary artery disease in patients with AS versus non-AS controls. They showed that AS was associated with a 1.41-fold increased risk of coronary artery disease compared with non-AS participants (pooled risk ratio 1.41 [95% CI: 1.29–1.54]) (Ungprasert et al., 2015) (Table 15.2).

4. CARDIOVASCULAR RISK FACTORS IN ANKYLOSING SPONDYLITIS

There are several modifiable and nonmodifiable risk factors associated with CV disease. The five leading modifiable risk factors including hypertension (HT), diabetes mellitus type-2 (DM), hypercholesterolemia, obesity, and smoking are estimated to be responsible for more than half of CV mortality in US adults aged 45–79 years (Patel et al., 2015). The aforementioned epidemiological studies have demonstrated an increased CV morbidity and mortality in AS. However, limited information is available regarding the CV risk factors in AS.

There are several case-control studies focused on the association of AS and CV risk factors. Unfortunately, small sample size and other methodological issues make it difficult to interpret the results of these studies. More robust data are available from large-scale epidemiological studies. Han et al. (2006) showed an increase in the prevalence of comorbidities including HT (RR: 1.3 [95% CI: 1.1–1.4]) and hyperlipidemia (HL; RR: 1.2 [95% CI: 1.1–1.3]) in AS. On the other hand, DM was not different compared to controls (RR: 1.2 [95% CI: 1.0–1.4]) (Han et al., 2006). Similar observation was documented by a study from Taiwan (HT; OR: 1.87 [95% CI: 1.75–1.99], HL; OR: 1.46 [95% CI: 1.35–1.57] and DM; OR: 1.11 [95% CI: 0.98–1.22]) (Kang et al., 2010). Brophy et al. (2012) revealed an increase in the frequency of HT (OR: 1.65 [95% CI: 1.47–1.85]) and type II diabetes (OR: 1.27 [95% CI: 1.09–1.49]) but not in HL (OR: 1.12 [95% CI: 0.95–1.33]). A Swedish study also reported higher prevalence of HT (SMR: 1.98 [95% CI: 1.72–2.28]) and DM (SMR: 1.41 [95% CI: 1.1–1.78]) and unchanged frequency of HL (SMR: 1.26 [95% CI: 0.89–1.22]) in the AS group compared to controls (Bremander et al., 2011). In their mortality study, Exarchou et al. (2015) showed that presence of DM predicted mortality in the AS group with an age- and sex-adjusted HR of 1.92 (95% CI: 1.51–2.45). Haroon et al. (2015) found that enhanced vascular mortality in AS patients was independent of HT and DM. In a meta-analysis, there were no differences in terms of blood pressure, glucose levels, and atherogenic index (the ratio of total cholesterol/HDL cholesterol) between AS and control groups (Mathieu et al., 2011) (Table 15.3).

TABLE 15.2 Summary of the Studies Reporting Cardiovascular and Cerebrovascular Morbidity in Ankylosing Spondylitis (AS)

	AS (n)	Male (%)	IHD		MI	Cerebrovascular Disease/Stroke
Han[a], USA (Han et al., 2006)	1,843	61	1.2 (NS)			1.7
Peters[b], Netherlands (Peters et al., 2010)	593	76	Male		1.60 (NS)	
			Female		5.75	
			Total		1.94	
Kang[b], Taiwan, (Kang et al., 2010)	11,701	79	Male	2.32		1.01 (NS)
			Female	4.49		1 (NS)
			Total	2.74		1.01 (NS)
Bremander[c], Sweden (Bremander et al., 2011)	935	67	Male	2.18	1.29 (NS)	
			Female	2.27	1.45 (NS)	
			Total	2.20	1.32 (NS)	
Szabo[d], Canada (Szabo et al., 2011)	8,616	56	1.37			1.25
Brophy[e], Wales (Brophy et al., 2012)	1,686	76	1.28 (NS)			1.0 (NS)
Huang[e], Taiwan (Huang et al., 2013)	4,794	74	1.47			

Numbers indicate significant values unless NA (data not available) or NS (not significant) present. *IHD*, ischemic heart disease; *MI*, myocardial infarction.
[a]*Relative risk.*
[b]*Odds ratio.*
[c]*Standardized mortality ratio.*
[d]*Standardized prevalence ratio.*
[e]*Hazard ratio.*

TABLE 15.3 Summary of Epidemiologic Studies Focusing on Cardiovascular Risk Factors

	N	Male (%)	Hypertension		Diabetes Mellitus Type 2	Hyperlipidemia
Han[a], USA (Han et al., 2006)	1,843	61	1.3		1.2 (NS)	1.2
Kang[b], Taiwan (Kang et al., 2010)	11,701	79	Male	2.02	1.09 (NS)	1.42
			Female	1.45	1.15 (NS)	1.57
			Total	1.87	1.11 (NS)	1.46
Bremander[c], Sweden (Bremander et al., 2011)	935	67	Male	2.02	1.35	1.27 (NS)
			Female	1.9	1.83 (NS)	1.23 (NS)
			Total	1.98	1.41	1.26 (NS)
Brophy[b], Wales (Brophy et al., 2012)	1,686	76	1.65		1.27	1.12 (NS)

Numbers indicate significant values unless NA (data not available) or NS (not significant) present.
[a]*Relative risk.*
[b]*Odds ratio.*
[c]*Standardized mortality ratio.*

Smoking and its association with various aspects of AS have been studied extensively. Based on the available data, smoking has an unfavorable impact on disease activity, function, and treatment responses in AS. Some studies also suggested smokers have earlier disease onset, increased acute phase proteins, and higher syndesmophyte formation (Poddubnyy et al., 2012; Ciurea and Finckh, 2013; Wendling and Prati, 2013; Glintborg et al., 2015). However, many of the large epidemiological studies provided limited information regarding lifestyle variables (e.g., smoking) making it difficult to assess their role on the development of CV disease in AS. In addition, the lack of such data also preclude us from estimating whether or not smoking frequency is increased in AS.

Obesity, defined by excessive fat mass, is a global epidemic that affects all age groups in both developed and developing countries. There are several methods for determining obesity. The most commonly used ones are the calculation of the body mass index (BMI) and the waist circumference. More reliable but sophisticated methods are skinfold thickness measurement, bioelectric impedance analysis, dual energy X-ray absorptiometry, computerized tomography, and magnetic resonance imaging modalities (Cornier et al., 2011). There are contradictory results regarding the prevalence of obesity in AS.

Two epidemiological studies from Taiwan studied several CV risk factors as well as obesity in AS. Kang et al. (2010) reported that patients with (n = 11,701) or without (n = 58,505) AS had comparable frequencies of obesity. In another study, among 2895 AS patients, Keller et al. (2014) reported significantly lower obesity rate in AS compared to 11,580 non-AS subjects. However, both studies had considerably lower number of subjects with obesity (n = 123 and 31, respectively) suggesting an effect of underreporting or missing information, which may possibly contribute a bias when interpreting the results (Kang et al., 2010; Keller et al., 2014). In a meta-analysis, comparison of CV risk profiles in case-control studies showed no significant difference between BMI of AS patients and comparators (Mathieu et al., 2011). Studies on body composition in AS provided conflicting results with some suggesting altered body fat distribution in AS (Sari et al., 2007; Toussirot et al., 2013) while others not (Dos Santos et al., 2001; Toussirot et al., 2001; Plasqui et al., 2012). Based on the available information it is currently not possible to provide a link between obesity and excess CV morbidity/mortality in AS.

The metabolic syndrome (MetS) is a cluster of metabolic abnormalities including obesity, insulin resistance, glucose intolerance, hypertension, and dyslipidemia. It is an important risk factor for the subsequent development of type 2 diabetes and/or CV disease. Some studies proposed an increased prevalence of MetS in AS. In a rather small group of 24 patients, Malesci et al. (2007) reported that nearly half had MetS according to the NCEP-ATP III criteria. In a subsequent study, Papadakis et al. (2009) showed that MetS was significantly higher in men with AS compared to controls (34.9% vs. 19.0%). Meta-analysis of the published studies also suggested an increased relative risk of MetS in AS (RR: 2.13 [95% CI: 1.48–3.06]) (Mathieu et al., 2011).

In conclusion, there is no clear association between CV risk factors and increased CV mortality and morbidity in AS. It is more likely that multifactorial interactions such as inflammation, CV risk factors, genetic predisposition, and possibly environmental agents are responsible for the increased risk of CV morbidity and mortality in AS.

5. AORTIC DISEASE IN ANKYLOSING SPONDYLITIS

Aortitis and insufficiency of the aortic valve are among the most important and earliest defined CV manifestation of AS. Histologically, aortitis is defined by the presence of inflammatory infiltrates in the medial and/or intimal layers of the tissue. If inflammatory burden is restricted to the adventitia, the term periaortitis is more apt (Stone et al., 2015). Postmortem studies have provided detailed information about the nature of aortic involvement in AS. Bulkley and Roberts (1973), in an autopsy study of eight male patients with AS and severe aortic insufficiency (AI), found that aortic valve cusps and the proximal aortic wall behind and above the sinuses of Valsalva were thickened. Another finding was a subaortic fibrous ridge resulting from adventitial scar tissue that extended to the left ventricle, just below the aortic valve. In some patients, this scarring extended to the base of the mitral valve and into the intraventricular septum (Bulkley and Roberts, 1973). Intimal proliferation, advential scarring with thickening, and medial scarring were seen in histology. Obliterative vessel disease was seen with the infiltration of plasma cells and lymphocytes (Bulkley and Roberts, 1973). The histological pattern of aortitis in AS is thus lymphoplasmacytic (Stone et al., 2015). Although rare, thoracic or abdominal aorta may also be affected (Hull et al., 1984; Grewal et al., 2014).

One of the most important consequences of aortic involvement is the development of "lone" AI, which refers to aortic incompetency without accompanying stenosis (Bergfeldt, 1997). Dilatation of the aortic root, fibrotic thickening, and downward retraction of the bases of the cusps, and inward rolling of the edges or margins of the cusps can cause aortic valve incompetency (Bulkley and Roberts, 1973; Bergfeldt, 1997). Before the advent of echocardiography the estimated prevalence of AI was around 1−10%. In a survey of 222 AS patients Ansell et al. (1958) reported 2 patients had AI with a frequency of 0.9%. A study with 75 AS patients revealed 8 (10.7%) of them had AI (Weed et al., 1966). Another report, among 97 AS patients, showed that AI was present in 10 patients (10.3%) (Kinsella et al., 1974)

Later studies using echocardiography, provided more detailed information regarding prevalence and the affected anatomical structures in AS. Johnsen et al. studied the prevalence of AI in the Norwegian Sami population. Among 349 volunteers who underwent echocardiography 8.8% had AI compared to 18% in AS patients (Johnsen et al., 2009). This prevalence figure was replicated in a recent study with 187 patients, which showed 18% of the group had varying degrees of AI (Klingberg et al., 2015). In a study of 88 AS patients and 31 controls, Yildirir et al. (2002) showed 9 patients (20%) but none of the controls had AI.

There are also some reports based on transesophageal echocardiography. In a study with 44 AS patients and 30 age- and sex-matched controls, 16% of the patients showed AI whereas none of the controls had aortic involvement (Roldan et al., 1998). In contrast, Park et al. (2012) showed only 1 patient with AI in a group of 70 AS patients and 25 healthy controls. In a different methodology, Hollingworth et al. (1979) studied 20 "lone" AI patients and did not find any patient with sacroiliitis or HLA-B27 positivity. With the same approach Qaiyumi et al. (1985) evaluated 100 consecutive cases of "lone" AI for the prevalence of spondyloarthritis. Four patients were found to have AS and three had Reiter syndrome. Overall 7 (7%) patients had sacroiliitis (Qaiyumi et al., 1985). Another study in patients undergoing aortic valve replacement surgery for AI noted that among 887 patients, 3 (0.3%) had a background of AS (Kawasuji et al., 1982). In a Swedish study Bergfeldt et al. (1988) investigated several group of patients to identify HLA-B27−associated disease and its relation with "lone" AI. In the first group, authors focused on patients with pacemakers. In that group, among 479 patients (5 had also cardiac valve surgery) there were 24 patients with "lone" AI of whom 7 were diagnosed as AS (1.5% of the total pacemaker group). In the second group they also identified patients who underwent cardiac valve surgery (n = 59) because of "lone" AI. They reported that 4 out of 59 patients (6.8%) had a diagnosis of AS. In their third group, among 14 outpatient "lone" AI patients the prevalence of AS was found to be 14.2% (Bergfeldt et al., 1988). Olson et al. (1984) found that 3 (1.3%) out of 225 patients who received surgical aortic intervention because of "lone" AI indeed had AS. The etiology of the AI was evaluated in 160 patients in Finland. There were only 2 (1.3%) patients with a diagnosis of AS (Uusimaa et al., 2006).

Echocardiographic assessment of AS patients allows the visualization of aortic structures in detail. Roldan et al. (1998) reported that 82% of their patients had some degree of aortic root and/or valve involvement as compared with 27% of controls. Thickening of the aortic valve (41% vs. 10%), dilatation of aortic root (25% vs. 7%), and increased aortic stiffness (61% vs. 10%) were significantly different from controls. They also showed 25% of their patients had a subaortic bump (none present in controls), which is indicative of subaortic ridges (Roldan et al., 1998). In a small study, aortic root dilatation (ARD) was present in 6 (26%) out of 23 patients (Thomas et al., 1982). In contrast, none of the 22 controls had ARD. In that study the prevalence of AI was 4.3% (Thomas et al., 1982). Similarly, Yildirir et al. (2002) reported that aortic root dimensions of the AS patients were significantly higher than in controls. In a group of 35 patients and 20 controls, investigators did not find any AI and the ARD were similar between the patients and the controls. However, 17% of the AS patients had subaortic bump (Tucker et al., 1982). LaBresh et al. (1985) studied 36 patients (26 were diagnosed as AS) and reported that subaortic fibrous ridging and aortic valve thickening was present in 31% and 2.8% of the patients, respectively. The ARD were not different between patient and control groups (LaBresh et al., 1985). In a study including 57 consecutive patients with AS and 78 healthy subjects, researchers showed aortic diameter and strain were significantly higher in the patient group (Moyssakis et al., 2009). Another study also showed impaired aortic elasticity in a group of 35 AS patients compared to 30 controls (Demiralp et al., 2004). The aortic systolic and diastolic diameters were not different between the groups (Demiralp et al., 2004).

Aortic and valvular disease appears to occur more commonly in patients with a longer disease duration. Graham and Smythe (1958) reported that the prevalence of AI was noted in 3.5% of AS patients with <15 years of disease duration and in 10% with 30 years of disease. Roldan et al. noted that age and disease duration were the factors related with the aortic disease in AS. In their study, during follow-up of nearly 4 years, 24% of the patients developed new aortic root or valve abnormalities, in 12% existing valve regurgitation worsened significantly and in 20% previously observed abnormalities were resolved (Roldan et al., 1998). In another study, researchers reported that AI was related to increasing age and longstanding disease and the frequency of AI was increased from 20% in the 50s to 56% in the 70s (Klingberg et al., 2015). In that study, disease duration was an independent predictor of the AI (OR: 1.05; 95% CI, 1.01–1.8) (Klingberg et al., 2015). In a group of 95 subjects (AS = 70, controls = 25), Park et al. (2012) reported that 77% of the AS patients and 30% of the controls had aortic valve thickening. They also showed increased aortic stiffness and ARD, which were significant only in patients with >10 years of disease duration (Park et al., 2012). However, other studies did not support this relationship with aortic disease. O'Neill et al (1992) studied 24 AS patients who had at least 10 years of disease duration and 24 healthy controls. The frequency of AI was 8.3% and comparison of patients with or without cardiac disease was not different in terms of age and disease duration (O'Neill et al., 1992). In addition, some studies highlighted the presence of aortic disease in patients with short disease duration (Tucker et al., 1982). The involvement of the aortic structures seems not restricted to the adult AS patients. Studies in juvenile patients showed young age patients are also at risk. In a study of 20 juvenile onset SpA, 4 (20%) of them had AI (Gerster et al., 1987). Further study with 36 juvenile SpA and 33 healthy controls showed that 3 patients (8%) had AI (Stamato et al., 1995). None of the patients and controls had ARD. In that study there were no relation with disease duration and AI (Stamato et al., 1995). A third study included 20 juvenile onset AS, 31 adult AS, and 20 controls (Jimenez-Balderas et al., 2001). Based on their data ARD was present in 58% of the adult AS patients, in 30% of the juvenile AS patients, and in 0% in the control group. None of the patients and controls had an AI in that study (Jimenez-Balderas et al., 2001).

The relationship between clinical parameters, disease activity and aortic involvement is also of interest. In the former studies higher prevalence of peripheral arthritis, HLA-B27, and AI have been suggested (Ansell et al., 1958; Graham and Smythe, 1958; Bulkley and Roberts, 1973; Kinsella et al., 1974). However, further studies did not replicate this finding (Sukenik et al., 1987; O'Neill et al., 1992; Klingberg et al., 2015). Unlike with the HLA-B27 and uveitis association, HLA-B27 antigen and its relation with aortic disease is also controversial. Hollingworth et al. (1979) studied 20 patients with "lone" AI and did not find any patient with HLA-B27 positivity. None of these patients had X-ray–defined sacroiliitis also (Hollingworth et al., 1979). In the aforementioned study among Norwegian Sami population, regression analysis failed to show HLA-B27 and its predictive role in AI (Johnsen et al., 2009). In their study, Qaiyumi et al. (1985) typed 96 cases for HLA-B27 antigen, and it was found to be present in a total of 12 cases (7 with spondylitis). They suggested that in nonspondylitis AI patients there was no excess of HLA-B27 (Qaiyumi et al., 1985). Some studies suggested a relation between aortic disease and disease activity. Park et al (2012) showed that BASDAI, ESR, and CRP are correlated with aortic valve thickness. Radiographic disease severity, assessed by modified stoke ankylosing spondylitis spinal score, has been documented as one of the predictors of AI (Klingberg et al., 2015). In another study it has been shown that BASDAI was independently predicting the aortic distensibility (Moyssakis et al., 2009). In contrast, Roldan et al. (1998) showed there were no differences in terms of disease activity index and spinal mobility measures between ARD and non-ARD groups.

In summary, AS can affect various segments of the aorta, particularly ascending aorta. Inflammation may cause dilatation and reduced arterial elasticity. Dilatation of the proximal aorta along with the thickened cusps may cause valvular regurgitation nearly up to 20% of the patients. In general, many of the cases are subclinical but some of the patients may require surgical interventions. Longer disease duration and aging are likely to increase the aortic lesions. There is currently no single variable that may predict the development of aortic disease. It is more possible that combination of several factors including higher disease activity, HLA-B27 positivity, and extraspinal features such as peripheral arthritis may predispose certain patients who are susceptible to aortic disease.

6. MITRAL VALVE INVOLVEMENT IN ANKYLOSING SPONDYLITIS

Insufficiency of the mitral valve (MI) is less defined entity compared to AI in AS. Data on this subject are mostly based on case series with literature review. It may be a result of previously described subaortic bump and its extension to the anterior leaflet of the mitral cusp. Left ventricular dilatation secondary to AI may be another reason for MI (Roldan, 2008). The prevalence of mitral valve involvement varies between the studies. Yildirir et al. (2002) reported that 5 of 88 AS patients (5.7%) had evidence of mitral valve prolapse (MVP), 6 (6.8%) had thick mitral valves, and 5 (5.7%) had mild mitral regurgitation. In their control group none of the controls had MI and only 1 subject (3.2%) had MVP (Yildirir et al., 2002). Roldan et al. (1998) reported that mitral valve thickness (34% vs. 3%) and MI (32% vs. 3%) were significantly higher in the AS group than in controls. In a cohort of 77 AS patients, the reported prevalence of MI was 10.4% (Lange et al., 2007). High prevalence of MI has been reported in a recent echocardiography study consisting of 187 AS patients (Klingberg et al., 2015). According to that 73% of the patients had mild and 1% had severe mitral valve regurgitation (Klingberg et al., 2015). In a series of 97 patients, there was only 1 patient with MI (Kinsella et al., 1974). Park et al. (2012) showed increased mitral valve thickness in both groups of patients stratified according to the disease duration (<10 and >10 years) compared to controls. However, the prevalence of MI (<10 years, 4% and >10 years, 10%) was not different than in the controls (4%) (Park et al., 2012). Brunner et al. (2006) studied 100 male AS patients with a disease duration >15 years and showed that 29% of the group had MI. They compared their results with the normal population (22%), which retrieved from the literature review and the difference between the groups was not significant (Brunner et al., 2006). In a study of 40 AS patients, the prevalence of MVP was 10% (Alves et al., 1988). In another study consisting of 24 patients with long-standing AS and 24 controls, MVP was reported to be not different between the groups (AS: 4.2% and controls: 8.3%) (O'Neill et al., 1992). Data from juvenile AS patients showed that prevalence is around 20% for MVP (Gerster et al., 1987) and 5% for MI (Stamato et al., 1995).

In summary, mitral valve involvement (thickening, MVP, and MI) in AS can be seen in variable frequencies and it is usually mild in severity. Its relation with disease characteristics and clinical significance is poorly studied and additional data are required in that field.

7. CONDUCTION ABNORMALITIES IN ANKYLOSING SPONDYLITIS

One of the well-known cardiac complications of AS is conduction system abnormalities. Chronic inflammation originating from the proximal aorta may extend into the membranous part of interventricular (IV) septum and atrioventricular (AV) nodal area (Bulkley and Roberts, 1973). Diffuse increase of myocardial interstitial connective tissue may also be a possible offending factor leading to conduction disturbances (Brewerton et al., 1987). Direct or indirect injuries such as the involvement of blood vessels and decreasing blood supply to the related structures may cause conduction system pathologies. Several types of conduction abnormalities have been reported with varying frequencies. Isolated involvement of the sinoatrial (SA) node, AV node, His bundle or its branches as well as combinations of the above can be seen in AS. The most frequently reported conduction abnormality is AV block, particularly type 1. In the first systematic study on this subject, investigators examined routine electrocardiograms (ECGs) from 190 patients with AS. They found that 29 (15%) had first-degree and 3 (1.6%) had third-degree (complete) AV block (Bernstein and Broch, 1949). Graham and Smythe (1958) in a group of 519 AS patients, reported that prolonged PR interval was found in 0.6%, 1.2%, 2.7%, and 8.5% of patients whose disease durations were 5, 10, 15, and 30 years, respectively. Besides, the frequency of AV block was considerably higher in patients with peripheral arthritis (Graham and Smythe, 1958). In a study of 68 AS patients, 33% of subjects developed conduction disturbances during a 25-year follow-up (Bergfeldt et al., 1982a). The most frequent conduction abnormalities were AV block type 1 (21%), left anterior fascicular block (LAFB, 12%), AV block type 3 (9%), AV block type 2 (7%), left bundle branch block (LBBB, 6%), and right bundle branch block (RBBB, 6%). Atrial fibrillation (AF) was present in 3% of AS patients (Bergfeldt et al., 1982a). Similar to the previous study, subgroup analysis showed that the prevalence of conduction disturbances was significantly higher in patients with peripheral arthritis (Bergfeldt et al., 1982a). In a retrospective study of 40 AS patients, Sukenik et al. (1987) reported 3 (7.5%) had AV block (one case with a third-degree block), 5 (12.5%) had bundle branch block, 1 (2.5%) had Wolff-Parkinson-White (WPW) syndrome, and 1 (2.5%) had short PR interval. In a cross-sectional study of 210 AS patients, the prevalence of conduction abnormalities was 15%. First-degree AV block was present in 9% and LAFB in 6%. AF was present in 1% and pacemaker requirement in total group was 0.5%. None of the patients in that group had second- or third-degree AV block (Forsblad-d'Elia et al., 2013). A recent study reported that 25 of 187 patients (13%) had AV or IV conduction abnormalities (Klingberg et al., 2015). In a large retrospective cohort study including 641 AS patients the prevalence of paroxysmal supraventricular tachycardia (PSVT) and WPW syndrome was studied. 14 (2.2%) were identified as having PSVT, and 3 (0.5%) with WPW (Ho et al., 2012). The observed numbers in the study were considerably higher when compared with the normal population figures (PSVT: 0.62%, WPW: 0.09−0.15%) (Ho et al., 2012).

To obtain more detailed information, an ambulatory 24-h Holter ECG monitoring was also performed in some of the studies. Thomsen et al. (1986) studied 54 AS patients and showed that AV block (all had first-degree and 1 additionally had intermittent third-degree) and severe arrhythmias were present in 7% and 4% of the patients, respectively. Yildirir et al. (2002) studied 88 AS and 31 healthy controls. About 7.9% of AS group had conduction disturbances. The observed abnormalities were AV block (first-degree: 3.4%, second-degree: 1.1%, and third-degree: 1.1%), RBBB (1.1%), and LBBB (1.1%). In contrast, only one patient (3.2%) in the control group had AV block type II (Yildirir et al., 2002). The frequencies of supraventricular and ventricular ectopic beats were significantly higher in the patients group compared to the controls (Yildirir et al., 2002). A later study with 31 AS patients and 22 controls did not find a difference regarding atrial and ventricular arrhythmias between the groups (Kazmierczak et al., 2007).

In contrast, some studies did not find any increase in terms of conduction disturbances. In a comparative study, 97 AS, 81 RA, and 99 healthy controls were studied. In this study 5% of AS (4 first-degree and 1 third-degree AV block), 4% of RA (2 first-degree and 1 third-degree AV block), and 3% of controls (3 first-degree AV block) had conduction abnormalities (Kinsella et al., 1974). A study of 100 male subjects with AS (more than 15 years disease duration) showed that the prevalence of arrhythmia and conduction abnormalities was 7% and 5%, respectively. AF was observed in 2% of the cases. LBBB was present in 19% and AV block (8 with first-degree and 1 with third-degree) was found in 9%. Authors suggested that these were not different when compared with the numbers obtained from general population (Brunner et al., 2006).

Association of AS and conduction abnormalities were also studied in a different methodology. A population of 223 men who had permanently implanted pacemakers was screened. Sacroiliitis was found in 19 (8.5%), 15 (6.7%) of whom fulfilled the diagnostic criteria for AS (Bergfeldt et al., 1982b). Similarly, 35 men with permanent pacemaker without alternative causes for conduction disturbances were studied. The AS and inflammatory back pain prevalence were 3% and 23%, respectively. HLA B27 was present in five (14%) patients, which is a significantly higher prevalence than in healthy controls (17/292, 6%) (Peeters et al., 1991).

The observed abnormalities seem to be more frequent among male subjects. A recent prospective nationwide population-based cohort study from Sweden reported that age- and sex-adjusted HRs for AV block (2.75, 95% CI [2.05−3.69]), AF (1.43, 95% CI [1.25−1.65]), and pacemaker implantation (2.19, 95% CI [1.73−2.79]) were significantly increased in AS group compared to the general population. The HRs were also significant when compared to the patients with psoriatic arthritis. Importantly, the excess HRs were particularly higher in male AS patients (Bengtsson et al., 2015).

Conduction disturbances in the general population were studied in previous studies. De Bacquer et al. (2000) studied 47,358 men and women. The prevalence of AV block, bundle branch block, AF/flutter, and WPW syndrome was 0.2%, 1.6%, 0.55%, and 0.11% in men and 0.1%, 0.8%, 0.33%, and 0.04% in women, respectively (De Bacquer et al., 2000). In another study, Hingorani et al. (2012) analyzed baseline ECGs in healthy normal volunteers participating in phase I studies. Conduction abnormalities were present in 5.9% of 3978 healthy volunteers. First-degree AV block, RBBB, and WPW syndrome were reported in 2.2%, 0.2%, and 0.1% of the subjects (Hingorani et al., 2012). Cheng et al. (2009) investigated 7575 individuals from the Framingham Heart Study and reported that 1.6% of the individuals had first-degree AV block. In a French study, the global prevalence of IV block was 3.09% in 69,186 patients (Monin et al., 2015). In their large study, Hiss and Lamb (1962) examined 122,043 male subjects from the US Air Force personnel and noted that second- and third-degree AV block was present in 4 (0.003%) and 3 (0.002%) subjects, respectively.

In summary, several forms of arrhythmias and conduction blocks can be seen during the course of AS. When compared with the general population the most prevalent form of block is AV, which is predominantly localized in the suprahisian region (Bergfeldt et al., 1984). SA node dysfunction, WPW syndrome, tachycardia, bradycardia, or IV conduction abnormalities have also been described (Palazzi et al., 2008). Male sex and HLA-B27 seems to be more frequent but it should be noted that these abnormalities have also been reported in women or HLA-B27 negative AS (Bergfeldt, 1997). Clinical manifestations may range from asymptomatic patients to severe pacemaker requiring condition (Table 15.4).

TABLE 15.4 Summary of the Conduction Disturbances in Ankylosing Spondylitis (AS) and General Population

	AV Block	Type 1	Type 2	Type 3	BBB	RBBB	LBBB	AF	WPW
Bernstein and Broch (1949)		15		1.6					
Bergfeldt et al. (1982a)		21	7	9		6	6	3	
Sukenik et al. (1987)	7.5	5	0	2.5	12.5				2.5
Forsblad-d'Elia et al. (2013)		9	0	0				1	
Ho et al. (2012)									0.5
Thomsen et al. (1986)	7	7	0	2					
Yildirir et al. (2002)		3.4	1.1	1.1		1.1	1.1		
Brunner et al. (2006)	9	8	0	1			19	2	
General Population Frequencies									
Males, De Bacquer et al. (2000)	0.2				1.6			0.55	0.11
Hingorani et al. (2012)		2.2				0.2			0.1
Cheng et al. (2009)		1.6							
Hiss and Lamb (1962)			0.003	0.002					

Numbers indicate percentages.
AF, atrial fibrillation; *BBB*, bundle branch block; *LBBB*, left bundle branch block; *RBBB*, right bundle branch block; *WPW*, Wolff-Parkinson-White syndrome.

8. MYOCARDIUM AND PERICARDIUM IN ANKYLOSING SPONDYLITIS

After the application of echocardiography there has been increased recognition of myocardial disease in AS. Brewerton et al. (1987) reported that 53% of AS patients who had no cardiorespiratory symptoms or known cardiac abnormalities had diastolic left ventricular (LV) dysfunction. In that study, researchers also examined postmortem biopsies and found a mild increase of the interstitial connective tissue in the myocardium of AS patients. Computerized image analysis showed a significantly greater amount of interstitial reticulin in patients than in age- and sex-matched controls, which might be responsible from the observed abnormality (Brewerton et al., 1987). LV diastolic dysfunction (DD) has been reported in 10–50% of AS patients in different studies, which is also supported by a recent systematic review and meta-analysis (Brewerton et al., 1987; Okan et al., 2008; Heslinga et al., 2014). The varying incidences between studies may be related to the use of different imaging modalities and cut-off criteria. Clinical significance of asymptomatic DD in AS is not yet entirely clear. Some studies from general population suggest LV DD may be a precursor to chronic heart failure and may cause morbidity and mortality (Kuznetsova et al., 2014). Thus, further studies are needed to determine whether impaired diastolic function may be one of the underlying factors from the increased CV mortality in AS.

Involvement of the pericardium in AS is relatively less defined. Thickening of the pericardium or evidence of pericardial effusion have been reported in several studies. In a descriptive study of 40 AS patients, signs of pericardial disease (thickening or effusion) were found in 12.5% of the cases (Alves et al., 1988). In another study, with 40 AS patients, only 1 (2.5%) patient had pericarditis (Sukenik et al., 1987). In a study, assessing 24 patients with AS of 10 or more years duration showed that only one (7%) patient had small pericardial effusion (O'Neill et al., 1992). Yildirir et al. (2002) compared 88 AS patients and 31 healthy controls. In the AS group, three patients (3.4%) had minimal pericardial effusion and two (2.3%) had pericardial thickening, whereas one subject (3.2%) in the control group had minimal pericardial effusion. The difference in terms of pericardial disease was not different between patients and controls statistically (Yildirir et al., 2002). In a juvenile study of 20 AS patients, researchers noted that none of the subjects had pericardial effusion or thickening (Gerster et al., 1987). In a relatively recent study, Lange et al. (2007) showed that pericardial effusion was present in 1.5% of the AS patients. In summary, pericardium may be involved in AS. However, there is limited information regarding its clinical importance and association with disease characteristics.

9. SUBCLINICAL VASCULAR INVOLVEMENT IN ANKYLOSING SPONDYLITIS

Progress in imaging modalities made it possible to identify atherosclerosis-related changes at its earliest stages. Several invasive and noninvasive techniques are used to identify early arterial wall alterations. Intima-media thickness (IMT) of common carotid arteries (CCA) and assessment of flow-mediated dilatation (FMD) by ultrasound are the most widely used noninvasive methods. IMT of CCA is a reproducible marker of generalized atherosclerosis that allows evaluating the earliest structural changes in the arterial wall. On the other hand, FMD is used to detect endothelial dysfunction, which precedes morphological changes and is believed to be the initial step in the development of atherosclerosis. Impaired endothelial function have been reported in various studies in AS. Sari et al. (2006) evaluated 54 relatively young age AS patients and 31 controls. They showed that endothelium-dependent vasodilatation was impaired in the AS group. There were no correlation between disease activity measures and FMD (Sari et al., 2006). This observation was also supported by a further research, which included 43 patients with AS and 40 matched healthy controls (Bodnar et al., 2011). In a more recent study, Syngle et al. (2013) reported that FMD values of anti-TNF-naive AS patients with high disease activity ($n = 20$) was significantly lower compared to the healthy controls ($n = 10$), which is accordance with the results of the above mentioned data. In contrast with FMD studies, there are some discrepancies between the studies regarding IMT in AS. There are two meta-analysis on this subject. In the former one, Mathieu et al. (2011) analyzed six studies and reported an increased IMT in the AS group. In a more recent and extensive study, Arida et al. (2015) showed that carotid IMT, but not plaque burden, was significantly increased in AS compared to controls. Notably, this increase in IMT was present only in the active disease patients (based on BASDAI ≥ 4) (Arida et al., 2015). In summary, results of the previously published data show that patients with AS without clinically evident CV disease have a high prevalence of subclinical vascular involvement. Further studies are needed to define its pathogenic potential in the development of macrovascular disease in AS.

10. TREATMENT AND ITS IMPLICATIONS IN ATHEROSCLEROSIS IN ANKYLOSING SPONDYLITIS

Management of AS consists of pharmacological and nonpharmacological treatment strategies. The pharmacological treatment options are limited; however, with the introduction of biological drugs, remarkable improvements have been reported in this field. Nonsteroidal antiinflammatory drugs (NSAIDs) are the mainstay treatment for AS (Sari et al., 2015). One of the most important issues with the use of NSAIDs is the possible adverse effect on CV system. The increased CV toxicity was initially reported with rofecoxib, a selective cyclooxygenase 2 inhibitor (coxib), but it is also documented with the use of other NSAIDs including conventional ones except naproxen (Bhala et al., 2013). However, it should be noted that most studies assessing the cardiac risk of NSAIDs have been done in non-AS patients groups. In a population-based study in AS, Haroon et al. (2015) suggested a protective effect of traditional NSAID usage on vascular mortality in patients above 65 years of age. Additionally they also reported Coxibs were not associated with an increased risk for vascular mortality (Haroon et al., 2015). In another study, Bakland et al. (2011) showed that there was a significant negative association between overall mortality and use of NSAIDs at the time of follow-up, and patients who reported taking NSAIDs less frequently than on a monthly basis were at increased risk of premature overall mortality (OR 4.35). A large-scale population study from Taiwan suggested that nonfrequent, short-term NSAID users carry high risk for CV disease (for 6 months: OR, 1.41; 95% CI, 1.07−1.86) (Tsai et al., 2015). The risk tended to decline with long-term use. In frequent NSAID users, there was no significant risk of CV disease in both short and long terms. Interestingly longer NSAID use was associated with lower CV risk. Additionally, long-term frequent use of coxibs had a strong protective CV effect (Tsai et al., 2015). In summary, NSAIDs possess CV risk but data from AS studies suggest a favorable CV risk profile of long-term NSAID usage in addition to reducing pain and improving mobility. Clearly individual risk assessment including age and consideration of comorbidities is required before making a decision on long-term NSAID use.

Biologic drugs, especially tumor necrosis factor alpha (TNF-α) inhibitors, have given new treatment options in the management of AS. Several studies documented their effectiveness in the management of AS. On the other hand, researchers showed particular attention to safety issues especially infections. However, less is known about TNF inhibitory (TNFi) usage and its relation with CV disease. Available data provides indirect information that is obtained mainly from small sample-size studies. Mathieu et al. (2008) analyzed 18 patients who received TNFi. The augmentation index, a measure of systemic arterial stiffness, did not change when compared to baseline after 14 weeks of biologic therapy (Mathieu et al., 2008). Capkin et al. (2012) studied 28 active AS patients with carotid/femoral pulse wave velocity (PWV) analysis, a measure of arterial stiffness. Results from that study showed that after 24 weeks of TNFi therapy there was no significant difference in PWV between the pretreatment and posttreatment patients (Capkin et al., 2012). In another study compromising 49 patients with long-standing and active AS, researchers reported that arterial stiffness was not improved after 6 and 12 months of TNFi (Mathieu et al., 2013). In a randomized controlled trial comparing the vascular effect of placebo with golimumab, investigators reported that 6 months of treatment with golimumab was effective in preventing the progression of arterial stiffness in AS patients with active disease (Tam et al., 2014). In comparison, placebo group showed significant progression of PWV (Tam et al., 2014). In a prospective study with a long-term follow-up (median 4.9 years), AS patients who continued treatment with TNFi (n = 56) exhibited a slower progression of carotid IMT compared to those who discontinued anti-TNF (n = 9) (van Sijl et al., 2015). In summary, although there are some signals regarding a positive impact on vascular function, available data are not supporting a direct beneficial effect of anti-TNF treatments on CV disease.

11. CONCLUSIONS

Available data suggests that AS is associated with several cardiac and vascular abnormalities. Structural abnormalities, such as aortic and valvular involvement, conduction disturbances, myocardial disease, and vascular wall alterations are well defined now with the advent of imaging modalities. The defined abnormalities are mostly subclinical but it is clear that there is increased CV mortality and morbidity risk in AS. It is more likely that inflammation-driven mechanisms along with comorbidities may trigger the pathological alterations in this disease. Further studies with larger sample size and long-term follow-up are needed to identify the underlying mechanisms and the consequences of observed abnormalities. Considering the increased CV disease risk, there is a need for developing prevention and treatment strategies in AS. Another requirement is to develop guidelines and a standardized approach for CV examination and laboratory workup in routine clinical care of AS patients.

REFERENCES

Alves, M.G., Espirito-Santo, J., Queiroz, M.V., et al., 1988. Cardiac alterations in ankylosing spondylitis. Angiology 39, 567.

Ansell, B.M., Bywaters, E.G., Doniach, I., 1958. The aortic lesion of ankylosing spondylitis. Br. Heart J. 20, 507.

Arida, A., Protogerou, A.D., Konstantonis, G., et al., 2015. Subclinical atherosclerosis is not accelerated in patients with ankylosing spondylitis with low disease activity: new data and metaanalysis of published studies. J. Rheumatol. 42, 2098.

Bakland, G., Gran, J.T., Nossent, J.C., 2011. Increased mortality in ankylosing spondylitis is related to disease activity. Ann. Rheum. Dis. 70, 1921.

Bengtsson, K., Forsblad-d'Elia, H., Lie, E., et al., 2015. Increased risk of atrioventricular block, atrial fibrillation and pacemaker implantation in ankylosing spondylitis, undifferentiated spondylarthritis and psoriatic arthritis compared to the general population [abstract]. Arthritis Rheumatol. 67 (Suppl. 10).

Bergfeldt, L., 1997. HLA-B27-associated cardiac disease. Ann. Intern. Med. 127, 621.

Bergfeldt, L., Edhag, O., Vallin, H., 1982a. Cardiac conduction disturbances, an underestimated manifestation in ankylosing spondylitis. A 25-year follow-up study of 68 patients. Acta Med. Scand. 212, 217.

Bergfeldt, L., Edhag, O., Vedin, L., et al., 1982b. Ankylosing spondylitis: an important cause of severe disturbances of the cardiac conduction system. Prevalence among 223 pacemaker-treated men. Am. J. Med. 73, 187.

Bergfeldt, L., Vallin, H., Edhag, O., 1984. Complete heart block in HLA B27 associated disease. Electrophysiological and clinical characteristics. Br. Heart J. 51, 184.

Bergfeldt, L., Insulander, P., Lindblom, D., et al., 1988. HLA-B27: an important genetic risk factor for lone aortic regurgitation and severe conduction system abnormalities. Am. J. Med. 85, 12.

Bernstein, L., Broch, O.J., 1949. Cardiac complications in spondylarthritis ankylopoietica. Acta Med. Scand. 185.

Bhala, N., Emberson, J., Merhi, A., et al., 2013. Vascular and upper gastrointestinal effects of non-steroidal anti-inflammatory drugs: meta-analyses of individual participant data from randomised trials. Lancet 382, 769.

Bodnar, N., Kerekes, G., Seres, I., et al., 2011. Assessment of subclinical vascular disease associated with ankylosing spondylitis. J. Rheumatol. 38, 723.

Braun, J., Pincus, T., 2002. Mortality, course of disease and prognosis of patients with ankylosing spondylitis. Clin. Exp. Rheumatol. 20, S16.

Bremander, A., Petersson, I.F., Bergman, S., et al., 2011. Population-based estimates of common comorbidities and cardiovascular disease in ankylosing spondylitis. Arthritis Care Res. (Hoboken) 63, 550.

Brewerton, D.A., Gibson, D.G., Goddard, D.H., et al., 1987. The myocardium in ankylosing spondylitis. A clinical, echocardiographic, and histopathological study. Lancet 1, 995.

Brophy, S., Cooksey, R., Atkinson, M., et al., 2012. No increased rate of acute myocardial infarction or stroke among patients with ankylosing spondylitis-a retrospective cohort study using routine data. Semin. Arthritis Rheum. 42, 140.

Brunner, F., Kunz, A., Weber, U., et al., 2006. Ankylosing spondylitis and heart abnormalities: do cardiac conduction disorders, valve regurgitation and diastolic dysfunction occur more often in male patients with diagnosed ankylosing spondylitis for over 15 years than in the normal population? Clin. Rheumatol. 25, 24.

Bulkley, B.H., Roberts, W.C., 1973. Ankylosing spondylitis and aortic regurgitation. Description of the characteristic cardiovascular lesion from study of eight necropsy patients. Circulation 48, 1014.

Capkin, E., Karkucak, M., Kiris, A., et al., 2012. Anti-TNF-alpha therapy may not improve arterial stiffness in patients with AS: a 24-week follow-up. Rheumatology (Oxford) 51, 910.

Cheng, S., Keyes, M.J., Larson, M.G., et al., 2009. Long-term outcomes in individuals with prolonged PR interval or first-degree atrioventricular block. JAMA 301, 2571.

Chou, C.H., Lin, M.C., Peng, C.L., et al., 2014. A nationwide population-based retrospective cohort study: increased risk of acute coronary syndrome in patients with ankylosing spondylitis. Scand. J. Rheumatol. 43, 132.

Ciurea, A., Finckh, A., 2013. Smoking and spondyloarthritis. Jt. Bone Spine 80, 234.

Cornier, M.A., Despres, J.P., Davis, N., et al., 2011. Assessing adiposity: a scientific statement from the American Heart Association. Circulation 124, 1996.

De Bacquer, D., De Backer, G., Kornitzer, M., 2000. Prevalences of ECG findings in large population based samples of men and women. Heart 84, 625.

Demiralp, E., Kardesoglu, E., Kiralp, M.Z., et al., 2004. Aortic elasticity in patients with ankylosing spondylitis. Acta Cardiol. 59, 630.

Dos Santos, F.P., Constantin, A., Laroche, M., et al., 2001. Whole body and regional bone mineral density in ankylosing spondylitis. J. Rheumatol. 28, 547.

Exarchou, S., Lie, E., Lindstrom, U., et al., 2015. Mortality in ankylosing spondylitis: results from a nationwide population-based study. Ann. Rheum. Dis.

Forsblad-d'Elia, H., Wallberg, H., Klingberg, E., et al., 2013. Cardiac conduction system abnormalities in ankylosing spondylitis: a cross-sectional study. BMC Musculoskelet. Disord. 14, 237.

Gerster, J.C., Payot, M., Piccinin, P., 1987. Clinical and echocardiographic assessment in juvenile-onset spondyloarthropathy. Br. J. Rheumatol. 26, 155.

Glintborg, B., Hojgaard, P., Lund Hetland, M., et al., 2015. Impact of tobacco smoking on response to tumour necrosis factor-alpha inhibitor treatment in patients with ankylosing spondylitis: results from the Danish nationwide DANBIO registry. Rheumatology (Oxford).

Graham, D.C., Smythe, H.A., 1958. The carditis and aortitis of ankylosing spondylitis. Bull. Rheum. Dis. 9, 171.

Grewal, G.S., Leipsic, J., Klinkhoff, A.V., 2014. Abdominal aortitis in HLA-B27$^+$ spondyloarthritis: case report with 5-year follow-up and literature review. Semin. Arthritis Rheum. 44, 305.

Han, C., Robinson Jr., D.W., Hackett, M.V., et al., 2006. Cardiovascular disease and risk factors in patients with rheumatoid arthritis, psoriatic arthritis, and ankylosing spondylitis. J. Rheumatol. 33, 2167.

Haroon, N.N., Paterson, J.M., Li, P., et al., 2014. Increasing proportion of female patients with ankylosing spondylitis: a population-based study of trends in the incidence and prevalence of AS. BMJ Open 4, e006634.

Haroon, N.N., Paterson, J.M., Li, P., et al., 2015. Patients with ankylosing spondylitis have increased cardiovascular and cerebrovascular mortality: a population-based study. Ann. Intern. Med. 163, 409.

Heslinga, S.C., Van Dongen, C.J., Konings, T.C., et al., 2014. Diastolic left ventricular dysfunction in ankylosing spondylitis—a systematic review and meta-analysis. Semin. Arthritis Rheum. 44, 14.

Hingorani, P., Natekar, M., Deshmukh, S., et al., 2012. Morphological abnormalities in baseline ECGs in healthy normal volunteers participating in phase I studies. Indian J. Med. Res. 135, 322.

Hiss, R.G., Lamb, L.E., 1962. Electrocardiographic findings in 122,043 individuals. Circulation 25, 947.

Ho, H.H., Yeh, S.J., Tsai, W.P., et al., 2012. Paroxysmal supraventricular tachycardia and Wolff-Parkinson-White syndrome in ankylosing spondylitis: a large cohort observation study and literature review. Semin. Arthritis Rheum. 42, 246.

Hollingworth, P., Hall, P.J., Knight, S.C., et al., 1979. Lone aortic regurgitation, sacroiliitis, and HLA B27. Case history and frequency of association. Br. Heart J. 42, 229.

Huang, Y.P., Wang, Y.H., Pan, S.L., 2013. Increased risk of ischemic heart disease in young patients with newly diagnosed ankylosing spondylitis—a population-based longitudinal follow-up study. PLoS One 8, e64155.

Hull, R.G., Asherson, R.A., Rennie, J.A., 1984. Ankylosing spondylitis and an aortic arch syndrome. Br. Heart J. 51, 663.

Jimenez-Balderas, F.J., Garcia-Rubi, D., Perez-Hinojosa, S., et al., 2001. Two-dimensional echo Doppler findings in juvenile and adult onset ankylosing spondylitis with long-term disease. Angiology 52, 543.

Johnsen, K., Mahonen, M., Lunde, P., 2009. Prevalence estimation and follow-up of aortic regurgitation subjects in a Norwegian Sami population. Scand. Cardiovasc. J. 43, 176.

Kang, J.H., Chen, Y.H., Lin, H.C., 2010. Comorbidity profiles among patients with ankylosing spondylitis: a nationwide population-based study. Ann. Rheum. Dis. 69, 1165.

Kaprove, R.E., Little, A.H., Graham, D.C., et al., 1980. Ankylosing spondylitis: survival in men with and without radiotherapy. Arthritis Rheum. 23, 57.

Kawasuji, M., Hetzer, R., Oelert, H., et al., 1982. Aortic valve replacement and ascending aorta replacement in ankylosing spondylitis: report of three surgical cases and review of the literature. Thorac. Cardiovasc. Surg. 30, 310.

Kazmierczak, J., Peregud-Pogorzelska, M., Biernawska, J., et al., 2007. Cardiac arrhythmias and conduction disturbances in patients with ankylosing spondylitis. Angiology 58, 751.

Keller, J.J., Hsu, J.L., Lin, S.M., et al., 2014. Increased risk of stroke among patients with ankylosing spondylitis: a population-based matched-cohort study. Rheumatol. Int. 34, 255.

Khan, M.A., Khan, M.K., Kushner, I., 1981. Survival among patients with ankylosing spondylitis: a life-table analysis. J. Rheumatol. 8, 86.

Kinsella, T.D., Johnson, L.G., Ian, R., 1974. Cardiovascular manifestations of ankylosing spondylitis. Can. Med. Assoc. J. 111, 1309.

Klingberg, E., Svealv, B.G., Tang, M.S., et al., 2015. Aortic regurgitation is common in ankylosing spondylitis: time for routine echocardiography evaluation? Am. J. Med. 128, 1244.

Kuznetsova, T., Thijs, L., Knez, J., et al., 2014. Prognostic value of left ventricular diastolic dysfunction in a general population. J. Am. Heart Assoc. 3, e000789.

LaBresh, K.A., Lally, E.V., Sharma, S.C., et al., 1985. Two-dimensional echocardiographic detection of preclinical aortic root abnormalities in rheumatoid variant diseases. Am. J. Med. 78, 908.

Lange, U., Stapfer, G., Ditting, T., et al., 2007. Pathologic alterations of the heart and the kidney in patients with ankylosing spondylitis. Eur. J. Med. Res. 12, 573.

Lehtinen, K., 1993. Mortality and causes of death in 398 patients admitted to hospital with ankylosing spondylitis. Ann. Rheum. Dis. 52, 174.

Malesci, D., Niglio, A., Mennillo, G.A., et al., 2007. High prevalence of metabolic syndrome in patients with ankylosing spondylitis. Clin. Rheumatol. 26, 710.

Mathieu, S., Joly, H., Baron, G., et al., 2008. Trend towards increased arterial stiffness or intima-media thickness in ankylosing spondylitis patients without clinically evident cardiovascular disease. Rheumatology (Oxford) 47, 1203.

Mathieu, S., Gossec, L., Dougados, M., et al., 2011. Cardiovascular profile in ankylosing spondylitis: a systematic review and meta-analysis. Arthritis Care Res. (Hoboken) 63, 557.

Mathieu, S., Pereira, B., Couderc, M., et al., 2013. No significant changes in arterial stiffness in patients with ankylosing spondylitis after tumour necrosis factor alpha blockade treatment for 6 and 12 months. Rheumatology (Oxford) 52, 204.

Mathieu, S., Pereira, B., Soubrier, M., 2015. Cardiovascular events in ankylosing spondylitis: an updated meta-analysis. Semin. Arthritis Rheum. 44, 551.

Mok, C.C., Kwok, C.L., Ho, L.Y., et al., 2011. Life expectancy, standardized mortality ratios, and causes of death in six rheumatic diseases in Hong Kong, China. Arthritis Rheum. 63, 1182.

Monin, J., Bisconte, S., Nicaise, A., et al., 2015. Prevalence of intraventricular conduction disturbances in a large French population. Ann. Noninvasive Electrocardiol.

Moyssakis, I., Gialafos, E., Vassiliou, V.A., et al., 2009. Myocardial performance and aortic elasticity are impaired in patients with ankylosing spondylitis. Scand. J. Rheumatol. 38, 216.

Nurmohamed, M.T., van der Horst-Bruinsma, I., Maksymowych, W.P., 2012. Cardiovascular and cerebrovascular diseases in ankylosing spondylitis: current insights Curr. Rheumatol. Rep. 14, 415.

Okan, T., Sari, I., Akar, S., et al., 2008. Ventricular diastolic function of ankylosing spondylitis patients by using conventional pulsed wave Doppler, myocardial performance index and tissue Doppler imaging. Echocardiography 25, 47.

O'Neill, T.W., King, G., Graham, I.M., et al., 1992. Echocardiographic abnormalities in ankylosing spondylitis. Ann. Rheum. Dis. 51, 652.

Olson, L.J., Subramanian, R., Edwards, W.D., 1984. Surgical pathology of pure aortic insufficiency: a study of 225 cases. Mayo Clin. Proc. 59, 835.

Palazzi, C., D'Angelo, S., Lubrano, E., et al., 2008. Aortic involvement in ankylosing spondylitis. Clin. Exp. Rheumatol. 26, S131.

Papadakis, J.A., Sidiropoulos, P.I., Karvounaris, S.A., et al., 2009. High prevalence of metabolic syndrome and cardiovascular risk factors in men with ankylosing spondylitis on anti-TNFalpha treatment: correlation with disease activity. Clin. Exp. Rheumatol. 27, 292.

Park, S.H., Sohn, I.S., Joe, B.H., et al., 2012. Early cardiac valvular changes in ankylosing spondylitis: a transesophageal echocardiography study. J. Cardiovasc. Ultrasound 20, 30.

Patel, S.A., Winkel, M., Ali, M.K., et al., 2015. Cardiovascular mortality associated with 5 leading risk factors: national and state preventable fractions estimated from survey data. Ann. Intern. Med. 163, 245.

Peeters, A.J., Ten Wolde, S., Sedney, M.I., et al., 1991. Heart conduction disturbance: an HLA-B27 associated disease. Ann. Rheum. Dis. 50, 348.

Peters, M.J., Visman, I., Nielen, M.M., et al., 2010. Ankylosing spondylitis: a risk factor for myocardial infarction? Ann. Rheum. Dis. 69, 579.

Plasqui, G., Boonen, A., Geusens, P., et al., 2012. Physical activity and body composition in patients with ankylosing spondylitis. Arthritis Care Res. (Hoboken) 64, 101.

Poddubnyy, D., Sieper, J., 2012. Radiographic progression in ankylosing spondylitis/axial spondyloarthritis: how fast and how clinically meaningful? Curr. Opin. Rheumatol. 24, 363.

Poddubnyy, D., Haibel, H., Listing, J., et al., 2012. Baseline radiographic damage, elevated acute-phase reactant levels, and cigarette smoking status predict spinal radiographic progression in early axial spondylarthritis. Arthritis Rheum. 64, 1388.

Qaiyumi, S., Hassan, Z.U., Toone, E., 1985. Seronegative spondyloarthropathies in lone aortic insufficiency. Arch. Intern. Med. 145, 822.

Radford, E.P., Doll, R., Smith, P.G., 1977. Mortality among patients with ankylosing spondylitis not given X-ray therapy. N. Engl. J. Med. 297, 572.

Roldan, C.A., 2008. Valvular and coronary heart disease in systemic inflammatory diseases: systemic disorders in heart disease. Heart 94, 1089.

Roldan, C.A., Chavez, J., Wiest, P.W., et al., 1998. Aortic root disease and valve disease associated with ankylosing spondylitis. J. Am. Coll. Cardiol. 32, 1397.

Sari, I., Okan, T., Akar, S., et al., 2006. Impaired endothelial function in patients with ankylosing spondylitis. Rheumatology (Oxford) 45, 283.

Sari, I., Demir, T., Kozaci, L.D., et al., 2007. Body composition, insulin, and leptin levels in patients with ankylosing spondylitis. Clin. Rheumatol. 26, 1427.

Sari, I., Ozturk, M.A., Akkoc, N., 2015. Treatment of ankylosing spondylitis. Turk J. Med. Sci. 45, 416.

Smith, P.G., Doll, R., Radford, E.P., 1977. Cancer mortality among patients with ankylosing spondylitis not given X-ray therapy. Br. J. Radiol. 50, 728.

Stamato, T., Laxer, R.M., de Freitas, C., et al., 1995. Prevalence of cardiac manifestations of juvenile ankylosing spondylitis. Am. J. Cardiol. 75, 744.

Stone, J.R., Bruneval, P., Angelini, A., et al., 2015. Consensus statement on surgical pathology of the aorta from the society for cardiovascular pathology and the association for European cardiovascular pathology: I. Inflammatory diseases. Cardiovasc. Pathol. 24, 267.

Sukenik, S., Pras, A., Buskila, D., et al., 1987. Cardiovascular manifestations of ankylosing spondylitis. Clin. Rheumatol. 6, 588.

Syngle, A., Vohra, K., Khichi, D., et al., 2013. Spironolactone improves endothelial dysfunction in ankylosing spondylitis. Clin. Rheumatol. 32, 1029.

Szabo, S.M., Levy, A.R., Rao, S.R., et al., 2011. Increased risk of cardiovascular and cerebrovascular diseases in individuals with ankylosing spondylitis: a population-based study. Arthritis Rheum. 63, 3294.

Tam, L.S., Shang, Q., Kun, E.W., et al., 2014. The effects of golimumab on subclinical atherosclerosis and arterial stiffness in ankylosing spondylitis-a randomized, placebo-controlled pilot trial. Rheumatology (Oxford) 53, 1065.

Thomas, D., Hill, W., Geddes, R., et al., 1982. Early detection of aortic dilatation in ankylosing spondylitis using echocardiography. Aust. N. Z. J. Med. 12, 10.

Thomsen, N.H., Horslev-Petersen, K., Beyer, J.M., 1986. Ambulatory 24-hour continuous electrocardiographic monitoring in 54 patients with ankylosing spondylitis. Eur. Heart J. 7, 240.

Toussirot, E., Michel, F., Wendling, D., 2001. Bone density, ultrasound measurements and body composition in early ankylosing spondylitis. Rheumatology (Oxford) 40, 882.

Toussirot, E., Grandclement, E., Gaugler, B., et al., 2013. Serum adipokines and adipose tissue distribution in rheumatoid arthritis and ankylosing spondylitis. A comparative study. Front Immunol. 4, 453.

Tsai, W.C., Ou, T.T., Yen, J.H., et al., 2015. Long-term frequent use of non-steroidal anti-inflammatory drugs might protect patients with ankylosing spondylitis from cardiovascular diseases: a nationwide case-control study. PLoS One 10, e0126347.

Tucker, C.R., Fowles, R.E., Calin, A., et al., 1982. Aortitis in ankylosing spondylitis: early detection of aortic root abnormalities with two dimensional echocardiography. Am. J. Cardiol. 49, 680.

Ungprasert, P., Srivali, N., Kittanamongkolchai, W., 2015. Risk of coronary artery disease in patients with ankylosing spondylitis: a systematic review and meta-analysis. Ann. Transl Med. 3, 51.

Uusimaa, P., Krogerus, M.L., Airaksinen, J., et al., 2006. Aortic valve insufficiency in patients with chronic rheumatic diseases. Clin. Rheumatol. 25, 309.

van Sijl, A.M., van Eijk, I.C., Peters, M.J., et al., 2015. Tumour necrosis factor blocking agents and progression of subclinical atherosclerosis in patients with ankylosing spondylitis. Ann. Rheum. Dis. 74, 119.

Weed, C.L., Kulander, B.G., Massarella, J.A., et al., 1966. Heart block in ankylosing spondylitis. Arch. Intern. Med. 117, 800.

Wendling, D., Prati, C., 2013. Spondyloarthritis and smoking: towards a new insight into the disease. Expert Rev. Clin. Immunol. 9, 511.

Yildirir, A., Aksoyek, S., Calguneri, M., et al., 2002. Echocardiographic evidence of cardiac involvement in ankylosing spondylitis. Clin. Rheumatol. 21, 129.

Zochling, J., Braun, J., 2009. Mortality in rheumatoid arthritis and ankylosing spondylitis. Clin. Exp. Rheumatol. 27, S127.

FURTHER READING

Ross, R., 1993. The pathogenesis of atherosclerosis: a perspective for the 1990s. Nature 362, 801.

Chapter 16

Cardiovascular Involvement in Psoriatic Arthritis

F. Atzeni,* F. Caso,§ I.F. Masala¶ and P. Sarzi-Puttini||
**IRCCS Galeazzi Orthopedic Institute, Milan, Italy; §Rheumatology Unit, Department of Clinical Medicine and Surgery, University Federico II, Naples, Italy; ¶Santissima Trinità Hospital, Cagliari, Italy; ||Rheumatology Unit, L. Sacco University Hospital, Milan, Italy*

Key points

- Psoriatic arthritis (PsA) is a chronic inflammatory condition associated with a high prevalence of cardiovascular disease and risk factors.
- In comparison with the general population, PsA patients are at significantly increased risk of cardiovascular (CV) risk factors, CV events, and mortality.
- The prevalence of at least one CV event (8%) and coronary heart disease (9%) is significantly higher in PsA patients than in those with psoriasis alone or the general population.
- The relationship between PsA and cardiovascular events is complex. The increased CV risk can be explained by the increased prevalence of cardiovascular risk factors but the chronic underlining inflammatory state seems to play a crucial role.
- Instrumental investigations have shown a high prevalence of macrovascular disease, endothelial dysfunction, arterial stiffness, and left ventricle diastolic dysfunction in PsA patients without any clinically evident signs of atherosclerosis or its complications.
- Various studies have shown the potentially beneficial role of DMARD-induced immunosuppression on cardiovascular diseases. A number of studies have found that anti-TNF drugs can also have a positive effect on carotid IMT and endothelial dysfunction.
- Physicians should take cardiovascular risk into account when assessing patients with psoriatic arthritis patients, even in the absence of a clinically evident cardiovascular disease, mainly by identifying and modifying cardiovascular risk factors.

1. INTRODUCTION

Psoriatic arthritis (PsA) is a chronic inflammatory condition in which unbalanced inflammatory pathways act as key drivers of a wide range of manifestations at the level of axial and peripheral joints, entheses, the synovial sheaths of tendons, and skin (Moll and Wright, 1973; Duarte et al., 2012). Its diagnosis is based on anamnestic and clinical criteria such as the presence or a family history of psoriasis, dactylitis, enthesitis, inflammatory low-back pain, and rheumatoid factor (RF) seronegativity (Gladman, 2012; Marchesoni et al., 2012; Caso et al., 2014). The Classification Criteria for Psoriatic Arthritis (CASPAR) are highly specific (98.7%) and sensitive (91.4%) and can be useful in differential diagnosis (Taylor et al., 2006; Tillett et al., 2012).

PsA has long been considered a disease with a mild clinical and low inflammatory profile (Scarpa et al., 2015), but recent studies have provided growing evidence of its multisystemic nature and association with extra-articular involvement in the form of colitis, uveitis, metabolic syndrome (MetS), and atherosclerosis (Scarpa et al., 2000; Egeberg et al., 2015; Costa et al., 2012), and this has led to the concept of psoriatic disease (PsoD) as a systemic condition that is not exclusively confined to joints and the skin (Scarpa et al., 2006).

2. EPIDEMIOLOGY

The global frequency of psoriasis is 1–5%, and arthritis occurs in 10–40% of patients with psoriasis as against up to 1% of the general population (Ogdie and Weiss, 2015). The highest estimated annual incidence in Europe is 23/100,000 (Liu et al., 2014).

The prevalence of cardiovascular (CV) comorbidities is high, which inevitably leads to greater use of healthcare resources and high costs (Feldman et al., 2015; Sitia et al., 2009).

In comparison with the general population, PsA patients are at significantly increased risk of CV risk factors, CV events, and mortality (Jamnitski et al., 2013; Horreau et al., 2013; Gladman et al., 2009). The prevalence of at least one CV event (8%) and coronary heart disease (9%) is significantly higher in PsA patients than in those with psoriasis alone or the general population (Husted et al., 2011). However, the relative risk (RR) of developing major CV events varies widely from 1.17 to 3.47, mainly because of the heterogeneity of the studied cohorts and general populations (Eder et al., 2015a). The risk of major adverse CV events is also higher in PsA patients who have not been treated with disease-modifying antirheumatic drugs (DMARDs) [hazard ratio (HR) 1.24, 95% CI 1.03–1.49] (Ogdie et al., 2015a). A 35-year follow-up study of 1091 PsA patients reported >100 CV events affecting 20% of the patients by the age of 70 years and 30% by the age of 80 years (Eder et al., 2015a). The same study found that the erythrocyte sedimentation rate (ESR) was a significant predictor among women (RR 1.83, $p = .02$), and that the independent predictors of major CV events were hypertension (RR 1.81, $p = .0159$), diabetes mellitus (DM: RR 2.7, $p < .001$), and the number of dactylitic digits (RR 1.20, $p < .001$) (Eder et al., 2015a).

It has also been reported that the increased rate of CV events in PsA patients is associated with PsA severity and traditional CV risk factors such as MetS and its components (Eder and Gladman, 2015; Han et al., 2006; Haroon et al., 2014; Tam et al., 2008a). PsA patients have a very high prevalence of MetS: 58.1% versus 35.2% in the Third National Health and Nutrition Examination Survey (NHANES III) (Raychaudhuri et al., 2010), and the prevalence of MetS components, dyslipidemia (21−61%), obesity (30−60%), hypertension (33−37%), and DM (12−14%) is significantly higher in PsA patients than in these with psoriasis alone and the general population (Lin et al., 2014; Mok et al., 2011; Husted et al., 2011; Khraishi et al., 2014; Edson-Heredia et al., 2015); and the high prevalence of MetS in PsA patients predisposes them to an increased risk of developing atherosclerotic cardiovascular disease and type II DM (Raychaudhuri et al., 2010). PsA patients with MetS are at higher risk of having atherosclerotic risk factors than patients with other arthritides (Mok et al., 2011). Significant CV comorbidity has also been associated with the early phases of PsA, with obesity being the most frequent CV risk factor among male patients (Khraishi et al., 2014).

In a study of 3066 PsA patients in a large health plan data set, the prevalence rates of hypertension (28.5%), hyperlipidemia (27.8%), type II DM (11.3%), cerebrovascular disease (3.1%), ischemic heart disease (3.1%), peripheral vascular disease (2.9%), and congestive heart failure (1.9%) were all significantly higher in the patients than in the controls ($p < .05$) (Han et al., 2006). The patients were also at increased risk of developing CV diseases: ischemic heart disease (RR: 1.3), atherosclerosis (RR: 1.4), congestive heart failure (RR: 1.5), peripheral vascular disease (RR: 1.6), cerebrovascular disease (RR: 1.3), type II DM (RR: 1.5), hyperlipidemia (RR: 1.2), and hypertension (RR: 1.3) (Han et al., 2006). Finally, they used more drugs (ACE inhibitors, calcium channel blockers, diuretics, nitrates/vasodilators, anticoagulants, and antihyperlipidemia agents) for CV comorbidities than the controls (Han et al., 2006).

It has also been shown that PsA patients with subclinical atherosclerosis also have more traditional risk factors, such as high glucose, total triglyceride, and total and high-density cholesterol levels, high white cell counts, and higher patient global assessment scores than those without subclinical atherosclerosis (Tam et al., 2008b).

However, there are conflicting data concerning the risk of CV mortality in PsA patients (Gladman et al., 2009), although the majority of studies have shown that they are at greater risk (Gladman et al., 1998; Gonzalez-Juanatey et al., 2007a, 2007b; Miller et al., 2013), some have found that they are not (Ogdie et al., 2014). One investigation of the causes of death in 428 PsA patients showed that the principal causes were diseases of the circulatory system, which were associated with a 1.3 increase in mortality (Wong et al., 1997). Another study of more than 680 PsA patients and almost 40,000 controls showed an increase in the standardized prevalence ratios of hypertension [1.90 (1.59–2.27)], angina [1.97 (1.24–3.12)], and myocardial infarction [2.57 (95%CI, 1.73–3.80)] (Gladman et al., 2009), and it has also been found that increased CV mortality in PsA patients is associated with the previous use of medications, a high ESR at the time of presentation, and radiological damage (Gladman et al., 1998).

PsA itself has been shown to be a predictor of CV events mainly due to increased subclinical atherosclerosis, regardless of the presence of traditional CV risk factors (Gonzalez-Juanatey et al., 2007a, 2007b).

3. ETIOLOGY/PATHOGENESIS

The increased CV risk can be explained by the increased prevalence of cardiovascular risk factors such as type II DM and insulin resistance, hyperlipidemia and hypertension, as well as by concomitant smoking, reduced physical activity, hypercoagulability, increased fibrinogen levels, and higher platelet counts (Gladman et al., 1998; Peters et al , 2004), but the chronic underlining inflammatory state seems to play a crucial role (Ross, 1999; Tam et al., 2008a).

Atherosclerosis, psoriasis, and other rheumatic diseases share a number of pathogenetic mechanisms (Eder and Gladman, 2015; Sarzi-Puttini et al., 2010; Matsuura et al., 2014). Atherosclerosis, the underlying mechanism of peripheral artery, coronary, and cerebrovascular diseases, is due to a chronic low-grade inflammatory state involving the arterial walls and seems to be mainly determined by alterations in the homeostatic state between immune mechanisms and lipid metabolism (Liehn et al., 2006; Weber and Noels, 2011; Ramji and Davies, 2015). It begins with endothelium activation and the consequent recruitment of immune cells mediated by cytokines and chemokines (Liehn et al., 2006; Weber and Noels, 2011; Ramji and Davies, 2015). This first step leads leukocytes adhering on the surface of endothelial cells expressing adhesion molecules, an interaction that is influenced by dysregulated pro- and antiinflammatory cytokines, chemokines, and their receptors, which also influence the translocation of leukocytes from the blood through the endothelial layer and into the vessel wall intima (Liehn et al., 2006; Weber and Noels, 2011; Ramji and Davies, 2015). Cholesterol efflux is also altered, and modified lipoproteins are taken up to form foam cells and fatty accumulation (Liehn et al., 2006; Weber and Noels, 2011; Ramji and Davies, 2015).

During the atherosclerotic process, cytokines and chemokines continue to promote the recruitment of monocytes and T cells, the lysis of foam cells releasing degradation products, the proliferation of vascular smooth muscle cells, and the development and formation of atheromatous plaques (Liehn et al., 2006; Weber and Noels, 2011; Ramji and Davies, 2015). These can remain stabilized by the vessel extracellular matrix, synthesized by smooth muscle cells or, when the plaques are destabilized by the metalloproteinase synthesized by macrophages, become unstable and break leading to thrombosis (Liehn et al., 2006; Weber and Noels, 2011; Ramji and Davies, 2015).

In patients with PsA, the precise pathogenetic mechanism of CV involvement has still to be clarified, but certain inflammatory cytokines play a key role in the atherosclerotic process (Eder and Gladman, 2015). It has been shown that proinflammatory cytokines, especially tumor necrosis factor (TNF)-α, interleukin (IL)-1β, and IL-6, are upregulated in peripheral blood, the skin, and synovial membranes and fluid (Fiocco et al., 2015a, 2015b; Fiocco et al., 2014; Goodman et al., 2009; van Kuijk et al., 2006). In particular, TNFα is the main factor involved in the intricate pathogenesis of psoriatic disease, and has often been considered a pivotal factor linking its different expressions, including CV involvement (Caso et al., 2015; Anandarajah and Ritchlin, 2004). TNFα arouses protective action of the host against microbial agents and tumor cytotoxicity by regulating cell apoptosis and proliferation, and is therefore a key mediator of inflammation (Pfeffer, 2003). During the course of synovitis, its overexpression (mainly by macrophages but also by other cells) promotes and generates the unbalanced inflammation leading to articular damage in various arthritides, including in PsA (Pfeffer, 2003). TNFα induces macrophage activation, superoxide production, and neutrophil chemotaxis, thus leading to endothelial inflammation and dysfunction and arterial damage (Widlansky et al., 2003; Sarzi-Puttini et al., 2005a, 2005b); furthermore, it acts as an adipokine by stimulating lipolysis and adipocyte apoptosis, increasing plasma triglyceride levels and promoting insulin resistance (Prins et al., 1997; Hotamisligil et al., 1996; Sethi and Hotamisligil, 1999; Rydén et al., 2004; Peraldi and Spiegelman, 1998). It has been suggested that the insulin resistance generated by chronic systemic inflammation is a key determinant of the high prevalence of MetS, endothelial dysfunction, and atherosclerosis during the course of PsA, even in the absence of clinically evident CV risk factors or disease (Boehncke et al., 2011; Sitia et al., 2010; Gonzalez-Juanatey et al., 2007a; Sharma et al., 2014; Yilmazer et al., 2015).

Finally, TNFα promotes the synthesis of other proinflammatory adipokines such as IL-6, and inhibits the synthesis of antiinflammatory adipokines such as adiponectin (Trayhurn and Wood, 2004). IL-6 promotes the hepatic production of many acute phase reactants (Atzeni et al., 2012), induces insulin resistance, and reduces adiponectin secretion by adipocytes (Trayhurn and Wood, 2004). Adiponectin is an antiinflammatory molecule and, by determining an increase in insulin sensitivity, the stimulation of fatty acid oxidation, the suppression of gluconeogenesis, and the regulation of food intake negatively correlates with obesity, type II DM, atherosclerosis, and MetS (Choi et al., 2007; Trayhurn and Wood, 2004). It has also been reported that, on the contrary in PsA and rheumatoid arthritis (RA), adiponectin promotes inflammation through cytokine synthesis and correlates with a higher burden of joint inflammation and damage (Eder et al., 2013).

Another adipokine is leptin, which is exclusively synthesized in adipose tissue and acts mainly on the hypothalamus. It plays an important role in body energy balance and adipose tissue deposition, and plasma leptin levels positively correlate with body fat mass (Trayhurn and Wood, 2004). Leptin levels are higher in women with PsA than in those with psoriasis, and positively correlate with the homeostasis model assessment of insulin resistance and BMI (Eder et al., 2013).

4. CLINICAL MANIFESTATIONS

Spondylitis, symmetrical polyarthritis, asymmetrical oligoarthritis, distal interphalangeal arthritis, and arthritis mutilans are the five clinical subsets of PsA (Moll and Wright, 1973), which can change over time, and peripheral articular involvement may overlap with axial disease (Jones et al., 1994). Furthermore, PsA can also occur in the absence of clinically evident psoriasis but in the presence of a family history of psoriasis (the "sine psoriasis" subset) (Taylor et al., 2006).

PsA patients experience CV events such as coronary heart disease (myocardial angina and infarction) more frequently than the general population (Husted et al., 2011; Gladman et al., 2009), because of the simultaneous presence of traditional CV risk factors and chronic inflammation (Eder and Gladman, 2015). Severe psoriasis is associated with an increased burden of CV risk and the presence of active arthritis may be an important predictor of CV disease (Gelfand et al., 2007; Wong et al., 1997; Gladman et al., 2009; Eder et al., 2015a). Furthermore, it is necessary to investigate the presence of classical risk factors hypercholesterolemia, hyperlipidemia, DM, hypertension, and obesity in PsA patients, all of which can increase the burden of CV comorbidities (Gladman et al., 2009; Yeung et al., 2013; Eder et al., 2015a; Atzeni et al., 2011a; Tobin et al., 2010), and hypertension and DM in particular may predict major cardiovascular events (Eder et al., 2015a).

Although some studies have found that cerebrovascular disease and heart failure are not more prevalent in PsA patients than in the general population (Gladman et al., 2009), there have been reports of a higher prevalence heart failure (RR: 1.5) and cerebrovascular diseases (RR: 1.3) among PsA patients with concomitant diabetes, hyperlipidemia, and hypertension (Han et al., 2006).

Given the high prevalence of MetS and its components in PsA patients (Mok et al., 2011; Raychaudhuri et al., 2010), waist circumference, blood pressure, and serum triglyceride, high-density lipoprotein (HDL) cholesterol and fasting glucose levels should be routinely evaluated. It should also be borne in mind that modifiable risk factors such as physical activity and smoking may be crucial in reducing the risk of CV events.

PsA itself is a potential risk factor for CV disease, and so patients should also be screened for subclinical CV involvement (Khraishi et al., 2014). Possible indicators of subclinical atherosclerosis and arterial stiffness have been clearly demonstrated in PsA patients, and it could be particularly useful to investigate them even in the absence of clinically evident CV disease (Costa et al., 2012; Jamnitski et al., 2013; Atzeni et al., 2011b). In particular, instrumental investigations have shown a high prevalence of macrovascular disease, endothelial dysfunction, arterial stiffness, and left ventricle diastolic dysfunction in PsA patients without any clinically evident signs of atherosclerosis or its complications (Gonzalez-Juanatey et al., 2007a, 2007b; Costa et al., 2012; Milaniuk et al., 2015). For this reason it could be useful to look for the subclinical presence of CV risk factors.

5. DIAGNOSTIC INVESTIGATIONS

5.1 Echocardiography

Echocardiography uses ultrasounds to visualize the structures of the heart and assess hemodynamic heart parameters using the Doppler method (Milaniuk et al., 2015). In comparison with healthy controls, patients with PsA seem to have higher prevalence of echocardiographic abnormalities, mainly left ventricle diastolic dysfunction, even in the absence of CV risk factors (Milaniuk et al., 2015). It has recently been estimated that subclinical findings of left ventricle diastolic function can be observed in 8–27% of patients with psoriasis and 28–63% of those with PsA (Milaniuk et al., 2015). Subclinical myocardial involvement in PsA can be detected by means of speckle tracking echocardiography (Shang et al., 2014), and other echocardiographic findings may include alterations in aortic elasticity, pulmonary hypertension, mitral and aortal valves insufficiency, and left ventricle hypertrophy with concomitant hypertension (Milaniuk et al., 2015).

One study did not find any silent subclinical echocardiographic abnormalities in 50 treated PsA patients without CV risk factors or clinically evident CV disease (Gonzalez-Juanatey et al., 2006), but others have demonstrated more frequent diastolic dysfunction in PsA patients than in healthy controls, and this significantly correlated with the presence of arthritis and the duration of psoriasis ($p < .05$) (Saricaoglu et al., 2003). A high prevalence of subclinical systolic and/or diastolic dysfunction has also been found in PsA patients with or without CV risk factors (Shang et al., 2014), and a Doppler echocardiography study of 94 PsA patients and 63 healthy controls found that 64% of the patients showed signs of subclinical left ventricular dysfunction (38% diastolic dysfunction, 4% systolic dysfunction, and 22% both) as defined by means of the myocardial peak systolic velocity (Sm) of cardiac segments, even in the absence of established CV disease or traditional CV risk factors (Shang et al., 2011). In this study, an age of >40 years at the time of the diagnosis of PsA (OR 3.388, 95% CI 1.065−10.777; $p = .039$) and hypertension (OR 4.732, 95% CI 1.345−16.639; $p = .015$) were independent predictors of subclinical left ventricular dysfunction (Shang et al., 2011).

Even in the presence of a normal left ventricular ejection fraction, subclinical myocardial deformation in multidimensional planes are highly frequent in PsA patients, including those with no CV risk factors, and a relationship has been found between apical rotation and PsA disease activity ($r = 0.299$, $p = .011$) and the ESR ($r = 0.309$, $p = .008$) (Shang et al., 2014). Increased left ventricular and arterial stiffness can also be seen in PsA patients even in the absence of hypertension and left ventricular remodeling, and a long PsA duration can increase the risk (Shang et al., 2012).

5.2 Coronary Flow Reserve

Coronary flow reserve (CFR) is a very sensitive (>90%) diagnostic marker of coronary artery disease and, when less than 2, predicts severe coronary stenosis. Transthoracic Doppler-derived CFR has been used to identify patients with known or suspected coronary artery disease, and it has a high prognostic value in RA patients (Atzeni et al., 2007).

CFR is significantly reduced in PsA patients, thus indicating endothelial dysfunction and early subclinical atherosclerosis (Atzeni et al., 2011b).

Only a few studies have investigated electrocardiographic signs during the course of psoriatic disease. However, in comparison with healthy controls, heart rate is significantly higher in patients with psoriasis ($p < .0001$), and there is a positive correlation between this and the severity of cutaneous involvement. Single supraventricular beats are also significantly more frequent in PsA patients than in healthy controls ($p < .0001$) (Markuszeski et al., 2007).

Another study found decreased heart rate variability in PsA patients in comparison with healthy controls, as verified by the decrease in the standard deviation of normal R-R intervals (65.1 ± 66.8 vs. 83.2 ± 43.3 ms; $p = .011$), the percentage of normal R-R intervals differing by more than 50 ms ($12.9 \pm 15.4\%$ vs. $20.6 \pm 17.1\%$; $p = .035$), and total power (2069.4 ± 1537.8 vs. 2942.5 ± 1734.2 ms(2); $p = .006$). The heart rate variability parameters also correlated with PsA duration and severity (Gaydukova et al., 2012).

5.3 Intima-Media Thickness

PsA patients have a higher prevalence of subclinical atherosclerosis as measured by means of carotid ultrasonography and the average values of carotid artery intima-media thickness (IMT) (Kimhi et al., 2007; Gonzalez-Juanatey et al., 2007a, 2007b; Tam et al., 2008b; Eder et al., 2008). Higher IMT values of the common carotid artery wall have been found in PsA patients with and without CV risk factors or cardiovascular disease than in healthy controls (Kimhi et al., 2007; Gonzalez-Juanatey et al., 2007a, 2007b; Tam et al., 2008b; Eder et al., 2008).

IMT directly correlates with various features of PsA, such as the duration of psoriasis and arthritis, spine involvement, and fibrinogen concentrations. It may also correlate with conventional atherosclerosis risk factors, including age, BMI, serum glucose levels, and arterial pressure (Kimhi et al., 2007).

Gonzalez-Juanatey et al. found that patients with PsA and no conventional CV risk factors or clinically evident CV disease have a higher prevalence of greater carotid artery IMT and endothelial dysfunction than matched controls (Gonzalez-Juanatey et al., 2007a, 2007b), and significantly greater carotid IMT values and a higher prevalence of MetS have been found in PsA patients in comparison with patients with psoriasis alone (Lin et al., 2014). Furthermore, higher IMT values were found in the PsA patients with MetS than in those without or in psoriasis patients with or without MetS (Lin et al., 2014).

The presence of carotid plaque is associated with the severity of PsA, age, and triglyceride levels (Eder et al., 2008).

Various studies have shown that, in comparison with healthy controls, PsA patients also have increased aortic stiffness (a marker of atherosclerotic disease) as determined by assessing central hemodynamic parameters and aortic pulse wave velocity by tonometry (Costa et al., 2012; Shen et al., 2015). This has also been found in patients without CV risk factors and is directly associated with the duration of arthritis (Costa et al., 2012).

5.4 Laboratory Investigations

During the course of PsA, inflammatory markers such as ESR are important predictors of major CV events, and the processes involving lipid metabolism may be impaired (Eder et al., 2015a). In 1992, Lazarevic et al. reported the presence of dyslipoproteinemia (similar to that observe in patients with RA) in PsA patients with active disease; the dyslipoproteinemia seemed to normalize as the disease improved (Lazarevic et al., 1992). PsA-related dyslipoproteinemia (increased triglyceride concentrations and decreased levels of total cholesterol, low-density lipoprotein (LDL) cholesterol, and HDL-cholesterol) has also been reported by others (Jones et al., 2000; Ma et al., 2013). A proatherogenic lipid profile in the form of an increase in LDL-cholesterol (mainly LDL_3) and a decrease in HDL-cholesterol has also been found in PsA patients (Jones et al., 2000).

Furthermore, a nuclear magnetic resonance spectroscopy study has shown that patients with psoriasis and a normal laboratory lipid profile can have an abnormal lipoprotein particle composition and decreased HDL efflux capacity, thus suggesting a link between psoriasis and CV disease (Mehta et al., 2012).

A recent study showed the presence of CV involvement in PsA patients on the basis of increased IMT values; the independent factors associated with subclinical atherosclerosis were increased glucose and total triglyceride levels (Tam, 2008a,b).

5.5 Plasma Asymmetric Dimethylarginine

Plasma asymmetric dimethylarginine (ADMA), a major endogenous inhibitor of all of the isoforms of nitric oxide (NO) synthase, is a risk factor for the endothelial dysfunction associated with atherosclerosis (Böger, 2004). Increased levels have been found in patients with atherosclerosis and contribute to its progression (Böger, 2004). Increased ADMA levels have also been shown in RA patients, thus suggesting progressive subclinical atherosclerosis (Turiel et al., 2009; Atzeni et al., 2007). This is supported by the fact that a 2011 study investigating coronary flow reserve and ADMA levels found that patients with PsA without any clinically evident cardiovascular disease or CV risk factors also had significantly higher plasma ADMA concentrations than healthy controls (Atzeni et al., 2011b).

A significant correlation has been found between increased ADMA concentrations and reduced CFR levels in PsA patients, thus supporting the possible role of endothelial dysfunction and impaired coronary microcirculation during the course of the disease (Atzeni et al., 2011b). ADMA levels therefore seem to be useful independent markers of endothelial dysfunction and early subclinical atherosclerosis in PsA patients, but the data need to be corroborated, particularly in relation to the possible influence of blood pressure, blood glucose, cholesterol levels, and antiinflammatory therapies (Atzeni et al., 2011b).

6. TREATMENT

Diagnostic delay and marked joint damage are factors favoring a poor long-term outcome in patients with PsA or other arthritides, and correlate with reduced physical function and disability (Eder and Gladman, 2014; Haroon et al., 2015). In the case of nonsevere articular involvement, the treatment of PsA is based on cycles of nonsteroidal antiinflammatory drugs (NSAIDs) and intraarticular steroid injections (Ash et al., 2012).

Traditional DMARDs such as sulfasalazine, methotrexate (MTX), cyclosporine (CSA), and leflunomide (LFN) are efficacious in treating various aspects of PsA, but the level of clinical and radiological evidence supporting their use is less than that supporting the use of anti-TNF drugs (Ash et al., 2012). It has been shown that, in comparison with NSAIDs and traditional

DMARDs, drugs targeting specific molecules such as TNFα and IL17/23R are more efficacious in treating cutaneous lesions, axial involvement, enthesitis, dactylitis, joint pain and swelling, and in inhibiting radiographic progression (Ash et al., 2012; Scarpa et al., 2013).

The recognition of CV risk factors is an important aspect when considering the best therapeutic approach to PsA as NSAIDs, LFN, and CSA can have hypertensive effects, and anti-TNF drugs are contraindicated in the case of New York Heart Association functional class III and IV congestive heart failure (Ash et al., 2012). Furthermore, modifying CV risk factors such as hypertension, dyslipidemia, and DM by means of targeted therapy, and making lifestyle changes such as stopping smoking or adopting a healthier diet, are useful means of improving CV outcomes, the quality of life, and the prognosis of PsA (Husni, 2015; Ogdie et al., 2015b).

However, patients with PsA may be at CV risk event in the absence of traditional CV risk factors because chronic inflammation plays a key role in determining articular and cutaneous manifestations, atherosclerosis, and dysmetabolism, and this may also be important when making therapeutic decisions (Husni, 2015; Ogdie et al., 2015b).

As in the case of other inflammatory arthopathies (Atzeni et al., 2010; Turiel et al., 2010), various studies have shown the potentially beneficial role of DMARD-induced immunosuppression on cardiovascular diseases. For example, the risk of hospitalization because of ischemic heart disease in patients with PsA or psoriasis is comparable on patients starting treatment with MTX and those starting treatment with other nonbiological antipsoriatic drugs (Chen et al., 2012), whereas it has been shown that anti-TNF drugs reduce the incidence of CV events (Sattar et al., 2007; Hürlimann et al., 2002).

A number of studies have found that anti-TNF drugs can also have a positive effect on carotid IMT and endothelial dysfunction (Jamnitski et al., 2013; Popa et al., 2009). However, there are also reports of progressive atherosclerosis (as measured by IMT) in PsA patients receiving anti-TNF drugs, the vascular effects of which need to be clarified (Ramonda et al., 2014).

Furthermore, biological agents can influence various aspects of MetS (lipid and glucose levels), possibly because of the articular improvements that they induce (da Silva et al., 2010; Costa et al., 2014; Costa et al., 2015), and it has been found that there is an inverse correlation between the presence of MetS and the probability of achieving minimal disease activity (MDA) in PsA patients regardless of the use of anti-TNF drugs (Costa et al., 2015).

Obesity is a negative predictor of MDA in PsA patients (Eder et al., 2015b), and it has been reported that anti-TNF drugs improve lipoprotein patterns (Popa et al., 2009).

CV risk should be considered in all PsA patients, regardless of the presence of cardiovascular risk factors or cardiovascular disease (Ogdie et al., 2015a), and so rheumatologists should identify and try to modify any CV risk factors in collaboration with other appropriate specialists (Peters et al., 2004).

Finally, to identify an algorithm for assessing and managing CV disease in PsA patients could be useful in clinical practice in order to improve their survival and quality of the life.

REFERENCES

Anandarajah, A.P., Ritchlin, C.T., 2004. Pathogenesis of psoriatic arthritis. Curr. Opin. Rheumatol. 16, 338.

Ash, Z., Gaujoux-Viala, C., Gossec, L., Hensor, E.M., FitzGerald, O., Winthrop, K., van der Heijde, D., Emery, P., Smolen, J.S., Marzo-Ortega, H., 2012. A systematic literature review of drug therapies for the treatment of psoriatic arthritis: current evidence and meta-analysis informing the EULAR recommendations for the management of psoriatic arthritis. Ann. Rheum. Dis. 71, 319.

Atzeni, F., Ventura, D., Batticciotto, A., Boccassini, L., Sarzi-Puttini, P., 2012. Interleukin 6 blockade: tocilizumab in psoriatic arthritis. J. Rheumatol. Suppl. 89, 97.

Atzeni, F., Turiel, M., Boccassini, L., Sitia, S., Tomasoni, L., Battellino, M., Marchesoni, A., De Gennaro Colonna, V., Sarzi-Puttini, P., 2011a. Cardiovascular involvement in psoriatic arthritis. Reumatismo 63, 148.

Atzeni, F., Sarzi-Puttini, P., Sitia, S., Tomasoni, L., Gianturco, L., Battellino, M., Boccassini, L., De Gennaro Colonna, V., Marchesoni, A., Turiel, M., 2011b. Coronary flow reserve and asymmetric dimethylarginine levels: new measurements for identifying subclinical atherosclerosis in patients with psoriatic arthritis. J. Rheumatol. 38, 1661.

Atzeni, F., Turiel, M., Caporali, R., Cavagna, L., Tomasoni, L., Sitia, S., Sarzi-Puttini, P., 2010. The effect of pharmacological therapy on the cardiovascular system of patients with systemic rheumatic diseases. Autoimmun. Rev. 9, 835.

Atzeni, F., Sarzi-Puttini, P., De Blasio, G., Delfino, L., Tomasoni, L., Turiel, M., 2007. Preclinical impairment of coronary flow reserve in patients with rheumatoid arthritis. Ann. N Y Acad. Sci. 1108, 392.

Böger, R.H., 2004. Asymmetric dimethylarginine, an endogenous inhibitor of nitric oxide synthase, explains the "L-arginine paradox" and acts as a novel cardiovascular risk factor. J. Nutr. 134, 2842S.

Boehncke, W.H., Boehncke, S., Tobin, A.M., Kirby, B., 2011. The 'psoriatic march': a concept of how severe psoriasis may drive cardiovascular comorbidity. Exp. Dermatol. 20, 303.

Caso, F., Costa, L., Atteno, M., Del Puente, A., Cantarini, L., Lubrano, E., Scarpa, R., 2014. Simple clinical indicators for early psoriatic arthritis detection. Springerplus 3, 759.

Caso, F., Lubrano, E., Del Puente, A., Caso, P., Peluso, R., Foglia, F., Benigno, C., Girolimetto, N., Bottiglieri, P., Scarpa, R., Costa, L., 2015. Progress in understanding and utilizing TNF-α inhibition for the treatment of psoriatic arthritis. Expert Rev. Clin. Immunol. http://dx.doi.org/10.1586/1744666X.2016.1117941.

Chen, Y.J., Chang, Y.T., Shen, J.L., Chen, T.T., Wang, C.B., Chen, C.M., Wu, C.Y., 2012. Association between systemic antipsoriatic drugs and cardiovascular risk in patients with psoriasis with or without psoriatic arthritis: a nationwide cohort study. Arthritis Rheum. 64, 1879.

Choi, K.M., Ryu, O.H., Lee, K.W., Kim, H.Y., Seo, J.A., Kim, S.G., Kim, N.H., Choi, D.S., Baik, S.H., 2007. Serum adiponectin, interleukin-10 levels and inflammatory markers in the metabolic syndrome. Diabetes Res. Clin. Pract. 75, 235.

Costa, L., Caso, F., D'Elia, L., Atteno, M., Peluso, R., Del Puente, A., Strazzullo, P., Scarpa, R., 2012. Psoriatic arthritis is associated with increased arterial stiffness in the absence of known cardiovascular risk factors: a case control study. Clin. Rheumatol. 31, 711.

Costa, L., Caso, F., Ramonda, R., Del Puente, A., Cantarini, L., Darda, M.A., Caso, P., Lorenzin, M., Fiocco, U., Punzi, L., Scarpa, R., 2015. Metabolic syndrome and its relationship with the achievement of minimal disease activity state in psoriatic arthritis patients: an observational study. Immunol. Res. 61, 147.

Costa, L., Caso, F., Atteno, M., Del Puente, A., Darda, M.A., Caso, P., Ortolan, A., Fiocco, U., Ramonda, R., Punzi, L., Scarpa, R., 2014. Impact of 24-month treatment with etanercept,adalimumab, or methotrexate on metabolic syndrome components in a cohort of 210 psoriatic arthritis patients. Clin. Rheumatol. 33, 833.

da Silva, B.S., Bonfá, E., de Moraes, J.C., Saad, C.G., Ribeiro, A.C., Gonçalves, C.R., de Carvalho, J.F., 2010. Effects of anti-TNF therapy on glucose metabolism in patients with ankylosing spondylitis, psoriatic arthritis or juvenile idiopathic arthritis. Biologicals 38, 567.

Duarte, G.V., Faillace, C., Freire de Carvalho, J., 2012. Psoriatic arthritis. Best Pract. Res. Clin. Rheumatol. 26, 147.

Eder, L., Zisman, D., Barzilai, M., Laor, A., Rahat, M., Rozenbaum, M., Bitterman, H., Feld, J., Rimar, D., Rosner, I., 2008. Subclinical atherosclerosis in psoriatic arthritis: a case-control study. J. Rheumatol. 35, 877.

Eder, L., Wu, Y., Chandran, V., Cook, R., Gladman, D.D., 2015a. Incidence and predictors for cardiovascular events in patients with psoriatic arthritis. Ann. Rheum. Dis. http://dx.doi.org/10.1136/annrheumdis-2015-207980.

Eder, L., Gladman, D.D., 2015. Atherosclerosis in psoriatic disease: latest evidence and clinical implications. Ther. Adv. Musculoskelet. Dis. 7, 187.

Eder, L., Thavaneswaran, A., Chandran, V., Cook, R.J., Gladman, D.D., 2015b. Obesity is associated with a lower probability of achieving sustained minimal disease activity state among patients with psoriatic arthritis. Ann. Rheum. Dis. 74, 813.

Eder, L., Gladman, D.D., 2014. Predictors for clinical outcome in psoriatic arthritis - what have we learned from cohort studies? Expert Rev. Clin. Immunol. 10, 763.

Eder, L., Jayakar, J., Pollock, R., Pellett, F., Thavaneswaran, A., Chandran, V., Rosen, C.F., Gladman, D.D., 2013. Serum adipokines in patients with psoriatic arthritis and psoriasis alone and their correlation with disease activity. Ann. Rheum. Dis. 72, 1956.

Edson-Heredia, E., Zhu, B., Lefevre, C., Wang, M., Barrett, A., Bushe, C.J., Cox, A., Wu, J.J., Maeda-Chubachi, T., 2015. Prevalence and incidence rates of cardiovascular, autoimmune, and other diseases in patients with psoriatic or psoriatic arthritis: a retrospective study using Clinical Practice Research Datalink. J. Eur. Acad. Dermatol. Venereol. 29, 955.

Egeberg, A., Khalid, U., Gislason, G.H., Mallbris, L., Skov, L., Hansen, P.R., 2015. Association of psoriatic disease with uveitis: a Danish nationwide cohort study. JAMA Dermatol. http://dx.doi.org/10.1001/jamadermatol.2015.1986.

Feldman, S.R., Zhao, Y., Shi, L., Tran, M.H., Lu, J., 2015. Economic and comorbidity burden among moderate-to-severe psoriasis patients with comorbid psoriatic arthritis. Arthritis Care Res. (Hoboken) 67, 708.

Fiocco, U., Martini, V., Accordi, B., Caso, F., Costa, L., Oliviero, F., Scanu, A., Felicetti, M., Frallonardo, P., Facco, M., Boso, D., Molena, B., Zambello, R., Ramonda, R., Cozzi, F., Scarpa, R., Basso, G., Semenzato, G., Dayer, J.M., Doria, A., Punzi, L., 2015a. Ex vivo signaling protein mapping in T lymphocytes in the psoriatic arthritis joints. J. Rheumatol. Suppl. 93, 48.

Fiocco, U., Martini, V., Accordi, B., Caso, F., Costa, L., Oliviero, F., Scanu, A., Facco, M., Boso, D., Gatto, M., Felicetti, M., Frallonardo, P., Ramonda, R., Piva, L., Zambello, R., Agostini, C., Scarpa, R., Basso, G., Semenzato, G., Dayer, J.M., Punzi, L., Doria, A., 2015b. Transcriptional network profile on synovial fluid T cells in psoriatic arthritis. Clin. Rheumatol. 34, 1571.

Fiocco, U., Accordi, B., Martini, V., Oliviero, F., Facco, M., Cabrelle, A., Piva, L., Molena, B., Caso, F., Costa, L., Scanu, A., Pagnin, E., Atteno, M., Scarpa, R., Basso, G., Semenzato, G., Punzi, L., Doria, A., Dayer, J.M., 2014. JAK/STAT/PKCδ molecular pathways in synovial fluid T lymphocytes reflect the in vivo T helper-17 expansion in psoriatic arthritis. Immunol. Res. 58, 61.

Gaydukova, I., Rebrov, A., Nikitina, N., Poddubnyy, D., 2012. Decreased heart rate variability in patients with psoriatic arthritis. Clin. Rheumatol. 31, 1377.

Gelfand, J.M., Troxel, A.B., Lewis, J.D., Kurd, S.K., Shin, D.B., Wang, X., Margolis, D.J., Strom, B.L., 2007. The risk of mortality in patients with psoriasis: results from a population-based study. Arch. Dermatol. 143, 1493.

Gladman, D.D., Farewell, V.T., Wong, K., Husted, J., 1998. Mortality studies in psoriatic arthritis: results from a single outpatient center. II. Prognostic indicators for death. Arthritis Rheum. 41, 1103.

Gladman, D.D., 2012. Early psoriatic arthritis. Rheum. Dis. Clin. North Am. 38, 373.

Gladman, D.D., Ang, M., Su, L., Tom, B.D., Schentag, C.T., Farewell, V.T., 2009. Cardiovascular morbidity in psoriatic arthritis. Ann. Rheum. Dis. 68, 1131.

Goodman, W.A., Levine, A.D., Massari, J.V., Sugiyama, H., McCormick, T.S., Cooper, K.D., 2009. IL-6 signaling in psoriasis prevents immune suppression by regulatory T cells. J. Immunol. 183, 3170.

Gonzalez-Juanatey, C., Llorca, J., Miranda-Filloy, J.A., Amigo-Diaz, E., Testa, A., Garcia-Porrua, C., Martin, J., Gonzalez-Gay, M.A., 2007a. Endothelial dysfunction in psoriatic arthritis patients without clinically evident cardiovascular disease or classic atherosclerosis risk factors. Arthritis Rheum. 57, 287.

Gonzalez-Juanatey, C., Llorca, J., Amigo-Diaz, E., Dierssen, T., Martin, J., Gonzalez-Gay, M.A., 2007b. High prevalence of subclinical atherosclerosis in psoriatic arthritis patients without clinically evident cardiovascular disease or classic atherosclerosis risk factors. Arthritis Rheum. 57, 1074.

Gonzalez-Juanatey, C., Amigo-Diaz, E., Miranda-Filloy, J.A., Testa, A., Revuelta, J., Garcia-Porrua, C., Martin, J., Llorca, J., Gonzalez-Gay, M.A., 2006. Lack of echocardiographic and Doppler abnormalities in psoriatic arthritis patients without clinically evident cardiovascular disease or classic atherosclerosis risk factors. Semin. Arthritis Rheum. 35, 333.

Han, C., Robinson Jr., D.W., Hackett, M.V., Paramore, L.C., Fraeman, K.H., Bala, M.V., 2006. Cardiovascular disease and risk factors in patients with rheumatoid arthritis, psoriatic arthritis, and ankylosing spondylitis. J. Rheumatol. 33, 2167.

Haroon, M., Gallagher, P., Heffernan, E., FitzGerald, O., 2014. High prevalence of metabolic syndrome and of insulin resistance in psoriatic arthritis is associated with the severity of underlying disease. J. Rheumatol. 41, 1357.

Haroon, M., Gallagher, P., FitzGerald, O., 2015. Diagnostic delay of more than 6 months contributes to poor radiographic and functional outcome in psoriatic arthritis. Ann. Rheum. Dis. 74, 1045.

Horreau, C., Pouplard, C., Brenaut, E., Barnetche, T., Misery, L., Cribier, B., Jullien, D., Aractingi, S., Aubin, F., Joly, P., Le Maître, M., Ortonne, J.P., Paul, C., Richard, M.A., 2013. Cardiovascular morbidity and mortality in psoriasis and psoriatic arthritis: a systematic literature review. J. Eur. Acad. Dermatol. Venereol. 27, 12.

Hotamisligil, G.S., Peraldi, P., Budavari, A., Ellis, R., White, M.F., Spiegelman, B.M., 1996. IRS-1-mediated inhibition of insulin receptor tyrosine kinase activity in TNF-alpha- and obesity-induced insulin resistance. Science 271, 665.

Hürlimann, D., Forster, A., Noll, G., Enseleit, F., Chenevard, R., Distler, O., Béchir, M., Spieker, L.E., Neidhart, M., Michel, B.A., Gay, R.E., Lüscher, T.F., Gay, S., Ruschitzka, F., 2002. Anti-tumor necrosis factor-alpha treatment improves endothelial function in patients with rheumatoid arthritis. Circulation 106, 2184.

Husni, M.E., 2015. Comorbidities in psoriatic arthritis. Rheum. Dis. Clin. North Am. 41, 677.

Husted, J.A., Thavaneswaran, A., Chandran, V., Eder, L., Rosen, C.F., Cook, R.J., Gladman, D.D., 2011. Cardiovascular and other comorbidities in patients with psoriatic arthritis: a comparison with patients with psoriasis. Arthritis Care Res. (Hoboken) 63, 1729.

Jamnitski, A., Symmons, D., Peters, M.J., Sattar, N., McInnes, I., Nurmohamed, M.T., 2013. Cardiovascular comorbidities in patients with psoriatic arthritis: a systematic review. Ann. Rheum. Dis. 72, 211.

Jones, S.M., Armas, J.B., Cohen, M.G., Lovell, C.R., Evison, G., McHugh, N.J., 1994. Psoriatic arthritis: outcome of disease subsets and relationship of joint disease to nail and skin disease. Br. J. Rheumatol. 33, 834.

Jones, S.M., Harris, C.P., Lloyd, J., Stirling, C.A., Reckless, J.P., McHugh, N.J., 2000. Lipoproteins and their subfractions in psoriatic arthritis: identification of an atherogenic profile with active joint disease. Ann. Rheum. Dis. 59, 904.

Khraishi, M., Aslanov, R., Rampakakis, E., Pollock, C., Sampalis, J.S., 2014. Prevalence of cardiovascular risk factors in patients with psoriatic arthritis. Clin. Rheumatol. 33, 1495.

Kimhi, O., Caspi, D., Bornstein, N.M., Maharshak, N., Gur, A., Arbel, Y., Comaneshter, D., Paran, D., Wigler, I., Levartovsky, D., Berliner, S., Elkayam, O., 2007. Prevalence and risk factors of atherosclerosis in patients with psoriatic arthritis. Semin. Arthritis Rheum. 36, 203.

Lazarevic, M.B., Vitic, J., Mladenovic, V., Myones, B.L., Skosey, J.L., Swedler, W.I., 1992. Dyslipoproteinemia in the course of active rheumatoid arthritis. Semin. Arthritis Rheum. 22, 172.

Liehn, E.A., Zernecke, A., Postea, O., Weber, C., 2006. Chemokines: inflammatory mediators of atherosclerosis. Arch. Physiol. Biochem. 112, 229.

Lin, Y.C., Dalal, D., Churton, S., Brennan, D.M., Korman, N.J., Kim, E.S., Husni, M.E., 2014. Relationship between metabolic syndrome and carotid intima-media thickness: cross-sectional comparison between psoriasis and psoriatic arthritis. Arthritis Care Res. (Hoboken) 66, 97.

Liu, J.T., Yeh, H.M., Liu, S.Y., Chen, K.T., 2014. Psoriatic arthritis: epidemiology, diagnosis, and treatment. World J. Orthop. 5, 537.

Ma, C., Harskamp, C.T., Armstrong, E.J., Armstrong, A.W., 2013. The association between psoriasis and dyslipidemia: a systematic review. Br. J. Dermatol. 168, 486.

Marchesoni, A., Atzeni, F., Spadaro, A., Lubrano, E., Provenzano, G., Cauli, A., Olivieri, I., Melchiorre, D., Salvarani, C., Scarpa, R., Sarzi-Puttini, P., Montepaone, M., Porru, G., D'Angelo, S., Catanoso, M., Costa, L., Manara, M., Varisco, V., Rotunno, L., DE Lucia, O., DE Marco, G., 2012. Identification of the clinical features distinguishing psoriatic arthritis and fibromyalgia. J. Rheumatol. 39, 849.

Markuszeski, L., Bissinger, A., Janusz, I., Narbutt, J., Jedrzejowska, A.S., Zalewska, A., 2007. Heart rate and arrhythmia in patients with psoriasis vulgaris. Arch. Med. Res. 38, 64.

Matsuura, E., Atzeni, F., Sarzi-Puttini, P., Turiel, M., Lopez, L.R., Nurmohamed, M.T., 2014. Is atherosclerosis an autoimmune disease? BMC Med. 12, 47.

Mehta, N.N., Li, R., Krishnamoorthy, P., Yu, Y., Farver, W., Rodrigues, A., Raper, A., Wilcox, M., Baer, A., DerOhannesian, S., Wolfe, M., Reilly, M.P., Rader, D.J., VanVoorhees, A., Gelfand, J.M., 2012. Abnormal lipoprotein particles and cholesterol efflux capacity in patients with psoriasis. Atherosclerosis 224, 218.

Milaniuk, S., Pietrzak, A., Mosiewicz, B., Mosiewicz, J., Reich, K., 2015. Influence of psoriasis on circulatory system function assessed in echocardiography. Arch. Dermatol. Res. 307, 855.

Miller, I.M., Ellervik, C., Yazdanyar, S., Jemec, G.B., 2013. Meta-analysis of psoriasis, cardiovascular disease, and associated risk factors. J. Am. Acad. Dermatol. 69, 1014.

Moll, J.M., Wright, V., 1973. Psoriatic arthritis. Semin. Arthritis Rheum. 3, 55.

Mok, C.C., Ko, G.T., Ho, L.Y., Yu, K.L., Chan, P.T., To, C.H., 2011. Prevalence of atherosclerotic risk factors and the metabolic syndrome in patients with chronic inflammatory arthritis. Arthritis Care Res. (Hoboken) 63, 195.

Ogdie, A., Haynes, K., Troxel, A.B., Love, T.J., Hennessy, S., Choi, H., Gelfand, J.M., 2014. Risk of mortality in patients with psoriatic arthritis, rheumatoid arthritis and psoriasis: a longitudinal cohort study. Ann. Rheum. Dis. 73, 149.

Ogdie, A., Weiss, P., 2015. The epidemiology of psoriatic arthritis. Rheum. Dis. Clin. North Am. 41, 545.

Ogdie, A., Yu, Y., Haynes, K., Love, T.J., Maliha, S., Jiang, Y., Troxel, A.B., Hennessy, S., Kimmel, S.E., Margolis, D.J., Choi, H., Mehta, N.N., Gelfand, J.M., 2015a. Risk of major cardiovascular events in patients with psoriatic arthritis, psoriasis and rheumatoid arthritis: a population-based cohort study. Ann. Rheum. Dis. 74, 326.

Ogdie, A., Schwartzman, S., Husni, M.E., 2015b. Recognizing and managing comorbidities in psoriatic arthritis. Curr. Opin. Rheumatol. 27, 118.

Peraldi, P., Spiegelman, B., 1998. TNF-alpha and insulin resistance: summary and future prospects. Mol. Cell Biochem. 182, 169.

Pfeffer, K., 2003. Biological functions of tumor necrosis factor cytokines and their receptors. Cytokine Growth Factor Rev. 14, 185.

Peters, M.J., van der Horst-Bruinsma, I.E., Dijkmans, B.A., Nurmohamed, M.T., 2004. Cardiovascular risk profile of patients with spondylarthropathies, particularly ankylosing spondylitis and psoriatic arthritis. Semin. Arthritis Rheum. 34, 585.

Popa, C., van Tits, L.J., Barrera, P., Lemmers, H.L., van den Hoogen, F.H., van Riel, P.L., Radstake, T.R., Netea, M.G., Roest, M., Stalenhoef, A.F., 2009. Anti-inflammatory therapy with tumour necrosis factor alpha inhibitors improves high-density lipoprotein cholesterol antioxidative capacity in rheumatoid arthritis patients. Ann. Rheum. Dis. 68, 868.

Prins, J.B., Niesler, C.U., Winterford, C.M., Bright, N.A., Siddle, K., O'Rahilly, S., Walker, N.I., Cameron, D.P., 1997. Tumor necrosis factor-alpha induces apoptosis of human adipose cells. Diabetes 46, 1939.

Ramji, D.P., Davies, T.S., 2015. Cytokines in atherosclerosis: key players in all stages of disease and promising therapeutic targets. Cytokine Growth Factor Rev. http://dx.doi.org/10.1016/j.cytogfr.2015.04.003.

Ramonda, R., Puato, M., Punzi, L., Rattazzi, M., Zanon, M., Balbi, G., Ortolan, A., Frallonardo, P., Faggin, E., Plebani, M., Zaninotto, M., Lorenzin, M., Pauletto, P., Doria, A., 2014. Atherosclerosis progression in psoriatic arthritis patients despite the treatment with tumor necrosis factor-alpha blockers: a two-year prospective observational study. Jt. Bone Spine 81, 421.

Raychaudhuri, S.K., Chatterjee, S., Nguyen, C., Kaur, M., Jialal, I., Raychaudhuri, S.P., 2010. Increased prevalence of the metabolic syndrome in patients with psoriatic arthritis. Metab. Syndr. Relat. Disord. 8, 331.

Rydén, M., Arvidsson, E., Blomqvist, L., Perbeck, L., Dicker, A., Arner, P., 2004. Targets for TNF-alpha-induced lipolysis in human adipocytes. Biochem. Biophys. Res. Commun. 318, 168.

Ross, R., 1999. Atherosclerosis—an inflammatory disease. N. Engl. J. Med. 340, 115.

Saricaoglu, H., Güllülü, S., Bülbül Baskan, E., Cordan, J., Tunali, S., 2003. Echocardiographic findings in subjects with psoriatic arthropathy. J. Eur. Acad. Dermatol. Venereol. 17, 414.

Sarzi-Puttini, P., Atzeni, F., Shoenfeld, Y., Ferraccioli, G., 2005a. TNF-alpha, rheumatoid arthritis, and heart failure: a rheumatological dilemma. Autoimmun. Rev. 4, 153.

Sarzi-Puttini, P., Atzeni, F., Doria, A., Iaccarino, L., Turiel, M., 2005b. Tumor necrosis factor-alpha, biologic agents and cardiovascular risk. Lupus 14, 780.

Sarzi-Puttini, P., Atzeni, F., Gerli, R., Bartoloni, E., Doria, A., Barskova, T., Matucci-Cerinic, M., Sitia, S., Tomasoni, L., Turiel, M., 2010. Cardiac involvement in systemic rheumatic diseases: an update. Autoimmun. Rev. 9, 849.

Sattar, N., Crompton, P., Cherry, L., Kane, D., Lowe, G., McInnes, I.B., 2007. Effects of tumor necrosis factor blockade on cardiovascular risk factors in psoriatic arthritis: a double-blind, placebo-controlled study. Arthritis Rheum. 56, 831.

Scarpa, R., Manguso, F., D'Arienzo, A., D'Armiento, F.P., Astarita, C., Mazzacca, G., Ayala, F., 2000. Microscopic inflammatory changes in colon of patients with both active psoriasis and psoriatic arthritis without bowel symptoms. J. Rheumatol. 27, 1241.

Scarpa, R., Ayala, F., Caporaso, N., Olivieri, I., 2006. Psoriasis, psoriatic arthritis, or psoriatic disease? J. Rheumatol. 33, 210.

Scarpa, R., Costa, L., Atteno, M., Del Puente, A., Caso, F., Moll, J.M., 2013. Psoriatic arthritis: advances in pharmacotherapy based on molecular target. Expert Opin. Pharmacother. 14, 2311.

Scarpa, R., Caso, F., Costa, L., Peluso, R., Spanò, A., Lubrano, E., Del Puente, A., Moll, J.M., 2015. Psoriatic disease: clinical staging. J. Rheumatol. Suppl. 93, 24.

Sethi, J.K., Hotamisligil, G.S., 1999. The role of TNF alpha in adipocyte metabolism. Semin. Cell Dev. Biol. 10, 19.

Shang, Q., Tam, L.S., Yip, G.W., Sanderson, J.E., Zhang, Q., Li, E.K., Yu, C.M., 2011. High prevalence of subclinical left ventricular dysfunction in patients with psoriatic arthritis. J. Rheumatol. 38, 1363.

Shang, Q., Tam, L.S., Sanderson, J.E., Lee, A.P., Li, E.K., Yu, C.M., 2014. Impaired left ventricular apical rotation is associated with disease activity of psoriatic arthritis. J. Rheumatol. 41, 706.

Shang, Q., Tam, L.S., Sanderson, J.E., Sun, J.P., Li, E.K., Yu, C.M., 2012. Increase in ventricular-arterial stiffness in patients with psoriatic arthritis. Rheumatology (Oxford) 51, 2215.

Sharma, A., Reddy, M.H., Sharma, K., Dogra, S., Vijayvergiya, R., 2014. Study of endothelial dysfunction in patients of psoriatic arthritis by flow mediated and nitroglycerine mediated dilatation of brachial artery. Int. J. Rheum. Dis. http://dx.doi.org/10.1111/1756-185X.12336.

Shen, J., Shang, Q., Li, E.K., Leung, Y.Y., Kun, E.W., Kwok, L.W., Li, M., Li, T.K., Zhu, T.Y., Yu, C.M., Tam, L.S., 2015. Cumulative inflammatory burden is independently associated with increased arterial stiffness in patients with psoriatic arthritis: a prospective study. Arthritis Res. Ther. 17, 75.

Sitia, S., Atzeni, F., Sarzi-Puttini, P., Di Bello, V., Tomasoni, L., Delfino, L., Antonini-Canterin, F., Di Salvo, G., De Gennaro Colonna, V., La Carrubba, S., Carerj, S., Turiel, M., 2009. Cardiovascular involvement in systemic autoimmune diseases. Autoimmun. Rev. 8, 281.

Sitia, S., Tomasoni, L., Atzeni, F., Ambrosio, G., Cordiano, C., Catapano, A., Tramontana, S., Perticone, F., Naccarato, P., Camici, P., Picano, E., Cortigiani, L., Bevilacqua, M., Milazzo, L., Cusi, D., Barlassina, C., Sarzi-Puttini, P., Turiel, M., 2010. From endothelial dysfunction to atherosclerosis. Autoimmun. Rev. 9, 830.

Taylor, W., Gladman, D., Helliwell, P., Marchesoni, A., Mease, P., Mielants, H., CASPAR Study Group, 2006. Classification criteria for psoriatic arthritis: development of new criteria from a large international study. Arthritis Rheum. 54, 2665.

Tam, L.S., Tomlinson, B., Chu, T.T., Li, M., Leung, Y.Y., Kwok, L.W., Li, T.K., Yu, T., Zhu, Y.E., Wong, K.C., Kun, E.W., Li, E.K., 2008a. Cardiovascular risk profile of patients with psoriatic arthritis compared to controls—the role of inflammation. Rheumatol. Oxford 47, 718.

Tam, L.S., Shang, Q., Li, E.K., Tomlinson, B., Chu, T.T., Li, M., Leung, Y.Y., Kwok, L.W., Wong, K.C., Li, T.K., Yu, T., Zhu, T.Y., Kun, E.W., Yip, G.W., Yu, C.M., 2008b. Subclinical carotid atherosclerosis in patients with psoriatic arthritis. Arthritis Rheum. 59, 1322.

Tillett, W., Costa, L., Jadon, D., Wallis, D., Cavill, C., McHugh, J., Korendowych, E., McHugh, N., 2012. The ClASsification for Psoriatic ARthritis (CASPAR) criteria—a retrospective feasibility, sensitivity, and specificity study. J. Rheumatol. 39, 154.

Tobin, A.M., Veale, D.J., Fitzgerald, O., Rogers, S., Collins, P., O'Shea, D., Kirby, B., 2010. Cardiovascular disease and risk factors in patients with psoriasis and psoriatic arthritis. J. Rheumatol. 37, 1386.

Trayhurn, P., Wood, I.S., 2004. Adipokines: inflammation and the pleiotropic role of white adipose tissue. Br. J. Nutr. 92, 347.

Turiel, M., Sitia, S., Atzeni, F., Tomasoni, L., Gianturco, L., Giuffrida, M., De Gennaro Colonna, V., Sarzi-Puttini, P., 2010. The heart in rheumatoid arthritis. Autoimmun. Rev. 9, 414.

Turiel, M., Atzeni, F., Tomasoni, L., de Portu, S., Delfino, L., Bodini, B.D., Longhi, M., Sitia, S., Bianchi, M., Ferrario, P., Doria, A., De Gennaro Colonna, V., Sarzi-Puttini, P., 2009. Non-invasive assessment of coronary flow reserve and ADMA levels: a case-control study of early rheumatoid arthritis patients. Rheumatology (Oxford) 48, 834.

van Kuijk, A.W., Reinders-Blankert, P., Smeets, T.J., Dijkmans, B.A., Tak, P.P., 2006. Detailed analysis of the cell infiltrate and the expression of mediators of synovial inflammation and joint destruction in the synovium of patients with psoriatic arthritis: implications for treatment. Ann. Rheum. Dis. 65, 1551.

Weber, C., Noels, H., 2011. Atherosclerosis: current pathogenesis and therapeutic options. Nat. Med. 17, 1410.

Widlansky, M.E., Gokce, N., Keaney Jr., J.F., Vita, J.A., 2003. The clinical implications of endothelial dysfunction. J. Am. Coll. Cardiol. 42, 1149.

Wong, K., Gladman, D.D., Husted, J., Long, J.A., Farewell, V.T., 1997. Mortality studies in psoriatic arthritis: results from a single outpatient clinic. I: causes and risk of death. Arthritis Rheum. 40, 1868.

Yilmazer, B., Sahin, T., Unlu, B.Ö., Kir, H.M., Cefle, A., 2015. Investigation of subclinical atherosclerosis in psoriatic arthritis patients with minimal disease activity. Rheumatol. Int. 35, 1385.

Yeung, H., Takeshita, J., Mehta, N.N., Kimmel, S.E., Ogdie, A., Margolis, D.J., Shin, D.B., Attor, R., Troxel, A.B., Gelfand, J.M., 2013. Psoriasis severity and the prevalence of major medical comorbidity: a population-based study. JAMA Dermatol. 149, 1173.

Chapter 17

Cardiovascular Involvement in Primary Sjögren's Syndrome

P. Brito-Zerón,[*,§] M. Pérez-de-Lis,[¶] I. Sánchez Berná,[||]
R. Pérez-Álvarez,[¶] A. Sisó-Almirall[#,**] and M. Ramos-Casals[§§]

**Hospital CIMA-Sanitas, Barcelona, Spain; [§]Laboratory of Autoimmune Diseases Josep Font, CELLEX-IDIBAPS, Department of Autoimmune Diseases, ICMiD, Hospital Clínic, Barcelona, Spain; [¶]Department of Internal Medicine, Hospital Alvaro Cunqueiro, Vigo, Spain; [||]Department of Internal Medicine, Hospital Virgen de las Nieves, Granada, Spain; [#]Consorci d'Atenció Primària de Salut Barcelona Esquerre (CAPS-BE). Transversal Group for Research in Primary Care. Institut d'Investigacions Biomèdiques August Pi i Sunyer, (IDIBAPS) Barcelona, Spain; **University of Barcelona, Barcelona, Spain; [§§]Sjögren Syndrome Research Group (AGAUR), Laboratory of Autoimmune Diseases Josep Font, CELLEX-IDIBAPS, Department of Autoimmune Diseases, ICMiD, University of Barcelona, Hospital Clínic, Barcelona, Spain*

1. INTRODUCTION

Sjögren syndrome (SjS) is a systemic autoimmune disease that mainly affects the exocrine glands and causes dryness of the main mucosal surfaces (Ramos-Casals et al., 2012). When symptoms appear in a previously healthy person, the disease is classified as primary SjS. However, the clinical spectrum of SjS extends from dryness to systemic involvement (extraglandular manifestations) and includes a large number of organ-specific manifestations. Cardiovascular involvement is one of the extraglandular involvements less frequently studied in primary SjS, although a growing interest on investigating cardiovascular features in SjS patients has emerged from studies reported in the last 10 years.

2. RAYNAUD PHENOMENON

Raynaud phenomenon, with a prevalence of 10–20%, is probably the most common vascular feature of SjS, and may be the first sign of the disease. We reported in 2002 (Garcia-Carrasco et al., 2002) that Raynaud phenomenon preceded the onset of sicca symptoms in 75% of our patients with primary SjS. In comparison with other systemic autoimmune diseases such as systemic sclerosis, the clinical course of Raynaud phenomenon in primary SjS is milder, and vascular complications (digital ischemia, fingertip infarctions) are uncommon, with pharmacologic interventions being necessary in less than 40% of cases.

In patients with primary SjS presenting with Raynaud phenomenon, a capillaroscopic study is highly recommended, together with the determination of serum anticentromere antibodies (ACAs), especially in those with negative anti-Ro/La antibodies presenting with severe vascular features. Two recent studies (Nakamura et al., 2010; Bournia et al., 2010) have reported a prevalence of ACAs of 4–11% in primary SjS patients; these patients had a differentiated clinical and immunological profile, including a higher frequency of Raynaud phenomenon and dysphagia and a lower frequency of hypergammaglobulinemia and positive Ro/La autoantibodies; some SjS-ACA + patients finally developed an overt systemic sclerosis during the follow-up.

3. CARDIOVASCULAR DISEASE

Cardiovascular disease has emerged as a major cause of morbidity and mortality in patients with autoimmune diseases such as systemic lupus erythematosus and rheumatoid arthritis, and it has been associated with both traditional and autoimmune cardiovascular risk factors (Pérez-De-Lis et al., 2010). In 2005, two case-control studies suggested that primary SjS may be associated with a higher frequency of cardiovascular and metabolic abnormalities. Lodde et al. (2006) reported an abnormal lipid serum profile in 46 patients with primary SjS, while Vaudo et al. (2005) found a higher rate of subclinical atherosclerosis in 37 female SjS patients who were studied by femoral and carotid ultrasonography.

3.1 Cardiovascular Risk Factors

In 2007, we reported the first case-control study that analyzed the main cardiovascular risk factors in a large series of unselected patients with primary SjS (Pérez-De-Lis et al., 2010). In our SjS patients, the most prevalent cardiovascular risk factors were hypercholesterolemia (30%), hypertension (30%), diabetes mellitus (27%), and hypertriglyceridemia (22%). We found a high frequency of diabetes mellitus and hypertriglyceridemia and a lower frequency of hypertension and smoking in comparison with an age- and sex-matched control population from a primary care center. The frequency of diabetes mellitus was 10% higher than that of our primary care patients, reinforcing the association between diabetes and SjS reported in experimental studies using the NOD mouse, a murine model of diabetes that develops an exocrine disease similar to human SjS (Tran et al., 2007). The prevalence of cardiovascular risk factors in our patients with primary SjS was lower in those treated with antimalarials, a finding confirmed in a recently published multicenter registry (Gheitasi et al., 2015).

Three recent case-control studies from UK (Juarez et al., 2014) and Italy (Bartoloni et al., 2015; Augusto et al., 2015) have confirmed a higher frequency of the main cardiovascular risk factors in patients with primary SjS in comparison with those without autoimmune diseases, including a higher frequency of hypertension, dyslipidemia, and metabolic syndrome.

3.2 Subclinical Cardiovascular Disease

Vaudo et al. (2005) published the first study that evaluated the presence of subclinical carotid disease in patients with primary SjS. Table 17.1 summarizes the main results obtained in studies in patients with primary SjS. Two studies reported a higher frequency of carotid plaques in SjS patients in comparison with controls, although the difference was not statistically significant (Vaudo et al., 2005; Gravani et al., 2015). Five studies studied the intima-media thickness (IMT) with no homogeneous results: two studies found an increased IMT in SjS patients (Gravani et al., 2015; Vaudo et al., 2005) and the other three found no significant differences in comparison with the control group (Akyel et al., 2012; Atzeni et al., 2014; Zardi et al., 2014). Other studies have reported an abnormal ankle-brachial index (Rachapalli et al., 2009) or an increased arterial stiffness (Atzeni et al., 2014; Sabio et al., 2015) in patients with primary SjS.

3.3 Cardiovascular Events and Mortality

Reported mortality rates in primary SjS cohorts have decreased progressively during the last four decades: Kassan et al. (1978) reported a rate of 40%, a figure that was reduced to 20–26% in studies in the 1990s and 5–15% in studies in the 2000s (Brito-Zeron et al., 2014). Mortality is mainly attributed to systemic disease and lymphoma, although all the studies mentioned included all causes of mortality in their analyses. But as occurs with other systemic autoimmune diseases, mortality in primary SjS is not only related to the autoimmune disease itself. In our recent study (Brito-Zeron et al., 2014), the main cause of death in the largest cohorts of patients with primary SjS is cardiovascular diseases (30% of deaths), followed by infections, systemic disease, and hematological neoplasia. A recent systematic review that analyzed 10 studies including nearly 8000 patients with primary SjS (Singh et al., 2015) have confirmed cardiovascular disease as the leading cause of mortality in SjS. Bartoloni et al. (2015) have retrospectively evaluated a cohort of 1343 Italian patients with primary SjS and reported an increased risk of cardiovascular events in primary SjS patients in comparison with the control group, including a higher frequency of cerebrovascular events (2.5% vs. 1.4%) and myocardial infarction (1.0% vs. 0.4%); the authors identified central nervous system involvement, leukopenia, and the use of immunosuppressive therapy as SjS-related factors associated with a higher risk of cardiovascular events.

TABLE 17.1 Carotid Ultrasound in Primary Sjögren Syndrome (SjS) (Akyel et al., 2012; Atzeni et al., 2014; Gravani et al., 2015; Vaudo et al., 2005; Zardi et al., 2014)

Author (Ref), Year. Country	Study Group	Groups Size (n); Women (%)	Age (Years)	Carotid Mean ITM (mm)	*P* value	Carotid Plaques (n (%))	*P* value
Vaudo et al. (2005). Italy	SjS	37; 100	48 ± 14	0.82 ± 0.24	≤0.001	9 (24)	0.44
	Control	35; 100	51 ± 16	0.63 ± 0.2		7 (20)	
Akyel et al. (2012). Turkey	SjS	35; 88.6	47.6 ± 8	0.53 ± 0.08	0.345	–	–
	Control	20; 85	48.1 ± 7.8	0.5 ± 0.1		–	
Atzeni et al. (2014). Italy	SjS	22; 72.7	60.14 ± 7.81	0.6 (0.55–0.7)	NS	–	–
	Control	22; 72.7	59.25 ± 2.08	0.57 (0.5–0.6)		–	
Zardi et al. (2014). Italy	SjS	18; 100	65 ± 5.93	0.7 (0.6–0.95)	0.85	10 (56)	0.74
	Control	18; 100	66 ± 5.94	0.7 (0.6–1.1)		8 (44)	
Gravani et al. (2015). Greece	SjS	64; 93.7	57.2 ± 12.4	1 ± 0.3	<0.05	44 (68.8)	NS
	Control	60; 92.8	56.4 ± 7.8	0.9 ± 0.2		34 (56.9)	

ITM, intima-media thickness; *NS*, not significant.

4. AUTONOMIC CARDIOVASCULAR FEATURES

Several studies have reported autonomic cardiovascular disturbances in patients with primary SjS, including orthostatic intolerance, secretomotor dysfunction, male sexual dysfunction, urinary dysfunction, gastroparesis, pupillomotor dysfunction, vasomotor dysfunction, or sleep disorders. Table 17.2 summarizes the main case-control studies published in the last 10 years (Newton et al., 2012; Barendregt et al., 2002; Cai et al., 2008; Mandl et al. 2001, 2007, 2008, 2010; Niemela et al., 2003; Ng et al., 2012; Kovács et al., 2004): four studies found a higher rate of autonomic involvement using standardized scores (COMPASS, AN, and ASP), and the remaining studies demonstrated differences in the results of a wide list of objective tests that

TABLE 17.2 Autonomic Cardiovascular Abnormalities in Patients With Primary Sjögren Syndrome (SjS) (Newton et al., 2012; Barendregt et al., 2002; Cai et al., 2008; Mandl et al. 2001, 2007, 2008, 2010; Niemela et al., 2003; Ng et al., 2012; Kovács et al., 2004)

Author (Ref), Year	Study Design	SjS Patients (n)	Control Groups (n)	Abnormal Scores	Abnormal Tests
Newton et al. (2012)	Case-control	317	317	COMPASjS subscales	–
Barendregt et al. (2002)	Case-control	43	30	–	HRV, SPB, IBI, DBP, BSR
Cai et al. (2008)	Case-control	25	25	COMPASjS subscales	SPB, HRV
Mandl et al. (2001)	Case-control	30	80/50	–	VAC, DBT, SBP, DBP
Niemela et al. (2003)	Case-control	30	30	–	None
Mandl et al. (2007)	Case-control	46	56/238/80	–	DBT, SBP, DBP, VAC
Ng et al. (2012)	Case-control	21	21	–	SBP
Kovács et al. (2004)	Case-control	51	559	AN score	HRV, BP
Mandl et al. (2008)	Case-control	38	200	ASP score	DBT, VAC, SBP, DBP

BSR, baro-reflex sensitivity; *DBP*, diastolic blood pressure; *DBT*, deep-breathing test (expiratory/inspiratory ratio); *HRV*, heart rate variability; *IBI*, interbeat interval; *SBP*, systolic blood pressure; *VAC*, vasoconstrictory index.

evaluate autonomic dysfunction (Table 17.2), except the study reported by Niemela et al. (2003) in which no significant differences were found in comparison with the control group. Mandl et al. (2010) analyzed the progression of autonomic dysfunction in 27 patients observed for a mean of 5 years and reported that only one parameter (the diastolic blood pressure ratio) worsened at the end of follow-up; these authors also reported a significant association between autonomic symptoms and general symptoms (fatigue, anxiety, and depression).

5. PULMONARY ARTERIAL HYPERTENSION

Pulmonary arterial hypertension (PAH) is a vascular disease of the small pulmonary arteries that causes a progressive increase in pulmonary vascular resistance leading to right ventricular failure and, potentially, death. PAH is one of the main vascular complications of the limited form of systemic sclerosis, although recent studies have reported PAH in patients with other systemic autoimmune diseases, including primary SjS (Ahmed and Palevsky, 2014).

A total of eight studies have analyzed the prevalence of PAH in patients with primary SjS (Lin et al., 2010; Vassiliou et al., 2008; Ye et al., 2008; Taouli et al., 2002; Parambil et al., 2006; Yan et al., 2008; Lei et al., 2009; Launay et al., 2007; Leone et al., 1996; Kobak et al., 2014) and identified 170 cases (14%) in 1205 patients, with a prevalence ranging from 4% to 44%. We have identified 35 additional reported cases (Chen et al., 2006a,b; Launay et al., 2007; Luo et al., 2011; Biyajima et al., 1994; Gallerani et al., 1996; Usui et al., 1998; Aoki et al., 2000; Ohnishi et al., 2000; Nakagawa et al., 2003; Tatsukawa et al., 2003; Aslaksen and Nossent, 2004; Vallalta Morales et al., 2004; Bertoni et al., 2005; Chen et al., 2006a,b; Thiam et al., 2006; Seck et al., 2007; Zhu et al., 2007; Yasuda et al., 2009; Szturmowicz et al., 2010; Arca Barca et al., 2011; Naniwa and Takeda, 2011). Nearly 75% of the total cases (141/194) were reported in Asian countries (China, Japan and Taiwan). Epidemiological features were detailed in 30 cases, with a mean age of 49 years (range 21−71 years) and a female: male ratio of 29:1. Death was reported in 10 out of 30 cases.

The clinical presentation of PAH in patients with primary SjS was detailed in 30 cases and consisted of dyspnea in all reported cases, accompanied by a history of right heart failure in 23% and syncope in 10%. The main extraglandular features associated with PAH were Raynaud phenomenon (52%) and interstitial lung disease (31%). The majority of patients had anti-Ro/SjS-A (20/26, 77%) or anti-La/SjS-B (12/21, 57%) antibodies; none of the reported patients who were tested for scleroderma-related autoantibodies were positive, although anti-RNP antibodies were positive in 6/11 (55%) patients.

PAH should be suspected in primary SjS patients presenting with unexplained dyspnea and normal chest radiography. Cardiac echo-Doppler is a noninvasive PAH screening technique. However, PAH should be confirmed by right-heart catheterization, demonstrating an elevated mean pulmonary artery pressure (mPAP) > 25 mm Hg at rest or >30 mm Hg during exercise. In half the detailed cases in primary SjS, diagnosis of PAH preceded or coincided with the diagnosis of SjS, with a delay between the first symptom and the diagnosis of PAH of >1 year in two-thirds of cases (Launay et al., 2007). Right-heart catheterization confirmed PAH in all but two of the isolated reported cases with primary SjS, with a mean mPAP of 54 mm Hg (range, 36–100 mm Hg) and with one patient diagnosed with an mPAP of 33 mm Hg during exercise. Prevalence studies using echocardiography found that only 11/45 (24%) patients had an estimated PAP >50 mm Hg.

The principal causes of PAH unrelated to primary SjS (mainly congenital heart disease, chronic pulmonary/liver disease, and HIV infection) should first be ruled out. In addition, the emergence of associated systemic diseases (mainly scleroderma and SLE) should also be investigated in all SjS patients with PAH; PAH may also be related to complications that can develop in some patients with SjS, such as cirrhosis related to liver involvement (hepatitis C infection, primary biliary cirrhosis), pulmonary fibrosis, or lymphoma.

6. ARRHYTHMIAS

6.1 Ro-Associated Congenital Heart Block

Ro-associated or autoimmune congenital heart block (CHB) is included among the manifestations induced by maternal antibodies against the Ro/La autoantigens that cross the placenta (collectively referred to as neonatal lupus). These autoantibodies damage the conduction tissues during fetal development of the heart inducing inflammation, calcification, and fibrosis, which leads to blocking signal conduction at the atrioventricular (AV) node in an otherwise structurally normal heart (Brito-Zerón et al., 2015). The great majority of the affected pregnancies present with complete (third-degree) AV block resulting in ventricular heart rates often ranging between 50 and 70 beats per minute. Analysis of underlying maternal autoimmune diseases showed that nearly half of mothers had some clinical autoimmune features or were asymptomatic carriers of Ro antibodies, not fulfilling the classification criteria for a specific systemic autoimmune disease; for the remaining mothers, SjS and SLE (alone or reported together) accounted for 95% of cases with a well-defined systemic autoimmune disease (Brito-Zerón et al., 2015).

In primary SjS, the identification of CHB during pregnancy may be the first clue to the disease in women of childbearing age. In these asymptomatic pregnant women, the diagnosis of fetal CHB in a structurally normal heart, especially during weeks 16–24 of gestation, should immediately trigger an evaluation of the maternal sera for antibodies reactive overwhelmingly against the Ro antigen. In a recent systematic review, 113 (13%) out of 856 CHB-affected mothers had an underlying primary SjS at the diagnosis of fetal heart block (Brito-Zerón et al., 2015). Table 17.3 summarizes the data of three studies in which mothers were followed-up searching for the development of a defined SAD after a diagnosis of autoimmune CHB (Press et al., 1996; Julkunen and Eronen, 2001; Rivera et al., 2009); after a mean follow-up ranging between 7 and 10 years, the disease more frequently diagnosed was SjS in 16% of cases followed by SLE in 8%. These data suggest that a positive immunological result may lead to an early diagnosis of primary SjS, either at the diagnosis of CHB or, in some cases, several years before the onset of overt sicca syndrome.

6.2 Ro-Associated Arrhythmias in Adults

Recent studies have suggested that the adult heart, classically considered invulnerable to the effect of anti-Ro antibodies, may be a potential target for the development of arrhythmias in patients carrying these autoantibodies. The prolongation of the QTc interval is the most frequent abnormality observed in adults carrying anti-Ro antibodies, together with an increased risk of ventricular arrhythmias that could be life-threatening (Lazzerini et al., 2010). A recent study has tested the hypothesis that anti-Ro Abs target the HERG-K(+) channel in an animal model of autoimmune-associated QTc prolongation (Yue et al., 2015). The authors have reported that anti-Ro antibodies from patients with autoimmune diseases inhibit IKr by cross-reacting with the HERG channel likely at the pore region, probably related to the molecular homology between the anti-52-kDa Ro antigen and the HERG channel. The authors proposed that adult patients carrying anti-Ro antibodies may benefit from routine ECG screening to detect QTc prolongation syndrome (Lazzerini et al., 2011).

Table 17.4 summarizes the main features of five isolated cases of cardiac arrhythmias reported in adult Ro + patients with primary SjS (Lee et al., 1996; Baumgart et al., 1998; Sung et al., 2011; Liang et al., 2015). Theander et al. (1999) also reported a 55-year old woman diagnosed with primary SjS who suddenly developed AV-block III and was finally diagnosed with systemic sarcoidosis.

7. PERICARDITIS

Pericarditis is caused by inflammation of the pericardium; pericardial effusion complicates pericarditis in two-thirds of cases, and effusions are classified as small (<1 cm), moderate (1–2 cm), or large (>2 cm). In primary SjS, pericardial effusion was reported in 87/655 (13%) patients evaluated by echography (Gyongyosi et al., 1996; Manganelli et al., 1997; Ye et al., 2008; Vassiliou et al., 2008), while pericarditis was reported in 9/456 (2%) patients included in clinical SjS cohorts (Gyongyosi et al., 1996; Kruize et al., 1996; Skopouli et al., 2000; Pertovaara et al., 2001); one study (Brucato et al., 2006)

TABLE 17.3 Studies in Which Mothers Were Followed-up Searching for the Development of a Defined SAD After a Diagnosis of Autoimmune Congenital Heart Block (CHB)

Author (Ref), Year	Mothers	Maternal SjS at CHB Diagnosis	Asymptomatic/UAD Mothers	New SjS at Follow-up	New SLE at Follow-up	Follow-up (Years)
Press et al. (1996)	64	1	54	2/54	4/54	10
Julkunen and Eronen (2001)	83	3	74	33/74	9/74	9.9
Rivera et al. (2009)	229	65	151	10/151	10/151	7
TOTAL	**376**	**69**	**279**	**45/279 (16%)**	**23/279 (8%)**	

TABLE 17.4 Main Features of Five Isolated Sases of Cardiac Arrhythmias Reported in Adult Ro + Patients With Primary Sjögren Syndrome (SjS)

Author (Ref), Year	Arrhythmia	Ro/La Autoantibodies
Lee et al. (1996)	Complete AV block	Ro52+, Ro60+
Baumgart et al. (1998)	Complete AV block	Ro60+, La+
Sung et al. (2011)	Complete AV block	Ro/SjSA+
Liang et al. (2015)	Premature ventricular contraction + intraventricular conduction block	Ro52+
Liang et al. (2015)	Intra-atrial & intraventricular conduction block	Ro52+

reported primary SjS in 4/48 (8%) patients with "idiopathic" recurrent pericarditis, and four additional isolated cases have been reported (Kau et al., 2004; Mutsukura et al., 2007; Yoong et al., 2007; Chen et al., 2009).

Epidemiological features have been detailed in only 4 of the 17 reported cases of pericarditis in primary SjS (all were female, with a mean age of 57 years). Clinically, pericarditis was the initial manifestation of primary SjS in two of the four detailed cases. Clinical features included dyspnea (n = 4), chest pain (n = 2), fever (n = 2), pericardial effusion (n = 2), and heart failure (n = 2). All four patients had positive ANA and anti-Ro/SjS-A antibodies and all had associated diseases or conditions (primary cardiac lymphoma, thrombotic thrombocytopenic purpura, systemic cryoglobulinemic vasculitis, and pregnancy, respectively). Complications such as cardiac tamponade, constrictive pericarditis, or purulent pericarditis, or the need for invasive procedures (pericardiocentesis/pericardial window) have not been reported in primary SjS patients.

Pericarditis should be diagnosed clinically, with the following features being highly suggestive: characteristic chest pain, pericardial friction rub, suggestive electrocardiographic (ECG) changes, and new/worsening pericardial effusion. The standard diagnostic approach should include complete blood cell count, cardiac enzymes, and measurement of sedimentation rate/C-reactive protein concentration, together with ECG and echocardiography to evaluate pericardial effusion. The pericardial fluid in SjS-related pericarditis was exudative in all reported cases (Gyongyosi et al., 1996; Vassiliou et al., 2008; Ye et al., 2008). Finally, investigation underlying autoimmune diseases in patients with idiopathic recurrent pericarditis is mandatory (one study identified SjS in nearly 10% of patients) (Brucato et al., 2006).

Due to the very-low frequency of pericarditis in primary SjS, the main causes of pericarditis in the general population should first be ruled out, especially viruses and other nonautoimmune causes such as cardiac disease (myocardial infarction, history of cardiac surgery), tuberculosis, chronic heart/liver/renal failure, and neoplasia (lymphoma). In addition, the possible emergence of an associated autoimmune disease (mainly SLE but also systemic sclerosis) should also be evaluated.

8. MYOCARDITIS

Autoimmune myocarditis is an infrequent cause of cardiac involvement in patients with SAD. This life-threatening clinical presentation has been mainly reported in patients with SLE, with a frequency lower than 10%. In patients with primary SjS, myocarditis has been reported in only four patients (Yoshioka et al., 1999; Levin et al., 1999), including patients with associated cryoglobulinemic vasculitis (Kau et al., 2004) or who presented with severe arrhythmias (Liang et al., 2015).

REFERENCES

Ahmed, S., Palevsky, H.I., 2014. Pulmonary arterial hypertension related to connective tissue disease: a review. Rheum. Dis. Clin. North Am. 40 (1), 103–124.

Akyel, A., et al., 2012. Endothelial dysfunction in primary Sjögren syndrome. Int. J. Immunopathol. Pharmacol. 61 (9), 870–872.

Aoki, A., et al., 2000. Pulmonary hypertension in a patient with primary Sjogren's syndrome, Hashimoto's disease, and primary biliary cirrhosis. Nihon Rinsho Men'eki Gakkai Kaishi 23 (5), 462–469.

Arca Barca, B., Paredes Vila, S., Mazaira Riocabo, A., 2011. Primary pulmonary hypertension in Sjogren's syndrome: a rare association. Reumatol. Clin. 7 (3), 212.

Aslaksen, H.K., Nossent, H.C., 2004. Fatal pulmonary hypertension in primary Sjogren's syndrome. Clin. Exp. Rheumatol. 22 (4), 507.

Atzeni, F., et al., 2014. New parameters for identifying subclinical atherosclerosis in patients with primary Sjogren's syndrome: a pilot study. Clin. Exp. Rheumatol. 32 (3), 361–368.

Augusto, K.L., et al., 2015. Metabolic syndrome in Sjogren's syndrome patients: a relevant concern for clinical monitoring. Clin. Rheumatol.

Barendregt, P.J., et al., 2002. Spectral analysis of heart rate and blood pressure variability in primary Sjogren's syndrome. Ann. Rheum. Dis. 61 (3), 232–236.

Bartoloni, E., et al., 2015. Cardiovascular disease risk burden in primary Sjogren's syndrome: results of a population-based multicentre cohort study. J. Intern. Med.

Baumgart, D.C., Gerl, H., Dorner, T., 1998. Complete heart block caused by primary Sjogren's syndrome and hypopituitarism. Ann. Rheum. Dis. 57 (10), 635.

Bertoni, M., et al., 2005. Pulmonary hypertension in primary Sjogren's syndrome: report of a case and review of the literature. Clin. Rheumatol. 24 (4), 431–434.

Biyajima, S., et al., 1994. Pulmonary hypertension and antiphospholipid antibody in a patient with Sjogren's syndrome. Intern. Med. (Tokyo, Japan) 33 (12), 768–772.

Bournia, V.-K.K., et al., 2010. Anticentromere antibody positive Sjogren's Syndrome: a retrospective descriptive analysis. Arthritis Res. Ther. 12 (2), R47.

Brito-Zeron, P., et al., 2014. Systemic activity and mortality in primary Sjogren syndrome: predicting survival using the EULAR-SS Disease Activity Index (ESSDAI) in 1045 patients. Ann. Rheum. Dis.

Brito-Zerón, P., et al., 2015. The clinical spectrum of autoimmune congenital heart block. Nat. Rev. Rheumatol. 11 (5), 301–312. Available at: http://www.ncbi.nlm.nih.gov/pubmed/25800217.

Brucato, A., et al., 2006. Long-term outcomes in difficult-to-treat patients with recurrent pericarditis. Am. J. Cardiol. 98 (2), 267–271.

Cai, F.Z.J., et al., 2008. Mild autonomic dysfunction in primary Sjögren's syndrome: a controlled study. Arthritis Res. Ther. 10 (2), R31. Available at: http://www.pubmedcentral.nih.gov/articlerender.fcgi?artid=2453776&tool=pmcentrez&rendertype=abstract.

Chen, C.-H., et al., 2006a. Clinical features and endothelin receptor antagonist in primary Sjogren's syndrome with pulmonary arterial hypertension. Scand. J. Rheumatol. 35 (3), 245–247.

Chen, C.-H., et al., 2006b. Pulmonary arterial hypertension in autoimmune diseases: an analysis of 19 cases from a medical center in northern Taiwan. J. Microbiol. Immunol. Infect. 39 (2), 162–168.

Chen, H.-A., Chen, C.-H., Cheng, H.-H., 2009. Hemolytic uremic syndrome and pericarditis as early manifestations of primary Sjogren's syndrome. Clin. Rheumatol. 28 (Suppl 1), S43–S46.

Gallerani, M., et al., 1996. A 49-year-old woman with dyspnoea, palpitations and syncope. Int. J. Cardiol. 55 (1), 67–78.

Garcia-Carrasco, M., et al., 2002. Raynaud's phenomenon in primary Sjogren's syndrome. Prevalence and clinical characteristics in a series of 320 patients. J. Rheumatol. 29 (4), 726–730.

Gheitasi, H., et al., 2015. How we are treating our systemic patients with primary Sjögren syndrome? Analysis of 1120 patients. Int. Immunopharmacol. Available at: http://www.sciencedirect.com/science/article/pii/S1567576915001290.

Gravani, F., et al., 2015. Subclinical atherosclerosis and impaired bone health in patients with primary Sjogren's syndrome: prevalence, clinical and laboratory associations. Arthritis Res. Ther. 17, 99. Available at: http://www.pubmedcentral.nih.gov/articlerender.fcgi?artid=4416325&tool=pmcentrez&rendertype=abstract.

Gyongyosi, M., et al., 1996. Cardiac manifestations in primary Sjogren's syndrome. Ann. Rheum. Dis. 55 (7), 450–454.

Juarez, M., et al., 2014. Cardiovascular risk factors in women with primary Sjogren's syndrome: United Kingdom primary Sjogren's syndrome registry results. Arthritis Care Res. 66 (5), 757–764. Available at: http://ovidsp.ovid.com/ovidweb.cgi?T=JS&PAGE=reference&D=medl&NEWS=N&AN=24877201.

Julkunen, H., Eronen, M., 2001. Long-term outcome of mothers of children with isolated heart block in Finland. Arthritis Rheum. 44 (3), 647–652.

Kassan, S.S., et al., 1978. Increased risk of lymphoma in sicca syndrome. Ann. Intern. Med. 89 (6), 888–892.

Kau, C.-K., et al., 2004. Primary Sjogren's syndrome complicated with cryoglobulinemic glomerulonephritis, myocarditis, and multi-organ involvement. J. Formos. Med. Assoc. 103 (9), 707–710.

Kobak, S., et al., 2014. Pulmonary arterial hypertension in patients with primary Sjogren's syndrome. Autoimmune. Dis. 2014, 710401.

Kovács, L., et al., 2004. Cardiovascular autonomic dysfunction in primary Sjögren's syndrome. Rheumatology (Oxford, England) 43 (1), 95–99.

Kruize, A.A., et al., 1996. Long-term followup of patients with Sjogren's syndrome. Arthritis Rheum. 39 (2), 297–303.

Launay, D., et al., 2007. Pulmonary arterial hypertension: a rare complication of primary Sjogren syndrome: report of 9 new cases and review of the literature. Medicine 86 (5), 299–315.

Lazzerini, P.E., et al., 2011. Anti-Ro/SSA-associated corrected QT interval prolongation in adults: the role of antibody level and specificity. Arthritis Care Res. 63 (10), 1463–1470.

Lazzerini, P.E., Capecchi, P.L., Laghi-Pasini, F., 2010. Anti-Ro/SSA antibodies and cardiac arrhythmias in the adult: facts and hypotheses. Scand. J. Immunol. 72 (3), 213–222.

Lee, L.A., Pickrell, M.B., Reichlin, M., 1996. Development of complete heart block in an adult patient with Sjogren's syndrome and anti-Ro/SS-A autoantibodies. Arthritis Rheum. 39 (8), 1427–1429.

Lei, Y., et al., 2009. Clinical analysis of 79 pulmonary arterial hypertension cases from 1892 connective tissue disease patients. Zhonghua Yi Xue Za Zhi 89 (41), 2934–2937.

Leone, J., et al., 1996. Pulmonary manifestations of primary Gougerot-Sjogren syndrome. Apropos of 8 cases in a series of 35 patients. Rev. Med. Interne. 17 (4), 291–299.

Levin, M.D., Zoet-Nugteren, S.K., Markusse, H.M., 1999. Myocarditis and primary Sjogren's syndrome. Lancet (London, England) 354 (9173), 128–129.

Liang, M., et al., 2015. Cardiac arrhythmias as the initial manifestation of adult primary Sjogren's syndrome: a case report and literature review. Int. J. Rheum. Dis. 18 (7), 800–806.

Lin, D.-F., et al., 2010. Clinical and prognostic characteristics of 573 cases of primary Sjogren's syndrome. Chin. Med. J. 123 (22), 3252–3257.

Lodde, B.M., et al., 2006. Serum lipid levels in Sjogren's syndrome. Rheumatology (Oxford, England) 45 (4), 481–484.

Luo, Y., et al., 2011. Frequency of pleural effusions in patients with pulmonary arterial hypertension associated with connective tissue diseases. Chest 140 (1), 42–47.

Mandl, T., et al., 2007. Autonomic and orthostatic dysfunction in primary Sjogren's syndrome. J. Rheumatol. 34 (9), 1869–1874. Available at: http://ovidsp.ovid.com/ovidweb.cgi?T=JS&PAGE=reference&D=med5&NEWS=N&AN=17659755.

Mandl, T., et al., 2010. Autonomic nervous dysfunction development in patients with primary Sjogren's syndrome: a follow-up study. Rheumatology (Oxford, England) 49 (6), 1101–1106. Available at: http://www.ncbi.nlm.nih.gov/pubmed/20219783.

Mandl, T., et al., 2008. Autonomic nervous symptoms in primary Sjogren's syndrome. Rheumatology (Oxford, England) 47 (6), 914–919. Available at: http://ovidsp.ovid.com/ovidweb.cgi?T=JS&PAGE=reference&D=med5&NEWS=N&AN=18411214.

Mandl, T., et al., 2001. Sympathetic dysfunction in patients with primary {Sjogren}'s syndrome. J. Rheumatol. 28 (2), 296–301. Available at://000166973300014.

Manganelli, P., et al., 1997. Echocardiographic findings in primary Sjogren's syndrome. Ann. Rheum. Dis. 56 (9), 568.

Mutsukura, K., et al., 2007. Successful treatment of a patient with primary Sjogren's syndrome complicated with pericarditis during pregnancy. Intern. Med. (Tokyo, Japan) 46 (14), 1143–1147.

Nakagawa, N., et al., 2003. Severe pulmonary hypertension associated with primary Sjogren's syndrome. Intern. Med. (Tokyo, Japan) 42 (12), 1248–1252.

Nakamura, H., et al., 2010. Anti-centromere antibody-seropositive Sjogren's syndrome differs from conventional subgroup in clinical and pathological study. BMC Musculoskelet. Dis. 11, 140.

Naniwa, T., Takeda, Y., 2011. Long-term remission of pulmonary veno-occlusive disease associated with primary Sjogren's syndrome following immunosuppressive therapy. Mod. Rheumatol. 21 (6), 637–640.

Newton, J.L., et al., 2012. Autonomic symptoms are common and are associated with overall symptom burden and disease activity in primary Sjogren's syndrome. Ann. Rheum. Dis. 71 (12), 1973–1979. Available at: http://www.pubmedcentral.nih.gov/articlerender.fcgi?artid=3488764&tool=pmcentrez&rendertype=abstract.

Ng, W.F., et al., 2012. Primary Sjogrens syndrome is associated with impaired autonomic response to orthostasis and sympathetic failure. QJM 105, 1191–1199. September.

Niemela, R.K., et al., 2003. Comprehensive study of autonomic function in a population with primary Sjogren's syndrome. No evidence of autonomic involvement. J. Rheumatol. 30 (1), 74–79. Available at: http://www.ncbi.nlm.nih.gov/pubmed/12508393.

Ohnishi, H., et al., 2000. Sjogren's syndrome with malignant lymphoma, interstitial pneumonia, and pulmonary hypertension. Nihon Kokyuki Gakkai Zasshi 38 (3), 190–194.

Parambil, J.G., et al., 2006. Interstitial lung disease in primary Sjogren syndrome. Chest 130 (5), 1489–1495.

Pérez-De-Lis, M., et al., 2010. Cardiovascular risk factors in primary Sjögren's syndrome: a case-control study in 624 patients. Lupus 19 (8), 941–948. Available at: http://www.ncbi.nlm.nih.gov/pubmed/20581017.

Pertovaara, M., et al., 2001. A longitudinal cohort study of Finnish patients with primary Sjogren's syndrome: clinical, immunological, and epidemiological aspects. Ann. Rheum. Dis. 60 (5), 467–472.

Press, J., et al., 1996. Long-term outcome of mothers of children with complete congenital heart block. Am. J. Med. 100 (3), 328–332.

Rachapalli, S.M., Kiely, P.D., Bourke, B.E., 2009. Prevalence of abnormal ankle brachial index in patients with primary Sjogren's syndrome. Clin. Rheumatol. 28 (5), 587–590.

Ramos-Casals, M., et al., 2012. Primary Sjogren syndrome. BMJ 344, e3821. Available at: http://www.ncbi.nlm.nih.gov/pubmed/22700787.

Rivera, T.L., et al., 2009. Disease progression in mothers of children enrolled in the research registry for neonatal lupus. Ann. Rheum. Dis. 68 (6), 828–835.

Sabio, J.M., et al., 2015. Prevalence of and factors associated with increased arterial stiffness in patients with primary Sjogren's syndrome. Arthritis Care Res. (Hoboken) 67 (4), 554–562.

Seck, S.M., et al., 2007. Pulmonary hypertension revealing systemic diseases: two Senegalese case reports. Dakar Med. 52 (3), 175–179.

Singh, A.G., Singh, S., Matteson, E.L., 2015. Rate, risk factors and causes of mortality in patients with Sjogren's syndrome: a systematic review and meta-analysis of cohort studies. Rheumatology (Oxford, England).

Skopouli, F.N., et al., 2000. Clinical evolution, and morbidity and mortality of primary Sjögren's syndrome. Semin. Arthritis Rheum. 29 (5), 296–304.

Sung, M.J., et al., 2011. Complete atrioventricular block in adult Sjogren's syndrome with anti-Ro autoantibody. Korean J. Intern. Med. 26 (2), 213–215.

Szturmowicz, M., et al., 2010. Primary Sjogren's Syndrome with two extraglandular sites involvement - case report. Pneumonol. Alergol. Polska 78 (6), 445–450.

Taouli, B., et al., 2002. Thin-section chest CT findings of primary Sjogren's syndrome: correlation with pulmonary function. Eur. Radiol. 12 (6), 1504–1511.

Tatsukawa, H., et al., 2003. A case of primary Sjogren's syndrome with severe pulmonary hypertension and glomerular damage. Ryumachi 43 (3), 564–568.

Theander, E., et al., 1999. AV-block III in a patient with sarcoidosis mimicking Sjogren's syndrome. Scand. J. Rheumatol. 28 (6), 377–379.

Thiam, M., et al., 2006. Pulmonary arterial hypertension revealing pseudolymphoma associated with Sjogren's syndrome. Dakar Med. 51 (3), 178–180.

Tran, S.D., et al., 2007. Reversal of Sjogren's-like syndrome in non-obese diabetic mice. Ann. Rheum. Dis. 66 (6), 812–814.

Usui, K., et al., 1998. Primary Sjogren's syndrome with pulmonary hypertension. Nihon Kokyuki Gakkai Zasshi 36 (5), 478–481.

Vallalta Morales, M., et al., 2004. Pulmonary arterial hypertension and Sjogren's syndrome: and uncommon association. Med. Clin. 123 (19), 758–759.

Vassiliou, V.A., et al., 2008. Is the heart affected in primary Sjogren's syndrome? An echocardiographic study. Clin. Exp. Rheumatol. 26 (1), 109–112.

Vaudo, G., et al., 2005. Precocious intima-media thickening in patients with primary Sjögren's syndrome. Arthritis Rheum. 52 (12), 3890–3897. Available at: http://www.ncbi.nlm.nih.gov/pubmed/16320337.

Yan, S.-M., et al., 2008. Lung involvement of primary Sjogren's syndrome. Zhonghua Jie He He Hu Xi Za Zhi 31 (7), 513–516.

Yasuda, T., et al., 2009. Pulmonary hypertension in a patient on chronic hemodialysis. Nihon Kokyuki Gakkai Zasshi 47 (1), 52–56.

Ye, Y., et al., 2008. Cardiac manifestations in Sjogren syndrome. Zhonghua Xin Xue Guan Bing Za Zhi 36 (4), 327–331.

Yoong, J.K.-C., et al., 2007. Cardiac lymphoma in primary Sjogren syndrome: a novel case established by targeted imaging and pericardial window. J. Thorac. Cardiovasc. Surg. 134 (2), 513–514.

Yoshioka, K., et al., 1999. Myocarditis and primary Sjogren's syndrome. Lancet (London, England) 354 (9194), 1996.

Yue, Y., et al., 2015. Pathogenesis of the novel autoimmune-associated long-QT syndrome. Circulation 132 (4), 230–240.

Zardi, E.M., et al., 2014. Subclinical carotid atherosclerosis in elderly patients with primary Sjogren syndrome: a duplex Doppler sonographic study. Int. J. Immunopathol. Pharmacol. 27 (4), 645–651.

Zhu, F., Deng, C.-X., Li, Z.-Q., 2007. Pulmonary hypertension caused by Sjogren's Syndrome: a case report. Zhonghua Xin Xue Guan Bing Za Zhi 35 (5), 465.

Chapter 18

Gout and Heart Disease: A Two-Way Street?

M. Heslinga, M. Nurmohamed and M. Gerritsen
Amsterdam Rheumatology and Immunology Center and Reade, Amsterdam, The Netherlands

Key Points

- Gout is the most common inflammatory rheumatic disease with an increasing incidence.
- Traditional cardiovascular risk factors such as hypertension, diabetes mellitus, and chronic kidney disease are more prevalent in patients with gout.
- Hyperuricemia and gout seem to be independent cardiovascular risk factors.
- A link between hyperuricemia and gout and cardiovascular disease is provided by the inflammatory status in which inflammasome activation plays an important role.
- Physicians treating patients with gout should be aware of the increased cardiovascular risk; cardiovascular risk factors should be identified and treated.

1. INTRODUCTION

Gout is the most common inflammatory rheumatic disease, with an estimated prevalence ranging between 1% and 3% (Zhu et al., 2011). In addition, the incidence is rising (Smith et al., 2014). Gout is a disease characterized by the deposition of monosodium urate (MSU) crystals in the joints, skin, and kidneys. Crystal deposition in the joints can result in acute gouty arthritis and chronic arthropathy while depositions in soft tissue may result in the presence of tophi (tophaceous gout). As in other inflammatory diseases, for example, rheumatoid arthritis (RA), gout is considered a condition associated with an

The Heart in Systemic Autoimmune Diseases.

increased cardiovascular risk (Kuo et al., 2016). The origin of this increase appears to be two-fold; first, traditional risk factors such as such as dyslipidemia, hypertension, smoking, obesity, and diabetes mellitus (DM) are more prevalent in gout patients compared with the general population. Secondly there is mounting evidence that gout and hyperuricemia are independent risk factors for cardiovascular disease. In this chapter, associations between gout, hyperuricemia, and cardiovascular comorbidities will be discussed. The focus will be on atherosclerotic cardiovascular disease, but nonischemic heart disease will also be discussed.

2. GOUT—OVERVIEW

In humans, uric acid is derived from xanthine by the action of xanthine oxidase, and it is the end product of purine metabolism (Fig. 18.1). Uric acid is mainly excreted by the kidneys, and therefore serum levels increase when renal function is impaired. Uric acid levels increase in case of excessive intake of purine rich foods, fructose, or alcohol. Other causes of hyperuricemia are conditions associated with high cell turnover, that is, lymphoproliferative

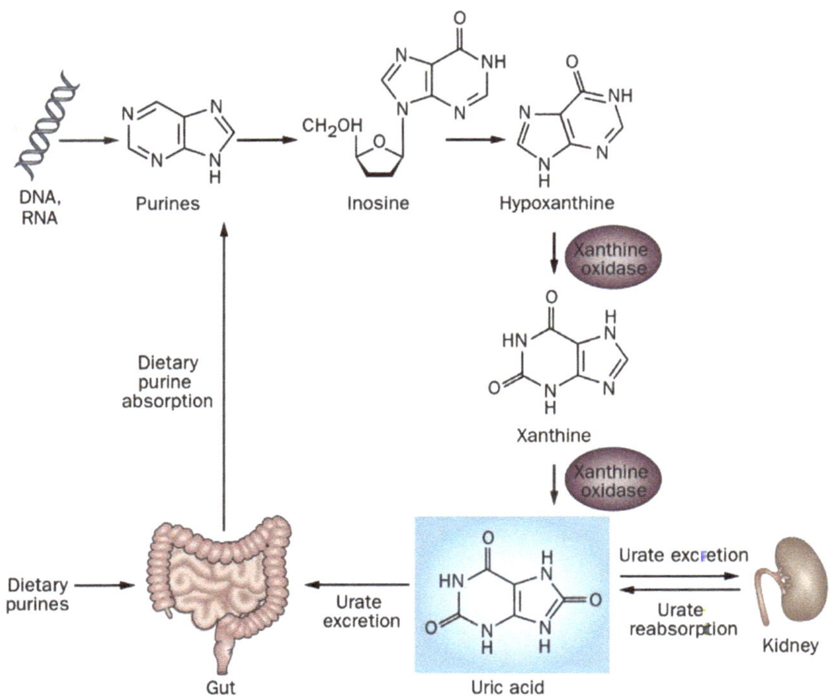

FIGURE 18.1 Uric acid metabolism (Rock et al., 2013).

disease. Hyperuricemia is usually defined as an uric acid level >6.5 or 7.0 mg/dL (>416 μmol/L) in men and >6.0 mg/dL (>360 μmol/L) in women; however, thresholds varying between 6 and 8 mg/dL are used in clinical studies (Khanna et al., 2012).

Clinical manifestations of gout may include acute attacks of arthritis, which are often recurrent, chronic arthropathy, or tophaceous deposits. In addition, gout may present as nephrolithiasis, and also nephropathy is common as gout. Although all patients with gout have hyperuricemia, not all hyperuricemic patients develop gout.

Gout is more common in males than females, although this difference diminishes at older age, and prevalences in males and postmenopausal females are similar. Estimates of the prevalence of gout range between 1% and 3% (Zhu et al., 2011) and increases (Smith et al. 2014) in parallel with the increased prevalence of risk factors for gout: obesity, hypertension, hyperlipidemia, and DM.

Acute gouty arthritis is typically monoarticular and occurs most often in, but is not limited to, the lower extremities. An acute gout attack may also be polyarticular; this is more likely to occur in patients with long-standing disease and is characterized by intense inflammation, and clinical features include redness, severe pain, swelling, and warmth. Maximum inflammation develops within one day and the attack often fades within a couple of days to weeks.

Gout can be diagnosed by the presence of intracellular MSU crystals (visualized by polarized light microscopy) in synovial fluid or material aspirated from tophi. When crystal confirmation is not possible, a clinical diagnosis based on history, physical examination, and laboratory tests can be made. Laboratory evaluation shows inflammatory changes: elevation of the erythrocyte sedimentation rate or C-reactive protein and leukocytosis. Serum uric acid during an acute attack might be low, normal, or high. Imaging modalities can be used to diagnose gout and include radiography or magnetic resonance imaging to assess the presence of subcortical cysts and ultrasound (US) were signs of arthritis can be seen as well as tophaceous deposits in joints or tendons. Dual-energy computed tomography is a new technique able to visualize urate deposits in the joints and periarticular locations (Ogdie et al., 2015).

For the diagnosis and classification of gout, there are several sets of criteria (Janssens et al., 2010; Wallace et al., 1977). Until recently, the 1977 American Rheumatism Association [now the American College of Rheumatology (ACR)] preliminary criteria were used most frequently. Since then new imaging modalities have been developed, and an increasing number of trials on gout have led to the need for more sensitive and specific criteria. Therefore, the ACR and the European League Against Rheumatism (EULAR) recently developed classification criteria for gout with a stepwise diagnostic approach (Table 18.1) (Neogi et al., 2015). These criteria include the occurrence of at least one episode of peripheral joint or bursal swelling, pain, or tenderness, combined with specified clinical characteristics (pattern of joint/bursa involvement,

TABLE 18.1 The ACR/EULAR Gout Classification Criteria

	Categories	
Step 1: Entry criterion (only apply criteria below to those meeting this entry criterion)	At least 1 episode of swelling, pain, or tenderness in a peripheral joint or bursa	
Step 2: Sufficient criterion (if met, can classify as gout without applying criteria below)	Presence of MSU crystals in a symptomatic joint or bursa or tophus	
Step 3: Criteria (to be used if sufficient criterion not met)		
Clinical		**Score**
Pattern of joint/bursa involvement during symptomatic episode(s) ever	Ankle or mid-foot	1
	Involvement of the first metatarsophalangeal joint	2
Characteristics of symptomatic episode(s) ever • Erythema overlying affected joint • Can't bear touch or pressure to affected joint • Great difficulty with walking or inability to use affected joint	One characteristic	1
	Two characteristics	2
	Three characteristics	3
Time course of episode(s) ever presence (ever) of ≥2, irrespective of antiinflammatory treatment: • Time to maximal pain <24 h • Resolution of symptoms in ≤14 days • Complete resolution (to baseline level) between symptomatic episodes	One typical episode	1
	Recurrent typical episodes	2
Clinical evidence of tophus Draining or chalk-like subcutaneous nodule under transparent skin, often with overlying vascularity, located in typical locations: joints, ears, olecranon bursae, finger pads, tendons	Present	4
Laboratory		
Serum urate:	<4 mg/dL (<0.24 mmol/L)	−4
	6–<8 mg/dL (0.36–<0.48 mmol/L)	2
	8–<10 mg/dL (0.48–<0.60 mmol/L)	3
	≥10 mg/dL (≥0.60 mmol/L)	4
Synovial fluid analysis of a symptomatic (ever) joint or bursa	MSU negative	−2

TABLE 18.1 The ACR/EULAR Gout Classification Criteria—cont'd

Clinical		Score
Imaging		
Imaging evidence of urate deposition in symptomatic (ever) joint or bursa: ultrasound evidence of double-contour sign or DECT demonstrating urate deposition	Present (either modality)	4
Imaging evidence of gout-related joint damage: conventional radiography of the hands and/or feet demonstrates at least 1 erosion	Present	4

Adapted from the ACR/EULAR gout classification criteria (Neogi et al., 2015).

characteristics, and time course of symptomatic episodes), laboratory results (serum urate, MSU negative synovial fluid aspirate), and imaging (double contour sign on US or urate on dual-energy computed tomography, radiographic gout-related erosion).

3. CARDIOVASCULAR DISEASE

The association between uric acid, gout, and an increased cardiovascular risk has been long recognized: however, if uric acid and/or gout are causal to this increased risk for cardiovascular disease has been under debate. Evidence supporting that gout and serum uric acid level are independent risk factors has emerged in the last decades. This section will discuss the association between gout and cardiovascular disease. In addition to atherosclerotic heart disease, data on the association between hyperuricemia and other cardiac diseases have been reported. These include atrial fibrillation (AF), diastolic dysfunction, and ventricular hypertrophy.

3.1 Gout and Atherosclerotic Cardiovascular Disease

Cardiovascular disease comprises a range of clinical manifestations including angina pectoris, myocardial infarction, cerebral vascular disease (ischemic stroke), heart failure, and peripheral arterial disease. Hyperuricemia was found to be a predictor of poor prognosis in several (cardiovascular) diseases, for example, in stroke and myocardial infarction.

The Framingham Heart Study was one of the first large studies reporting the association between serum urate with cardiovascular morbidity and mortality (Abbott et al., 1988). After correction for known cardiovascular risk factors, no association was found between serum uric acid and cardiovascular disease, suggesting that the association is confounded by other cardiovascular risk factors. Since then, other studies investigating this association reported conflicting results, although a recent meta-analysis suggests that an elevated serum uric acid level is indeed an independent cardiovascular risk factor (Kim et al., 2009, 2010; Li et al., 2014, 2016). Kim et al. performed two systematic reviews, analyzing the association between hyperuricemia and coronary heart disease and stroke, respectively. In the first systematic review, 17 prospective cohort studies reporting the incidence of both fatal and nonfatal cardiovascular disease and cardiac mortality as outcomes were included. In all included studies, associations were corrected for traditional cardiovascular risk factors, and this meta-analysis showed an increased risk for cardiovascular disease (RR = 1.09; 95% BI = [1.03; 1.16]) and mortality (RR = 1.16 [1.01; 1.30]). In subgroup analyses, the association between hyperuricemia and cardiovascular disease and mortality was only significant in women (RR = 1.07 [0.82; 1.32] and 1.67 [1.30; 2.04], respectively). The second systematic review investigating the association between hyperuricemia and stroke was a meta-analysis comprising 10 prospective cohort studies, corrected for traditional cardiovascular risk factors. Hyperuricemia was significantly associated with stroke (RR = 1.47 [1.19; 1.76]) and stroke mortality (RR = 1.26 [1.12; 1.39]). Interestingly, a study by Kuo et al. (2013) demonstrated that individuals with serum uric acid levels at both lowest and highest strata were associated with a higher risk for all-cause and cardiovascular mortality.

For gout, data on the association with cardiovascular disease are more sparse, although this topic has received increasing attention over the last decade. A meta-analysis based on four studies showed that gout increases cardiovascular risk by 38% (CI 1.23; 1.56) (Nederlandse Vereniging voor Reumatologie, 2013). These results were confirmed by a more recent meta-analysis, reporting that patients with gout have an increased risk for nonfatal myocardial infarction (RR 1.29, 95% CI 1.19−1.39) (Liu et al., 2015). In a large cohort of primary care patients with gout multivariable analysis showed an increased risk of cardiovascular events, which differed between men and women (HR 1.06, 95% CI 1.01−1.12 and HR 1.25, 95% CI 1.15−1.35, respectively) (Clarson et al., 2015).

In conclusion, evidence suggesting that hyperuricemia and gout are independent cardiovascular risk factors is mounting, and physicians treating patients with gout should be aware of the increased cardiovascular risk.

3.2 Gout and Nonatherosclerotic Cardiovascular Disease

3.2.1 Atrial Fibrillation

An UK population-based study assessed the prevalence of AF in gout patients and matched controls and found a twofold higher prevalence in gout patients. After correction for known risk factors for AF, gout was still independently associated with AF (Kuo et al., 2015). An US cohort study compared the risk of AF in gout patients to the risk in osteoarthritis patients, and also reported a higher risk of AF in gout after adjusting for other risk factors (Kim et al.,

2015). Of all cardiac arrhythmias, AF is the most prevalent. Risk factors for AF include (among others) hypertension, obesity, and heavy alcohol intake and it is no coincidence that these risk factors are also risk factors for gout. Hypertension can affect cardiac structure, that is, enlargement of the left atrium, slowing atrial conduction, which favor the development of AF. In light of these findings, it is interesting to consider the potential benefit of colchicine and allopurinol on reducing the risk of AF, either as a direct effect or by decreasing blood pressure (Imazio et al., 2011). In the COPPS (Colchicine for the Prevention of the Postpericardiotomy Syndrome) trial, the administration of colchicine after cardiac surgery was associated with a 45% reduction in the incidence of postoperative AF 45% (Imazio et al., 2011).

3.2.2 Diastolic Dysfunction and Ventricular Hypertrophy

Raised serum uric acid levels are associated with left ventricular hypertrophy (Fujita et al., 2013; Mitsuhashi et al., 2009), and this also seems true for gout (Lin et al., 2015). In addition, elevated uric acid has been associated with diastolic dysfunction (Cicoira et al., 2002). Remodeling of the left ventricle plays a major part in the development of heart failure. Reactive oxygen species in the myocardium are key mediators in this process by activating signaling pathways that lead to ventricular hypertrophy and ultimately dysfunction of the left ventricle. Some studies have reported an increased expression of xanthine oxidation in heart failure. Reactive oxidant species from xanthine oxidase directly induce hypertrophy and dysfunction in vitro. This process has also been demonstrated in rats: rats with hyperuricemia had increased oxidant and superoxide production post myocardial infarction, which was associated with increased left ventricular dysfunction and myocardial hypertrophy (Chen et al., 2011). Treatment with allopurinol attenuated this process (Chen et al., 2011). Similar results were found in a study in mice. These results represent allopurinol as a possible strategy to prevent LV remodeling and dysfunction after myocardial infarction (Engberding et al., 2004).

4. GOUT AND TRADITIONAL CARDIOVASCULAR RISK FACTORS

Although both hyperuricemia and gout are independent risk factors for cardiovascular disease, there is undoubtedly an association with the traditional cardiovascular risk factors. This section will discuss these risk factors and how these relate to gout.

4.1 Hypertension

The relationship between hyperuricemia and the incidence of hypertension has been noticed in many observational studies. A recent meta-analysis assessed the association between uric acid levels and the risk of developing hypertension and reported a dose-responsive relationship: a 1 mg/dL increase in uric acid level was associated with a 15% adjusted risk increase for incident hypertension (95% CI 1.06–1.26) (van et al., 2014). Unfortunately, this meta-analysis did not include studies in gout patients. However, other published data show an increased prevalence of hypertension in patients with gout: in a Chinese population of gout patients, the risk of developing hypertension was increased by 18% compared to participants without gout (95% CI 1.02–1.37) (Pan et al., 2015). A population-based study from Stockholm reported an increased risk for hypertension in patients with gout (OR 4.02, 95% CI 3.69–4.37 in women and OR 3.21, 95% CI 3.06–3.37 in men) (Wandell et al., 2015). In addition, serum uric acid level seems to predict the development of hypertension (Sundstrom et al., 2005). Mechanisms by which uric acid might induce hypertension have been studied in animal models and include activation of the renin-angiotensin system and reduction of nitric oxide (NO) production (Mazzali et al., 2001).

4.2 Metabolic Syndrome and Diabetes Mellitus

Metabolic syndrome (MetS) is defined by the clustering of overweight, high blood pressure, high blood glucose, and dyslipidemia and is of major importance because of its increasing incidence and close relation to DM type 2 and cardiovascular disease. The prevalence of MetS in gout patients is more than doubled compared to the general population (62.8% vs. 25.4%) (Choi et al., 2007). A possible connection between hyperuricemia and MetS might be insulin resistance, as hyperuricemia can lead to elevated insulin levels. Moreover, hyperinsulinemia can increase reabsorption of uric acid in the kidneys, leading to hyperuricemia. Data on hyperuricemia and DM is abundant, showing an increased prevalence of DM in hyperuricemic subjects and in patients with gout (Krishnan et al., 2013; Rho et al., 2016).

4.3 Chronic Kidney Disease

Hyperuricemia is associated with chronic kidney disease, although a causal role has not been established (Borghi et al., 2015). In chronic kidney disease, urate excretion is diminished leading almost inevitable to hyperuricemia. Persistent hyperuricemia can also result in the deposition of urate in the renal interstitium, leading to progressive tubular injury. Patients with chronic kidney disease have a markedly increased cardiovascular risk compared with the general population.

5. ETIOLOGY AND PATHOGENESIS

5.1 Uric Acid

The role of uric acid in gout has been known since the 1850s, when the first papers on levels of uric acid and gout were published (Garrod, 1854). More recently, it was discovered that uric acid also has a role in hypertension and cardiovascular disease, as hyperuricemia is a common finding in these patients.

As discussed in the previous sections, evidence linking hyperuricemia to cardiovascular disease is ample, and hyperuricemia may be considered an independent cardiovascular risk factor. This implies a causative role between uric acid and cardiovascular disease, but the mechanisms on how uric acid accelerates atherosclerosis still need further unraveling.

Uric acid plays a dual role as both an antioxidant and prooxidant (Krishnan, 2010). As antioxidant, uric acid scavenges peroxynitrite, which is a toxic substance produced by the reaction of NO and superoxide (Squadrito et al., 2000). In addition to its antioxidant scavenging properties, uric acid also has the ability to oxidize and form radicals, acting as a prooxidant particularly in endothelial cells. The role of uric acid in atherosclerosis is supported by the association between serum uric and the presence of vulnerable atherosclerotic plaques and the finding of uric acid in the atherosclerotic plaque (Li et al., 2015; Patetsios et al., 2001). The presence of uric acid may induce microvascular changes, such as proliferation of smooth muscle cells and the production of inflammatory and oxidative factors, and promote prothrombotic phenomena by increasing platelet adhesiveness (Battelli et al., 2014a). Regarding cardiovascular mortality, the association between serum uric acid levels and cardiovascular mortality has a U-shaped curve, and optimal levels of uric acid are in the mid-range (Kuo et al., 2013). This U-shaped relation is possibly also applicable to the balance between the pro- and antioxidant effects of uric acid; in different concentrations, the effects might be either more pro- or antioxidant. Oxidized low-density lipoprotein (LDL), an important factor in the pathogenesis of atherosclerosis, has an interesting role in this balance. Uric acid can act both as an antioxidant and as a prooxidant, depending on the oxidative state of LDL (Patterson et al., 2003).

5.2 Chronic Inflammation

Monocytes and synoviocytes release a range of cytokines in response to MSU crystals in the joint: these include interleukin (IL) 1, IL-6, IL-8, and tumor necrosis factor. Increased levels of these cytokines are found in gouty tissue (Busso and So, 2010). The acute phase of a gout flare usually lasts for a couple of days, but MSU crystals remain in the joints during the intercritical phase, causing an ongoing low-grade inflammation (Pascual and Sivera, 2007). A 2015 study by Kienhorst et al. (2015) demonstrated that proinflammatory cytokines were present in patients with intercritical gout, and this was associated with the co-occurrence of DM.

The molecular mechanisms underlying the activation of the immune system by MSU crystals have been further unraveled with the discovery of inflammasomes: a component of the innate immune system that consists of multimeric protein complexes. Several inflammasomes exist dependent of the stimulus to the immune system; canonical inflammasomes collectively activate the caspase-1 cascade, which ultimately leads to the production and release of IL-1 beta and IL-18. IL-1 beta is a critical cytokine in gout, which is also demonstrated by the efficacy of IL-1 antagonists in treatment of acute gout flares. The link between inflammation and cardiovascular disease has long been established, and inflammasomes have been linked to a range of diseases, including gout, DM, obesity, and atherosclerosis (Coll et al., 2015). The role of IL-18 in atherosclerosis has been demonstrated by the presence of IL-18 in the atherosclerotic plaque. Elevated lipid levels can be a stimulus for inflammasome activation, and there is evidence that intracellular cholesterol crystals can activate certain types of inflammasomes. Another possibility is the direct activation of inflammasomes by urate depositions in the vascular walls. In conclusion, the activation of the inflammasome by cytokines in response to MSU crystals provides us with a strong connection between gout and hyperuricemia and increased cardiovascular risk.

5.3 Xanthine Oxidase

Another important mechanism causing atherosclerosis is oxidative stress, an imbalance between the production of reactive oxygen species and antioxidants. Xanthine oxidoreductase (XOR) is the enzyme that is responsible for uric acid metabolism, and generates oxidative stress that may induce endothelial dysfunction, leading to atherosclerosis and ultimately clinically overt cardiovascular disease (Battelli et al., 2014a; Battelli et al., 2014b). Treatment with xanthine oxidase inhibitors might thus reduce cardiovascular risk not only by lowering serum uric acid levels, but also by reducing oxidative stress and improving endothelial function (Landmesser et al., 2007).

6. DIAGNOSTIC INTERVENTIONS

6.1 Estimation of Cardiovascular Risk in Gout Patients

The increased cardiovascular risk in gout patients implies that nearly all of these patients are eligible for cardiovascular risk management. This includes screening for cardiovascular risk factors in gout patients with no history of cardiovascular disease. Although gout is not mentioned as an independent risk factor for cardiovascular disease in current guidelines, it is plausible that multiple cardiovascular risk factors are present in gout patients; thus patients qualify for cardiovascular risk management including screening for hypertension and dyslipidemia, according to local standards.

6.2 Diagnosis of Cardiovascular Disease

The presence and degree of severity of cardiovascular disease can be assessed using many different diagnostic investigations. In research and also in clinical practice, surrogate markers of cardiovascular risk or cardiovascular disease are frequently used. An example is the detection of subclinical atherosclerosis; gout patients more often have subclinical atherosclerosis compared to patients with asymptomatic hyperuricemia, reflected by an increased carotid intima-media thickness and an increased presence of plaques (Li et al., 2015). Another interesting marker is arterial stiffness, measured by carotid-femoral pulse wave velocity (PWV) (Laurent et al., 2006). This surrogate endpoint relates with cardiovascular endpoints: an increased PWV is an independent predictor of cardiovascular disease in several populations (Willum-Hansen et al., 2006) and is currently investigated in patients with gout (CT Identifier NCT02500641). Uric acid has been associated with arterial stiffness in several studies (Hsu et al., 2013).

7. TREATMENT

7.1 Acute Gouty Arthritis

Acute gouty arthritis does resolve spontaneously within a few days to weeks, but treatment with antiinflammatory drugs leads to more rapid resolution of symptoms. First-line therapy consist of colchicine or nonsteroidal antiinflammatory drugs, and for patients who do not tolerate these, glucocorticosteroids can be used, either as oral prednisone or an intraarticular injection. In patients with refractory gout attacks an IL-1 inhibitor, such as anakinra or canakinumab is a treatment option.

7.2 Chronic (Tophaceous) Gout

In patients with severe established gout, including tophaceous gout, radiographic changes of gout, or associated uric acid nephrolithiasis, urate-lowering therapy is indicated, consisting of nonpharmacological urate-lowering lifestyle advices such as dietary advices on one hand and pharmacological therapy on the other (Zhang et al., 2006). Allopurinol is considered the first-line treatment, although other urate-lowering treatments can be started in patients hypersensitive to allopurinol. The goal of urate-lowering therapy is to prevent urate crystal formation, for which an SUA in the range of 300–360 μmol/L needs to be achieved (Zhang et al., 2006).

7.3 Cardiovascular Effects of Urate-Lowering Therapy

Treatment of gout aims at lowering the uric acid level in the blood and preventing further gout attacks. Since the level of uric acid is associated with the risk of cardiovascular disease, it would be a logical consequence that proper treatment of gout would also reduce the risk of cardiovascular disease. Up to now, no randomized clinical trials investigating the effect of urate-lowering therapy on cardiovascular endpoints have been published; however, observational cohort studies indicate a favorable effect of allopurinol on cardiovascular disease risk. A Scottish cohort study using a record-linkage database assessed the association between urate levels, dispensed allopurinol, and cardiovascular hospitalization and mortality, and found no difference in cardiovascular disease risk between users of allopurinol and nonusers. However, they did find differences within the allopurinol use cohort: compared with low-dose (100 mg) users, high-dose ($\geq$300 mg) users had a lower risk of both cardiovascular events and mortality: with an adjusted HR of 0.69 (95% CI 0.50–0.94) and 0.75 (95% CI 0.59–0.94), respectively (Wei et al., 2011). Another cohort study including a population of hyperuricemic veterans showed an association between allopurinol treatment and lower mortality risk, but did not report cause specific mortality data (Luk et al., 2009). A recent population-based retrospective matched-cohort study from Taiwan studied the association with allopurinol use and cardiovascular outcomes in gout patients and reported a negative effect of allopurinol on cardiovascular outcomes, but they did not correct for conventional cardiovascular risk factors (Kok et al., 2014). In contrast, a large Danish cohort study reported an HR of 0.89 (95% CI 0.81–0.97) for cardiovascular mortality among allopurinol treated compared with nonusers of allopurinol (Larsen et al., 2015). A possible mechanism is the inhibition of the oxidation of LDL cholesterol by allopurinol. Oxidized LDL cholesterol is an important mediator of atherosclerosis, and small studies have demonstrated a beneficial effect of allopurinol on endothelial function (Dawson et al., 2007).

Treatment with urate-lowering therapy might also improve cardiovascular outcomes through beneficial effects on cardiovascular risk factors. Clinical trials with allopurinol and febuxostat have shown favorable effects on blood pressure (Agarwal et al., 2013; Kim et al., 2014).

7.4 Treatment of Traditional Cardiovascular Risk Factors

As gout is associated with an increased cardiovascular risk, identifying and treating traditional risk factors is crucial. To date, no studies have been carried out to assess the effect of treatment of traditional cardiovascular risk factors in patients with gout or hyperuricemia specifically. Regardless, it is well established that treatment of hypertension, hypercholesterolemia, and DM leads to a reduction in cardiovascular risk. As gout is considered to be both an independent cardiovascular risk factor and a condition associated with the presence of multiple cardiovascular risk factors, qualify for cardiovascular risk management including screening for and treatment of, for example, hypertension and dyslipidemia, in line with local standards.

8. FUTURE PERSPECTIVES

The expanding knowledge regarding the pathophysiological link between gout and cardiovascular disease provides us with the opportunity to develop preventive and treatment strategies. Observational data suggest a beneficial effect of urate-lowering therapy on cardiovascular risk; however, it is not possible to conclude whether the protective effect of allopurinol is the result of uric acid lowering per se, or other biological activities of allopurinol, or if the favorable effect is mediated by effects on cardiovascular risk factors such as blood pressure. In order to address this question, a therapeutic trial should be conducted using clinical cardiovascular outcomes. This will be challenging as large patients numbers are needed as well as several years of follow-up.

9. CONCLUSION

Gout is the most common inflammatory rheumatic disease, with a rising incidence. Traditional cardiovascular risk factors such as hypertension, DM, and chronic kidney disease are more prevalent in patients with gout compared to the general population. In addition, evidence on the association between uric acid, gout, and an increased cardiovascular risk has emerged in the last decades revealing that hyperuricemia and gout seem to be independent cardiovascular risk factors. Although a causative role between uric acid and cardiovascular disease has been implied, the mechanisms behind this are still not completely clear. Uric acid has both antioxidant and prooxidant functions and in different concentrations its vascular effects might be either more pro- or antioxidant. XOR is the enzyme that is responsible for uric acid metabolism and generates oxidative stress that may induce endothelial dysfunction, leading to atherosclerosis and ultimately clinically overt cardiovascular disease. Another link between hyperuricemia and gout and cardiovascular disease is provided by the inflammatory status. This link has long been established in several other inflammatory diseases. In gout there is also an ongoing low-grade inflammation between attacks. The activation of the inflammasome by cytokines in response to MSU crystals provides a strong connection between inflammation and the increased cardiovascular risk in gout and hyperuricemia.

Treatment with urate-lowering therapy might improve cardiovascular outcomes by both lowering the uric acid level, inhibition of xanthine oxidase activity, and additional beneficial effects on cardiovascular risk factors such as a reduction in blood pressure. Identifying and treating traditional risk factors in gout patients is of great importance.

REFERENCES

Abbott, R.D., Brand, F.N., Kannel, W.B., Castelli, W.P., 1988. Gout and coronary heart disease: the Framingham Study. J. Clin. Epidemiol. 41 (3), 237–242. Available from: PM: 3339376.

Agarwal, V., Hans, N., Messerli, F.H., 2013. Effect of allopurinol on blood pressure: a systematic review and meta-analysis. J. Clin. Hypertens. (Greenwich) 15 (6), 435–442. Available from: PM: 23730993.

Battelli, M.G., Bolognesi, A., Polito, L., 2014a. Pathophysiology of circulating xanthine oxidoreductase: new emerging roles for a multi-tasking enzyme. Biochim. Biophys. Acta 1842 (9), 1502–1517. Available from: PM: 24882753.

Battelli, M.G., Polito, L., Bolognesi, A., 2014b. Xanthine oxidoreductase in atherosclerosis pathogenesis: not only oxidative stress. Atherosclerosis 237 (2), 562–567. Available from: PM: 25463089.

Borghi, C., Rosei, E.A., Bardin, T., Dawson, J., Dominiczak, A., Kielstein, J.T., Manolis, A.J., Perez-Ruiz, F., Mancia, G., 2015. Serum uric acid and the risk of cardiovascular and renal disease. J. Hypertens. 33 (9), 1729–1741. Available from: PM: 26136207.

Busso, N., So, A., 2010. Mechanisms of inflammation in gout. Arthritis Res. Ther. 12 (2), 206. Available from: PM: 20441605.

Chen, C.C., Hsu, Y.J., Lee, T.M., 2011. Impact of elevated uric acid on ventricular remodeling in infarcted rats with experimental hyperuricemia. Am. J. Physiol. Heart Circ. Physiol. 301 (3), H1107–H1117. Available from: PM: 21622823.

Choi, H.K., Ford, E.S., Li, C., Curhan, G., 2007. Prevalence of the metabolic syndrome in patients with gout: the Third National Health and Nutrition Examination Survey. Arthritis Rheum. 57 (1), 109–115. Available from: PM: 17266099.

Cicoira, M., Zanolla, L., Rossi, A., Golia, G., Franceschini, L., Brighetti, G., Zeni, P., Zardini, P., 2002. Elevated serum uric acid levels are associated with diastolic dysfunction in patients with dilated cardiomyopathy. Am. Heart J. 143 (6), 1107–1111. Available from: PM: 12075270.

Clarson, L.E., Hider, S.L., Belcher, J., Heneghan, C., Roddy, E., Mallen, C.D., 2015. Increased risk of vascular disease associated with gout: a retrospective, matched cohort study in the UK clinical practice research datalink. Ann. Rheum. Dis. 74 (4), 642–647. Available from: PM: 25165032.

Coll, R.C., Robertson, A.A., Chae, J.J., Higgins, S.C., Munoz-Planillo, R., Inserra, M.C., Vetter, I., Dungan, L.S., Monks, B.G., Stutz, A., Croker, D.E., Butler, M.S., Haneklaus, M., Sutton, C.E., Nunez, G., Latz, E., Kastner, D.L., Mills, K.H., Masters, S.L., Schroder, K., Cooper, M.A., O'Neill, L.A., 2015. A small-molecule inhibitor of the NLRP3 inflammasome for the treatment of inflammatory diseases. Nat. Med. 21 (3), 248–255. Available from: PM: 25686105.

Dawson, J., Quinn, T., Walters, M., 2007. Uric acid reduction: a new paradigm in the management of cardiovascular risk? Curr. Med. Chem. 14 (17), 1879–1886. Available from: PM: 17627523.

Engberding, N., Spiekermann, S., Schaefer, A., Heineke, A., Wiencke, A., Muller, M., Fuchs, M., Hilfiker-Kleiner, D., Hornig, B., Drexler, H., Landmesser, U., 2004. Allopurinol attenuates left ventricular remodeling and dysfunction after experimental myocardial infarction: a new action for an old drug? Circulation 110 (15), 2175–2179. Available from: PM: 15466649.

Fujita, S., Okamoto, Y., Shibata, K., Morita, H., Ito, T., Sohmiya, K., Hoshiga, M., Ishizaka, N., 2013. Serum uric acid is associated with left ventricular hypertrophy independent of serum parathyroid hormone in male cardiac patients. PLoS One 8 (12), e82735. Available from: PM: 24340056.

Garrod, A.B., 1854. On the blood and effused fluids in gout, rheumatism, and Bright's disease. Med. Chir. Trans. 37, 49–60. Available from: PM: 20896032.

Hsu, P.F., Chuang, S.Y., Cheng, H.M., Sung, S.H., Ting, C.T., Lakatta, E.G., Yin, F.C., Chou, P., Chen, C.H., 2013. Associations of serum uric acid levels with arterial wave reflections and central systolic blood pressure. Int. J. Cardiol. 168 (3), 2057–2063. Available from: PM: 23453449.

Imazio, M., Brucato, A., Ferrazzi, P., Rovere, M.E., Gandino, A., Cemin, R., Ferrua, S., Belli, R., Maestroni, S., Simon, C., Zingarelli, E., Barosi, A., Sansone, F., Patrini, D., Vitali, E.,

Trinchero, R., Spodick, D.H., Adler, Y., 2011. Colchicine reduces postoperative atrial fibrillation: results of the Colchicine for the Prevention of the Postpericardiotomy Syndrome (COPPS) atrial fibrillation substudy. Circulation 124 (21), 2290–2295. Available from: PM: 22090167.

Janssens, H.J., Fransen, J., van de Lisdonk, E.H., van Riel, P.L., van, W.C., Janssen, M., 2010. A diagnostic rule for acute gouty arthritis in primary care without joint fluid analysis. Arch. Intern. Med. 170 (13), 1120–1126. Available from: PM: 20625017.

Khanna, D., Fitzgerald, J.D., Khanna, P.P., Bae, S., Singh, M.K., Neogi, T., Pillinger, M.H., Merill, J., Lee, S., Prakash, S., Kaldas, M., Gogia, M., Perez-Ruiz, F., Taylor, W., Liote, F., Choi, H., Singh, J.A., Dalbeth, N., Kaplan, S., Niyyar, V., Jones, D., Yarows, S.A., Roessler, B., Kerr, G., King, C., Levy, G., Furst, D.E., Edwards, N.L., Mandell, B., Schumacher, H.R., Robbins, M., Wenger, N., Terkeltaub, R., 2012. 2012 American College of Rheumatology guidelines for management of gout. Part 1: systematic nonpharmacologic and pharmacologic therapeutic approaches to hyperuricemia. Arthritis Care Res. (Hoboken) 64 (10), 1431–1446. Available from: PM: 23024028.

Kienhorst, L.B., van, L.E., Kievit, W., Dalbeth, N., Merriman, M.E., Phipps-Green, A., Loof, A., van, H.W., Vermeulen, S., Stamp, L.K., van, K.E., de, G.J., Holzinger, D., Roth, J., Janssens, H.J., Merriman, T.R., Broen, J.C., Janssen, M., Radstake, T.R., 2015. Gout is a chronic inflammatory disease in which high levels of Interleukin-8 (CXCL8), myeloid-related protein 8/Myeloid-Related protein 14 complex, and an altered proteome are associated with diabetes mellitus and cardiovascular disease. Arthritis Rheumatol. 67 (12), 3303–3313. Available from: PM: 26248007.

Kim, H.A., Seo, Y.I., Song, Y.W., 2014. Four-week effects of allopurinol and febuxostat treatments on blood pressure and serum creatinine level in gouty men. J. Korean Med. Sci. 29 (8), 1077–1081. Available from: PM: 25120316.

Kim, S.C., Liu, J., Solomon, D.H., 2015. Risk of incident atrial fibrillation in gout: a cohort study. Ann. Rheum. Dis. Available from: PM: 26324846.

Kim, S.Y., Guevara, J.P., Kim, K.M., Choi, H.K., Heitjan, D.F., Albert, D.A., 2009. Hyperuricemia and risk of stroke: a systematic review and meta-analysis. Arthritis Rheum. 61 (7), 885–892. Available from: PM: 19565556.

Kim, S.Y., Guevara, J.P., Kim, K.M., Choi, H.K., Heitjan, D.F., Albert, D.A., 2010. Hyperuricemia and coronary heart disease: a systematic review and meta-analysis. Arthritis Care Res. (Hoboken) 62 (2), 170–180. Available from: PM: 20191515.

Kok, V.C., Horng, J.T., Chang, W.S., Hong, Y.F., Chang, T.H., 2014. Allopurinol therapy in gout patients does not associate with beneficial cardiovascular outcomes: a population-based matched-cohort study. PLoS One 9 (6), e99102. Available from: PM: 24897240.

Krishnan, E., 2010. Inflammation, oxidative stress and lipids: the risk triad for atherosclerosis in gout. Rheumatology (Oxford) 49 (7), 1229–1238. Available from: PM: 20202928.

Krishnan, E., Akhras, K.S., Sharma, H., Marynchenko, M., Wu, E.Q., Tawk, R., Liu, J., Shi, L., 2013. Relative and attributable diabetes risk associated with hyperuricemia in US veterans with gout. QJM 106 (8), 721–729. Available from: PM: 23620537.

Kuo, C.F., Grainge, M.J., Mallen, C., Zhang, W., Doherty, M., 2015. Impact of gout on the risk of atrial fibrillation. Rheumatology (Oxford). Available from: PM: 26683193.

Kuo, C.F., Grainge, M.J., Mallen, C., Zhang, W., Doherty, M., 2016. Comorbidities in patients with gout prior to and following diagnosis: case-control study. Ann. Rheum. Dis. 75 (1), 210–217. Available from: PM: 25398375.

Kuo, C.F., See, L.C., Yu, K.H., Chou, I.J., Chiou, M.J., Luo, S.F., 2013. Significance of serum uric acid levels on the risk of all-cause and cardiovascular mortality. Rheumatology (Oxford) 52 (1), 127–134. Available from: PM: 22923756.

Landmesser, U., Spiekermann, S., Preuss, C., Sorrentino, S., Fischer, D., Manes, C., Mueller, M., Drexler, H., 2007. Angiotensin II induces endothelial xanthine oxidase activation: role for endothelial dysfunction in patients with coronary disease. Arterioscler. Thromb. Vasc. Biol. 27 (4), 943–948. Available from: PM: 17234726.

Larsen, K.S., Pottegard, A., Lindegaard, H.M., Hallas, J., 2015. Effect of allopurinol on cardiovascular outcomes in hyperuricemic patients: a cohort study. Am. J. Med Available from: PM: 26589484.

Laurent, S., Cockcroft, J., Van, B.L., Boutouyrie, P., Giannattasio, C., Hayoz, D., Pannier, B., Vlachopoulos, C., Wilkinson, I., Struijker-Boudier, H., 2006. Expert consensus document on arterial stiffness: methodological issues and clinical applications. Eur. Heart J. 27 (21), 2588–2605. Available from: PM: 17000623.

Li, M., Hou, W., Zhang, X., Hu, L., Tang, Z., 2014. Hyperuricemia and risk of stroke: a systematic review and meta-analysis of prospective studies. Atherosclerosis 232 (2), 265–270. Available from: PM: 24468137.

Li, M., Hu, X., Fan, Y., Li, K., Zhang, X., Hou, W., Tang, Z., 2016. Hyperuricemia and the risk for coronary heart disease morbidity and mortality a systematic review and dose-response meta-analysis. Sci. Rep. 6, 19520. Available from: PM: 26814153.

Li, Q., Zhou, Y., Dong, K., Wang, A., Yang, X., Zhang, C., Zhu, Y., Wu, S., Zhao, X., 2015. The association between serum uric acid levels and the prevalence of vulnerable atherosclerotic carotid plaque: a cross-sectional study. Sci. Rep. 5, 10003. Available from: PM: 25961501.

Lin, J.C., Lin, C.L., Chen, M.C., Chang, P.J., Chang, S.T., Chung, C.M., Pan, K.L., 2015. Gout, not hyperuricemia alone, impairs left ventricular diastolic function. Arthritis Res. Ther. 17 (1), 323. Available from: PM: 26568484.

Liu, S.C., Xia, L., Zhang, J., Lu, X.H., Hu, D.K., Zhang, H.T., Li, H.J., 2015. Gout and risk of myocardial infarction: a systematic review and meta-analysis of cohort studies. PLoS One 10 (7), e0134088. Available from: PM: 26230580.

Luk, A.J., Levin, G.P., Moore, E.E., Zhou, X.H., Kestenbaum, B.R., Choi, H.K., 2009. Allopurinol and mortality in hyperuricaemic patients. Rheumatology (Oxford) 48 (7), 804–806. Available from: PM: 19447769.

Mazzali, M., Hughes, J., Kim, Y.G., Jefferson, J.A., Kang, D.H., Gordon, K.L., Lan, H.Y., Kivlighn, S., Johnson, R.J., 2001. Elevated uric acid increases blood pressure in the rat by a novel crystal-independent mechanism. Hypertension 38 (5), 1101–1106 Available from: PM: 11711505.

Mitsuhashi, H., Yatsuya, H., Matsushita, K., Zhang, H., Otsuka, R., Muramatsu, T., Takefuji, S., Hotta, Y., Kondo, T., Murohara, T., Toyoshima, H., Tamakoshi, K., 2009. Uric acid and left ventricular hypertrophy in Japanese men. Circ. J. 73 (4), 667–672. Available from: PM: 19225200.

Nederlandse Vereniging voor Reumatologie, 2013. Richtlijn Jicht. Ref Type: Generic.

Neogi, T., Jansen, T.L., Dalbeth, N., Fransen, J., Schumacher, H.R., Berendsen, D., Brown, M., Choi, H., Edwards, N.L., Janssens, H.J., Liote, F., Naden, R.P., Nuki, G., Ogdie, A., Perez-Ruiz, F., Saag, K., Singh, J.A., Sundy, J.S., Tausche, A.K., Vaquez-Mellado, J., Yarows, S.A., Taylor, W.J., 2015. 2015 Gout classification criteria: an American College of Rheumatology/European League Against Rheumatism collaborative initiative. Ann. Rheum. Dis. 74 (10), 1789–1798. Available from: PM: 26359487.

Ogdie, A., Taylor, W.J., Weatherall, M., Fransen, J., Jansen, T.L., Neogi, T., Schumacher, H.R., Dalbeth, N., 2015. Imaging modalities for the classification of gout: systematic literature review and meta-analysis. Ann. Rheum. Dis. 74 (10), 1868–1874. Available from: PM: 24915980.

Pan, A., Teng, G.G., Yuan, J.M., Koh, W.P., 2015. Bidirectional association between self-reported hypertension and gout: the Singapore Chinese Health Study. PLoS One 10 (10), e0141749. Available from: PM: 26510154.

Pascual, E., Sivera, F., 2007. Time required for disappearance of urate crystals from synovial fluid after successful hypouricaemic treatment relates to the duration of gout. Ann. Rheum. Dis. 66 (8), 1056–1058. Available from: PM: 17223663.

Patetsios, P., Song, M., Shutze, W.P., Pappas, C., Rodino, W., Ramirez, J.A., Panetta, T.F., 2001. Identification of uric acid and xanthine oxidase in atherosclerotic plaque. Am. J. Cardiol. 88 (2), 188–191, A6 Available from: PM: 11448423.

Patterson, R.A., Horsley, E.T., Leake, D.S., 2003. Prooxidant and antioxidant properties of human serum ultrafiltrates toward LDL: important role of uric acid. J. Lipid Res. 44 (3), 512–521. Available from: PM: 12562831.

Rho, Y.H., Lu, N., Peloquin, C.E., Man, A., Zhu, Y., Zhang, Y., Choi, H.K., 2016. Independent impact of gout on the risk of diabetes mellitus among women and men: a population-based, BMI-matched cohort study. Ann. Rheum. Dis. 75 (1), 91–95. Available from: PM: 25277955.

Rock, K.L., Kataoka, H., Lai, J.J., 2013. Uric acid as a danger signal in gout and its comorbidities. Nat. Rev. Rheumatol. 9 (1), 13–23. Available from: PM: 22945591.

Smith, E., Hoy, D., Cross, M., Merriman, T.R., Vos, T., Buchbinder, R., Woolf, A., March, L., 2014. The global burden of gout: estimates from the Global Burden of Disease 2010 study. Ann. Rheum. Dis. 73 (8), 1470–1476. Available from: PM: 24590182.

Squadrito, G.L., Cueto, R., Splenser, A.E., Valavanidis, A., Zhang, H., Uppu, R.M., Pryor, W.A., 2000. Reaction of uric acid with peroxynitrite and implications for the mechanism of neuroprotection by uric acid. Arch. Biochem. Biophys. 376 (2), 333–337. Available from: PM: 10775420.

Sundstrom, J., Sullivan, L., D'Agostino, R.B., Levy, D., Kannel, W.B., Vasan, R.S., 2005. Relations of serum uric acid to longitudinal blood pressure tracking and hypertension incidence. Hypertension 45 (1), 28–33. Available from: PM: 15569852.

van, D.C., van Echteld, I.A., Falzon, L., Aletaha, D., van der Heijde, D.M., Landewe, R.B., 2014. Cardiovascular risk factors and comorbidities in patients with hyperuricemia and/or gout: a systematic review of the literature. J. Rheumatol. Suppl. 92, 9–14. Available from: PM: 25180123.

Wallace, S.L., Robinson, H., Masi, A.T., Decker, J.L., McCarty, D.J., Yu, T.F., 1977. Preliminary criteria for the classification of the acute arthritis of primary gout. Arthritis Rheum. 20 (3), 895–900. Available from: PM: 856219.

Wandell, P., Carlsson, A.C., Ljunggren, G., 2015. Gout and its comorbidities in the total population of Stockholm. Prev. Med. 81, 387–391. Available from: PM: 26500085.

Wei, L., Mackenzie, I.S., Chen, Y., Struthers, A.D., MacDonald, T.M., 2011. Impact of allopurinol use on urate concentration and cardiovascular outcome. Br. J. Clin. Pharmacol. 71 (4), 600–607. Available from: PM: 21395653.

Willum-Hansen, T., Staessen, J.A., Torp-Pedersen, C., Rasmussen, S., Thijs, L., Ibsen, H., Jeppesen, J., 2006. Prognostic value of aortic pulse wave velocity as index of arterial stiffness in the general population. Circulation 113 (5), 664–670. Available from: PM: 16461839.

Zhang, W., Doherty, M., Bardin, T., Pascual, E., Barskova, V., Conaghan, P., Gerster, J., Jacobs, J., Leeb, B., Liote, F., McCarthy, G., Netter, P., Nuki, G., Perez-Ruiz, F., Pignone, A., Pimentao, J., Punzi, L., Roddy, E., Uhlig, T., Zimmermann-Gorska, I., 2006. EULAR evidence based recommendations for gout. Part II: management. Report of a task force of the EULAR

Standing Committee for International Clinical Studies Including Therapeutics (ESCISIT). Ann. Rheum. Dis. 65 (10), 1312–1324. Available from: PM: 16707532.

Zhu, Y., Pandya, B.J., Choi, H.K., 2011. Prevalence of gout and hyperuricemia in the US general population: the National Health and Nutrition Examination Survey 2007–2008. Arthritis Rheum. 63 (10), 3136–3141. Available from: PM: 21800283.

Chapter 19

Heart Involvement in Osteoarthritis

A. Courties*[,§] and J. Sellam*[,§]
*Department of Rheumatology, DHU i2B, Saint-Antoine hospital, Assistance Publique—Hôpitaux de Paris (AP-HP), Paris, France; [§]Sorbonnes Universités UPMC, Paris, France

Key Points

- Prevalence of cardiovascular disease (CVD) and mortality is increased in osteoarthritis (OA) patients.
- Age, obesity, and metabolic syndrome are risk factors for OA and CVD.
- OA is now considered a low-grade inflammation disease.
- Inflammaging and metainflammation could be the cornerstone of OA and CVD.
- An independent association between OA and CVD has been reported and could be due to a direct effect of atheroma on joint tissues but needs to be investigated.
- Chronic use of NSAIDs and disability strengthens the association and need to be considered as aggravating factors by rheumatologists and cardiologists.

1. INTRODUCTION

Osteoarthritis (OA) is the main musculoskeletal disease leading to articular pain and stiffness. It is one of the leading causes of disability after 65 years of age. Longtime set aside and associated with inevitable aging, OA is also associated with obesity, female gender, joint injury, and trauma as well as metabolic diseases such as type 2 diabetes. Furthermore, OA may be associated with excess cardiovascular diseases (CVD) (Barbour et al., 2015; Hall et al., 2015; Liu et al., 2015; Nüesch et al., 2011; Ong et al., 2013; Veronese et al., 2016). Greater occurrence of CVD and CV mortality in OA compared to the non-OA population of the same age and sex raises many issues.

First, this association could be due to the common risk factors of OA and CVD: age, obesity but also metabolic syndrome (MetS), a new OA risk factor with a cumulative, and negative effect of each of its components on OA occurrence and progression (Dahaghin et al., 2007; Tomi et al., 2016; Visser et al., 2014; Yoshimura et al., 2012). Beyond this epidemiological association, basic research has suggested that overweight or obesity and their metabolic complications could have a direct systemic harmful effect on joint tissues (Laiguillon et al., 2015; Lippiello et al., 1991; Triantaphyllidou et al., 2013). Second, because an independent association between coronary, carotid, or popliteal atherosclerosis and OA has been reported (Jonsson et al., 2011, 2009), another and more hypothetical hypothesis could be that once installed, atheroma may directly affect OA by low-grade inflammation and/or defective vascularization (Courties et al., 2015). Finally, the last hypothesis could be an indirect artifactual association due to functional disability with OA and long-term prescription of analgesics or nonsteroidal antiinflammatory drugs (NSAIDs), which may themselves promote CVD (Coxib and traditional NSAID Trialists' (CNT) Collaboration et al., 2013; Hoeven et al., 2014).

In this chapter, we review the available literature on the association of OA and CVD and the possible mechanisms (i.e., shared risk factors, direct inflammatory influence, or indirect artifactual association).

2. PREREQUISITES: PATHOPHYSIOLOGY OF OSTEOARTHRITIS

OA is a chronic joint disease leading to cartilage degradation that also involves synovial inflammation and subchondral bone remodeling (Sellam and Berenbaum, 2010; Loeser et al., 2012). Articular cartilage is composed of a single cell type, the chondrocyte, which is responsible for both the production and degradation of the extracellular matrix (ECM). ECM contains mostly type II collagen, proteoglycans, and water, and plays an essential role in absorption of mechanical stresses. Under physiologic conditions, the ECM features an equilibrium between anabolism and catabolism. The cartilage is not innervated, is avascular and, receives nutrients through the subchondral bone and the synovial fluid, which participate in joint homeostasis.

In OA, an initial mechanical or biological stress disrupts this homeostasis in the ECM, which generates the production of proinflammatory mediators such as cytokines (interleukin [IL]-1β, IL-6, IL-17, tumor necrosis factor [TNF]-α); lipid mediators (prostaglandin E_2 (PGE_2); and reactive oxygen species (ROS) by chondrocytes, synoviocytes, and subchondral osteoblasts. Locally, these mediators promote the production of matrix metalloproteases (MMPs) and aggrecanases, responsible for cartilage degradation, which in turn amplify proinflammatory cytokine release, thereby creating a vicious circle leading to joint destruction. Furthermore, innate immunity is implicated in OA-related cytokine production via macrophage recruitment and activation in the synovium (Bondeson et al., 2006; Kraus et al., 2016), toll-like receptor 2 (TLR-2), and TLR-4 (Gómez et al., 2015) expressed by chondrocytes and synoviocytes, but also complement activation (Wang et al., 2011). Moreover, beyond this local joint inflammation, a systemic low-grade inflammation occurs in OA and can be assessed by blood biomarker measurements (Punzi et al., 2005).

3. EPIDEMIOLOGIC DATA: OSTEOARTHRITIS AND CARDIOVASCULAR DISEASES, TWO ENDEMIC DISEASES

OA is the most frequent disease and affects principally the knee, hip, hand, and lumbar spine. According to the World Health Organization, symptomatic OA affects 10% of men and 18% of women worldwide (Woolf and Pfleger, 2003). Radiographic OA is much more common than symptomatic OA. In a population-based study such as the Framingham OA study, over 70% of subjects had radiographic hand OA (Haugen et al., 2011) and about 35–45% older than 70 years had knee OA (Felson et al., 1987). Because of the aging of the population and the increasing prevalence of obesity, OA prevalence is expected to increase and could become the leading cause of disability in 2020.

Along this line, CVD represents the first worldwide cause of mortality, responsible for 17.5 million deaths every year (including ischemic cardiac disease, stroke, arteritis, and heart failure)—31% of the mortality causes (McAloon et al., 2016).

The CVD-induced mortality is significantly increased in the OA population (Nüesch et al., 2011; Liu et al., 2015). The two intuitive explanations are walking disability and NSAID intake. However, other mechanisms may occur because metabolic disturbances and OA both exhibit low-grade inflammation and are closely linked to CVD.

4. ASSOCIATION BETWEEN OSTEOARTHRITIS AND CARDIOVASCULAR DISEASES: SHARED RISK FACTORS

The first assumption of the high frequency of CVD in the OA population is that the two diseases share several risk factors.

4.1 Nonmodifiable Risk Factors

4.1.1 Age and "Inflammaging"

Age is certainly the nonmodifiable risk factor with the greatest effect on CV events and OA occurrence. In the Framingham population-based cohort, the prevalence of radiographic hand OA was $<10\%$ before 40 years and $>70\%$ after 70 years (Haugen et al., 2011). Similarly, the risk of CVD increases linearly with age (Driver et al., 2008). Similar mechanisms related to aging occur during OA and atherosclerosis. OA chondrocytes such as endothelial atherosclerosis cells showed both markers of cellular senescence such as shortened telomerase and increased beta-galactosidase expression but also a senescence-associated secretory phenotype, which is responsible for the release of cytokines and MMPs (Forsyth et al., 2005; Gorenne et al., 2006; Greene and Loeser, 2015). Furthermore, tissue aging is associated with increased posttranslational modifications of protein such as glycation and oxidation leading to the overproduction of ROS and advanced glycation end products (AGEs) both in the endothelium and cartilage. ROS and AGEs promote an inflammatory process and modulate mechanical tissue properties (Brüel and Oxlund, 1996; Verzijl et al., 2000; Rodríguez-Mañas et al., 2009). All these inflammatory processes in aging tissues are responsible for "inflammaging," defined as the inflammatory state established during physiological aging. For example, the blood level of IL-6 increases with age in healthy subjects (Wei et al., 1992; Hager et al., 1994) and is a predictor of hospitalization or mortality in older patients (Adriaensen et al., 2015). This inflammatory state, which is due to cellular senescence and a concomitant reduction in the naive cell pool, is recognized as a pathogenic factor in the development of several age-related diseases including Alzheimer disease and CVD and possibly OA.

4.1.2 Genetic Factors

Genetic factors are associated with OA and CVD. From studies of twins, the contribution of genetics has been estimated at between 39% and 65% in OA, especially hand OA (Spector et al., 1996). As well, a family history of CVD events increases the risk of CVD to 45% for a single patient, independent of all other risk factors (Yusuf et al., 2004). Genetic factors for CVD are partly due to the genetic susceptibility of CV risk factors. Indeed, studies of twins and siblings showed that genetic factors are involved in fat mass repartition, hypertension, or type 2 diabetes (Medici et al., 1999; Rankinen et al., 2015; Karaderi et al., 2015).

Genetic risk of polygenic diseases such as CVD and OA is related to genetic polymorphisms. Several single nucleotide polymorphisms (SNPs) found associated with CVD include those located in apolipoprotein E (Chaudhary et al., 2012) and NO synthase (Carreras-Torres et al., 2014) and proinflammatory cytokines (IL-6 promoter gene or TNF) (Hernández-Díaz et al., 2015; Wang et al., 2015). As well, the same SNP of the IL-6 promoter gene (IL-6 -174G/C, rs1800795) was associated with increased risk of knee OA (Honsawek et al., 2011), but this association was not confirmed in two meta-analysis (Valdes et al., 2010; Ai et al., 2014). Some other SNPs associated with OA include vascular endothelial growth factor, collagen 11A1, and growth differentiation factor 5 (Pan et al., 2014; Rodriguez-Fontenla et al., 2014). However, to date, no robust genetic factor is common to both OA and CVD.

4.1.3 Gender

Gender differences seem to affect OA and CVD prevalence because OA is more prevalent in women than men, especially after menopause (Srikanth et al., 2005). However, the role of hormones still remains unclear in OA because it is closely associated with aging (de Klerk et al., 2009). Similarly, after menopause, the risk of atherosclerosis strongly increases in women (Witteman et al., 1989), possibly because of visceral adiposity (Nedungadi and Clegg, 2009), which is also involved in obesity-related OA pathophysiology.

4.2 Modifiable Risk Factors

4.2.1 Obesity and "Metainflammation"

Obesity and overweight are among the most important modifiable risk factors of OA and CVD. For many years, obesity and overweight were considered associated with only lower-limb OA and solely attributed to excessive mechanical stress. This theory was broadly confirmed with basic research because mechanoreceptors are expressed by chondrocytes and osteoblasts. Furthermore, ex vivo studies demonstrated that mechanical stress is transduced through these specific receptors into a biological proinflammatory and prodegradative signal (Millward-Sadler and Salter, 2004; Gosset et al., 2006; McGlashan et al., 2008; Sanchez et al., 2009).

However, obesity also affects hand OA, which cannot be explained by mechanical stress. This paradigm has been debated because epidemiological studies have found risk of hand OA increased by two-fold in obese or overweight patients (Yusuf et al., 2010). To explain the association, the systemic harmful role of excess fat mass on joint tissues has been raised. Interestingly, this systemic effect of fat tissue (especially visceral adiposity) also has an impact on endothelium in CVD.

The first demonstration that inflammation occurs in obese tissues came from the Hotamisligil et al. studies of humans (Hotamisligil et al., 1995) and mice (Hotamisligil et al., 1993). In both models, adipose tissue was a major source of TNF-α in obese rather than nonobese people, for a concept of metainflammation. Moreover, local TNF-α level was associated with metabolic features such as blood glucose and insulin resistance. It is now appreciated that not only the levels of TNF-α but also a range of cytokines such as IL-6 or IL-1β are increased in adipose tissue from obese patients (Park et al., 2005). The increased levels are responsible for obesity-related complications such as type 2 diabetes but also CVD. This association with atherosclerosis could be largely explained by the implication of these cytokines in plaque development and disruption. Indeed, in atherogenic mice with deficient apolipoprotein E (apoE$^{-/-}$), the inhibition of TNF-α and IL-1β significantly reduced the size of the plaque via a decrease in adhesion molecular molecule levels (e.g., vascular cell adhesion molecule 1, monocyte chemoattractant protein-1) (Elhage et al., 1998; Merhi-Soussi et al., 2005; Ohta et al., 2005). The IL-6 level in this model seems to enhance the fatty lesions (Huber et al., 1999), but its role seems more ambivalent because older IL-6–deficient apoE$^{-/-}$mice showed increased plaque formation (Schieffer et al., 2004).

Features of the inflammatory state of obesity beyond cytokines are increased local production of adipokines and free fatty acids (FFAs) by adipose tissue, associated with infiltration of immune cells. Among all the adipokines, leptin, visfatin, and adiponectin are the most studied. They also directly affect atherosclerotic plaque formation (Scotece et al., 2012).

Leptin was the first adipokine discovered, in 1994. It is a 16-kDa non-glycosylated hormone mainly produced by white adipose tissue and its serum rate is correlated with the amount of fat (Zhang et al., 1994). Its concentration is also associated with myocardial infarction and stroke history independent of other risk factors (Sierra-Johnson et al., 2007). Leptin is able to induce hypertrophy of vascular smooth muscle (Zeidan et al., 2005), enhance the production of MMPs (Park et al., 2001) and cytokines by endothelial cells, and stimulate the secretion of proatherogenic factors such as lipoprotein lipase (Maingrette and Renier, 2003) or caveolin-1 (Singh et al., 2011). In vivo, leptin-deficient (*ob/ob*) obese mice are protected against atherosclerosis, so leptin is an important factor of the noxious effect of fat mass (Taleb et al., 2007; Chiba et al., 2008).

Visfatin expression was first found in visceral fat and is associated with fat mass, metabolic disease, and CV events in patients (Chang et al., 2011). Visfatin is also known as nicotinamide phosphoribosyltransferase or pre-B cell colony-enhancing factor. It seems to play an important role in atherogenesis because it is expressed especially by perivascular adipose tissue and macrophages of carotid and coronary atherosclerotic plaque (Dahl et al., 2007). Visfatin is also able to activate endothelial cells and angiogenesis (Adya et al., 2009; Kim et al., 2012) and promotes plaque destabilization. In vivo, the overexpression of visfatin in apoE$^{-/-}$ mice promoted lipid accumulation in macrophages, MMP production, and decreased collagen level (Li et al., 2016) and overall increased plaque vulnerability.

Unlike most adipose-derived hormones, adiponectin has a protective antiinflammatory role in the CV system. Serum adiponectin level is decreased in obese patients (Arita et al., 1999; Matsubara et al., 2002) and its level has a strong inverse relationship with fat mass (Kern et al., 2003). It appears to be a protective adipokine in obesity and related complications such as type 2 diabetes and CVD (Kadowaki et al., 2006). Adiponectin enhances insulin sensitivity (Yamauchi et al., 2001) and has a direct action in the vascular system: inhibition of adhesion molecules such as vascular cell adhesion molecule 1, intercellular adhesion molecule 1, and E-selectin (Ouchi et al.,

1999); antiinflammatory properties on endothelial cells suppressing macrophage activation; and limiting plaque rupture via tissue inhibitor of metalloproteinase 1 production (Kumada et al., 2004). In vivo, adiponectin deficiency induces a vascular loss of response to vasodilatory signals and a higher production of ROS in vessels (Cao et al., 2009), whereas adding adiponectin to apoE$^{-/-}$ mice blocked oxidative stress and reduced atherosclerotic lesions (Cai et al., 2015).

Some of these cytokines and adipokines are also involved in OA pathophysiology and could explain the systemic association of obesity and hand OA.

The expression of cytokines is increased in joint tissue during OA as their spontaneous production in vitro by OA chondrocytes, osteoblasts, or synoviocytes (Tsuchida et al., 2012, 2014). In vitro, IL-1β and TNF-α themselves induce other proinflammatory cytokines, chemokines, or bioactive lipids (IL-6 and IL-8, PGE_2) and MMP chondrocyte production (Henrotin et al., 1996; Kunisch et al., 2014) but they also decrease collagen levels (Lefebvre et al., 1990), modulate mitochondrial function (López-Armada et al., 2006), and increase chondrocyte apoptosis (Fischer et al., 2000). During OA, TNF receptor-1 (or p55-TNF receptor) and IL-1 receptor expression is increased in chondrocytes, which leads to greater susceptibility of their catabolic effects (Martel-Pelletier et al., 1992; Webb et al., 1997). Another major source of cytokines in knee OA is the infrapatellar fat pad, a local source of IL-6, IL-8, and TNF-α that can induce synovial proinflammatory activation (Clockaerts et al., 2012; Eymard et al., 2014). However, although a murine model of OA treated with TNF-α blockers was encouraging (Ma et al., 2015), phase 3 clinical trials reported no effects on hand OA (Verbruggen et al., 2012; Chevalier et al., 2015). IL-6 involvement is more ambivalent because the results may depend on the model studied. In normal human chondrocytes, IL-6 increases GAG production, whereas under OA conditions, chondrocytes do not respond to IL-6 and lose this ability of GAG production (Tsuchida et al., 2012). Conversely, in other studies, IL-6 induced MMP-1 and MMP-13 expression by normal human chondrocytes (Aida et al., 2012). Despite a global procatabolic effect on cartilage, this cytokine needs further studies because, surprisingly, IL-6—knockout mice show more severe OA than do wild-type mice (de Hooge et al., 2005).

Adipokine involvement in OA was recently observed and may also explain the systemic effect of obesity on joint tissue. Leptin is increased in OA cartilage as compared to non-OA cartilage (Dumond et al., 2003) and its level in synovial fluid or expression in cartilage is associated with OA severity (Ku et al., 2009; Simopoulou et al., 2007a). In vitro, leptin synergizes with IL-1β and enhances IL-6, PGE_2, MMP-9, and MMP-13 production, thereby leading to a low-grade inflammatory state and cartilage proteolysis (Simopoulou et al., 2007b; Vuolteenaho et al., 2009; Koskinen et al., 2011). During OA, visfatin serum rate is increased as compared to controls (Chen et al., 2010). In vitro, it inhibits the anabolic action of insulin growth-factor 1 and promotes proinflammatory cytokine release by chondrocytes and osteoblasts (Laiguillon et al., 2014; Yammani and Loeser, 2012). Finally, it showed catabolic activity in mechanical induction of OA in mice (Yang et al., 2015). Despite a systemic antiinflammatory role, adiponectin function seems more complex in OA. In vitro, adiponectin induces proinflammatory activation of chondrocytes and synoviocytes (Frommer et al., 2012; Lago et al., 2008) but also has anticatabolic properties (Chen et al., 2006). Furthermore, studies of the association of OA and serum adiponectin level seem contradictory: some have described a higher adiponectin level associated with slower OA progression (Yusuf et al., 2011) and others found a higher level associated with erosive hand OA (Filková et al., 2009). Potential explanations for this discrepancy include different isoforms of adiponectin (globular, full length) (Francin et al., 2014) and different receptors of adiponectin having diverse biological effects (Tong et al., 2011; Zuo et al., 2011).

However, despite all these studies, we cannot conclude that systemic inflammation related to obesity is directly implicated in the pathophysiology of OA. Likewise, these diseases may not affect each other simply because the same mediators are involved in both. Evidence of the systemic association of OA and obesity come from more recent in vivo studies exploring obesity-related inflammation and OA. First, Griffin et al. demonstrated that leptin-deficient mice (*ob/ob*) did not show OA, despite their major obesity, which illustrates that mechanical factors are not enough to promote OA (Griffin et al., 2009). The authors also showed that knee OA, spontaneously developed in high-fat diet-induced obese mice, was correlated with the levels of leptin and adiponectin independent of fat mass and weight gain (Griffin et al., 2010). In the same murine model, the wheel running exercise, which increases mechanical stress without reducing body fat, did not worsen OA but disrupted cytokine production and reduced OA progression (Griffin et al., 2012).

4.2.2 Metabolic Syndrome

MetS is an accumulation of metabolic disorders [abdominal obesity, increased blood pressure, impaired glucose tolerance, and lipid abnormalities such as high triglycerides level and low high-density lipoprotein cholesterol (HDL-C) level] associated with increased risk of stroke, type 2 diabetes mellitus, and CVD (Grundy et al., 2004; Alberti et al., 2005, 2009; Hari et al., 2012; Hajat and Shather, 2012). An association of MetS, beyond obesity, and OA has been reported numerous times, even after adjustment on age, which itself is a strong risk factor of MetS (Dahaghin et al., 2007; Puenpatom and Victor, 2009; Yoshimura et al., 2012; Visser et al., 2014; Tomi et al., 2016). Discovery of the association between OA and MetS, beyond the link with obesity, has delineated a wide and frequent subtype of OA called metabolic OA (Bijlsma et al., 2011).

MetS is frequent in the OA population. In the NHANES cohort, MetS was present in 59% of OA patients as compared to 23% of non-OA patients of the same age (Puenpatom and Victor, 2009). Besides its high prevalence, MetS independently increased the risk of knee (Yoshimura et al., 2012; Monira Hussain et al., 2014), hip, hand (Dahaghin et al., 2007; Visser et al., 2014), and lumbar spine OA (Gandhi et al., 2014). Indeed, unhealthy metabolic obesity was suggested to confer increased risk of OA as compared with healthy metabolic obesity (Sowers et al., 2009; Ahima and Lazar, 2013). Since the definition of MetS lacks consensus, some studies have investigated the cumulative effect of components of MetS on OA. The most illustrative finding comes from the Japanese ROAD study finding that risk of occurrence and progression of knee OA increased with number of metabolic components (Yoshimura et al., 2012). A similar observation was from the Rotterdam cohort for hand OA (Dahaghin et al., 2007).

Besides the cumulative harmful effect of MetS, some MetS components are independently associated with OA. The most relevant evidence is probably for type 2 diabetes or hyperglycemia (Berenbaum, 2011; Yoshimura et al., 2012); a recent meta-analysis reported increased OA in patients with diabetes mellitus as compared to nondiabetic patients (Louati et al., 2015). Type 2 diabetes seems to promote OA progression as well as OA severity: diabetic patients have a two-fold greater indication for hip and knee arthroplasty and a higher rate of joint space narrowing by year than nondiabetics whatever the patient's age or body mass index (BMI) (Eymard et al., 2015; Schett et al., 2013). As well, hand OA has been found associated with type 2 diabetes (Dahaghin et al., 2007; Magnusson et al., 2015). These epidemiological findings are supported by recent basic research insights. In the setting of diabetes mellitus, high glucose concentration, insulin resistance, or AGEs was found to have noxious effects on joint cells, as for endothelium.

Type 2 diabetic OA cartilage explants are more responsive to IL-1β inflammatory stress, probably because of excess oxidative stress induced by a high glucose environment (Laiguillon et al., 2015). Type 2 synoviocytes from diabetic patients are insulin resistant. In an inflammatory condition, insulin has an anabolic function on joints, which supports that insulin resistance may promote the catabolic process (Hamada et al., 2015). Finally, diabetes could have a noxious role through AGEs because their production is also highly related to glycemia (Day et al., 1980). These AGEs are involved in diabetes onset and complications (Hirata and Kubo, 2004) and accumulate in diabetic OA joints, especially subchondral bone (Oren et al., 2011). In OA, in vitro studies demonstrated that via the receptor of AGE, AGEs may activate NF-kB and p38 mitogen-activated protein kinase signaling pathways leading to the production of proinflammatory cytokines, proteolytic enzymes, and ROS by chondrocytes and synoviocytes (Nah et al., 2008; Franke et al., 2009; Rasheed et al., 2011; Rasheed and Haqqi, 2012). AGEs also induce chondrocyte apoptosis and cartilage matrix vulnerability (Verzijl et al., 2002; Yamabe et al., 2013).

Prevalence of hypertension in OA population is also high, but studies showing an independent association after adjustment for confounding factors such as age or BMI are scarce (Sowers et al., 2009; Shin, 2014). Two recent studies demonstrated an independent but weak association regardless of BMI (Yoshimura et al., 2012; Monira Hussain et al., 2014). Likewise, hypertension is considered an aggravating factor for OA in people with obesity or other metabolic disturbances (Dahaghin et al., 2007). We have no experimental evidence of a direct pathological link between hypertension and OA. Hypertension could modify the vascularization of subchondral bone and lead to local ischemia via atherosclerosis (Conaghan et al., 2005).

Metabolic dyslipidemia, associated with obesity and CV complications, is characterized by elevated triglycerides level, reduced HDL-C level, plus increased level of low-density lipoprotein cholesterol (LDL-C) and circulating FFAs (Klop et al., 2013). Furthermore, LDL particles are oxidized in oxidized LDL (oxLDL), which promotes their uptake by tissue macrophages via their scavenger receptors. These macrophages become foam cells that participate in atherosclerotic lesions.

Several studies have suggested the involvement of lipid metabolism in OA: high cholesterol is associated with generalized OA (Stürmer et al., 1998; Addimanda et al., 2012) and hypertriglyceridemia or hypercholesterolemia are associated with bone marrow lesions of subchondral bone of the knee in asymptomatic women (Davies-Tuck et al., 2009). In addition, several studies support dysfunctional lipid metabolism in OA such as abnormalities in the cellular transport of cholesterol in OA chondrocytes as well as intracellular fat accumulation and especially arachidonic acid (Lippiello et al., 1991; Tsezou et al., 2010). Mice with decreased functional HDL-C particles by genetic modification show cartilage lesions but not weight gain (Triantaphyllidou et al., 2013). OxLDL is found in the synovial fluid of OA patients, and its expression as well as that of its receptors [lectin-like oxLDL receptor 1 (LOX-1)] is increased in OA cartilage as compared to healthy cartilage (Akagi et al., 2007; Simopoulou et al., 2007b). In vitro, the oxLDL/LOX-1 system induces vascular endothelial growth factor and MMPs, decreases the synthesis of proteoglycans and alters chondrocyte viability (Kakinuma et al., 2004). Besides apolipoprotein excess, FFA excess in obese people can also have a detrimental role in OA. In vitro, palmitate, a saturated FFA, induces proinflammatory activation of chondrocytes and synoviocytes via TLR-4 as well as apoptosis of chondrocytes (Alvarez-Garcia et al., 2014). Moreover, FFAs are known to activate macrophages present in the OA inflammatory synovium and involved in cartilage degradation (Nguyen et al., 2007).

4.2.3 *Smoking*

Smoking is another modifiable risk factor of CVD with a powerful noxious role on endothelial cells and a high proatherogenic effect. OA is inversely related to smoking, but in meta-analyses, only case-control findings reached significance and cohort findings were negative (Hui et al., 2011). Smoking may be associated with less radiographic OA but is associated with high painful OA (Felson and Zhang, 2015). Likewise, smoking is not usually considered a link between OA and CVD.

This indirect association between OA and CVD through MetS and its components could be sufficient, but beyond the association with CV risk factors, OA could be directly and independently associated with atherosclerosis lesions and CVD.

5. ASSOCIATION BETWEEN OSTEOARTHRITIS AND CARDIOVASCULAR DISEASES: DIRECT LINK BEYOND CV RISK FACTORS

Numerous reports, but not all, have been published in the last decade on an independent association between atherosclerotic lesions and OA. Popliteal wall thickness is increased in patients with generalized OA, including knee OA, independent of BMI (Kornaat et al., 2009). As well, carotid and coronary plaques are associated with hand OA and its progression independent of usual CV risk factors. This association is reinforced when hand OA occurs with other localizations (knee or hip) (Jonsson et al., 2009, 2011; Hoeven et al., 2013). Beyond anatomical lesions of atherosclerosis, CV events and CV mortality are more frequent in people with than without OA. In a large population-based study, the age- and sex-standardized overall mortality was increased by 55% in people with lower-limb OA (Nüesch et al., 2011). As well, hip OA increased CV mortality in women, which was only partially explained by disability (Barbour et al., 2015). Because hand OA is not disturbed by physical activity, studies of this OA localization are useful and have shown an association with cardiac events (Courties et al., 2014; Haugen et al., 2015) and mortality (Haara et al., 2003). A meta-analysis of 15 studies reported that the pooled overall prevalence of CVD in OA people was 38.4%, with almost a three-fold higher rate of heart failure [relative risk (RR) 2.80 (95% confidence interval 2.25–3.49)] and two-fold higher rate of ischemic heart disease [RR 1.78 (1.18–2.69)] compared to matched non-OA controls (Hall et al., 2015).

Because atherosclerosis has been found independently associated with OA, atherosclerotic plaque may affect OA occurrence and progression through its own production of inflammatory mediators (cytokines, ROS, or AGEs) and/or through the defect of subchondral bone vascularization. However, the effect of atherosclerosis on OA needs further investigation, as does the mutual aggravating role of CVD on OA and vice versa.

6. ASSOCIATION BETWEEN OSTEOARTHRITIS AND CARDIOVASCULAR DISEASES: AN EPIPHENOMENON?

The association between OA and CVD could be an artifact. First, the disability caused by OA itself could be responsible for inactivity, which is a CV risk factor. Such an association suggests that the problem is not OA but inactivity itself. Some authors reported an exclusive association between OA and CVD due to disability (Hoeven et al., 2014) and others found that disability was not the sole link between the two diseases (Rahman et al., 2013; Haugen et al., 2015). Although functional disability is an important factor to consider in the analysis of the link between OA and CVD, the association between hand OA and CVD supports the hypothesis that disability does not explain everything.

The other indirect link is the chronic intake of analgesics, including acetaminophen and NSAIDs, due to OA pain. Some NSAIDs (including coxib), which are especially prescribed for inflammatory OA flares, increase CVD events, especially with long-term use (Coxib and traditional NSAID Trialists' (CNT) Collaboration et al., 2013). Because of their selectivity, coxibs inhibit cyclo-oxygenase-2 (COX-2) more than COX-1, which leads to an imbalance in COX-1/COX-2 ratio (Kato et al., 2001) and a more potent inhibition of prostacyclin (normally promoted by COX-2) than thromboxane (promoted by COX-1), which could have a prothrombotic effect. The second mechanism is the potential increased blood pressure due to COX-2 renal long-term inhibition.

Furthermore, recent observational studies raised the question of CV risk with acetaminophen intake. Acetaminophen could have some antiinflammatory effects by inhibiting COX-2 (Hinz et al., 2008) and especially with frequent and repeated consumption could be associated with increased CV events (Chan et al., 2006; Roberts et al., 2015) potentially through increased blood pressure (Sudano et al., 2010). Consequently, bias of the prescription of NSAIDs and acetaminophen needs to be considered in the observational studies.

7. NEW PERSPECTIVES: THE ROLE OF MICROBIOTA

Aging and metabolic diseases represent two important conditions associated with excess risk of OA and CVD and are both associated with a systemic low-grade inflammation, inflammaging, and metainflammation, as discussed previously. In this context of both sources of low-grade inflammation states, the role of microbiota is particularly suspected and currently investigated. To date, abnormal microbiota has been well described in obesity (Cox et al., 2015; Hersoug et al., 2016), metabolic disturbances (Qin et al., 2012), and CVD (Tang and Hazen, 2014) as well as during aging (Claesson et al., 2012) with few studies of OA (Collins et al., 2015; Metcalfe et al., 2012). A study of an obese rat model of OA showed that together, the presence of *Lactobacillus species (spp.)* and *Methanobrevibacter spp.* associated with OA occurrence but could be related to obesity rather than OA (Collins et al., 2015). Finally, a new theory is that lipopolysaccharide could interact with TLR-4 or directly activate complement and thus enhance inflammation, which could promote OA as well as CVD (Huang and Kraus, 2016).

8. CONCLUSIONS

The association between OA and CVD is frequent and probably multifactorial. They both share an association with aging, obesity, and MetS, so the common background of systemic and low-grade inflammation related to aging and metabolic diseases could explain part of the association. OA and CVD may be associated regardless of these factors, which needs further investigation and might be due to a direct effect of atheroma on joint tissues. However, despite a probable true independent association, disability and NSAID intake represent aggravating factors, especially in OA patients with other CV risk factors (Fig. 19.1). Although we cannot conclude that OA is a CVD risk factor because we need to know how OA affects CVD outcomes, the association between OA and CVD needs to be considered in clinical practice by rheumatologists as well as cardiologists.

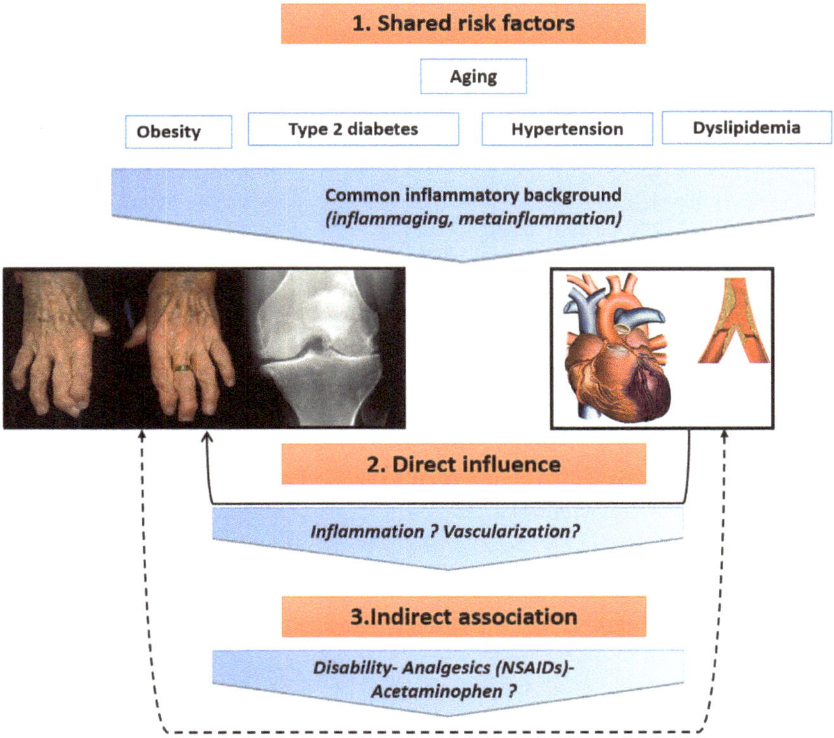

FIGURE 19.1 **Interrelationship between osteoarthritis (OA) and cardiovascular disease (CVD).** 1. OA and CVD share common risk factors that may explain their association by a direct effect but also via low-grade inflammation related to aging and metabolic disease. 2. An independent association between OA, atheroma, and CVD may be due to a direct effect of atheroma on joint tissues via inflammation or defective vascularization. 3. An indirect effect in this association must be considered, especially the effect of disability and intake of nonsteroidal antiinflammatory drugs (NSAIDs).

REFERENCES

Addimanda, O., Mancarella, L., Dolzani, P., Ramonda, R., Fioravanti, A., Brusi, V., Pignotti, E., Meliconi, R., 2012. Clinical associations in patients with hand osteoarthritis. Scand. J. Rheumatol. 41, 310–313. http://dx.doi.org/10.3109/03009742.2012.656699.

Adriaensen, W., Matheï, C., Vaes, B., van Pottelbergh, G., Wallemacq, P., Degryse, J.-M., 2015. Interleukin-6 as a first-rated serum inflammatory marker to predict mortality and hospitalization in the oldest old: a regression and CART approach in the BELFRAIL study. Exp. Gerontol. 69, 53–61. http://dx.doi.org/10.1016/j.exger.2015.06.005.

Adya, R., Tan, B.K., Chen, J., Randeva, H.S., 2009. Pre-B cell colony enhancing factor (PBEF)/visfatin induces secretion of MCP-1 in human endothelial cells: role in visfatin-induced angiogenesis. Atherosclerosis 205, 113–119. http://dx.doi.org/10.1016/j.atherosclerosis.2008.11.024.

Ahima, R.S., Lazar, M.A., 2013. Physiology. The health risk of obesity—better metrics imperative. Science 341, 856–858. http://dx.doi.org/10.1126/science.1241244.

Ai, Z., Ning, X., Shou, T., Tang, W., Luo, Y., Zhang, J., 2014. Association of interleukin-6 promoter polymorphism with knee osteoarthritis: a meta-analysis. Chin. Med. J. 127, 2492–2496.

Aida, Y., Honda, K., Tanigawa, S., Nakayama, G., Matsumura, H., Suzuki, N., Shimizu, O., Takeichi, O., Makimura, M., Maeno, M., 2012. IL-6 and soluble IL-6 receptor stimulate the production of MMPs and their inhibitors via JAK-STAT and ERK-MAPK signalling in human chondrocytes. Cell Biol. Int. 36, 367–376. http://dx.doi.org/10.1042/CBI20110150.

Akagi, M., Kanata, S., Mori, S., Itabe, H., Sawamura, T., Hamanishi, C., 2007. Possible involvement of the oxidized low-density lipoprotein/lectin-like oxidized low-density lipoprotein receptor-1 system in pathogenesis and progression of human osteoarthritis. Osteoarthr. Cartil. 15, 281–290. http://dx.doi.org/10.1016/j.joca.2006.07.010.

Alberti, K.G.M.M., Eckel, R.H., Grundy, S.M., Zimmet, P.Z., Cleeman, J.I., Donato, K.A., Fruchart, J.-C., James, W.P.T., Loria, C.M., Smith, S.C., International Diabetes Federation Task Force on Epidemiology and Prevention, Hational Heart, Lung, and Blood Institute, American Heart Association, World Heart Federation, International Atherosclerosis Society, International Association for the Study of Obesity, 2009. Harmonizing the metabolic syndrome: a joint interim statement of the International Diabetes Federation Task Force on Epidemiology and Prevention; National Heart, Lung, and Blood Institute; American Heart Association; World Heart Federation; International Atherosclerosis Society; and International Association for the Study of Obesity. Circulation 120, 1640–1645. http://dx.doi.org/10.1161/CIRCULATIONAHA.109.192644.

Alberti, K.G.M.M., Zimmet, P., Shaw, J., IDF Epidemiology Task Force Consensus Group, 2005. The metabolic syndrome—a new worldwide definition. Lancet 366, 1059–1062. http://dx.doi.org/10.1016/S0140-6736(05)67402-8.

Alvarez-Garcia, O., Rogers, N.H., Smith, R.G., Lotz, M.K., 2014. Palmitate has proapoptotic and proinflammatory effects on articular cartilage and synergizes with interleukin-1. Arthritis Rheumatol. (Hoboken, N.J.) 66, 1779–1788. http://dx.doi.org/10.1002/art.38399.

Arita, Y., Kihara, S., Ouchi, N., Takahashi, M., Maeda, K., Miyagawa, J., Hotta, K., Shimomura, I., Nakamura, T., Miyaoka, K., Kuriyama, H., Nishida, M., Yamashita, S., Okubo, K., Matsubara, K., Muraguchi, M., Ohmoto, Y., Funahashi, T., Matsuzawa, Y., 1999. Paradoxical decrease of an adipose-specific protein, adiponectin, in obesity. Biochem. Biophys. Res. Commun. 257, 79–83.

Barbour, K.E., Lui, L.-Y., Nevitt, M.C., Murphy, L.B., Helmick, C.G., Theis, K.A., Hochberg, M.C., Lane, N.E., Hootman, J.M., Cauley, J.A., Study of Osteoporotic Fractures Research Group, 2015. Hip osteoarthritis and the risk of all-cause and disease-specific mortality in older women: a population-based cohort study. Arthritis Rheumatol. (Hoboken, N.J.) 67, 1798–1805. http://dx.doi.org/10.1002/art.39113.

Berenbaum, F., 2011. Diabetes-induced osteoarthritis: from a new paradigm to a new phenotype. Ann. Rheum. Dis. 70, 1354–1356. http://dx.doi.org/10.1136/ard.2010.146399.

Bijlsma, J.W.J., Berenbaum, F., Lafeber, F.P.J.G., 2011. Osteoarthritis: an update with relevance for clinical practice. Lancet 377, 2115–2126. http://dx.doi.org/10.1016/S0140-6736(11)60243-2.

Bondeson, J., Wainwright, S.D., Lauder, S., Amos, N., Hughes, C.E., 2006. The role of synovial macrophages and macrophage-produced cytokines in driving aggrecanases, matrix metalloproteinases, and other destructive and inflammatory responses in osteoarthritis. Arthritis Res. Ther. 8, R187. http://dx.doi.org/10.1186/ar2099.

Brüel, A., Oxlund, H., 1996. Changes in biomechanical properties, composition of collagen and elastin, and advanced glycation endproducts of the rat aorta in relation to age. Atherosclerosis 127, 155–165.

Cai, X., Li, X., Li, L., Huang, X.-Z., Liu, Y.-S., Chen, L., Zhang, K., Wang, L., Li, X., Song, J., Li, S., Zhang, Y., Zhang, M., 2015. Adiponectin reduces carotid atherosclerotic plaque formation in ApoE-/- mice: roles of oxidative and nitrosative stress and inducible nitric oxide synthase. Mol. Med. Rep. 11, 1715–1721. http://dx.doi.org/10.3892/mmr.2014.2947.

Cao, Y., Tao, L., Yuan, Y., Jiao, X., Lau, W.B., Wang, Y., Christopher, T., Lopez, B., Chan, L., Goldstein, B., Ma, X.L., 2009. Endothelial dysfunction in adiponectin deficiency and its mechanisms involved. J. Mol. Cell. Cardiol. 46, 413–419. http://dx.doi.org/10.1016/j.yjmcc.2008.10.014.

Carreras-Torres, R., Kundu, S., Zanetti, D., Esteban, E., Via, M., Moral, P., 2014. Genetic risk score of NOS gene variants associated with myocardial infarction correlates with coronary incidence across Europe. PLoS One 9, e96504. http://dx.doi.org/10.1371/journal.pone.0096504.

Chan, A.T., Manson, J.E., Albert, C.M., Chae, C.U., Rexrode, K.M., Curhan, G.C., Rimm, E.B., Willett, W.C., Fuchs, C.S., 2006. Nonsteroidal antiinflammatory drugs, acetaminophen, and the risk of cardiovascular events. Circulation 113, 1578–1587. http://dx.doi.org/10.1161/CIRCULATIONAHA.105.595793.

Chang, Y.-H., Chang, D.-M., Lin, K.-C., Shin, S.-J., Lee, Y.-J., 2011. Visfatin in overweight/obesity, type 2 diabetes mellitus, insulin resistance, metabolic syndrome and cardiovascular diseases: a meta-analysis and systemic review. Diabetes Metab. Res. Rev. 27, 515–527. http://dx.doi.org/10.1002/dmrr.1201.

Chaudhary, R., Likidlilid, A., Peerapatdit, T., Tresukosol, D., Srisuma, S., Ratanamaneechat, S., Sriratanasathavorn, C., 2012. Apolipoprotein E gene polymorphism: effects on plasma lipids and risk of type 2 diabetes and coronary artery disease. Cardiovasc. Diabetol. 11, 36. http://dx.doi.org/10.1186/1475-2840-11-36.

Chen, T.-H., Chen, L., Hsieh, M.-S., Chang, C.-P., Chou, D.-T., Tsai, S.-H., 2006. Evidence for a protective role for adiponectin in osteoarthritis. Biochim. Biophys. Acta 1762, 711–718. http://dx.doi.org/10.1016/j.bbadis.2006.06.008.

Chen, W.-P., Bao, J.-P., Feng, J., Hu, P.-F., Shi, Z.-L., Wu, L.-D., 2010. Increased serum concentrations of visfatin and its production by different joint tissues in patients with osteoarthritis. Clin. Chem. Lab. Med. 48, 1141–1145. http://dx.doi.org/10.1515/CCLM.2010.230.

Chevalier, X., Ravaud, P., Maheu, E., Baron, G., Rialland, A., Vergnaud, P., Roux, C., Maugars, Y., Mulleman, D., Lukas, C., Wendling, D., Lafforgue, P., Loeuille, D., Foltz, V., Richette, P., French Section of Osteoarthritis, 2015. Adalimumab in patients with hand osteoarthritis refractory to analgesics and NSAIDs: a randomised, multicentre, double-blind, placebo-controlled trial. Ann. Rheum. Dis. 74, 1697–1705. http://dx.doi.org/10.1136/annrheumdis-2014-205348.

Chiba, T., Shinozaki, S., Nakazawa, T., Kawakami, A., Ai, M., Kaneko, E., Kitagawa, M., Kondo, K., Chait, A., Shimokado, K., 2008. Leptin deficiency suppresses progression of atherosclerosis in apoE-deficient mice. Atherosclerosis 196, 68–75. http://dx.doi.org/10.1016/j.atherosclerosis.2007.01.040.

Claesson, M.J., Jeffery, I.B., Conde, S., Power, S.E., O'Connor, E.M., Cusack, S., Harris, H.M.B., Coakley, M., Lakshminarayanan, B., O'Sullivan, O., Fitzgerald, G.F., Deane, J., O'Connor, M., Harnedy, N., O'Connor, K., O'Mahony, D., van Sinderen, D., Wallace, M., Brennan, L., Stanton, C., Marchesi, J.R., Fitzgerald, A.P., Shanahan, F., Hill, C., Ross, R.P., O'Toole, P.W., 2012. Gut microbiota composition correlates with diet and health in the elderly. Nature 488, 178–184. http://dx.doi.org/10.1038/nature11319.

Clockaerts, S., Bastiaansen-Jenniskens, Y.M., Feijt, C., De Clerck, L., Verhaar, J.a. N., Zuurmond, A.-M., Stojanovic-Susulic, V., Somville, J., Kloppenburg, M , van Osch, G.J.V.M., 2012. Cytokine production by infrapatellar fat pad can be stimulated by interleukin 1β and inhibited by peroxisome proliferator activated receptor α agonist. Ann. Rheum. Dis. 71, 1012–1018. http://dx.doi.org/10.1136/annrheumdis-2011-200688.

Collins, K.H., Paul, H.A., Reimer, R.A., Seerattan, R.A., Hart, D.A., Herzog, W., 2015. Relationship between inflammation, the gut microbiota, and metabolic osteoarthritis development: studies in a rat model. Osteoarthr. Cartil. 23, 1989–1998. http://dx.doi.org/10.1016/j.joca.2015.03.014.

Conaghan, P.G., Vanharanta, H., Dieppe, P.A., 2005. Is progressive osteoarthritis an atheromatous vascular disease? Ann. Rheum. Dis. 64, 1539–1541. http://dx.doi.org/10.1136/ard.2005.039263.

Courties, A., Gualillo, O., Berenbaum, F., Sellam, J., 2015. Metabolic stress-induced joint inflammation and osteoarthritis. Osteoarthr. Cartil.. http://dx.doi.org/10.1016/j.joca.2015.05.016.

Courties, A., Sellam, J., Maheu, E., Barthe, Y., Cadet, C., Carrat, F., Berenbaum, F., 2014. Association between Cardiometabolic Disorders and hand osteoarthritis severity: a cross sectionnal and longitudinal study. Arthritis Rheum. 66, S558. Poster 1275.

Cox, A.J., West, N.P., Cripps, A.W., 2015. Obesity, inflammation, and the gut microbiota. Lancet Diabetes Endocrinol. 3, 207–215. http://dx.doi.org/10.1016/S2213-8587(14)70134-2.

Coxib and Traditional NSAID Trialists' (CNT) Collaboration, Bhala, N., Emberson, J., Merhi, A., Abramson, S., Arber, N., Baron, J.A., Bombardier, C., Cannon, C., Farkouh, M.E., FitzGerald, G.A., Goss, P., Halls, H., Hawk, E., Hawkey, C., Hennekens, C., Hochberg, M., Holland, L.E., Kearney, P.M., Laine, L., Lanas, A., Lance, P., Laupacis, A., Oates, J., Patrono, C., Schnitzer, T.J., Solomon, S., Tugwell, P., Wilson, K., Wittes, J., Baigent, C., 2013. Vascular and upper gastrointestinal effects of non-steroidal anti-inflammatory drugs: meta-analyses of individual participant data from randomised trials. Lancet 382, 769–779. http://dx.doi.org/10.1016/S0140-6736(13)60900-9.

Dahaghin, S., Bierma-Zeinstra, S.M.A., Koes, B.W., Hazes, J.M.W., Pols, H.a. P., 2007. Do metabolic factors add to the effect of overweight on hand osteoarthritis? The Rotterdam Study. Ann. Rheum. Dis. 66, 916–920. http://dx.doi.org/10.1136/ard.2005.045724.

Dahl, T.B., Yndestad, A., Skjelland, M., Øie, E., Dahl, A., Michelsen, A., Damås, J.K., Tunheim, S.H., Ueland, T., Smith, C., Bendz, B., Tonstad, S., Gullestad, L., Frøland, S.S., Krohg-Sørensen, K., Russell, D., Aukrust, P., Halvorsen, B., 2007. Increased expression of visfatin in macrophages of human unstable carotid and coronary atherosclerosis: possible role in inflammation and plaque destabilization. Circulation 115, 972–980 http://dx.doi.org/10.1161/CIRCULATIONAHA.106.665893.

Davies-Tuck, M.L., Hanna, F., Davis, S.R., Bell, R.J., Davison, S.L., Wluka, A.E., Adams, J., Cicuttini, F.M., 2009. Total cholesterol and triglycerides are associated with the development of new bone marrow lesions in asymptomatic middle-aged women - a prospective cohort study. Arthritis Res. Ther. 11, R181. http://dx.doi.org/10.1186/ar2873.

Day, J.F., Ingebretsen, C.G., Ingebretsen, W.R., Baynes, J.W., Thorpe, S.R., 1980. Nonenzymatic glucosylation of serum proteins and hemoglobin: response to changes in blood glucose levels in diabetic rats. Diabetes 29, 524–527.

de Hooge, A.S.K., van de Loo, F.A.J., Bennink, M.B., Arntz, O.J., de Hooge, P., van den Berg, W.B., 2005. Male IL-6 gene knock out mice developed more advanced osteoarthritis upon aging. Osteoarthr. Cartil. 13, 66–73. http://dx.doi.org/10.1016/j.joca.2004.09.011.

de Klerk, B.M., Schiphof, D., Groeneveld, F.P.M.J., Koes, B.W., van Osch, G.J.V.M., van Meurs, J.B.J., Bierma-Zeinstra, S.M.A., 2009. No clear association between female hormonal aspects and osteoarthritis of the hand, hip and knee: a systematic review. Rheumatology (Oxford) 48, 1160–1165. http://dx.doi.org/10.1093/rheumatology/kep194.

Driver, J.A., Djoussé, L., Logroscino, G., Gaziano, J.M., Kurth, T., 2008. Incidence of cardiovascular disease and cancer in advanced age: prospective cohort study. BMJ 337, a2467.

Dumond, H., Presle, N., Terlain, B., Mainard, D., Loeuille, D., Netter, P., Pottie, P., 2003. Evidence for a key role of leptin in osteoarthritis. Arthritis Rheum. 48, 3118–3129. http://dx.doi.org/10.1002/art.11303.

Elhage, R., Maret, A., Pieraggi, M.T., Thiers, J.C., Arnal, J.F., Bayard, F., 1998. Differential effects of interleukin-1 receptor antagonist and tumor necrosis factor binding protein on fatty-streak formation in apolipoprotein E-deficient mice. Circulation 97, 242–244.

Eymard, F., Parsons, C., Edwards, M.H., Petit-Dop, F., Reginster, J.-Y., Bruyère, O., Richette, P., Cooper, C., Chevalier, X., 2015. Diabetes is a risk factor for knee osteoarthritis progression. Osteoarthr. Cartil. 23, 851–859. http://dx.doi.org/10.1016/j.joca.2015.01.013.

Eymard, F., Pigenet, A., Citadelle, D., Flouzat-Lachaniette, C.-H., Poignard, A., Benelli, C., Berenbaum, F., Chevalier, X., Houard, X., 2014. Induction of an inflammatory and prodegradative phenotype in autologous fibroblast-like synoviocytes by the infrapatellar fat pad from patients with knee osteoarthritis. Arthritis Rheumatol. (Hoboken, N.J.) 66, 2165–2174. http://dx.doi.org/10.1002/art.38657.

Felson, D.T., Naimark, A., Anderson, J., Kazis, L., Castelli, W., Meenan, R.F., 1987. The prevalence of knee osteoarthritis in the elderly. The Framingham Osteoarthritis Study. Arthritis Rheum. 30, 914–918.

Felson, D.T., Zhang, Y., 2015. Smoking and osteoarthritis: a review of the evidence and its implications. Osteoarthr. Cartil. 23, 331–333. http://dx.doi.org/10.1016/j.joca.2014.11.022.

Filková, M., Lisková, M., Hulejová, H., Haluzík, M., Gatterová, J., Pavelková, A., Pavelka, K., Gay, S., Müller-Ladner, U., Senolt, L., 2009. Increased serum adiponectin levels in female patients with erosive compared with non-erosive osteoarthritis. Ann. Rheum. Dis. 68, 295–296. http://dx.doi.org/10.1136/ard.2008.095737.

Fischer, B.A., Mundle, S., Cole, A.A., 2000. Tumor necrosis factor-alpha induced DNA cleavage in human articular chondrocytes may involve multiple endonucleolytic activities during apoptosis. Microsc. Res. Tech. 50, 236–242. http://dx.doi.org/10.1002/1097-0029(20000801)50:3<236::AID-JEMT7>3.0.CO;2-E.

Forsyth, C.B., Cole, A., Murphy, G., Bienias, J.L., Im, H.-J., Loeser, R.F., 2005. Increased matrix metalloproteinase-13 production with aging by human articular chondrocytes in response to catabolic stimuli. J. Gerontol. A Biol. Sci. Med. Sci. 60, 1118–1124.

Francin, P.-J., Abot, A., Guillaume, C., Moulin, D., Bianchi, A., Gegout-Pottie, P., Jouzeau, J.-Y., Mainard, D., Presle, N., 2014. Association between adiponectin and cartilage degradation in human osteoarthritis. Osteoarthr. Cartil. 22, 519–526. http://dx.doi.org/10.1016/j.joca.2014.01.002.

Franke, S., Sommer, M., Rüster, C., Bondeva, T., Marticke, J., Hofmann, G., Hein, G., Wolf, G., 2009. Advanced glycation end products induce cell cycle arrest and proinflammatory changes in osteoarthritic fibroblast-like synovial cells. Arthritis Res. Ther. 11, R136. http://dx.doi.org/10.1186/ar2807.

Frommer, K.W., Schäffler, A., Büchler, C., Steinmeyer, J., Rickert, M., Rehart, S., Brentano, F., Gay, S., Müller-Ladner, U., Neumann, E., 2012. Adiponectin isoforms: a potential therapeutic target in rheumatoid arthritis? Ann. Rheum. Dis. 71, 1724–1732. http://dx.doi.org/10.1136/annrheumdis-2011-200924.

Gandhi, R., Woo, K.M., Zywiel, M.G., Rampersaud, Y.R., 2014. Metabolic syndrome increases the prevalence of spine osteoarthritis. Orthop. Surg. 6, 23–27. http://dx.doi.org/10.1111/os.12093.

Gómez, R., Villalvilla, A., Largo, R., Gualillo, O., Herrero-Beaumont, G., 2015. TLR4 signalling in osteoarthritis–finding targets for candidate DMOADs. Nat. Rev. Rheumatol. 11, 159–170. http://dx.doi.org/10.1038/nrrheum.2014.209.

Gorenne, I., Kavurma, M., Scott, S., Bennett, M., 2006. Vascular smooth muscle cell senescence in atherosclerosis. Cardiovasc. Res. 72, 9–17. http://dx.doi.org/10.1016/j.cardiores.2006.06.004.

Gosset, M., Berenbaum, F., Levy, A., Pigenet, A., Thirion, S., Saffar, J.-L., Jacques, C., 2006. Prostaglandin E2 synthesis in cartilage explants under compression: mPGES-1 is a mechanosensitive gene. Arthritis Res. Ther. 8, R135. http://dx.doi.org/10.1186/ar2024.

Greene, M.A., Loeser, R.F., 2015. Aging-related inflammation in osteoarthritis. Osteoarthr. Cartil. 23, 1966–1971. http://dx.doi.org/10.1016/j.joca.2015.01.008.

Griffin, T.M., Fermor, B., Huebner, J.L., Kraus, V.B., Rodriguiz, R.M., Wetsel, W.C., Cao, L., Setton, L.A., Guilak, F., 2010. Diet-induced obesity differentially regulates behavioral, biomechanical, and molecular risk factors for osteoarthritis in mice. Arthritis Res. Ther. 12, R130. http://dx.doi.org/10.1186/ar3068.

Griffin, T.M., Huebner, J.L., Kraus, V.B., Guilak, F., 2009. Extreme obesity due to impaired leptin signaling in mice does not cause knee osteoarthritis. Arthritis Rheum. 60, 2935–2944. http://dx.doi.org/10.1002/art.24854.

Griffin, T.M., Huebner, J.L., Kraus, V.B., Yan, Z., Guilak, F., 2012. Induction of osteoarthritis and metabolic inflammation by a very high-fat diet in mice: effects of short-term exercise. Arthritis Rheum. 64, 443–453. http://dx.doi.org/10.1002/art.33332.

Grundy, S.M., Cleeman, J.I., Merz, C.N.B., Brewer, H.B., Clark, L.T., Hunninghake, D.B., Pasternak, R.C., Smith, S.C., Stone, N.J., Coordinating Committee of the National Cholesterol Education Program, 2004. Implications of recent clinical trials for the National Cholesterol Education Program Adult Treatment Panel III guidelines. Arterioscler. Thromb. Vasc. Biol. 24, e149–161. http://dx.doi.org/10.1161/01.ATV.0000133317.49796.0E.

Haara, M.M., Manninen, P., Kröger, H., Arokoski, J.P.A., Kärkkäinen, A., Knekt, P., Aromaa, A., Heliövaara, M., 2003. Osteoarthritis of finger joints in Finns aged 30 or over: prevalence, determinants, and association with mortality. Ann. Rheum. Dis. 62, 151–158.

Hager, K., Machein, U., Krieger, S., Platt, D., Seefried, G., Bauer, J., 1994. Interleukin-6 and selected plasma proteins in healthy persons of different ages. Neurobiol. Aging 15, 771–772.

Hajat, C., Shather, Z., 2012. Prevalence of metabolic syndrome and prediction of diabetes using IDF versus ATPIII criteria in a Middle East population. Diabetes Res. Clin. Pract. 98, 481–486. http://dx.doi.org/10.1016/j.diabres.2012.09.037.

Hall, A.J., Stubbs, B., Mamas, M.A., Myint, P.K., Smith, T.O., 2015. Association between osteoarthritis and cardiovascular disease: systematic review and meta-analysis. Eur. J. Prev. Cardiol.. http://dx.doi.org/10.1177/2047487315610663.

Hamada, D., Maynard, R., Schott, E., Drinkwater, C.J., Ketz, J.P., Kates, S.L., Jonason, J.H., Hilton, M.J., Zuscik, M.J., Mooney, R.A., 2015. Insulin suppresses TNF-dependent early osteoarthritic changes associated with obesity and type 2 diabetes. Arthritis Rheumatol. (Hoboken, N.J.). http://dx.doi.org/10.1002/art.39561.

Hari, P., Nerusu, K., Veeranna, V., Sudhakar, R., Zalawadiya, S., Ramesh, K., Afonso, L., 2012. A gender-stratified comparative analysis of various definitions of metabolic syndrome and cardiovascular risk in a multiethnic U.S. population. Metab. Syndr. Relat. Disord. 10, 47–55. http://dx.doi.org/10.1089/met.2011.0087.

Haugen, I.K., Englund, M., Aliabadi, P., Niu, J., Clancy, M., Kvien, T.K., Felson, D.T., 2011. Prevalence, incidence and progression of hand osteoarthritis in the general population: the Framingham Osteoarthritis Study. Ann. Rheum. Dis. 70, 1581–1586. http://dx.doi.org/10.1136/ard.2011.150078.

Haugen, I.K., Ramachandran, V.S., Misra, D., Neogi, T., Niu, J., Yang, T., Zhang, Y., Felson, D.T., 2015. Hand osteoarthritis in relation to mortality and incidence of cardiovascular disease: data from the Framingham heart study. Ann. Rheum. Dis. 74, 74–81. http://dx.doi.org/10.1136/annrheumdis-2013-203789.

Henrotin, Y.E., De Groote, D.D., Labasse, A.H., Gaspar, S.E., Zheng, S.X., Geenen, V.G., Reginster, J.Y., 1996. Effects of exogenous IL-1 beta, TNF alpha, IL-6, IL-8 and LIF on cytokine production by human articular chondrocytes. Osteoarthr. Cartil. 4, 163–173.

Hernández-Díaz, Y., Tovilla-Zárate, C.A., Juárez-Rojop, I., Baños-González, M.A., Torres-Hernández, M.E., López-Narváez, M.L., Yañez-Rivera, T.G., González-Castro, T.B., 2015. The role of gene variants of the inflammatory markers CRP and TNF-α in cardiovascular heart disease: systematic review and meta-analysis. Int. J. Clin. Exp. Med. 8, 11958–11984.

Hersoug, L.-G., Møller, P., Loft, S., 2016. Gut microbiota-derived lipopolysaccharide uptake and trafficking to adipose tissue: implications for inflammation and obesity. Obes. Rev. 17, 297–312. http://dx.doi.org/10.1111/obr.12370.

Hinz, B., Cheremina, O., Brune, K., 2008. Acetaminophen (paracetamol) is a selective cyclooxygenase-2 inhibitor in man. FASEB J. 22, 383–390. http://dx.doi.org/10.1096/fj.07-8506com.

Hirata, K., Kubo, K., 2004. Relationship between blood levels of N-carboxymethyl-lysine and pentosidine and the severity of microangiopathy in type 2 diabetes. Endocr. J. 51, 537–544.

Hoeven, T.A., Kavousi, M., Clockaerts, S., Kerkhof, H.J.M., van Meurs, J.B., Franco, O., Hofman, A., Bindels, P., Witteman, J., Bierma-Zeinstra, S., 2013. Association of atherosclerosis with presence and progression of osteoarthritis: the Rotterdam Study. Ann. Rheum. Dis. 72, 646–651. http://dx.doi.org/10.1136/annrheumdis-2011-201178.

Hoeven, T.A., Leening, M.J.G., Bindels, P.J., Castaño-Betancourt, M., van Meurs, J.B., Franco, O.H., Kavousi, M., Hofman, A., Ikram, M.A., Witteman, J.C.M., Bierma-Zeinstra, S.M., 2014. Disability and not osteoarthritis predicts cardiovascular disease: a prospective population-based cohort study. Ann. Rheum. Dis.. http://dx.doi.org/10.1136/annrheumdis-2013-204388.

Honsawek, S., Deepaisarnsakul, B., Tanavalee, A., Yuktanandana, P., Bumrungpanichthaworn, P., Malila, S., Saetan, N., 2011. Association of the IL-6 -174G/C gene polymorphism with knee osteoarthritis in a Thai population. Genet. Mol. Res. 10, 1674–1680.

Hotamisligil, G.S., Arner, P., Caro, J.F., Atkinson, R.L., Spiegelman, B.M., 1995. Increased adipose tissue expression of tumor necrosis factor-alpha in human obesity and insulin resistance. J. Clin. Invest. 95, 2409–2415. http://dx.doi.org/10.1172/JCI117936.

Hotamisligil, G.S., Shargill, N.S., Spiegelman, B.M., 1993. Adipose expression of tumor necrosis factor-alpha: direct role in obesity-linked insulin resistance. Science 259, 87–91.

Huang, Z., Kraus, V.B., 2016. Does lipopolysaccharide-mediated inflammation have a role in OA? Nat. Rev. Rheumatol. 12, 123–129. http://dx.doi.org/10.1038/nrrheum.2015.158.

Huber, S.A., Sakkinen, P., Conze, D., Hardin, N., Tracy, R., 1999. Interleukin-6 exacerbates early atherosclerosis in mice. Arterioscler. Thromb. Vasc. Biol. 19, 2364–2367.

Hui, M., Doherty, M., Zhang, W., 2011. Does smoking protect against osteoarthritis? Meta-analysis of observational studies. Ann. Rheum. Dis. 70, 1231–1237 http://dx.doi.org/10.1136/ard.2010.142323.

Jonsson, H., Helgadottir, G.P., Aspelund, T., Eiriksdottir, G., Sigurdsson, S., Ingvarsson, T., Harris, T.B., Launer, L., Gudnason, V., 2009. Hand osteoarthritis in older women is associated with carotid and coronary atherosclerosis: the AGES Reykjavik study. Ann. Rheum. Dis. 68, 1696–1700. http://dx.doi.org/10.1136/ard.2008.096289.

Jonsson, H., Helgadottir, G.P., Aspelund, T., Eiriksdottir, G., Sigurdsson, S., Siggeirsdottir, K., Ingvarsson, T., Harris, T.B., Launer, L., Gudnason, V., 2011. The presence of total knee or hip replacements due to osteoarthritis enhances the positive association between hand osteoarthritis and atherosclerosis in women: the AGES-Reykjavik study. Ann. Rheum. Dis. 70, 1087–1090. http://dx.doi.org/10.1136/ard.2010.144980.

Kadowaki, T., Yamauchi, T., Kubota, N., Hara, K., Ueki, K., Tobe, K., 2006. Adiponectin and adiponectin receptors in insulin resistance, diabetes, and the metabolic syndrome. J. Clin. Invest. 116, 1784–1792. http://dx.doi.org/10.1172/JCI29126.

Kakinuma, T., Yasuda, T., Nakagawa, T., Hiramitsu, T., Akiyoshi, M., Akagi, M., Sawamura, T., Nakamura, T., 2004. Lectin-like oxidized low-density lipoprotein receptor 1 mediates matrix metalloproteinase 3 synthesis enhanced by oxidized low-density lipoprotein in rheumatoid arthritis cartilage. Arthritis Rheum. 50, 3495–3503. http://dx.doi.org/10.1002/art.20581.

Karaderi, T., Drong, A.W., Lindgren, C.M., 2015. Insights into the genetic susceptibility to type 2 diabetes from genome-wide association studies of obesity-related traits. Curr. Diab. Rep. 15, 83. http://dx.doi.org/10.1007/s11892-015-0648-8.

Kato, M., Nishida, S., Kitasato, H., Sakata, N., Kawai, S., 2001. Cyclooxygenase-1 and cyclooxygenase-2 selectivity of non-steroidal anti-inflammatory drugs: investigation using human peripheral monocytes. J. Pharm. Pharmacol. 53, 1679–1685.

Kern, P.A., Di Gregorio, G.B., Lu, T., Rassouli, N., Ranganathan, G., 2003. Adiponectin expression from human adipose tissue: relation to obesity, insulin resistance, and tumor necrosis factor-alpha expression. Diabetes 52, 1779–1785.

Kim, S.-R., Jung, Y.-H., Park, H.-J., Kim, M.-K., Jeong, J.-W., Jang, H.-O. Yun, I., Bae, S.-K., Bae, M.-K., 2012. Upregulation of thromboxane synthase mediates visfatin-induced interleukin-8 expression and angiogenic activity in endothelial cells. Biochem. Biophys. Res. Commun. 418, 662–668. http://dx.doi.org/10.1016/j.bbrc.2012.01.072.

Klop, B., Elte, J.W.F., Cabezas, M.C., 2013. Dyslipidemia in obesity: mechanisms and potential targets. Nutrients 5, 1218–1240. http://dx.doi.org/10.3390/nu5041218.

Kornaat, P.R., Sharma, R., van der Geest, R.J., Lamb, H.J., Kloppenburg, M., Hellio le Graverand, M.-P., Bloem, J.L., Watt, I., 2009. Positive association between increased popliteal artery vessel wall thickness and generalized osteoarthritis: is OA also part of the metabolic syndrome? Skeletal Radiol. 38, 1147–1151. http://dx.doi.org/10.1007/s00256-009-0741-7.

Koskinen, A., Vuolteenaho, K., Nieminen, R., Moilanen, T., Moilanen, E., 2011. Leptin enhances MMP-1, MMP-3 and MMP-13 production in human osteoarthritic cartilage and correlates with MMP-1 and MMP-3 in synovial fluid from OA patients. Clin. Exp. Rheumatol. 29, 57–64.

Kraus, V.B., McDaniel, G., Huebner, J.L., Stabler, T.V., Pieper, C.F., Shipes, S.W., Petry, N.A., Low, P.S., Shen, J., McNearney, T.A., Mitchell, P., 2016. Direct in vivo evidence of activated macrophages in human osteoarthritis. Osteoarthr. Cartil. http://dx.doi.org/10.1016/j.joca.2016.04.010.

Ku, J.H., Lee, C.K., Joo, B.S., An, B.M., Choi, S.H., Wang, T.H., Cho, H.L., 2009. Correlation of synovial fluid leptin concentrations with the severity of osteoarthritis. Clin. Rheumatol. 28, 1431–1435. http://dx.doi.org/10.1007/s10067-009-1242-8.

Kumada, M., Kihara, S., Ouchi, N., Kobayashi, H., Okamoto, Y., Ohashi, K., Maeda, K., Nagaretani, H., Kishida, K., Maeda, N., Nagasawa, A., Funahashi, T., Matsuzawa, Y., 2004. Adiponectin specifically increased tissue inhibitor of metalloproteinase-1 through interleukin-10 expression in human macrophages. Circulation 109, 2046–2049. http://dx.doi.org/10.1161/01.CIR.0000127953.98131.ED.

Kunisch, E., Kinne, R.W., Alsalameh, R.J., Alsalameh, S., 2014. Pro-inflammatory IL-1beta and/or TNF-alpha up-regulate matrix metalloproteases-1 and -3 mRNA in chondrocyte subpopulations potentially pathogenic in osteoarthritis: in situ hybridization studies on a single cell level. Int. J. Rheum. Dis. http://dx.doi.org/10.1111/1756-185X.12431.

Lago, R., Gomez, R., Otero, M., Lago, F., Gallego, R., Dieguez, C., Gomez-Reino, J.J., Gualillo, O., 2008. A new player in cartilage homeostasis: adiponectin induces nitric oxide synthase type II and pro-inflammatory cytokines in chondrocytes. Osteoarthr. Cartil. 16, 1101–1109. http://dx.doi.org/10.1016/j.joca.2007.12.008.

Laiguillon, M.-C., Courties, A., Houard, X., Auclair, M., Sautet, A., Capeau, J., Fève, B., Berenbaum, F., Sellam, J., 2015. Characterization of diabetic osteoarthritic cartilage and role of high glucose environment on chondrocyte activation: toward pathophysiological delineation of diabetes mellitus-related osteoarthritis. Osteoarthr. Cartil. http://dx.doi.org/10.1016/j.joca.2015.04.026.

Laiguillon, M.-C., Houard, X., Bougault, C., Gosset, M., Nourissat, G., Sautet, A., Jacques, C., Berenbaum, F., Sellam, J., 2014. Expression and function of visfatin (Nampt), an adipokine-enzyme involved in inflammatory pathways of osteoarthritis. Arthritis Res. Ther. 16, R38. http://dx.doi.org/10.1186/ar4467.

Lefebvre, V., Peeters-Joris, C., Vaes, G., 1990. Modulation by interleukin 1 and tumor necrosis factor alpha of production of collagenase, tissue inhibitor of metalloproteinases and collagen types in differentiated and dedifferentiated articular chondrocytes. Biochim. Biophys. Acta 1052, 366–378.

Li, B., Zhao, Y., Liu, H., Meng, B., Wang, J., Qi, T., Zhang, H., Li, T., Zhao, P., Sun, H., Xu, J., Song, H., Dong, Z., An, F., 2016. Visfatin destabilizes atherosclerotic plaques in apolipoprotein e-deficient mice. PLoS One 11, e0148273. http://dx.doi.org/10.1371/journal.pone.0148273.

Lippiello, L., Walsh, T., Fienhold, M., 1991. The association of lipid abnormalities with tissue pathology in human osteoarthritic articular cartilage. Metab. Clin. Exp. 40, 571–576.

Liu, Q., Niu, J., Huang, J., Ke, Y., Tang, X., Wu, X., Li, R., Li, H., Zhi, X., Wang, K., Zhang, Y., Lin, J., 2015. Knee osteoarthritis and all-cause mortality: the Wuchuan Osteoarthritis Study. Osteoarthr. Cartil. 23, 1154–1157. http://dx.doi.org/10.1016/j.joca.2015.03.021.

Loeser, R.F., Goldring, S.R., Scanzello, C.R., Goldring, M.B., 2012. Osteoarthritis: a disease of the joint as an organ. Arthritis Rheum. 64, 1697–1707. http://dx.doi.org/10.1002/art.34453.

López-Armada, M.J., Caramés, B., Martín, M.A., Cillero-Pastor, B., Lires-Dean, M., Fuentes-Boquete, I., Arenas, J., Blanco, F.J., 2006. Mitochondrial activity is modulated by TNFalpha and IL-1beta in normal human chondrocyte cells. Osteoarthr. Cartil. 14, 1011–1022. http://dx.doi.org/10.1016/j.joca.2006.03.008.

Louati, K., Vidal, C., Berenbaum, F., Sellam, J., 2015. Association between diabetes mellitus and osteoarthritis: systematic literature review and meta-analysis. RMD Open 1, e000077. http://dx.doi.org/10.1136/rmdopen-2015-000077.

Ma, C.H., Lv, Q., Yu, Y.X., Zhang, Y., Kong, D., Niu, K.R., Yi, C.Q., 2015. Protective effects of tumor necrosis factor-α blockade by adalimumab on articular cartilage and subchondral bone in a rat model of osteoarthritis. Braz. J. Med. Biol. Res. 48, 863–870. http://dx.doi.org/10.1590/1414-431X20154407.

Magnusson, K., Hagen, K.B., Østerås, N., Nordsletten, L., Natvig, B., Haugen, I.K., 2015. Diabetes is associated with increased hand pain in erosive hand osteoarthritis: data from a population-based study. Arthritis Care Res. (Hoboken) 67, 187–195. http://dx.doi.org/10.1002/acr.22460.

Maingrette, F., Renier, G., 2003. Leptin increases lipoprotein lipase secretion by macrophages: involvement of oxidative stress and protein kinase C. Diabetes 52, 2121–2128.

Martel-Pelletier, J., McCollum, R., DiBattista, J., Faure, M.P., Chin, J.A., Fournier, S., Sarfati, M., Pelletier, J.P., 1992. The interleukin-1 receptor in normal and osteoarthritic human articular chondrocytes. Identification as the type I receptor and analysis of binding kinetics and biologic function. Arthritis Rheum. 35, 530–540.

Matsubara, M., Maruoka, S., Katayose, S., 2002. Inverse relationship between plasma adiponectin and leptin concentrations in normal-weight and obese women. Eur. J. Endocrinol. 147, 173–180.

McAloon, C.J., Boylan, L.M., Hamborg, T., Stallard, N., Osman, F., Lim, P.B., Hayat, S.A., 2016. The changing face of cardiovascular disease 2000–2012: an analysis of the world health organisation global health estimates data. Int. J. Cardiol. 224, 256–264.

McGlashan, S.R., Cluett, E.C., Jensen, C.G., Poole, C.A., 2008. Primary cilia in osteoarthritic chondrocytes: from chondrons to clusters. Dev. Dyn. 237, 2013–2020. http://dx.doi.org/10.1002/dvdy.21501.

Medici, F., Hawa, M., Ianari, A., Pyke, D.A., Leslie, R.D., 1999. Concordance rate for type II diabetes mellitus in monozygotic twins: actuarial analysis. Diabetologia 42, 146–150. http://dx.doi.org/10.1007/s001250051132.

Merhi-Soussi, F., Kwak, B.R., Magne, D., Chadjichristos, C., Berti, M., Pelli, G., James, R.W., Mach, F., Gabay, C., 2005. Interleukin-1 plays a major role in vascular inflammation and atherosclerosis in male apolipoprotein E-knockout mice. Cardiovasc. Res. 66, 583–593. http://dx.doi.org/10.1016/j.cardiores.2005.01.008.

Metcalfe, D., Harte, A.L., Aletrari, M.O., Al Daghri, N.M., Al Disi, D., Tripathi, G., McTernan, P.G., 2012. Does endotoxaemia contribute to osteoarthritis in obese patients? Clin. Sci. 123, 627–634. http://dx.doi.org/10.1042/CS20120073.

Millward-Sadler, S.J., Salter, D.M., 2004. Integrin-dependent signal cascades in chondrocyte mechanotransduction. Ann. Biomed. Eng. 32, 435–446.

Monira Hussain, S., Wang, Y., Cicuttini, F.M., Simpson, J.A., Giles, G.G., Graves, S., Wluka, A.E., 2014. Incidence of total knee and hip replacement for osteoarthritis in relation to the metabolic syndrome and its components: a prospective cohort study. Semin. Arthritis Rheum. 43, 429–436. http://dx.doi.org/10.1016/j.semarthrit.2013.07.013.

Nah, S.-S., Choi, I.-Y., Lee, C.K., Oh, J.S., Kim, Y.G., Moon, H.-B., Yoo, B., 2008. Effects of advanced glycation end products on the expression of COX-2, PGE2 and NO in human osteoarthritic chondrocytes. Rheumatology (Oxford) 47, 425–431. http://dx.doi.org/10.1093/rheumatology/kem376.

Nedungadi, T.P., Clegg, D.J., 2009. Sexual dimorphism in body fat distribution and risk for cardiovascular diseases. J. Cardiovasc. Transl Res. 2, 321–327. http://dx.doi.org/10.1007/s12265-009-9101-1.

Nguyen, M.T.A., Favelyukis, S., Nguyen, A.-K., Reichart, D., Scott, P.A., Jenn, A., Liu-Bryan, R., Glass, C.K., Neels, J.G., Olefsky, J.M., 2007. A subpopulation of macrophages infiltrates hypertrophic adipose tissue and is activated by free fatty acids via Toll-like receptors 2 and 4 and JNK-dependent pathways. J. Biol. Chem. 282, 35279–35292. http://dx.doi.org/10.1074/jbc.M706762200.

Nüesch, E., Dieppe, P., Reichenbach, S., Williams, S., Iff, S., Jüni, P., 2011. All cause and disease specific mortality in patients with knee or hip osteoarthritis: population based cohort study. BMJ 342, d1165.

Ohta, H., Wada, H., Niwa, T., Kirii, H., Iwamoto, N., Fujii, H., Saito, K., Sekikawa, K., Seishima, M., 2005. Disruption of tumor necrosis factor-alpha gene diminishes the development of atherosclerosis in ApoE-deficient mice. Atherosclerosis 180, 11–17. http://dx.doi.org/10.1016/j.atherosclerosis.2004.11.016.

Ong, K.L., Wu, B.J., Cheung, B.M.Y., Barter, P.J., Rye, K.-A., 2013. Arthritis: its prevalence, risk factors, and association with cardiovascular diseases in the United States, 1999 to 2008. Ann. Epidemiol. 23, 80–86. http://dx.doi.org/10.1016/j.annepidem.2012.11.008.

Oren, T.W., Botolin, S., Williams, A., Bucknell, A., King, K.B., 2011. Arthroplasty in veterans: analysis of cartilage, bone, serum, and synovial fluid reveals differences and similarities in osteoarthritis with and without comorbid diabetes. J. Rehabil. Res. Dev. 48, 1195–1210.

Ouchi, N., Kihara, S., Arita, Y., Maeda, K., Kuriyama, H., Okamoto, Y., Hotta, K., Nishida, M., Takahashi, M., Nakamura, T., Yamashita, S., Funahashi, T., Matsuzawa, Y., 1999. Novel modulator for endothelial adhesion molecules: adipocyte-derived plasma protein adiponectin. Circulation 100, 2473–2476.

Pan, F., Tian, J., Winzenberg, T., Ding, C., Jones, G., 2014. Association between GDF5 rs143383 polymorphism and knee osteoarthritis: an updated meta-analysis based on 23,995 subjects. BMC Musculoskelet. Disord. 15, 404. http://dx.doi.org/10.1186/1471-2474-15-404.

Park, H.S., Park, J.Y., Yu, R., 2005. Relationship of obesity and visceral adiposity with serum concentrations of CRP, TNF-alpha and IL-6. Diabetes Res. Clin. Pract. 69, 29–35. http://dx.doi.org/10.1016/j.diabres.2004.11.007.

Park, H.Y., Kwon, H.M., Lim, H.J., Hong, B.K., Lee, J.Y., Park, B.E., Jang, Y., Cho, S.Y., Kim, H.S., 2001. Potential role of leptin in angiogenesis: leptin induces endothelial cell proliferation and expression of matrix metalloproteinases in vivo and in vitro. Exp. Mol. Med. 33, 95–102. http://dx.doi.org/10.1038/emm.2001.17.

Puenpatom, R.A., Victor, T.W., 2009. Increased prevalence of metabolic syndrome in individuals with osteoarthritis: an analysis of NHANES III data. Postgrad. Med. 121, 9–20. http://dx.doi.org/10.3810/pgm.2009.11.2073.

Punzi, L., Ramonda, R., Oliviero, F., Sfriso, P., Mussap, M., Plebani, M., Podswiadek, M., Todesco, S., 2005. Value of C reactive protein in the assessment of erosive osteoarthritis of the hand. Ann. Rheum. Dis. 64, 955–957. http://dx.doi.org/10.1136/ard.2004.029892.

Qin, J., Li, Y., Cai, Z., Li, S., Zhu, J., Zhang, F., Liang, S., Zhang, W., Guan, Y., Shen, D., Peng, Y., Zhang, D., Jie, Z., Wu, W., Qin, Y., Xue, W., Li, J., Han, L., Lu, D., Wu, P., Dai, Y., Sun, X., Li, Z., Tang, A., Zhong, S., Li, X., Chen, W., Xu, R., Wang, M., Feng, Q., Gong, M., Yu, J., Zhang, Y., Zhang, M., Hansen, T., Sanchez, G., Raes, J., Falony, G., Okuda, S., Almeida, M., LeChatelier, E., Renault, P., Pons, N., Batto, J.-M., Zhang, Z., Chen, H., Yang, R., Zheng, W., Li, S., Yang, H., Wang, J., Ehrlich, S.D., Nielsen, R., Pedersen, O., Kristiansen, K., Wang, J., 2012. A metagenome-wide association study of gut microbiota in type 2 diabetes. Nature 490, 55–60. http://dx.doi.org/10.1038/nature11450.

Rahman, M.M., Kopec, J.A., Cibere, J., Goldsmith, C.H., Anis, A.H., 2013. The relationship between osteoarthritis and cardiovascular disease in a population health survey: a cross-sectional study. BMJ Open 3. http://dx.doi.org/10.1136/bmjopen-2013-002624.

Rankinen, T., Sarzynski, M.A., Ghosh, S., Bouchard, C., 2015. Are there genetic paths common to obesity, cardiovascular disease outcomes, and cardiovascular risk factors? Circ. Res. 116, 909–922. http://dx.doi.org/10.1161/CIRCRESAHA.116.302888.

Rasheed, Z., Akhtar, N., Haqqi, T.M., 2011. Advanced glycation end products induce the expression of interleukin-6 and interleukin-8 by receptor for advanced glycation end product-mediated activation of mitogen-activated protein kinases and nuclear factor-κB in human osteoarthritis chondrocytes. Rheumatology (Oxford) 50, 838–851. http://dx.doi.org/10.1093/rheumatology/keq380.

Rasheed, Z., Haqqi, T.M., 2012. Endoplasmic reticulum stress induces the expression of COX-2 through activation of eIF2α, p38-MAPK and NF-κB in advanced glycation end products stimulated human chondrocytes. Biochim. Biophys. Acta 1823, 2179–2189. http://dx.doi.org/10.1016/j.bbamcr.2012.08.021.

Roberts, E., Delgado Nunes, V., Buckner, S., Latchem, S., Constanti, M., Miller, P., Doherty, M., Zhang, W., Birrell, F., Porcheret, M., Dziedzic, K., Bernstein, I., Wise, E., Conaghan, P.G., 2015. Paracetamol: not as safe as we thought? A systematic literature review of observational studies. Ann. Rheum. Dis. http://dx.doi.org/10.1136/annrheumdis-2014-206914.

Rodriguez-Fontenla, C., Calaza, M., Evangelou, E., Valdes, A.M., Arden, N., Blanco, F.J., Carr, A., Chapman, K., Deloukas, P., Doherty, M., Esko, T., Garcés Aletá, C.M., Gomez-Reino Carnota, J.J., Helgadottir, H., Hofman, A., Jonsdottir, I., Kerkhof, H.J.M., Kloppenburg, M., McCaskie, A., Ntzani, E.E., Ollier, W.E.R., Oreiro, N., Panoutsopoulou, K., Ralston, S.H., Ramos, Y.F., Riancho, J.A., Rivadeneira, F., Slagboom, P.E., Styrkarsdottir, U., Thorsteinsdottir, U., Thorleifsson, G., Tsezou, A., Uitterlinden, A.G., Wallis, G.A., Wilkinson, J.M., Zhai, G., Zhu, Y., arcOGEN Consortium, Felson, D.T., Ioannidis, J.P.A., Loughlin, J., Metspalu, A., Meulenbelt, I., Stefansson, K., van Meurs, J.B., Zeggini, E., Spector, T.D., Gonzalez, A., 2014. Assessment of osteoarthritis candidate genes in a meta-analysis of nine genome-wide association studies. Arthritis Rheumatol. (Hoboken, N.J.) 66, 940–949. http://dx.doi.org/10.1002/art.38300.

Rodríguez-Mañas, L., El-Assar, M., Vallejo, S., López-Dóriga, P., Solís, J., Petidier, R., Montes, M., Nevado, J., Castro, M., Gómez-Guerrero, C., Peiró, C., Sánchez-Ferrer, C.F., 2009. Endothelial dysfunction in aged humans is related with oxidative stress and vascular inflammation. Aging Cell 8, 226–238. http://dx.doi.org/10.1111/j.1474-9726.2009.00466.x.

Sanchez, C., Gabay, O., Salvat, C., Henrotin, Y.E., Berenbaum, F., 2009. Mechanical loading highly increases IL-6 production and decreases OPG expression by osteoblasts. Osteoarthr. Cartil. 17, 473–481. http://dx.doi.org/10.1016/j.joca.2008.09.007.

Schett, G., Kleyer, A., Perricone, C., Sahinbegovic, E., Iagnocco, A., Zwerina, J., Lorenzini, R., Aschenbrenner, F., Berenbaum, F., D'Agostino, M.-A., Willeit, J., Kiechl, S., 2013. Diabetes is an independent predictor for severe osteoarthritis: results from a longitudinal cohort study. Diabetes Care 36, 403–409. http://dx.doi.org/10.2337/dc12-0924.

Schieffer, B., Selle, T., Hilfiker, A., Hilfiker-Kleiner, D., Grote, K., Tietge, U.J.F., Trautwein, C., Luchtefeld, M., Schmittkamp, C., Heeneman, S., Daemen, M.J.A.P., Drexler, H., 2004. Impact of interleukin-6 on plaque development and morphology in experimental atherosclerosis. Circulation 110, 3493–3500. http://dx.doi.org/10.1161/01.CIR.0000148135.08582.97.

Scotece, M., Conde, J., Gómez, R., López, V., Pino, J., González, A., Lago, F., Gómez-Reino, J.J., Gualillo, O., 2012. Role of adipokines in atherosclerosis: interferences with cardiovascular complications in rheumatic diseases. Mediators Inflamm. 2012, 125458. http://dx.doi.org/10.1155/2012/125458.

Sellam, J., Berenbaum, F., 2010. The role of synovitis in pathophysiology and clinical symptoms of osteoarthritis. Nat. Rev. Rheumatol. 6, 625–635. http://dx.doi.org/10.1038/nrrheum.2010.159.

Shin, D., 2014. Association between metabolic syndrome, radiographic knee osteoarthritis, and intensity of knee pain: results of a national survey. J. Clin. Endocrinol. Metab. 99, 3177–3183. http://dx.doi.org/10.1210/jc.2014-1043.

Sierra-Johnson, J., Romero-Corral, A., Lopez-Jimenez, F., Gami, A.S., Sert Kuniyoshi, F.H., Wolk, R., Somers, V.K., 2007. Relation of increased leptin concentrations to history of myocardial infarction and stroke in the United States population. Am. J. Cardiol. 100, 234–239. http://dx.doi.org/10.1016/j.amjcard.2007.02.088.

Simopoulou, T., Malizos, K.N., Iliopoulos, D., Stefanou, N., Papatheodorou, L., Ioannou, M., Tsezou, A., 2007a. Differential expression of leptin and leptin's receptor isoform (Ob-Rb) mRNA between advanced and minimally affected osteoarthritic cartilage; effect on cartilage metabolism. Osteoarthr. Cartil. 15, 872–883. http://dx.doi.org/10.1016/j.joca.2007.01.018.

Simopoulou, T., Malizos, K.N., Tsezou, A., 2007b. Lectin-like oxidized low density lipoprotein receptor 1 (LOX-1) expression in human articular chondrocytes. Clin. Exp. Rheumatol. 25, 605–612.

Singh, P., Peterson, T.E., Sert-Kuniyoshi, F.H., Jensen, M.D., Somers, V.K., 2011. Leptin upregulates caveolin-1 expression: implications for development of atherosclerosis. Atherosclerosis 217, 499–502. http://dx.doi.org/10.1016/j.atherosclerosis.2010.10.012.

Sowers, M., Karvonen-Gutierrez, C.A., Palmieri-Smith, R., Jacobson, J.A., Jiang, Y., Ashton-Miller, J.A., 2009. Knee osteoarthritis in obese women with cardiometabolic clustering. Arthritis Rheum. 61, 1328–1336. http://dx.doi.org/10.1002/art.24739.

Spector, T.D., Cicuttini, F., Baker, J., Loughlin, J., Hart, D., 1996. Genetic influences on osteoarthritis in women: a twin study. BMJ 312, 940–943.

Srikanth, V.K., Fryer, J.L., Zhai, G., Winzenberg, T.M., Hosmer, D., Jones, G., 2005. A meta-analysis of sex differences prevalence, incidence and severity of osteoarthritis. Osteoarthr. Cartil. 13, 769–781. http://dx.doi.org/10.1016/j.joca.2005.04.014.

Stürmer, T., Sun, Y., Sauerland, S., Zeissig, I., Günther, K.P., Puhl, W., Brenner, H., 1998. Serum cholesterol and osteoarthritis. The baseline examination of the Ulm Osteoarthritis Study. J. Rheumatol. 25, 1827–1832.

Sudano, I., Flammer, A.J., Périat, D., Enseleit, F., Hermann, M., Wolfrum, M., Hirt, A., Kaiser, P., Hurlimann, D., Neidhart, M., Gay, S., Holzmeister, J., Nussberger, J., Mocharla, P., Landmesser, U., Haile, S.R., Corti, R., Vanhoutte, P.M., Lüscher, T.F., Noll, G., Ruschitzka, F., 2010. Acetaminophen increases blood pressure in patients with coronary artery disease. Circulation 122, 1789–1796. http://dx.doi.org/10.1161/CIRCULATIONAHA.110.956490.

Taleb, S., Herbin, O., Ait-Oufella, H., Verreth, W., Gourdy, P., Barateau, V., Merval, R., Esposito, B., Clément, K., Holvoet, P., Tedgui, A., Mallat, Z., 2007. Defective leptin/leptin receptor signaling improves regulatory T cell immune response and protects mice from atherosclerosis. Arterioscler. Thromb. Vasc. Biol. 27, 2691–2698. http://dx.doi.org/10.1161/ATVBAHA.107.149567.

Tang, W.H.W., Hazen, S.L., 2014. The contributory role of gut microbiota in cardiovascular disease. J. Clin. Invest. 124, 4204–4211. http://dx.doi.org/10.1172/JCI72331.

Tomi, A.-L., Sellam, J., Lacombe, K., Fellahi, S., Sebire, M., Rey-Jouvin, C., Miquel, A., Bastard, J.-P., Maheu, E., Haugen, I.K., Felson, D.T., Capeau, J., Girard, P.-M., Berenbaum, F., Meynard, J.-L., 2016. Increased prevalence and severity of radiographic hand osteoarthritis in patients with HIV-1 infection associated with metabolic syndrome: data from the cross-sectional METAFIB-OA study. Ann. Rheum. Dis.. http://dx.doi.org/10.1136/annrheumdis-2016-209262.

Tong, K.-M., Chen, C.-P., Huang, K.-C., Shieh, D.-C., Cheng, H.-C., Tzeng, C.-Y., Chen, K.-H., Chiu, Y.-C., Tang, C.-H., 2011. Adiponectin increases MMP-3 expression in human chondrocytes through AdipoR1 signaling pathway. J. Cell. Biochem. 112, 1431–1440. http://dx.doi.org/10.1002/jcb.23059.

Triantaphyllidou, I.-E., Kalyvioti, E., Karavia, E., Lilis, I., Kypreos, K.E., Papachristou, D.J., 2013. Perturbations in the HDL metabolic pathway predispose to the development of osteoarthritis in mice following long-term exposure to western-type diet. Osteoarthr. Cartil. 21, 322–330. http://dx.doi.org/10.1016/j.joca.2012.11.003.

Tsezou, A., Iliopoulos, D., Malizos, K.N., Simopoulou, T., 2010. Impaired expression of genes regulating cholesterol efflux in human osteoarthritic chondrocytes. J. Orthop. Res. 28, 1033–1039. http://dx.doi.org/10.1002/jor.21084.

Tsuchida, A.I., Beekhuizen, M., Rutgers, M., van Osch, G.J.V.M., Bekkers, J.E.J., Bot, A.G.J., Geurts, B., Dhert, W.J.A., Saris, D.B.F., Creemers, L.B., 2012. Interleukin-6 is elevated in synovial fluid of patients with focal cartilage defects and stimulates cartilage matrix production in an in vitro regeneration model. Arthritis Res. Ther. 14, R262. http://dx.doi.org/10.1186/ar4107.

Tsuchida, A.I., Beekhuizen, M., 't Hart, M.C., Radstake, T.R.D.J., Dhert, W.J.A., Saris, D.B.F., van Osch, G.J.V.M., Creemers, L.B., 2014. Cytokine profiles in the joint depend on pathology, but are different between synovial fluid, cartilage tissue and cultured chondrocytes. Arthritis Res. Ther. 16, 441. http://dx.doi.org/10.1186/s13075-014-0441-0.

Valdes, A.M., Arden, N.K., Tamm, A., Kisand, K., Doherty, S., Pola, E., Cooper, C., Tamm, A., Muir, K.R., Kerna, I., Hart, D., O'Neil, F., Zhang, W., Spector, T.D., Maciewicz, R.A., Doherty, M., 2010. A meta-analysis of interleukin-6 promoter polymorphisms on risk of hip and knee osteoarthritis. Osteoarthr. Cartil. 18, 699–704. http://dx.doi.org/10.1016/j.joca.2009.12.012.

Verbruggen, G., Wittoek, R., Vander Cruyssen, B., Elewaut, D., 2012. Tumour necrosis factor blockade for the treatment of erosive osteoarthritis of the interphalangeal finger joints: a double blind, randomised trial on structure modification. Ann. Rheum. Dis. 71, 891–898. http://dx.doi.org/10.1136/ard.2011.149849.

Veronese, N., Trevisan, C., De Rui, M., Bolzetta, F., Maggi, S., Zambon, S., Musacchio, E., Sartori, L., Perissinotto, E., Crepaldi, G., Manzato, E., Sergi, G., 2016. Association of osteoarthritis with increased risk of cardiovascular diseases in the elderly: findings from the progetto veneto anziano study cohort. Arthritis Rheumatol. (Hoboken, N.J.) 68, 1136–1144. http://dx.doi.org/10.1002/art.39564.

Verzijl, N., DeGroot, J., Ben, Z.C., Brau-Benjamin, O., Maroudas, A., Bank, R.A., Mizrahi, J., Schalkwijk, C.G., Thorpe, S.R., Baynes, J.W., Bijlsma, J.W.J., Lafeber, F.P.J.G., TeKoppele, J.M., 2002. Crosslinking by advanced glycation end products increases the stiffness of the collagen network in human articular cartilage: a possible mechanism through which age is a risk factor for osteoarthritis. Arthritis Rheum. 46, 114–123. http://dx.doi.org/10.1002/1529-0131(200201)46:1<114::AID-ART10025>3.0.CO;2-P.

Verzijl, N., DeGroot, J., Oldehinkel, E., Bank, R.A., Thorpe, S.R., Baynes, J.W., Bayliss, M.T., Bijlsma, J.W., Lafeber, F.P., Tekoppele, J.M., 2000. Age-related accumulation of Maillard reaction products in human articular cartilage collagen. Biochem. J. 350 (2), 381–387.

Visser, A.W., de Mutsert, R., le Cessie, S., den Heijer, M., Rosendaal, F.R., Kloppenburg, M., for the NEO Study Group, 2014. The relative contribution of mechanical stress and systemic processes in different types of osteoarthritis: the NEO study. Ann. Rheum. Dis. http://dx.doi.org/10.1136/annrheumdis-2013-205012.

Vuolteenaho, K., Koskinen, A., Kukkonen, M., Nieminen, R., Päivärinta, U., Moilanen, T., Moilanen, E., 2009. Leptin enhances synthesis of proinflammatory mediators in human osteoarthritic cartilage—mediator role of NO in leptin-induced PGE2, IL-6, and IL-8 production. Mediators Inflamm. 2009, 345838. http://dx.doi.org/10.1155/2009/345838.

Wang, K., Dong, P.S., Zhang, H.F., Li, Z.J., Yang, X.M., Liu, H., 2015. Role of interleukin-6 gene polymorphisms in the risk of coronary artery disease. Genet. Mol. Res. 14, 3177—3183. http://dx.doi.org/10.4238/2015.April.10.29.

Wang, Q., Rozelle, A.L., Lepus, C.M., Scanzello, C.R., Song, J.J., Larsen, D.M., Crish, J.F., Bebek, G., Ritter, S.Y., Lindstrom, T.M., Hwang, I., Wong, H.H., Punzi, L., Encarnacion, A., Shamloo, M., Goodman, S.B., Wyss-Coray, T., Goldring, S.R., Banda, N.K., Thurman, J.M., Gobezie, R., Crow, M.K., Holers, V.M., Lee, D.M., Robinson, W.H., 2011. Identification of a central role for complement in osteoarthritis. Nat. Med. 17, 1674—1679. http://dx.doi.org/10.1038/nm.2543.

Webb, G.R., Westacott, C.I., Elson, C.J., 1997. Chondrocyte tumor necrosis factor receptors and focal loss of cartilage in osteoarthritis. Osteoarthr. Cartil. 5, 427—437.

Wei, J., Xu, H., Davies, J.L., Hemmings, G.P., 1992. Increase of plasma IL-6 concentration with age in healthy subjects. Life Sci. 51, 1953—1956.

Witteman, J.C., Grobbee, D.E., Kok, F.J., Hofman, A., Valkenburg, H.A., 1989. Increased risk of atherosclerosis in women after the menopause. BMJ 298, 642—644.

Woolf, A.D., Pfleger, B., 2003. Burden of major musculoskeletal conditions. Bull. World Health Organ. 81, 646—656.

Yamabe, S., Hirose, J., Uehara, Y., Okada, T., Okamoto, N., Oka, K., Taniwaki, T., Mizuta, H., 2013. Intracellular accumulation of advanced glycation end products induces apoptosis via endoplasmic reticulum stress in chondrocytes. FEBS J. 280, 1617—1629. http://dx.doi.org/10.1111/febs.12170.

Yamauchi, T., Kamon, J., Waki, H., Terauchi, Y., Kubota, N., Hara, K., Mori, Y., Ide, T., Murakami, K., Tsuboyama-Kasaoka, N., Ezaki, O., Akanuma, Y., Gavrilova, O., Vinson, C., Reitman, M.L., Kagechika, H., Shudo, K., Yoda, M., Nakano, Y., Tobe, K., Nagai, R., Kimura, S., Tomita, M., Froguel, P., Kadowaki, T., 2001. The fat-derived hormone adiponectin reverses insulin resistance associated with both lipoatrophy and obesity. Nat. Med. 7, 941—946. http://dx.doi.org/10.1038/90984.

Yammani, R.R., Loeser, R.F., 2012. Extracellular nicotinamide phosphoribosyltransferase (NAMPT/visfatin) inhibits insulin-like growth factor-1 signaling and proteoglycan synthesis in human articular chondrocytes. Arthritis Res. Ther. 14, R23. http://dx.doi.org/10.1186/ar3705.

Yang, S., Ryu, J.-H., Oh, H., Jeon, J., Kwak, J.-S., Kim, J.-H., Kim, H.A., Chun, C.-H., Chun, J.-S., 2015. NAMPT (visfatin), a direct target of hypoxia-inducible factor-2α, is an essential catabolic regulator of osteoarthritis. Ann. Rheum. Dis. 74, 595—602. http://dx.doi.org/10.1136/annrheumdis-2013-204355.

Yoshimura, N., Muraki, S., Oka, H., Tanaka, S., Kawaguchi, H., Nakamura, K., Akune, T., 2012. Accumulation of metabolic risk factors such as overweight, hypertension, dyslipidaemia, and impaired glucose tolerance raises the risk of occurrence and progression of knee osteoarthritis: a 3-year follow-up of the ROAD study. Osteoarthr. Cartil. 20, 1217—1226. http://dx.doi.org/10.1016/j.joca.2012.06.006.

Yusuf, E., Ioan-Facsinay, A., Bijsterbosch, J., Klein-Wieringa, I., Kwekkeboom, J., Slagboom, P.E., Huizinga, T.W.J., Kloppenburg, M., 2011. Association between leptin, adiponectin and resistin and long-term progression of hand osteoarthritis. Ann. Rheum. Dis. 70, 1282—1284. http://dx.doi.org/10.1136/ard.2010.146282.

Yusuf, E., Nelissen, R.G., Ioan-Facsinay, A., Stojanovic-Susulic, V., DeGroot, J., van Osch, G., Middeldorp, S., Huizinga, T.W.J., Kloppenburg, M., 2010. Association between weight or body mass index and hand osteoarthritis: a systematic review. Ann. Rheum. Dis. 69, 761—765. http://dx.doi.org/10.1136/ard.2008.106930.

Yusuf, S., Hawken, S., Ounpuu, S., Dans, T., Avezum, A., Lanas, F., McQueen, M., Budaj, A., Pais, P., Varigos, J., Lisheng, L., INTERHEART Study Investigators, 2004. Effect of potentially modifiable risk factors associated with myocardial infarction in 52 countries (the INTERHEART study): case-control study. Lancet 364, 937–952. http://dx.doi.org/10.1016/S0140-6736(04)17018-9.

Zeidan, A., Purdham, D.M., Rajapurohitam, V., Javadov, S., Chakrabarti, S., Karmazyn, M., 2005. Leptin induces vascular smooth muscle cell hypertrophy through angiotensin II- and endothelin-1-dependent mechanisms and mediates stretch-induced hypertrophy. J. Pharmacol. Exp. Ther. 315, 1075–1084. http://dx.doi.org/10.1124/jpet.105.091561.

Zhang, Y., Proenca, R., Maffei, M., Barone, M., Leopold, L., Friedman, J.M., 1994. Positional cloning of the mouse obese gene and its human homologue. Nature 372, 425–432. http://dx.doi.org/10.1038/372425a0.

Zuo, W., Wu, Z.-H., Wu, N., Duan, Y.-H., Wu, J.-T., Wang, H., Qiu, G.-X., 2011. Adiponectin receptor 1 mediates the difference in adiponectin- induced prostaglandin E2 production in rheumatoid arthritis and osteoarthritis synovial fibroblasts. Chin. Med. J. 124, 3919–3924.

Chapter 20

Cardiac Effects of Antirheumatic Drugs

Z. Szekanecz
Department of Rheumatology, Faculty of Medicine, University of Debrecen, Debrecen, Hungary

Key Points

- Increased cardio- and cerebrovascular morbidity and mortality have been associated with inflammatory rheumatic diseases.
- Systemic inflammation, as well as traditional risk factors account for accelerated atherosclerosis.
- There may be differences among nonsteroidal antiinflammatory drugs in causing cardiovascular complications.
- Corticosteroids may have both beneficial and detrimental effects on the vascular system.
- Traditional and biologic disease-modifying antirheumatic drugs may suppress systemic inflammation and thus they may have beneficial effects on atherosclerosis.
- Heart failure, arrhythmias, and hypertension should also be considered.

1. INTRODUCTION

Accelerated atherosclerosis, various other types of vasculopathies, and increased cardiovascular (CV) risk have become major factors of mortality in inflammatory rheumatic diseases. Such diseases include rheumatoid arthritis (RA), spondyloarthropathies (SpA) including ankylosing spondylitis (AS) and psoriatic arthritis (PsA), systemic lupus erythematosus (SLE), antiphospholipid syndrome (APS), systemic sclerosis (SSc, scleroderma), systemic vasculitides, and possibly other chronic conditions (Szekanecz et al., 2007; Shoenfeld et al., 2005; Kaplan, 2009). Both classical CV risk factors, as well as systemic inflammation have been implicated in atherosclerosis associated with these rheumatic diseases (Shoenfeld et al., 2005; Szekanecz et al., 2007; Giles et al., 2006; Kaplan, 2009; Choy et al., 2014).

As sustained autoimmunity and inflammatory disease activity may be the predominant risk factors for vascular diseases underlying rheumatic conditions, after risk assessment, optimal prevention and management are needed in order to minimize CV risk. First, vasculoprotective agents including aspirin, statins, angiotensin-converting enzyme (ACE) inhibitors, folate, or vitamin B12 could be introduced to rheumatic patients at a higher vascular risk (Bruce, 2005a; Maki-Petaja et al., 2007). Yet, the effective control of the underlying rheumatic disease may be even more important. Nonsteroidal antiinflammatory drugs (NSAIDs), corticosteroids, traditional disease-modifying antirheumatic drugs (DMARDs), and targeted therapies may attenuate systemic inflammation and they may also have effects on the vasculature (Table 20.1) (Atzeni et al., 2010; Turiel et al., 2010; Suissa et al., 2006; van Halm et al., 2006; Szekanecz et al., 2009; Gasparyan et al., 2012; Ketelhuth and Hansson, 2015).

For a long time, there have been no official recommendations for the prevention and treatment of vascular disease in autoimmune rheumatic diseases. After some preliminary recommendations in RA and SLE (Bruce, 2005a; Giles et al., 2006; Klareskog and Hamsten, 2004; Van Doornum et al., 2006; Atzeni et al., 2010), in 2009, the European League Against Rheumatism (EULAR) has set up a task force that has prepared 10 recommendations for CV risk management in arthritis including RA and SpA. Apart from other recommendations, the EULAR task force suggests that adequate control of disease activity is necessary to lower the CV disease (CVD) risk. These recommendations have recently been updated (Nurmohamed, 2015).

In this chapter, we summarize recent, sometimes controversial data on the CV and metabolic effects of antiinflammatory agents, traditional DMARDs, and targeted therapies. Most data have become available when these treatments were administered to rheumatic patients. However, a few larger trials have also been initiated in solely CV patients. We will also discuss other heart diseases, such as hypertension, arrhythmias, and congestive heart failure. Finally, we will briefly present the original and updated EULAR CV recommendations, as well as other national recommendations.

2. ATHEROSCLEROSIS AND METABOLIC SYNDROME

2.1 Nonsteroidal Antiinflammatory Drugs

After the withdrawal of rofecoxib from the market due to increased incidence of CVD, a lot of attention has been paid to both traditional NSAIDs and coxibs (Atzeni et al., 2010). Earlier reports suggested that not only coxibs, but nonselective NSAIDs might also increase CV risk (Liu et al., 2010; Kearney et al., 2006; McGettigan and Henry, 2006; Nurmohamed et al., 2002; Atzeni et al., 2010). In the meta-analysis of Kearney et al. (2006) coxibs were

TABLE 20.1 **Cardiovascular Effects of Antirheumatic Drugs (Gasparyan et al., 2012; Ketelhuth and Hansson, 2015)**

Drug	Preclinical	Clinical
NSAIDs		↑ Increased CV risk ↑ Hypertension ↑ Heart failure ↑ Arrhythmias
Corticosteroids		↑ CV risk ↑ Hypertension ↑ Hyperglycemia. Diabetes ↑ Heart failure ↑ Arrhythmias
Antimalarials		↓ CV risk ↑ Conduction disorders
Sulfasalazine		↑ Thrombocytopenia
Methotrexate	↓ Atherosclerosis in rabbits	↓ CV risk ↑ Hypotension ↑ Pericarditis
Leflunomide		↑ Hypertension
Cyclosporin A		↑ Hypertension
TNFα blockers	↓ Atherosclerosis in mice, rabbits	↓ CV risk ↓ Insulin resistance ↓ Platelet activation ↓ Endothelial cell adhesion molecules ↑ Heart failure (NYHA III-IV) ↑ Dyslipidaemia ↑ Hypertension ↑ Infusion-related (if intravenous)
Rituximab	↓ Atherosclerosis in mice	↑ Infusion-related
Tocilizumab		↑ Dyslipidemia ↑ Infusion-related
Abatacept	↓ Atherosclerosis in mice ↓ Blood pressure in mice	↑ Hypertension ↑ Infusion-related
Canakinumab	↓ Atherosclerosis in mice	↑ Endothelial function ↓ Proatherogenic biomarkers
Tofacitinib		↑ Dyslipidaemia

associated with a 42% relative increase in the incidence of serious vascular events in comparison to placebo. The overall incidence of serious CV complications was comparable between any coxib and any traditional NSAID. Among traditional NSAIDs, high doses of ibuprofen and diclofenac but not those of naproxen were associated with a moderate increase in the risk of vascular events. In the systematic review of McGettigan and Henry (2006) 17 case-control and six cohort studies were included. Here a dose-related, increased risk was associated with rofecoxib (RR of 1.33 and 2.19 at doses ≤25 mg/day and >25 mg/day, respectively). Among nonselective NSAIDs, diclofenac had the highest risk of 1.4, while naproxen, piroxicam, and ibuprofen had relative risks close to 1.0. Suissa et al. (2006) conducted a nested case-control analysis on more than 100,000 subjects. The use of nonselective NSAIDs or COX-2 inhibitors was not associated with increased myocardial infarction (MI) rates (RR 1.05 and 1.11, respectively). However, rofecoxib itself, but not celecoxib and naproxen, exerted an increased MI rate of 1.26. These analyses were published in 2006. In order to address this issue in more complexity, in 2008, Scott et al. (2007) performed a systematic review of 18 randomized controlled trials (RCTs) and 20 observational studies. The odds ratio (OR) for MI of all COX-2 inhibitors was 1.6; however, most of this risk was accounted for by rofecoxib. No or very modest increases in MI risk were observed with use of other NSAIDs (Table 20.1).

In 2015, Roubille et al. performed a meta-analysis of more than 15 large trials in order to determine the CV risk of NSAID use in RA, psoriasis, or PsA. The all-CV morbidity RR values of all NSAIDs, COX-2 inhibitors, or non-coxib NSAIDs were 1.18 (1.01; 1.38), 1.36 (1.10; 1.67), and 1.08 (0.94; 1.24), respectively. With respect to MI, stroke, and major CV events (MACE), RR values were 1.13 (0.93; 1.37), 2.15 (1.19; 3.87), and 1.56 (0.82; 2.97). Thus there is clear signal that NSAIDs, especially coxibs, increase the risk of all types of CV morbidity (Roubille et al., 2015a).

In contrast, Tsai et al. (2015) assessed CV risk in SpA patients undergoing long-term NSAID treatment. It has become clear, that some NSAIDs, contrary to RA, may exert disease-modifying action in SpA (Wanders et al., 2005; Ardoin and Sundy, 2006). As systemic inflammation is the major driver of atherosclerosis and CVD both in RA and in SpA, halting disease progression in SpA may have beneficial effects on the vasculature. Indeed, Tsai et al. (2015), longer versus shorter use of NSAIDs including coxibs in SpA resulted in decreased CV morbidity.

As seen above, there have been lots of controversies with respect to the CV effects of NSAIDs. Recent studies also suggested that the CV risk of NSAIDs may be different in inflammatory diseases, such as RA and the general population. Some studies suggest that NSAIDs that exert an unfavorable CV profile in otherwise healthy individuals may not increase CV risk in RA patients, where the antiinflammatory effects of NSAIDs may override their harmful CV effects (Sfikakis et al., 2014; Lindhardsen et al., 2013; Goodson et al., 2009). For example, in a Danish cohort, the CV risk associated with NSAID use was actually lower [RR 1.22 (1.09; 1.37)] than in controls [RR 1.51 (1.36; 1.66)] (Lindhardsen et al., 2013).

In addition, one should consider which NSAID is actually in question. Rofecoxib may be the only NSAID that equivocally increased CV risk in most studies. Studies on other NSAIDs, such as naproxen or diclofenac yielded to highly controversial results (Sfikakis et al., 2014; Ferraz-Amaro et al., 2009; Lindhardsen et al., 2013; van Walsem et al., 2015).

Another controversial issue is the possible interactions between NSAIDs and the cardioprotective effects of aspirin. Some studies suggested that ibuprofen might suppress the effects of aspirin by competing for the same COX-1—binding site on platelets (Li et al., 2010). This speculation was later confirmed in an epidemiologic study (Norris et al., 2010). This issue has not yet been addressed in meta-analyses and systematic reviews.

Therefore, from the CV perspective, long-term use of any NSAID is not recommended, especially in the elderly and in patients with history of CVD or in the presence of CV risk factors (Simmonds et al., 2009; Banfi et al., 2010; Zhang et al., 2005; Nurmohamed et al., 2002). According to the 2010 EULAR CV recommendations and the recent update, in RA and PsA, traditional NSAID and coxib use should be very cautious especially in patients with documented CV disease or in the presence of CV risk factors (Peters et al., 2010a; Nurmohamed, 2015). In AS, NSAIDs are recommended as first-line treatment in patients with pain and stiffness unless NSAIDs are contraindicated (Nurmohamed, 2015).

2.2 Corticosteroids

Half of UK patients with RA are prescribed corticosteroids in the primary care setting (Black et al., 2015)! Corticosteroids themselves are atherogenic by influencing body fat distribution, blood pressure, and glucose metabolism leading to obesity, dyslipidemia, hypertension, and diabetes mellitus (Table 20.1) (Bruce, 2005a; Roos et al., 2010; Maxwell et al., 1994; Atzeni et al., 2010; Buttgereit et al., 2009; Konijn et al., 2015). According to a very recent study, corticosteroid treatment exerted an unfavorable effect on body composition by increasing BMI and body fat mass in early RA patients (Konijn et al., 2015). On the other hand, pulsed corticosteroid treatment reduced the levels of the proatherogenic homocysteine in RA patients (Lazzerini et al., 2003). Controversy arises from the dual action of glucocorticoids, as they are atherogenic, but also antiinflammatory (Roos et al., 2010; Petri et al., 1994; Atzeni et al., 2010; Karp et al., 2008; Maxwell et al., 1994; Buttgereit et al., 2009). For example, in SLE, both inflammatory activity and recent corticosteroid use have been independently associated with CVD (Karp et al., 2008). In RA, combination therapy that included prednisolone rapidly improved the total cholesterol (TC)/HDL-C index in RA patients (Nurmohamed et al., 2002).

In a recent case-control study, 202 corticosteroid-treated RA patients were compared to 436 RA patients not treated with corticosteroids. Corticosteroids administered at ≥7.5 mg/day increased HDL-C levels, while LDL-C and the atherogenic index did not change (Schroeder et al., 2015). With respect to imaging, steroid pulse therapy impaired FMD in patients with IgA nephropathy (Uchida et al., 2006).

In an earlier systematic review that assessed the effects of corticosteroid use on the vasculature in RA, only a weak association between low-dose corticosteroid therapy and CV risk factors was established (Wu et al., 2004). Although it is rather difficult to determine, whether the favorable antiinflammatory effects of glucocorticoids would override their potential proatherogenic nature, there is a growing body of evidence that inflammatory factors associated with more active SLE or RA may exert higher risk for atherosclerosis than corticosteroid treatment (Karp et al., 2008; Roos et al., 2010; Maxwell et al., 1994; Nurmohamed et al., 2002). The net effect of corticosteroids may also be dose related. For example, low doses did not affect lipid levels, while a daily dose >10 mg increased serum triglyceride and LDL-C concentrations (Roos et al., 2010; Bruce, 2005a).

Ajeganova et al. (2014) assessed CV outcome in patients treated with 7.5 mg/day prednisone combined with DMARD versus DMARD alone during the first 2 years after RA diagnosis. In this inception cohort, the incidence of CVD was similar in the two groups; however, the long-term risk of ischemic cerebrovascular events was higher in the corticosteroid group. In addition, there was a tendency toward reduced survival in the prednisone group (Ajeganova et al., 2014).

In a recent real-life Dutch cohort, van Sijl et al. (2014) reported that corticosteroid use including longer duration of exposure or cumulative exposure was associated with elevated CV risk. However, adjustment for disease activity negated this association. Thus, stratification of corticosteroid use for disease activity may be crucial from the CV perspective. In a cohort of almost 400 RA patients, Toms et al. (2008) did not find any association between corticosteroid use and metabolic syndrome in RA. Thus, the beneficial effects of corticosteroids on inflammation may outweigh their harmful CV effects.

In the 2015 analysis of Roubille et al. described above, at least 10 large studies were included. Corticosteroids increased the risk of all CV events, MI, stroke, and MACE with RR values of 1.47 (134; 1.60), 1.41 (1.22; 1.63), 1.57 (1.05; 2.35), and 1.62 (1.22; 2.16), respectively. However, this meta-analysis was later criticized by Boers (2015) who in a meta-analysis of 4381 patients could not find increased CV risk. In this paper, Boers questioned that mostly observational data were included in the other study. Therefore, whether corticosteroids are harmful or beneficial from this aspect remains to be determined.

With respect to optimal corticosteroid dose, del Rincon et al. (2014) determined the daily threshold dose of 8 mg, above which the number of deaths increased in a dose-dependent manner. Thus, also from the CV point of view, glucocorticoid doses of <8 mg/day may be considered safe (del Rincon et al., 2014).

The EULAR CV recommendations suggest to use the lowest dose possible (Peters et al., 2010a). According to the latest update, glucocorticoid dosage should be kept to a minimum and tapering should be attempted in case of low disease activity and remission (Nurmohamed, 2015). Thus, although much controversy has arisen with respect to the atherogenic or atheroprotective effects of corticosteroids during the treatment of arthritides, these drugs should be used with caution. Yet, the potential CV risk associated with glucocorticoids should be different in inflammatory and noninflammatory states (Toms et al., 2008; van Sijl et al., 2014).

2.3 Traditional Disease-Modifying Drugs

2.3.1 Antimalarial Drugs

In contrast to corticosteroids, antimalarial drugs, such as chloroquine (CQ) and hydroxychloroquine (HCQ), may exert evident antiatherogenic properties (Table 20.1) (Petri et al., 1994; Tam et al., 2000; Apte, 2009; Borba and Bonfa, 2001; Espinola et al., 2002; Ruiz-Irastorza et al., 2010; van Halm et al., 2006; Choy et al., 2014). These agents are used to treat mild to moderate SLE and RA (Ruiz-Irastorza et al., 2010; van Halm et al., 2006). In RA, antimalarials are usually part of traditional DMARD combinations (Rainsford et al., 2015; Smolen et al., 2013). HCQ therapy has been associated with lower serum total cholesterol levels (Petri et al., 1994). Antimalarials may also reduce LDL-C, VLDL-C and, in corticosteroid-treated patients, triglyceride (TG) production (Tam et al., 2000; Apte, 2009; Borba and Bonfa, 2001; Bruce, 2005b; Morris et al., 2011). In a recent study, HCQ users exerted significantly lower TC, LDL-C, and TG levels, as well as TC/HDL-C ratio compared to HCQ nonusers. There was no difference between the two groups in HDL-C levels (Kerr et al., 2014). HCQ may also improve glucose homeostasis (Hage et al., 2014). In vitro studies also suggest that antimalarials may inhibit platelet aggregation and the thrombogenic effects of antiphospholipid antibodies (Espinola et al., 2002).

Thus, antimalarials may be vasculoprotective in various rheumatic diseases, especially when coprescribed with corticosteroids (Bruce, 2005b).

2.3.2 Sulfasalazine

There is very little information available regarding the possible vascular or metabolic effects of sulfasalazine (SASP). In a case-control study, SASP was associated with somewhat lower CVD risk compared to RA patients who never used SASP, HCQ, or MTX (van Halm et al., 2006). In animal studies, SASP prolonged graft survival and prevented ischemia reperfusion injury in cardiac transplants (Feeley et al., 1999). SASP may also exert its antiinflammatory activity by inducing the release of adenosine (Furuichi et al., 2000). Folate supplementation to SASP therapy may reduce homocysteine production and thus it may also be vasculoprotective in arthritis (Baskan et al., 2009).

Today, SASP is mainly used in combination, therefore it is very difficult to determine the net CV effects of this compound (Atzeni et al., 2010).

2.3.3 Methotrexate

The vascular effects of methotrexate (MTX) may also be somewhat controversial. MTX itself increases the production of the proatherogenic homocysteine. Homocysteine is toxic for endothelial cells and stimulates LDL oxidation. Folate supplementation suppresses the atherogenic effects of homocysteine. On the other hand, MTX, like corticosteroids, controls systemic inflammation and thus may exert beneficial CV effects (Van Doornum et al., 2002). In recent studies, MTX reduced, rather than aggravated CV risk (Table 20.1) (Micha et al., 2011; Marks and Edwards, 2012; Westlake et al., 2010).

MTX has several vascular and metabolic actions. It improves reverse cholesterol transport and inhibits the formation of foam cells (Reiss et al., 2008). In recent studies, MTX restored ABCG1-mediated, high disease activity—related impairment of cholesterol efflux in RA (Ronda et al., 2015; 2014). MTX does not increase lipid levels and exerts no effect on platelet function (Micha et al., 2011; Marks and Edwards, 2012). In a single, small study, MTX was able to reduce carotid atherosclerosis in RA (Kim et al., 2015).

It is well known that in RA MTX acts by increasing adenosine release. In a recent study carried out in an animal model of vasculopathy and in in vitro endothelial cell systems, MTX induced adenosine monophosphate—activated protein kinase (AMPK). MTX attenuated vasculopathy in the animal model. Furthermore, MTX also suppressed endothelial injury via the AMPK pathway (Thornton et al., 2016).

All-cause CVD morbidity was reduced by MTX in most studies. There was a trend toward reduced incidence of stroke, while data on MI and metabolic syndrome, were rather inconclusive (Micha et al., 2011; Marks and Edwards, 2012). In an earlier study, Suissa et al. (2006) reported that the use of MTX was associated with significantly lower rate of MI (RR 0.81) in comparison to RA patients not receiving MTX monotherapy.

Baseline inflammatory markers, carotid atherosclerosis and the number of CV risk factors may predict rapid progression of atherosclerosis in RA. MTX treatment significantly slowed down this progression (del Rincon et al., 2015).

Roubille et al. (2015a) have recently performed a meta-analysis of eight studies assessing CV risk of MTX in RA, psoriasis, and PsA. MTX reduced the risk of all CV events, MI, stroke, and MACE showing RR values of 0.72 (0.57; 0.91), 0.81 (0.68; 0.96), 0.78 (0.40; 1.50), and 0.38 (0.05; 2.84), respectively (Roubille et al., 2015a). In the 2015 meta-analysis of De Vecchis et al. (2016), MTX significantly decreased the risk of MACE with an OR of 0.73 (0.70; 0.77).

Studies described above have been carried out in arthritis patients. However, as most pathways inhibited by MTX are involved in the pathogenesis of atherosclerosis, some hard endpoint CV trials have also been initiated in patients with CVD. One of these trials that assesses the effects of MTX on CV outcome is the CIRT trial that is currently still recruiting (Ridker, 2014; Ridker and Luscher, 2014).

In conclusion, the net effects of MTX in arthritis may be vasculoprotective. The recent EULAR recommendations suggest the administration of MTX in order to suppress systemic inflammation and prevent CVD (Peters et al., 2010a).

2.3.4 Leflunomide

In general, leflunomide, similarly to other DMARDs, suppress systemic inflammation that may be beneficial with regards to CVD. Leflunomide inhibits the NFκB signal transduction pathway that is critically involved in both systemic inflammation and atherogenesis (Feng et al., 2005; Minoretti et al., 2007). Leflunomide also interferes with leukocyte-endothelial adhesion (Grisar et al., 2004; Minoretti et al., 2007). Leflunomide use was associated with a significantly lower rate of MI in comparison to RA patients receiving other medications (RR 0.28) (Suissa et al., 2006).

One additional proof for the vasculoprotective effect of this drug is the use of leflunomide-eluting stents in invasive cardiology. Leflunomide stents preserved endothelial proliferation, improved arterial healing, and were found to be safe in clinical studies (Tanaka et al., 2010).

Thus, in contrast to some earlier studies, leflunomide may be vasculoprotective in RA.

2.4 Targeted Therapies

2.4.1 Anti-TNF Biologics

Numerous reports have suggested that tumor necrosis factor α (TNFα) inhibitors may have variable effects on the vasculature and lipid profile in RA patients (Table 20.1) (Roubille et al., 2013; Szekanecz et al., 2009).

TNFα has been implicated in almost all stages of atherogenesis. It exerts major proinflammatory, metabolic, and proatherogenic effects suggesting that TNF blockade may have favorable effects on the vasculature. TNFα is released by inflammatory leukocytes, as well as vascular endothelial and smooth muscle cells. TNFα promotes the endothelial expression of cellular adhesion molecules and thus the migration of leukocytes into and through the vessel wall (Greenberg et al., 2011; Szekanecz, 2008; Ross, 1999; Popa et al., 2007a;

Szekanecz et al., 2016). TNFα has been associated with the incidence of insulin resistance, dyslipidemia, and obesity (Szekanecz, 2008; Popa et al., 2007a; Szekanecz et al., 2016). Very recently, high TNFα expression has been documented in the aortic adventitia of RA patients with CVD (Ahmed et al., 2016).

Regarding surrogate markers of vascular pathology, the first vascular imaging study was published in 2002. Here brachial artery flow-mediated vasodilation (FMD), a marker of endothelial function (Kerekes et al., 2012), was assessed in 11 patients with active RA before and after 12 weeks of infliximab therapy. Infliximab improved FMD, which was accompanied by decreased CRP levels (Hurlimann et al., 2002). In following short-term studies infliximab treatment also resulted in rapid but transient improvement of FMD (Bosello et al., 2008; Bilsborough et al., 2006; Gonzalez-Juanatey et al., 2004; Tremblay et al., 2005). Unfortunately, this effect was reversible and FMD returned to baseline some weeks after infusion (Bosello et al., 2008; Gonzalez-Juanatey et al., 2004). Regarding other TNF blockers, adalimumab treatment in RA resulted in a rapid increase of FMD, which was sustained for 12 weeks. Improvement of endothelial function was accompanied by decrease of clinical activity and systemic inflammation (Gonzalez-Juanatey et al., 2006; Sidiropoulos et al., 2009). In one long-term study, 18 months of infliximab or adalimumab therapy in RA resulted in sustained improvement of FMD (Baba et al., 2007). In a comparative study, infliximab, etanercept, and adalimumab therapy in RA yielded to long-term improvement (>2 years) of FMD in 25%, 60%, and 100% of patients, respectively (Capria et al., 2010). We have also reported that adalimumab treatment significantly improved FMD in early RA patients (Kerekes et al., 2011).

Manifest atherosclerosis may be assessed by common carotid artery intima-media thickness (ccIMT) and carotid plaque (Kerekes et al., 2012; Damjanov et al., 2014). TNFα has been associated with increased ccIMT (Skoog et al., 2002). In one study, infliximab or etanercept therapy significantly improved ccIMT on both after long-term treatment of RA patients. These vascular effects were preceded by an early and lasting decrease in disease activity markers (Del Porto et al., 2007). In our hands, adalimumab treatment significantly decreased ccIMT in patients with early RA (Kerekes et al., 2011). In contrast, in another studies, infliximab, adalimumab, or etanercept treatment of RA patients did not affect ccIMT at all (Wong et al., 2009; Takashima et al., 2005; Turiel et al., 2010). In a recent study in AS, after a mean 4.9 years of treatment duration, ccIMT did not progress in patients continuing anti-TNF therapy, while ccIMT further increased in those who discontinued treatment (van Sijl et al., 2015). Thus, data are rather conflicting regarding the effects of TNFα blockers on carotid atherosclerosis (Tam et al., 2014). It is possible that the effects of biologics on carotid atherosclerosis is more prominent in early compared to long-standing RA. In addition, changes in ccIMT may require longer follow-up (Szekanecz et al., 2009; Tam et al.,

2014). TNF blockade also significantly halted the progression of atherosclerosis as determined by ccIMT (del Rincon et al., 2015).

Infliximab, adalimumab, or etanercept therapy of RA patients significantly reduced arterial stiffness indicated by pulse-wave velocity (PWV) (Maki-Petaja et al., 2006; Cypiene et al., 2007; Galarraga et al., 2009; Kerekes et al., 2012; Damjanov et al., 2014; Kume et al., 2011; Tam et al., 2014; Vassilopoulos et al., 2015; Wong et al., 2009). In a long-term cohort, 56-week infliximab treatment in RA resulted in a significant decrease of PWV (Wong et al., 2009). We have also reported that adalimumab treatment significantly improved PWV in early RA patients (Kerekes et al., 2011). However, in another study, when RA patients were treated with either infliximab, etanercept, or adalimumab, despite significant clinical response and reduction of inflammation, there was no change in arterial stiffness (Van Doornum et al., 2005). Thus, results on arterial stiffness are also rather controversial. Biologic effects on PWV, similar to ccIMT may require more time in comparison to rapid FMD changes (Szekanecz et al., 2009). One recent study also suggests that the beneficial effect of TNF inhibition on arterial stiffness may also be independent of its effect on disease activity (Vassilopoulos et al., 2015).

Among metabolic effects, most anti-TNFs influence lipid profile but not the TC/HDL-C atherogenic index (AI) (Robertson et al., 2013; Kerekes et al., 2014; Choy et al., 2014). In most studies, short-term infliximab treatment of RA or SpA patients variably influenced HDL-C, LDL-C, TC, and TG levels; however, AI remained unchanged in all these studies (Kiortsis et al., 2006; Vis et al., 2005; Tam et al., 2007; Seriolo et al., 2006; Soubrier et al., 2008; Daien et al., 2012; Damjanov et al., 2014; Popa et al., 2005; 2007b). Adalimumab treatment resulted in significantly increased HDL-C levels, while LDL-C and TG levels did not change (Popa et al., 2005). In another cohort, adalimumab also reduced the AI in RA patients (Gonzalez-Juanatey et al., 2006). In a comparative study of RA and SpA patients, while infliximab treatment increased TC and LDL-C levels, etanercept significantly increased HDL-C, while had no effects on TC or LDL-C levels (Garces et al., 2008). In a 2012 meta-analysis, anti-TNF treatment significantly increased TC, HDL-C, and TG, but not LDL-C. AI was also unaffected (Daien et al., 2012). In a recent study, 6 months of adalimumab or etanercept treatment, contrary to tocilizumab, increased HDL-C only but not TC or LDL-C (Chen et al., 2015). These results suggest that there may be controversy with respect to the effects of anti-TNF biologics on lipids. In addition, there may be differences between the effects of various TNFα inhibitors on the lipid profile (Kerekes et al., 2009a; Szekanecz et al., 2009). Differences between infliximab and etanercept may be due to the fact that while etanercept inhibits the pro-atherogenic lymphotoxin-α, as well as TNFα, infliximab only blocks TNFα (Garces et al., 2008).

Lipid elevations associated with anti-TNF and other biological therapy may be explained by the "lipid paradox." In brief, an inverse correlation between CRP and lipid levels has been described. Biologics that suppress inflammation and thus CRP levels consequently increase basically all lipid fractions (TC, LDL-C, and HDL-C). Furthermore, in patients with higher disease activity and systemic inflammation, lower LDL-C levels have been associated with increased CV risk (Myasoedova et al., 2011; Choy et al., 2014; Robertson et al., 2013). Such lipid elevations with unchanged atherogenic index associated with improvement of inflammatory markers have been reported with respect to infliximab, adalimumab, etanercept, or golimumab (Kirkham et al., 2014; Szekanecz et al., 2009; Kerekes et al., 2014; Peters et al., 2007; Vis et al., 2005; Seriolo et al., 2006; Soubrier et al., 2008; Popa et al., 2005; Robertson et al., 2013). The inverse relationship between CRP and TC has recently been confirmed in healthy individuals as well (Johnsson et al., 2014).

RA has been associated with impaired cholesterol efflux capacity (CEC) of HDL and increased serum cell cholesterol-loading capacity (CLC) leading to foam cell formation. In a recent study, adalimumab improved CEC, reduced CLC, and inhibited macrophage cholesterol uptake (Ronda et al., 2015). Infliximab may also restore impaired cholesterol efflux in RA (Voloshyna et al., 2014).

Adipokines have been implicated in the pathogenesis of arthritides, as well as atherosclerosis. In the general population, leptin, resistin, and visfatin are proatherogenic, while adiponectin is rather antiatherogenic. The levels of all four adipokines are elevated in RA and all of them are highly proinflammatory. However, there have been highly conflicting results on the effects of biologics on adipokine release (Abella et al., 2014; Kerekes et al., 2014; Gomez et al., 2011; Peters et al., 2010b). Recently a novel adipokine, chemerin has attracted lots of interest. Chemerin may be a "master adipokine" regulating both inflammation and cardiometabolic comorbidities in arthritides (Giles, 2014; Dessein et al., 2014). Anti-TNF therapy reduces chemerin production (Herenius et al., 2013).

Insulin resistance has also been associated with chronic inflammatory diseases including RA and SLE (Chung et al., 2008). Anti-TNF therapy, primarily infliximab and etanercept, improved insulin sensitivity as indicated by reduction of homeostatic model assessment (HOMA) in a number of trials (Barbuio et al., 2007; Gonzalez-Gay et al., 2010; Ursini et al., 2010; Seriolo et al., 2008; Huvers et al., 2007; Tam et al., 2007), as well as in a recent meta-analysis (Burska et al., 2015).

Body composition is also very important when discussing CV risk. RA and other chronic inflammatory diseases have been associated with loss of weight ("rheumatoid cachexia") mainly due to systemic inflammation and TNFα (originally known as "cachectin"). Treated patients with low disease activity or in remission gain weight and may even become slightly obese. There is also a redistribution of body fat. In patients with high disease activity there is a loss of abdominal (subcutaneous) fat and muscle mass. In contrast, visceral fat mass is increased also resulting in increased CV risk (Kerekes et al., 2014;

Ferraz-Amaro et al., 2013; Challal et al., 2015). As TNFα is highly involved, anti-TNF therapy should alter body composition. Unfortunately, rheumatoid cachexia may persist in patients receiving biologic therapy even after the improvement of arthritis symptoms (Kerekes et al., 2014; Metsios et al., 2007). Furthermore, in three studies, TNF blockade including etanercept and infliximab failed to show effects on body composition (Challal et al., 2015; Marcora et al., 2006; Metsios et al., 2007). Anti-TNF biologics may also reduce epicardial adipose tissue thickness (Lima-Martinez et al., 2014).

Vasculogenesis is the formation of new capillaries from endothelial progenitor cells (EPCs) (Szekanecz et al., 2010; Szekanecz and Koch, 2010). There has been evidence that low EPC numbers and impaired EPC function are observed in arthritides (Szekanecz et al., 2010; Szekanecz and Koch, 2010; Ablin et al., 2006; Grisar et al., 2007, 2005). Vasculogenesis is very important in vascular repair associated with atherosclerosis (Szekanecz et al., 2010; Szekanecz and Koch, 2010). TNFα levels have been inversely correlated with the number of EPCs (Martini et al., 2015). Anti-TNF agents may stimulate EPCs and thus vasculogenesis in inflammatory states including RA and JIA (Ablin et al., 2006; Grisar et al., 2007; Martini et al., 2015).

Platelet activation is involved in thromboembolic processes and also in atherosclerosis and CVD. In a very recent study, anti-TNF treatment of RA patients inhibited platelet activation, as well as tissue factor production. TNF inhibitors also suppressed platelet-dependent leukocyte activation (Manfredi et al., 2016).

Regarding other molecular mechanisms underlying inflammation-associated atherosclerosis, infliximab treatment resulted in the suppression of soluble endothelial cell adhesion molecule (sE-selectin, sVCAM-1) production in RA and AS patients (Gonzalez-Gay et al., 2006; Genre et al., 2015). Anti-TNF therapy also improved the total oxidative/antioxidative status in AS patients (Karkucak et al., 2010). In one study, onercept significantly decreased Lp(a) and homocysteine levels, which was associated with reduced CRP levels (Sattar et al., 2007).

Based on these scientific data, TNF blockers may also influence vascular function and thus the epidemiology of CVD in the clinical setting (Westlake et al., 2011). For example, in a Swedish national registry, 531 RA patients received infliximab or etanercept therapy between 1999 and 2005 and the primary endpoint was the first CVD event. In the anti-TNF treated patients, the age- and sex-adjusted incidence rate of first CVD events was less than half of that observed in the anti-TNF nontreated patients (Jacobsson et al., 2005). In a 2011 systematic review, anti-TNF treatment appeared to decrease the likelihood of CVD (Westlake et al., 2011). In a recent study, etanercept significantly reduced the risk of CV diseases (HR 0.52) (Morgan et al., 2014). In a British cohort, RA patients treated with TNF blockers were compared to those on traditional DMARDs. There was no difference in the incidence of MI between the two patient groups. However, when anti-TNF responders and nonresponders were compared, the risk of MI was markedly reduced in patients exerting a good clinical response after 6 months of anti-TNF therapy in comparison to nonresponders (Dixon et al., 2007).

In 2011, Greenberg et al. performed a meta-analysis of five then available studies. Most of these studies published between 2005 and 2008 showed that anti-TNF therapy reduced CV risk. The overall RR was 0.46 (0.28; 0.77) (Greenberg et al., 2011). In the same year, Barnabe et al. (2011) carried out a systematic review of 16 studies. This analysis suggested that anti-TNF agents reduce the risk of all CV events [RR 0.46 (0.28; 0.70)] and MI [RR 0.81 (0.68; 0.96)] (Barnabe et al., 2011).

The longer duration and thus the cumulative dose of anti-TNF treatment may also be of great importance. In a recent study of Nurmohamed et al. (2015), every 6 months of treatment extension resulted in 12% decrease in CV risk. Furthermore, continuation of TNF-α blockade for 1, 2, or 3 years reduced CV risk by 21%, 38%, or 51%, respectively (Nurmohamed et al., 2015).

Ljung et al. (2014) assessed the incidence of acute coronary syndrome in the Swedish ARTIS registry. The event-free survival was better in RA patients receiving TNF inhibitors compared to biologic-naïve patients (Ljung et al., 2014).

In the recent meta-analysis of Roubille et al. (2015a) 16 studies published between 2005 and 2012 were included. TNF inhibitors definitely reduced CV risk. RR values for all CV events, MI, stroke, and MACE were 0.70 (0.54; 0.90), 0.59 (0.36; 0.97), 0.57 (0.35; 0.92), and 0.30 (0.15; 0.57), respectively (Roubille et al., 2015a).

Prospective studies with hard CV endpoints are lacking. The ENTRACTE study has been designed to assess CV outcome during biological therapy. The active comparator of this still running trial is etanercept so information will be obtained with regards to clinical CV effects of this TNF inhibitor (Ridker and Luscher, 2014; Ridker, 2014).

Certainly, more epidemiological data from large cohorts and more prospective studies are needed to determine how molecular and morphological effects of biologics translate to clinical changes of vascular morbidity and mortality. Yet, there has been a clearer picture from earlier times to recent years suggesting that anti-TNF treatment may indeed be beneficial with regards to CV risk. Most data have become available with respect to infliximab, etanercept, and adalimumab. There have been only scattered reports on golimumab or certolizumab pegol.

2.4.2 Rituximab

In a pilot study on vascular effects of rituximab, we included five RA patients. All exerted 22−112% of improvement in FMD by week 16 (Kerekes et al., 2009b). Others also observed the positive effects of rituximab on micro- and macrovascular endothelial function (Gonzalez-Juanatey et al., 2008; Hsue et al., 2014). Improvement of endothelial function was associated with suppression of systemic inflammation indicated by decreases in CRP levels and DAS28 scores, as well as with improved lipid profiles (Table 20.1) (Gonzalez-Juanatey et al., 2008; Kerekes et al., 2009b; Hsue et al., 2014).

Regarding carotid atherosclerosis, in our rituximab study described above, despite of the short follow-up time of 16 weeks, carotid atherosclerosis significantly improved in three out of five patients by the end of the observation period (Kerekes et al., 2009b). In another very recent study, rituximab reduced ccIMT, which was accompanied by decreased disease activity and CRP levels (Novikova et al., 2016). In a cohort of 24 RA patients, 12 months of rituximab therapy significantly improved PWV (Provan et al., 2015); recent rituximab treatment also decreased total cholesterol and increased HDL-C levels in four out of five patients (Kerekes et al., 2009b). Six months of rituximab therapy beneficially altered the composition of proatherogenic HDL (Raterman et al., 2013). However, no randomized controlled study has been conducted with respect to the effects of rituximab on lipid profile (Souto et al., 2015).

In clinical trials, rituximab treatment was associated with good CV safety (Gurcan et al., 2009). In a recent analysis of the Corrona registry, rituximab and anti-TNF treatments had comparable CV safety profile (Harrold et al., 2015).

2.4.3 Tocilizumab

IL-6, similarly to TNFα, is also a key proinflammatory cytokine, which also increases the hepatic production of CRP, an independent risk factor for atherosclerosis (Ross, 1999; Szekanecz, 2008; Tzoulaki et al., 2005; Sherer and Shoenfeld, 2006; Szekanecz et al., 2016). IL-6 induces endothelial dysfunction (Bhagat and Vallance, 1997) and has been implicated in CVD, as well as cerebrovascular events and peripheral atherosclerosis (Tzoulaki et al., 2005; Hoshi et al., 2008). IL-6 induces platelet aggregation and activation, stimulates endothelial activation and the expression of endothelial adhesion molecules (Tzoulaki et al., 2005). IL-6 also stimulates the formation of foam cells and decreases HDL-C production (Coca and Sanz, 2009). On the other hand, IL-6 is a main inducer of CRP release and both circulating CRP and IL-6 levels were correlated with the risk of MI in otherwise healthy, nonsmoking men (Ridker, 2004). We have correlated plasma IL-6 levels with abnormal FMD and increased ccIMT in RA patients (Kerekes et al., 2008). Thus, targeting IL-6 may have net beneficial effects on the vasculature.

Yet, no prospective, hard endpoint studies have been completed showing effects of IL-6 or IL-6 receptor blockade on CV outcomes. The only running prospective trial is ENTRACTE, described above, assessing CV outcome during tocilizumab versus etanercept therapy. This trial will finally determine the effects of IL-6R inhibition on clinical CV outcome (Ridker, 2014; Ridker and Luscher, 2014).

In a retrospective, post-hoc analysis of almost 4000 RA patients treated with tocilizumab, the frequency of MACE was 0.34 cases per 100 patient years. At baseline, future MACE was associated with age, positive CV history, disease activity (DAS28), and TC/HDL-C ratio (atherogenic index). However, during treatment, future MACE was only associated with effects on disease activity, but not with lipid changes (Rao et al., 2015). Although these findings should be confirmed in larger trials, these data also suggest that during biologic treatment, CV outcome is primarily dependent on changes of systemic inflammation and disease activity rather than traditional CV risk factors.

It has become clear already from clinical trials that the anti-IL-6 receptor antibody tocilizumab may increase plasma TC, LDL-C, and TG levels, while it may decrease HDL-C levels in some patients (Nakata et al., 2008; Genovese et al., 2008; Takacova et al., 2008; Chen et al., 2015; Robertson et al., 2013; Souto et al., 2015). These effects were reversible in most cases (Nakata et al., 2008). In a recent meta-analysis of randomized controlled trials, the RR of tocilizumab to increase TC, LDL-C, and HDL-C were 4.6, 4.8, and 2.25, respectively (Souto et al., 2015). Again, the effects of tocilizumab on RA-associated atherosclerosis may be dual, as this drug very effectively suppress systemic inflammation. As described above, the lipid paradox, the suppression of CRP with consequent elevation of lipid levels may explain this feature (Choy et al., 2014; Myasoedova et al., 2011). Tocilizumab may increase lipid levels to a higher extend compared to anti-TNF biologics (Kerekes et al., 2014; Gabay et al., 2016; McInnes et al., 2015; Chen et al., 2015; Genovese et al., 2008). However, although IL-6 blockade may result in dyslipidemia, inhibition of the highly proinflammatory IL-6 may also improve vascular function. In large post-marketing databases and meta-analyses, no increase of CV events was observed upon tocilizumab therapy (Curtis et al., 2015; Kawashiri et al., 2010; Steiner and Urowitz, 2009).

In the absence of hard CV endpoint trials, surrogate markers can be determined in order to predict the vascular effects of IL-6 blockade. Tocilizumab treatment may attenuate the production of several other vasculopathy-associated and metabolic biomarkers (McInnes et al., 2015; Gabay et al., 2016). Tocilizumab affects lipid subfractions. It decreases the production of lipoprotein a [Lp(a)], proinflammatory, serum amyloid A-containing HDL. On the other hand, it increases small HDL and paraoxonase activity (Gabay et al., 2016; McInnes et al., 2015; Schultz et al., 2010). Tocilizumab also attenuates the levels of HOMA, a marker of insulin resistance and diabetes mellitus (Bradham et al., 2014; Schultz et al., 2010). Tocilizumab suppresses fibrinogen and D-dimer levels (McInnes et al., 2015). Among adipokines, tocilizumab treatment reduced the production of chemerin, a key adipokine described above (Makrilakis et al., 2015a, 2015b). With respect to vascular imaging, IL-6 inhibition by tocilizumab improved endothelial function (FMD) and arterial stiffness (PWV) (Protogerou et al., 2011; Kume et al., 2011; Makrilakis et al., 2015a). When seven RA patients were treated with tocilizumab, PWV significantly improved as early as after 3 months of therapy (Provan et al., 2015).

Yet, larger studies and close adverse event reporting are needed in order to determine CV outcome in tocilizumab-treated patients.

2.4.4 *Abatacept*

T cells have been implicated in both arthritis and atherosclerosis (Sherer and Shoenfeld, 2006; Kobezda et al., 2014; Szekanecz et al., 2016). Specific autoreactive T lymphocytes trigger atherosclerosis, as well as RA (Sherer and Shoenfeld, 2006; Kobezda et al., 2014). Among T cell subsets, both atherogenesis and RA have been associated with a type 1 T helper cell response (Sherer and Shoenfeld, 2006; Kobezda et al., 2014; Szekanecz et al., 2016). Thus, T-cell blockade may have vascular, as well as antiinflammatory effects in RA.

There have been few reports on CV safety of this drug. In the meta-analysis of available phase III trial results, abatacept treatment was found to be safe. The occurrence of angina or MI was not more common in abatacept-treated patients (Maxwell and Singh, 2009). In a very recent study on insurance database, abatacept treatment may have a lower risk for MI than TNF blockers in elderly RA patients (Zhang et al., 2016).

With respect to surrogate markers of vascular pathophysiology, in a small study, five patients were treated with abatacept. Arterial stiffness indicated by PWV did not change after 12 months of therapy (Provan et al., 2015). There have been no controlled trials in order to determine the possible effects of abatacept on lipids (Souto et al., 2015). In a recent small study, abatacept improved insulin sensitivity in RA patients (Ursini et al., 2015).

2.4.5 *Canakinumab*

IL-1 blockade has been approved for the treatment of childhood autoinflammatory diseases and there have been promising results in gout (Lachmann et al., 2009; Schlesinger et al., 2012). IL-1 blockade resulted in better endothelial function in RA patients (Ikonomidis et al., 2014). In high-risk CVD patients, canakinumab reduced the plasma levels of inflammatory and atherosclerotic markers including CRP, IL-6, and fibrinogen (Ridker et al., 2012). Canakinumab appeared to be safe in clinical trials (Schlesinger et al., 2012; Lachmann et al., 2009; Howard et al., 2014).

As far as nonarthritis patients with CVD are concerned, a prospective, hard endpoint CV trial called CANTOS (Canakinumab Antiinflammatory Thrombosis Outcomes Study) has been initiated in thousands of patients with stable CVD but higher degree of inflammation indicated by elevated CRP levels. This trial is still recruiting (Ridker, 2014; Ridker and Luscher, 2014).

2.4.6 *Tofacitinib*

Janus kinases (JAK1 and JAK3) are involved in mediating the signaling of multiple cytokines in RA (Vyas et al., 2013; Yamaoka and Tanaka, 2013). In addition, JAKs may also be involved in atherosclerosis and CV disease. Inhibition of JAK3 in mice protects against myocardial ischemia and reperfusion injury (Oh et al., 2013). However, as no large study on CV outcome has been conducted yet, the possible effects of JAK inhibition on CVD have not yet been clarified.

The JAK3 and JAK1 inhibitor tofacitinib has been approved for the treatment of RA in a number of countries. Tofacitinib, similar to tocilizumab, produces great increases in both LDL-C (19–21%) and HDL-C (11–14%) levels (Robertson et al., 2013; Souto et al., 2015). According to the comparative phase III trial, tofacitinib increases lipid levels to a greater extent than adalimumab (Robertson et al., 2013). On the other hand, tofacitinib effectively suppresses systemic inflammation (Fleischmann et al., 2012; van Vollenhoven et al., 2012; Souto et al., 2015). Available data from clinical studies and databases do not suggest increased CV risk in RA patients (van Vollenhoven et al., 2012; Souto et al., 2015). Atorvastatin effectively reversed Tofacitinib-induced dyslipidemia in RA (McInnes et al., 2014).

2.4.7 Other Drugs

In this chapter, we summarize information on the CV and cardiometabolic effects of antirheumatic drugs. However, other compounds that are not primarily used to treat rheumatic diseases but are vasculoprotective may also be administered to arthritis patients.

Statin therapy significantly reduces the risk of CVD. In addition to their lipid-lowering effects, statins may also be atheroprotective by modulating cell signaling and inflammatory pathways. Statins reduce serum CRP levels, directly inhibit IFN-γ–induced MHC class II expression and thus suppress T-cell–driven autoimmunity. Statins also prevent endothelial dysfunction (Nissen et al., 2006; Timar et al., 2013; El-Barbary et al., 2010). The pleiotropic effects of statins on vascular and immune systems argue for their use in RA (Peters et al., 2010a). To date, the largest trial on statin therapy in RA has been the published Trial of Atorvastatin in RA (TARA) study. In this 6-month study on 116 RA patients, the disease activity score improved significantly in the atorvastatin-treated group versus the placebo group. There was also a decrease in erythrocyte sedimentation rate, as well as serum CRP and IL-6 levels (McCarey et al., 2004). In a recent Japanese study, atorvastatin significantly improved lipid profiles in RA (Akiyama et al., 2015). Rosuvastatin also improved FMD, resulted in carotid plaque regression, and decreased serum TNFα, IL-6, and ICAM-1 levels in RA and AS patients (Garg et al., 2015; Ikdahl et al., 2015; Rollefstad et al., 2015). In AS, rosuvastatin decreased Bath Ankylosing Spondylitis Disease Activity Index (BASDAI), Bath Ankylosing Spondylitis Metrology Index (BASMI), and pain, accompanied by reduced acute phase reaction (van Denderen et al., 2006). In our SSc cohort, 6 months of rosuvastatin treatment significantly decreased CRP, as well as TC, LDL-C, and TG levels. This was associated with improved FMD in these patients (Timar et al., 2013).

Aspirin has been used for a long time to prevent CVD in the general population. Daily aspirin reduces the risk of MI and reduces CVD-related mortality. There is no evidence from large clinical trials to support the efficacy of low-dose aspirin in RA, yet, aspirin use may be recommended to prevent CVD in RA (Peters et al., 2010a).

As described above, insulin resistance has been associated with arthritides (Kerekes et al., 2014). Peroxisome proliferator-activated receptor gamma agonists (glitazones) improve insulin resistance but they may also have other antiinflammatory and vasculoprotective effects. In one study, pioglitazone improved arterial stiffness and diastolic blood pressure, which was independent on its effect on insulin sensitivity (Ormseth et al., 2014).

The EULAR CV recommendations discussed later also deals with the great importance of using statins, ACE inhibitors, and AT-II blockers in arthritis patients (Peters et al., 2010a).

Folic acid supplementation is not only beneficial in order to neutralize MTX side effects, but also suppresses hyperhomocysteinemia and thus CV risk. However, large, hard endpoint trials are needed in order to determine the CV effects of folic acid in arthritis patients (Essouma and Noubiap, 2015).

A number of arthritis patients also have secondary osteoporosis. These patients may use oral calcium supplementation. A recent study has suggested that oral calcium may not increase vascular calcification in RA patients (Geraldino-Pardilla et al., 2015). Interestingly, low serum magnesium has been associated with hyperlipidemia and possibly increased CV risk in RA patients. This suggests the importance of magnesium supplementation to these patients (Chavan et al., 2015).

3. OTHER HEART DISEASES

3.1 Infusion Reactions

Infusion reactions may occur when administering IV biologics. It is very important to differentiate CV events occurring during or immediately after the infusion and are usually reversible and chronic CV events caused by long-term use of antirheumatic drugs (Gasparyan et al., 2012). Such events, including hypertension or hypotension, arrhythmias, angina, MI, or even sudden cardiac death may rarely occur during infliximab, rituximab, tocilizumab, or abatacept infusions (Gasparyan et al., 2012; Wasserman et al., 2004; Lazzerini et al., 2008; Maxwell and Singh, 2009; Gurcan et al., 2009; Patel and Moreland, 2010).

3.2 Hypertension and Renal Disease

Hypertension and blood pressure variability are often seen in RA patients and they contribute to all-cause mortality (Myasoedova et al., 2014). Among antirheumatic drugs, NSAIDs, corticosteroids, cyclosporine A, and leflunomide may increase blood pressure (Atzeni et al., 2010). The most common CV side effect of leflunomide is hypertension (2–10%) (Rozman et al., 2002). In addition to hypertension as infusion reaction described above, almost all biologics may increase blood pressure (Gasparyan et al., 2012).

Chronic kidney disease (CKD) has been associated with both RA and CVD. In a recent study, the role of antirheumatic drugs in the development of CKD was assessed. NSAIDs were clearly associated with CKD: the RR was 1.45 in infrequent users and 2.01 in frequent users. Frequent use of corticosteroids also increased the risk of CKD (RR: 1.75). The use of MTX, SASP, HCQ, LEF, or any biologics was not associated with the development of CKD (Chiu et al., 2015b). A recent meta-analysis of more than 30,000 cases provided supportive evidence that NSAID use was associated with higher risk of CKD in hypertensive subjects (Hsu et al., 2015).

3.3 Arrhythmias

QTc time prolongation on ECG has been associated with arrhythmias. Chronic systemic inflammation and proinflammatory cytokines play an important role in prolonged QTc. In addition, long QTc has been related to high disease activity, elevated hsCRP, and increased all-cause mortality in RA (Lazzerini et al., 2013, 2015; Panoulas et al., 2014). Arrhythmias have also been associated with psoriasis and PsA (Chiu et al., 2015a). In a recent study, tocilizumab treatment corrected QTc intervals by suppressing systemic inflammation in RA (Lazzerini et al., 2015).

Arrhythmias may also occur during intravenous biologic treatment; however, as discussed above, this is considered as an infusion reaction.

3.4 Left Ventricular Dysfunction and Congestive Heart Failure

About 45% of RA patients with no cardiac symptoms has left ventricular systolic dysfunction (Cioffi et al., 2015). Continuous corticosteroid use may double the risk of congestive heart failure (CHF) (Wright et al., 2014). Multiple meta-analyses confirmed that MTX reduced the incidence of CHF, possibly by 50% (Marks and Edwards, 2012; Micha et al., 2011; Wright et al., 2014). Infliximab increased left ventricular ejection fraction, which was accompanied by reduction of inflammation, as well as IL-6, endothelin 1, and NT-proBNP levels (Kotyla et al., 2012).

It has been traditionally accepted, mostly based on a single phase II trial that TNF blockers are contraindicated in patients with NYHA class III or IV CHF (Weisman, 2002). In a 20111 Cochrane review, however, the rate of CHF was not significantly different between patients treated with biologics and controls (Singh et al., 2011). In recent years, controversy have arisen as numerous reports indicated that TNF blockers may even have beneficial effects in rheumatic patients with nonsevere CHF (Sarzi-Puttini et al., 2005). TNF blocker therapy in RA significantly reduced the risk of heart failure in a large cohort of RA patients with preexisting CVD (Wolfe and Michaud, 2004). Etanercept improved endothelial vasodilation capacity in patients with preexisting CHF (Fichtlscherer et al., 2001). Recently, Heslinga et al. (2015) have performed a systematic review of 54 available studies. They concluded that TNF blockade may indeed exert harmful effects on CHF in elderly RA patients, which was not observed in other patients. TNFα inhibition may improve some echocardiographic parameters and it definitely reduces NT-proBNP levels.

NT-proBNP has become a biomarker of heart failure and CV mortality (Wright et al., 2014). BNP is produced in RA (George et al., 2014). It has been confirmed that NT-proBNP is a marker of CV and all-cause mortality in early polyarthritis (Mirjafari et al., 2014). Infliximab treatment may reduce NT-proBNP production (Kotyla et al., 2012; Heslinga et al., 2015). In our hands, 12 months of anti-TNF treatment including either etanercept or certolizumab pegol significantly decreased NT-proBNP levels both in RA and in SpA (Szekanecz et al., 2010, unpublished observations). In RA, NT-proBNP is associated with IL-6 production, and tocilizumab may have favorable effects on NT-proBNP production (Bradham et al., 2014).

In conclusion, arthritis patients with history of CHF and an indication for the use of biologics do not need a baseline cardiac evaluation to screen for CHF. Patients with well-compensated mild (NYHA class I or II) CHF should be closely monitored for any clinical signs of worsening of CHF during anti-TNF therapy. Finally, patients with NYHA class III or IV CHF should not be treated with biologics (Sarzi-Puttini et al., 2005).

4. RECOMMENDATIONS FOR CARDIOVASCULAR RISK MANAGEMENT IN ARTHRITIDES

In 2009, EULAR has set up an ad-hoc committee that prepared 10 recommendations for the prevention and management of CVD associated with RA, AS, and PsA. It has been stated that arthritis and diabetes mellitus may exert similar risks for CVD (Peters et al., 2009); therefore, all efforts should be made in order to assess CV risk early and prevent further damage. As systemic inflammation is the key factor accounted for increased CV risk, adequate control of disease activity using traditional DMARDs, primarily MTX and biologics is essential. Among traditional vasculoprotective agents, statins, ACE inhibitors, and AT-II blockers are preferred treatment options. As the role of coxibs and NSAIDs regarding the CV risk in not yet determined, we should be very cautious when prescribing these drugs. The lowest effective dose of corticosteroids should be used.

These recommendations have recently been updated, presented, and will be published soon (Nurmohamed, 2015). In comparison to the first set of recommendations, more data have become available in AS and PsA. Risk assessment performed every 5 years was recommended. Low dosage and tapering of NSAIDs and corticosteroids received even more attention.

Other recent British (Board, 2014), Spanish (Martin-Martinez et al., 2014), French (Tournadre et al., 2015; Pham et al., 2006), Dutch (van den Oever et al., 2013; Peters and Nurmohamed, 2013), Canadian (Anderson et al., 2013; Roubille et al., 2015b), or US (Barber et al., 2015; Goff et al., 2014; Kaplan, 2009) recommendations also include similar suggestions with respect to antirheumatic therapy and CV risk.

5. CONCLUSIONS

Accelerated atherosclerosis and increased CV and cerebrovascular morbidity and mortality have been associated with RA, as well as other inflammatory rheumatic diseases. It is likely, that sustained systemic inflammation and clinical activity of arthritis are major contributors to atherogenesis. Aspirin, statins, folic acid, ACE inhibitors, and AT-II blockers have been introduced to the prevention and therapy of vascular diseases in RA; however, they primarily treat traditional CV risk factors. Blood pressure control and vasculoprotection using ACE inhibitors and AT-II blockers is also essential. NSAIDs, primarily COX-2 inhibitors may increase CV risk; therefore, we should be cautious when prescribing these compounds. Yet, there have been lots of controversies with respect to CV risk of NSAIDs in inflammatory states versus in the general population. Also, there may be differences among the various NSAIDs. Corticosteroids may exert both beneficial and detrimental effects on the vasculature. Again, the CV risk of corticosteroids may be different in arthritides or in noninflammatory conditions. It is possible that the antiinflammatory action of NSAIDs and corticosteroids may override their potential atherogenic nature. Antimalarials and MTX have been found to be cardioprotective in most studies. Leflunomide may not increase atherosclerosis but it can cause hypertension. Biologics, primarily TNFα inhibitors, effectively suppress arthritis and they have various effects on the vascular system. Increased lipid levels observed in the case of all biologics may be explained by the "lipid paradox." Biologics may also have beneficial effects on other metabolic markers (insulin resistance, body composition, etc.), as well as vascular pathophysiology (carotid atherosclerosis, arterial stiffness, endothelial dysfunction). In most large trials, especially recent ones, anti-TNF biologics have been associated with reduced CV risk. More data are needed on rituximab, tocilizumab, and abatacept, as well as tofacitinib. In this context, there may be significant differences among various biologics. In addition to atherosclerosis and CVD, other cardiac diseases, such as heart failure, arrhythmias, and hypertension should also be considered when administering antirheumatic drugs. The net effects of antirheumatic drugs on the vasculature and on vascular diseases, variability between individual agents, and differences between short- and long-term effects should be determined by more detailed analysis of patient cohorts and large registries. In the clinical practice, EULAR and other recommendations may guide the rheumatologist how to prevent and manage CV comorbidities in rheumatic patients.

REFERENCES

Abella, V., Scotece, M., Conde, J., Lopez, V., Lazzaro, V., Pino, J., Gomez-Reino, J.J., Gualillo, O., 2014. Adipokines, metabolic syndrome and rheumatic diseases. J. Immunol. Res. 2014, 343746.

Ablin, J.N., Boguslavski, V., Aloush, V., Elkayam, O., Paran, D., Caspi, D., George, J., 2006. Effect of anti-TNFalpha treatment on circulating endothelial progenitor cells (EPCs) in rheumatoid arthritis. Life Sci. 79, 2364–2369.

Ahmed, A., Hollan, I., Curran, S.A., Kitson, S.M., Riggio, M.P., Mikkelsen, K., Almdahl, S.M., Aukrust, P., Mcinnes, I.B., Goodyear, C.S., 2016. Rheumatoid arthritis patients have a pro-atherogenic cytokine microenvironment in the aortic adventitia. Arthritis Rheumatol. 68, 1361–1366.

Ajeganova, S., Svensson, B., Hafstrom, I., Group, B.S., 2014. Low-dose prednisolone treatment of early rheumatoid arthritis and late cardiovascular outcome and survival: 10-year follow-up of a 2-year randomised trial. BMJ Open 4, e004259.

Akiyama, M., Mawatari, T., Nakashima, Y., Miyahara, H., Yamada, H., Okazaki, K., Fukushi, J., Kondo, M., Kishimoto, J., Hashimura, C., Iwamoto, Y., 2015. Prevalence of dyslipidemia in Japanese patients with rheumatoid arthritis and effects of atorvastatin treatment. Clin. Rheumatol. 34, 1867–1875.

Anderson, T.J., Gregoire, J., Hegele, R.A., Couture, P., Mancini, G.B., Mcpherson, R., Francis, G.A., Poirier, P., Lau, D.C., Grover, S., Genest Jr., J., Carpentier, A.C., Dufour, R., Gupta, M., Ward, R., Leiter, L.A., Lonn, E., Ng, D.S., Pearson, G.J., Yates, G.M., Stone, J.A., Ur, E., 2013. 2012 update of the Canadian Cardiovascular Society guidelines for the diagnosis and treatment of dyslipidemia for the prevention of cardiovascular disease in the adult. Can J. Cardiol. 29, 151–167.

Apte, S.S., 2009. A disintegrin-like and metalloprotease (reprolysin-type) with thrombospondin type 1 motif (ADAMTS) superfamily: functions and mechanisms. J. Biol. Chem. 284, 31493–31497.

Ardoin, S.P., Sundy, J.S., 2006. Update on nonsteriodal anti-inflammatory drugs. Curr. Opin. Rheumatol. 18, 221–226.

Atzeni, F., Turiel, M., Caporali, R., Cavagna, L., Tomasoni, L., Sitia, S., Sarzi-Puttini, P., 2010. The effect of pharmacological therapy on the cardiovascular system of patients with systemic rheumatic diseases. Autoimmun. Rev. 9, 835–839.

Baba, M., Miyake, H., Wang, X., Okamoto, M., Takashima, K., 2007. Isolation and characterization of human immunodeficiency virus type 1 resistant to the small-molecule CCR5 antagonist TAK-652. Antimicrob. Agents Chemother. 51, 707–715.

Banfi, G., Lombardi, G., Colombini, A., Melegati, G., 2010. Whole-body cryotherapy in athletes. Sports Med. 40, 509–517.

Barber, C.E., Smith, A., Esdaile, J.M., Barnabe, C., Martin, L.O., Faris, P., Hazlewood, G., Noormohamed, R., Alvarez, N., Mancini, G.B., Lacaille, D., Keeling, S., Avina-Zubieta, J.A., Marshall, D., 2015. Best practices for cardiovascular disease prevention in rheumatoid arthritis: a systematic review of guideline recommendations and quality indicators. Arthritis Care Res. (Hoboken) 67, 169–179.

Barbuio, R., Milanski, M., Bertolo, M.B., Saad, M.J., Velloso, L.A., 2007. Infliximab reverses steatosis and improves insulin signal transduction in liver of rats fed a high-fat diet. J. Endocrinol. 194, 539–550.

Barnabe, C., Martin, B.J., Ghali, W.A., 2011. Systematic review and meta-analysis: anti-tumor necrosis factor alpha therapy and cardiovascular events in rheumatoid arthritis. Arthritis Care Res. (Hoboken) 63, 522–529.

Baskan, B.M., Sivas, F., Aktekin, L.A., Dogan, Y.P., Ozoran, K., Bodur, H., 2009. Serum homocysteine level in patients with ankylosing spondylitis. Rheumatol. Int. 29, 1435–1439.

Bhagat, K., Vallance, P., 1997. Inflammatory cytokines impair endothelium-dependent dilatation in human veins in vivo. Circulation 96, 3042–3047.

Bilsborough, W., Keen, H., Taylor, A., O'driscoll, G.J., Arnolda, L., Green D.J., 2006. Anti-tumour necrosis factor-alpha therapy over conventional therapy improves endothelial function in adults with rheumatoid arthritis. Rheumatol. Int. 26, 1125–1131.

Black, R.J., Joseph, R.M., Brown, B., Movahedi, M., Lunt, M., Dixon, W.G. 2015. Half of UK patients with rheumatoid arthritis are prescribed oral glucocorticoid therapy in primary care: a retrospective drug utilisation study. Arthritis Res. Ther. 17, 375.

Board, J.B.S., 2014. Joint British Societies' consensus recommendations for the prevention of cardiovascular disease (JBS3). Heart 100 (Suppl. 2), ii1–ii67.

Boers, M., 2015. Drugs and cardiovascular risk in inflammatory arthritis: another case of glucocorticoid-bashing? Ann. Rheum. Dis. 74, e33.

Borba, E.F., Bonfa, E., 2001. Longterm beneficial effect of chloroquine diphosphate on lipoprotein profile in lupus patients with and without steroid therapy. J. Rheumatol. 28, 780–785.

Bosello, S., Santoliquido, A., Zoli, A., Di Campli, C., Flore, R., Tondi, P., Ferraccioli, G., 2008. TNF-alpha blockade induces a reversible but transient effect on endothelial dysfunction in patients with long-standing severe rheumatoid arthritis. Clin. Rheumatol 27, 833–839.

Bradham, W.S., Ormseth, M.J., Oeser, A., Solus, J.F., Gebretsadik, T., Shintani, A., Stein, C.M., 2014. Insulin resistance is associated with increased concentrations of NT-proBNP in rheumatoid arthritis: IL-6 as a potential mediator. Inflammation 37, 801–808.

Bruce, I.N., 2005a. Cardiovascular disease in lupus patients: should all patients be treated with statins and aspirin? Best Pract. Res. Clin. Rheumatol. 19, 823–838.

Bruce, I.N., 2005b. 'Not only...but also': factors that contribute to accelerated atherosclerosis and premature coronary heart disease in systemic lupus erythematosus. Rheumatology (Oxford) 44, 1492–1502.

Burska, A.N., Sakthiswary, R., Sattar, N., 2015. Effects of tumour necrosis factor antagonists on insulin sensitivity/resistance in rheumatoid arthritis: a systematic review and meta-analysis. PLoS One 10, e0128889.

Buttgereit, F., Burmester, G.R., Lipworth, B.J., 2009. Inflammation, glucocorticoids and risk of cardiovascular disease. Nat. Clin. Pract. Rheumatol. 5, 18–19.

Capria, A., De Nardo, D., Baffetti, F.R., Barbini, U., Violo, A., Tondo, T., Fontana, L., 2010. Long-term anti-TNF-alpha treatments reverse the endothelial dysfunction in rheumatoid arthritis: the biological coherence between synovial and endothelial inflammation. Int. J. Immunopathol. Pharmacol. 23, 255–262.

Challal, S., Minichiello, E., Boissier, M.C., Semerano, L., 2015. Cachexia and adiposity in rheumatoid arthritis. Relevance for disease management and clinical outcomes. Jt. Bone Spine 83, 127–133.

Chavan, V.U., Ramavataram, D., Patel, P.A., Rupani, M.P., 2015. Evaluation of serum magnesium, lipid profile and various biochemical parameters as risk factors of cardiovascular diseases in patients with rheumatoid arthritis. J. Clin. Diagn. Res. 9, BC01–5.

Chen, D.Y., Chen, Y.M., Hsieh, T.Y., Hsieh, C.W., Lin, C.C., Lan, J.L., 2015. Significant effects of biologic therapy on lipid profiles and insulin resistance in patients with rheumatoid arthritis. Arthritis Res. Ther. 17, 52.

Chiu, H.Y., Chang, W.L., Huang, W.F., Wen, Y.W., Tsai, Y.W., Tsai, T.F., 2015a. Increased risk of arrhythmia in patients with psoriatic disease: a nationwide population-based matched cohort study. J. Am. Acad. Dermatol. 73, 429–438.

Chiu, H.Y., Huang, H.L., Li, C.H., Chen, H.A., Yeh, C.L., Chiu, S.H., Lin, W.C., Cheng, Y.P., Tsai, T.F., Ho, S.Y., 2015b. Increased risk of chronic kidney disease in rheumatoid arthritis associated with cardiovascular complications - a national population-based cohort study. PLoS One 10, e0136508.

Choy, E., Ganeshalingam, K., Semb, A.G., Szekanecz, Z., Nurmohamed, M., 2014. Cardiovascular risk in rheumatoid arthritis: recent advances in the understanding of the pivotal role of inflammation, risk predictors and the impact of treatment. Rheumatology (Oxford) 53, 2143–2154. Epub 2014 Jun 8.

Chung, C.P., Oeser, A., Solus, J.F., Gebretsadik, T., Shintani, A., Avalos, I., Sokka, T., Raggi, P., Pincus, T., Stein, C.M., 2008. Inflammation-associated insulin resistance: differential effects in rheumatoid arthritis and systemic lupus erythematosus define potential mechanisms. Arthritis Rheum. 58, 2105–2112.

Cioffi, G., Viapiana, O., Ognibeni, F., Dalbeni, A., Gatti, D., Adami, S., Mazzone, C., Faganello, G., Di Lenarda, A., Rossini, M., 2015. Prevalence and factors related to left ventricular systolic dysfunction in asymptomatic patients with rheumatoid arthritis : a prospective tissue Doppler echocardiography study. Herz 40, 989–996.

Coca, A., Sanz, I., 2009. B cell depletion in lupus and Sjogren's syndrome: an update. Curr. Opin. Rheumatol. 21, 483–488.

Curtis, J.R., Perez-Gutthann, S., Suissa, S., Napalkov, P., Singh, N., Thompson, L., Porter-Brown, B., Actemra Pharmacoepidemiology Board, 2015. Tocilizumab in rheumatoid arthritis: a case study of safety evaluations of a large postmarketing data set from multiple data sources. Semin. Arthritis Rheum. 44, 381–388.

Cypiene, A., Laucevicius, A., Venalis, A., Ryliskyte, L., Dadoniene, J., Petrulioniene, Z., Kovaite, M., Laskova, V., Gintautas, J., 2007. Non-invasive assessment of arterial stiffness indices by applanation tonometry and pulse wave analysis in patients with rheumatoid arthritis treated with TNF-alpha blocker remicade (infliximab). Proc. West Pharmacol. Soc. 50, 119–122.

Daien, C.I., Duny, Y., Barnetche, T., Daures, J.P., Combe, B., Morel, J., 2012. Effect of TNF inhibitors on lipid profile in rheumatoid arthritis: a systematic review with meta-analysis. Ann. Rheum. Dis. 71, 862–868.

Damjanov, N., Nurmohamed, M.T., Szekanecz, Z., 2014. Biologics, cardiovascular effects and cancer. BMC Med. 12, 48.

De Vecchis, R., Baldi, C., Palmisani, L., 2016. Protective effects of methotrexate against ischemic cardiovascular disorders in patients treated for rheumatoid arthritis or psoriasis: novel therapeutic insights coming from a meta-analysis of the literature data. Anatol. J. Cardiol. 16, 2–9.

Del Porto, F., Lagana, B., Lai, S., Nofroni, I., Tinti, F., Vitale, M., Podesta, E., Mitterhofer, A.P., D'amelio, R., 2007. Response to anti-tumour necrosis factor alpha blockade is associated with reduction of carotid intima-media thickness in patients with active rheumatoid arthritis. Rheumatology (Oxford) 46, 1111–1115.

del Rincon, I., Battafarano, D.F., Restrepo, J.F., Erikson, J.M., Escalante, A., 2014. Glucocorticoid dose thresholds associated with all-cause and cardiovascular mortality in rheumatoid arthritis. Arthritis Rheumatol. 66, 264–272.

del Rincon, I., Polak, J.F., O'leary, D.H., Battafarano, D.F., Erikson, J.M., Restrepo, J.F., Molina, E., Escalante, A., 2015. Systemic inflammation and cardiovascular risk factors predict rapid progression of atherosclerosis in rheumatoid arthritis. Ann. Rheum. Dis. 74, 1118–1123.

Dessein, P.H., Tsang, L., Woodiwiss, A.J., Norton, G.R., Solomon, A., 2014. Circulating concentrations of the novel adipokine chemerin are associated with cardiovascular disease risk in rheumatoid arthritis. J. Rheumatol. 41, 1746–1754.

Dixon, W.G., Watson, K.D., Lunt, M., Hyrich, K.L., Silman, A.J., Symmons, D.P., 2007. Reduction in the incidence of myocardial infarction in patients with rheumatoid arthritis who respond to anti-tumor necrosis factor alpha therapy: results from the British Society for Rheumatology Biologics Register. Arthritis Rheum. 56, 2905–2912.

El-Barbary, A.M., Hussein, M.S., Rageh, E.M., Hamouda, H.E., Wagih, A.A., Ismail, R.G., 2010. Effect of atorvastatin on inflammation and modification of vascular risk factors in rheumatoid arthritis. J. Rheumatol. 38, 229–235.

Espinola, R.G., Pierangeli, S.S., Gharavi, A.E., Harris, E.N., 2002. Hydroxychloroquine reverses platelet activation induced by human IgG antiphospholipid antibodies. Thromb. Haemost. 87, 518–522.

Essouma, M., Noubiap, J.J., 2015. Therapeutic potential of folic acid supplementation for cardiovascular disease prevention through homocysteine lowering and blockade in rheumatoid arthritis patients. Biomark Res. 3, 24.

Feeley, B.T., Park, A.K., Hoyt, E.G., Robbins, R.C., 1999. Sulfasalazine inhibits reperfusion injury and prolongs allograft survival in rat cardiac transplants. J. Heart Lung Transplant. 18, 1088–1095.

Feng, H., Li, X.Y., Zheng, J.R., Gao, J.W., Xu, L.F., Tang, M.Y., 2005. Inhibition of the nuclear factor-kappaB signaling pathway by leflunomide or triptolide also inhibits the anthralin-induced inflammatory response but does not affect keratinocyte growth inhibition. Biol. Pharm. Bull. 28, 1597–1602.

Ferraz-Amaro, I., Gonzalez-Juanatey, C., Lopez-Mejias, R., Riancho-Zarrabeitia, L., Gonzalez-Gay, M.A., 2013. Metabolic syndrome in rheumatoid arthritis. Mediators Inflamm. 2013, 710928.

Ferraz-Amaro, I., Machin, S., Carmona, L., Gonzalez-Alvaro, I., Diaz-Gonzalez, F., Group, E.S., 2009. Pattern of use and safety of non-steroidal anti-inflammatory drugs in rheumatoid arthritis patients. A prospective analysis from clinical practice. Reumatol Clin. 5, 252–258.

Fichtlscherer, S., Rossig, L., Breuer, S., Vasa, M., Dimmeler, S., Zeiher, A.M., 2001. Tumor necrosis factor antagonism with etanercept improves systemic endothelial vasoreactivity in patients with advanced heart failure. Circulation 104, 3023–3025.

Fleischmann, R., Kremer, J., Cush, J., Schulze-Koops, H., Connell, C.A., Bradley, J.D., Gruben, D., Wallenstein, G.V., Zwillich, S.H., Kanik, K.S., Investigators, O.S., 2012. Placebo-controlled trial of tofacitinib monotherapy in rheumatoid arthritis. N. Engl. J. Med. 367, 495–507.

Furuichi, K., Wada, T., Sakai, N., Iwata, Y., Yoshimoto, K., Shimizu, M., Kobayashi, K., Takasawa, K., Kida, H., Takeda, S.I., Mukaida, N., Matsushima, K., Yokoyama, H., 2000. Distinct expression of CCR1 and CCR5 in glomerular and interstitial lesions of human glomerular diseases. Am. J. Nephrol. 20, 291–299.

Gabay, C., Mcinnes, I.B., Kavanaugh, A., Tuckwell, K., Klearman, M., Pulley, J., Sattar, N., 2016. Comparison of lipid and lipid-associated cardiovascular risk marker changes after treatment with tocilizumab or adalimumab in patients with rheumatoid arthritis. Ann. Rheum. Dis. 75, 1806–1812.

Galarraga, B., Khan, F., Kumar, P., Pullar, T., Belch, J.J., 2009. Etanercept improves inflammation-associated arterial stiffness in rheumatoid arthritis. Rheumatology (Oxford) 48, 1418–1423.

Garces, S.P., Parreira Santos, M.J., Vinagre, F.M., Roque, R.M., de Silva, J.A., 2008. Anti-tumour necrosis factor agents and lipid profile: a class effect? Ann. Rheum. Dis. 67, 895–896.

Garg, N., Krishan, P., Syngle, A., 2015. Rosuvastatin improves endothelial dysfunction in ankylosing spondylitis. Clin. Rheumatol. 34, 1065–1071.

Gasparyan, A.Y., Ayvazyan, L., Cocco, G., Kitas, G.D., 2012. Adverse cardiovascular effects of antirheumatic drugs: implications for clinical practice and research. Curr. Pharm. Des. 18, 1543–1555.

Genovese, M.C., Mckay, J.D., Nasonov, E.L., Mysler, E.F., da Silva, N.A., Alecock, E., Woodworth, T., Gomez-Reino, J.J., 2008. Interleukin-6 receptor inhibition with tocilizumab reduces disease activity in rheumatoid arthritis with inadequate response to disease-modifying antirheumatic drugs: the tocilizumab in combination with traditional disease-modifying antirheumatic drug therapy study. Arthritis Rheum. 58, 2968–2980.

Genre, F., Lopez-Mejias, R., Miranda-Filloy, J.A., Ubilla, B., Mijares, V., Carnero-Lopez, B., Gomez-Acebo, I., Dierssen-Sotos, T., Remuzgo-Martinez, S., Blanco, R., Pina, T., Gonzalez-Juanatey, C., Llorca, J., Gonzalez-Gay, M.A., 2015. Anti-TNF-alpha therapy reduces endothelial cell activation in non-diabetic ankylosing spondylitis patients. Rheumatol. Int. 35, 2069–2078.

George, J., Khan, F., Struthers, A.D., 2014. The source of BNP in rheumatoid arthritis. Int. J. Cardiol. 174, 740.

Geraldino-Pardilla, L., Dhaduvai, S., Giles, J.T., Bathon, J.M., 2015. Lack of association of oral calcium supplementation with coronary artery calcification in rheumatoid arthritis. Arthritis Rheumatol. 67, 1465–1473.

Giles, J.T., 2014. Adipokine mediators of inflammation and cardiometabolic comorbidity in rheumatoid arthritis: is there a master adipokine? J. Rheumatol. 41, 1725–1727.

Giles, J.T., Post, W., Blumenthal, R.S., Bathon, J.M., 2006. Therapy Insight: managing cardiovascular risk in patients with rheumatoid arthritis. Nat. Clin. Pract. Rheumatol. 2, 320–329.

Goff Jr., D.C., Lloyd-Jones, D.M., Bennett, G., Coady, S., D'agostino, R.B., Gibbons, R., Greenland, P., Lackland, D.T., Levy, D., O'donnell, C.J., Robinson, J.G., Schwartz, J.S., Shero, S.T., Smith Jr., S.C., Sorlie, P., Stone, N.J., Wilson, P.W., Jordan, H.S., Nevo, L., Wnek, J., Anderson, J.L., Halperin, J.L., Albert, N.M., Bozkurt, B., Brindis, R.G., Curtis, L.H., Demets, D., Hochman, J.S., Kovacs, R.J., Ohman, E.M., Pressler, S.J., Sellke, F.W., Shen, W.K., Smith JR., S.C., Tomaselli, G.F., American College of Cardiology/American Heart Association Task Force on Practice Guidelines, 2014. 2013 ACC/AHA guideline on the assessment of cardiovascular risk: a report of the American College of Cardiology/American Heart Association Task Force on Practice Guidelines. Circulation 129, S49–S73.

Gomez, R., Conde, J., Scotece, M., Gomez-Reino, J.J., Lago, F., Gualillo, O., 2011. What's new in our understanding of the role of adipokines in rheumatic diseases? Nat. Rev. Rheumatol. 7, 528–536.

Gonzalez-Gay, M.A., Garcia-Unzueta, M.T., De Matias, J.M., Gonzalez-Juanatey, C., Garcia-Porrua, C., Sanchez-Andrade, A., Martin, J., Llorca, J., 2006. Influence of anti-TNF-alpha infliximab therapy on adhesion molecules associated with atherogenesis in patients with rheumatoid arthritis. Clin. Exp. Rheumatol. 24, 373–379.

Gonzalez-Gay, M.A., Gonzalez-Juanatey, C., Vazquez-Rodriguez, T.R., Miranda-Filloy, J.A., Llorca, J., 2010. Insulin resistance in rheumatoid arthritis: the impact of the anti-TNF-alpha therapy. Ann. N. Y Acad. Sci. 1193, 153–159.

Gonzalez-Juanatey, C., Llorca, J., Sanchez-Andrade, A., Garcia-Porrua, C., Martin, J., Gonzalez-Gay, M.A., 2006. Short-term adalimumab therapy improves endo-thelial function in patients with rheumatoid arthritis refractory to infliximab. Clin. Exp. Rheumatol. 24, 309–312.

Gonzalez-Juanatey, C., Llorca, J., Vazquez-Rodriguez, T.R., Diaz-Varela, N., Garcia-Quiroga, H., Gonzalez-Gay, M.A., 2008. Short-term improvement of endothelial function in rituximab-treated rheumatoid arthritis patients refractory to tumor necrosis factor alpha blocker therapy. Arthritis Rheum. 59, 1821–1824.

Gonzalez-Juanatey, C., Testa, A., Garcia-Castelo, A., Garcia-Porrua, C., Llorca, J., Gonzalez-Gay, M.A., 2004. Active but transient improvement of endothelial function in rheumatoid arthritis patients undergoing long-term treatment with anti-tumor necrosis factor alpha antibody. Arthritis Rheum. 51, 447–450.

Goodson, N.J., Brookhart, A.M., Symmons, D.P., Silman, A.J., Solomon, D.H., 2009. Non-steroidal anti-inflammatory drug use does not appear to be associated with increased cardiovascular mortality in patients with inflammatory polyarthritis: results from a primary care based inception cohort of patients. Ann. Rheum. Dis. 68, 367–372.

Greenberg, J.D., Furer, V., Farkouh, M.E., 2011. Cardiovascular safety of biologic therapies for the treatment of RA. Nat. Rev. Rheumatol. 8, 13–21.

Grisar, J., Aletaha, D., Steiner, C.W., Kapral, T., Steiner, S., Saemann, M., Schwarzinger, I., Buranyi, B., Steiner, G., Smolen, J.S., 2007. Endothelial progenitor cells in active rheumatoid arthritis: effects of tumour necrosis factor and glucocorticoid therapy. Ann. Rheum. Dis. 66, 1284–1288.

Grisar, J., Aletaha, D., Steiner, C.W., Kapral, T., Steiner, S., Seidinger, D., Weigel, G., Schwarzinger, I., Wolozcszuk, W., Steiner, G., Smolen, J.S., 2005. Depletion of endothelial progenitor cells in the peripheral blood of patients with rheumatoid arthritis. Circulation 111, 204–211.

Grisar, J., Aringer, M., Koller, M.D., Stummvoll, G.H., Eselbock, D., Zwolfer, B., Steiner, C.W., Zierhut, B., Wagner, L., Pietschmann, P., Smolen, J.S., 2004. Leflunomide inhibits transendothelial migration of peripheral blood mononuclear cells. Ann. Rheum. Dis. 63, 1632–1637.

Gurcan, H.M., Keskin, D.B., Stern, J.N., Nitzberg, M.A., Shekhani, H., Ahmed, A.R., 2009. A review of the current use of rituximab in autoimmune diseases. Int. Immunopharmacol. 9, 10–25.

Hage, M.P., Al-Badri, M.R., Azar, S.T., 2014. A favorable effect of hydroxychloroquine on glucose and lipid metabolism beyond its anti-inflammatory role. Ther. Adv. Endocrinol. Metab. 5, 77–85.

Harrold, L.R., Reed, G.W., Magner, R., Shewade, A., John, A., Greenberg, J.D., Kremer, J.M., 2015. Comparative effectiveness and safety of rituximab versus subsequent anti-tumor necrosis factor therapy in patients with rheumatoid arthritis with prior exposure to anti-tumor necrosis factor therapies in the United States Corrona registry. Arthritis Res. Ther. 17, 256.

Herenius, M.M., Oliveira, A.S., Wijbrandts, C.A., Gerlag, D.M., Tak, P.P., Lebre, M.C., 2013. Anti-TNF therapy reduces serum levels of chemerin in rheumatoid arthritis: a new mechanism by which anti-TNF might reduce inflammation. PLoS One 8, e57802.

Heslinga, S.C., van Sijl, A.M., De Boer, K., van Halm, V.P., Nurmohamed, M.T., 2015. Tumor necrosis factor blocking therapy and congestive heart failure in patients with inflammatory rheumatic disorders: a systematic review. Curr. Med. Chem. 22, 1892–1902.

Hoshi, T., Kitagawa, K., Yamagami, H., Furukado, S., Hougaku, H., Hori, M., 2008. Relation between interleukin-6 level and subclinical intracranial large-artery atherosclerosis. Atherosclerosis 197, 326–332.

Howard, C., Noe, A., Skerjanec, A., Holzhauer, B., Wernsing, M., Ligueros-Saylan, M., Thuren, T., 2014. Safety and tolerability of canakinumab, an IL-1beta inhibitor, in type 2 diabetes mellitus patients: a pooled analysis of three randomised double-blind studies. Cardiovasc. Diabetol. 13, 94.

Hsu, C.C., Wang, H., Hsu, Y.H., Chuang, S.Y., Huang, Y.W., Chang, Y.K., Liu, J.S., Hsiung, C.A., Tsai, H.J., 2015. Use of nonsteroidal anti-inflammatory drugs and risk of chronic kidney disease in subjects with hypertension: nationwide longitudinal cohort study. Hypertension 66, 524–533.

Hsue, P.Y., Scherzer, R., Grunfeld, C., Imboden, J., Wu, Y., Del Puerto, G., Nitta, E., Shigenaga, J., Schnell Heringer, A., Ganz, P., Graf, J., 2014. Depletion of B-cells with rituximab improves endothelial function and reduces inflammation among individuals with rheumatoid arthritis. J. Am. Heart Assoc. 3, e001267.

Hurlimann, D., Forster, A., Noll, G., Enseleit, F., Chenevard, R., Distler, O., Bechir, M., Spieker, L.E., Neidhart, M., Michel, B.A., Gay, R.E., Luscher, T.F., Gay, S., Ruschitzka, F., 2002. Anti-tumor necrosis factor-alpha treatment improves endothelial function in patients with rheumatoid arthritis. Circulation 106, 2184–2187.

Huvers, F.C., Popa, C., Netea, M.G., Van den Hoogen, F.H., Tack, C.J., 2007. Improved insulin sensitivity by anti-TNFalpha antibody treatment in patients with rheumatic diseases. Ann. Rheum. Dis. 66, 558–559.

Ikdahl, E., Hisdal, J., Rollefstad, S., Olsen, I.C., Kvien, T.K., Pedersen, T.R., Semb, A.G., 2015. Rosuvastatin improves endothelial function in patients with inflammatory joint diseases, longitudinal associations with atherosclerosis and arteriosclerosis: results from the RORA-AS statin intervention study. Arthritis Res. Ther. 17, 279.

Ikonomidis, I., Tzortzis, S., Andreadou, I., Paraskevaidis, I., Katseli, C., Katsimbri, P., Pavlidis, G., Parissis, J., Kremastinos, D., Anastasiou-Nana, M., Lekakis, J., 2014. Increased benefit of interleukin-1 inhibition on vascular function, myocardial deformation, and twisting in patients with coronary artery disease and coexisting rheumatoid arthritis. Circ. Cardiovasc. Imaging 7, 619–628.

Jacobsson, L.T., Turesson, C., Gulfe, A., Kapetanovic, M.C., Petersson, I.F., Saxne, T., Geborek, P., 2005. Treatment with tumor necrosis factor blockers is associated with a lower incidence of first cardiovascular events in patients with rheumatoid arthritis. J. Rheumatol. 32, 1213–1218.

Johnsson, H., Panarelli, M., Cameron, A., Sattar, N., 2014. Analysis and modelling of cholesterol and high-density lipoprotein cholesterol changes across the range of C-reactive protein levels in clinical practice as an aid to better understanding of inflammation-lipid interactions. Ann. Rheum. Dis. 73, 1495–1499.

Kaplan, M.J., 2009. Management of cardiovascular disease risk in chronic inflammatory disorders. Nat. Rev. Rheumatol. 5, 208–217.

Karkucak, M., Capkin, E., Alver, A., Akyuz, A., Kiris, A., Ak, E., Topbas, M., Tosun, M., 2010. The effect of anti-TNF agent on oxidation status in patients with ankylosing spondylitis. Clin. Rheumatol. 29, 303–307.

Karp, I., Abrahamowicz, M., Fortin, P.R., Pilote, L., Neville, C., Pineau, C.A., Esdaile, J.M., 2008. Recent corticosteroid use and recent disease activity: independent determinants of coronary heart disease risk factors in systemic lupus erythematosus? Arthritis Rheum. 59, 169–175.

Kawashiri, S.Y., Kawakami, A., Yamasaki, S., Imazato, T., Iwamoto, N., Fujikawa, K., Aramaki, T., Tamai, M., Nakamura, H., Ida, H., Origuchi, T., Ueki, Y., Eguchi, K., 2010. Effects of the anti-interleukin-6 receptor antibody, tocilizumab, on serum lipid levels in patients with rheumatoid arthritis. Rheumatol. Int. 31, 451–456.

Kearney, P.M., Baigent, C., Godwin, J., Halls, H., Emberson, J.R., Patrono, C., 2006. Do selective cyclo-oxygenase-2 inhibitors and traditional non-steroidal anti-inflammatory drugs increase the risk of atherothrombosis? Meta-analysis of randomised trials. BMJ 332, 1302–1308.

Kerekes, G., Nurmohamed, M.T., Gonzalez-Gay, M.A., Seres, I., Paragh, G., Kardos, Z., Barath, Z., Tamasi, L., Soltesz, P., Szekanecz, Z., 2014. Rheumatoid arthritis and metabolic syndrome. Nat. Rev. Rheumatol. 10, 691–696.

Kerekes, G., Soltesz, P., Der, H., Veres, K., Szabo, Z., Vegvari, A., Shoenfeld, Y., Szekanecz, Z., 2009a. Effects of biologics on vascular function and atherosclerosis associated with rheumatoid arthritis. Ann. N. Y Acad. Sci. 1173, 814–821.

Kerekes, G., Soltesz, P., Der, H., Veres, K., Szabo, Z., Vegvari, A., Szegedi, G., Shoenfeld, Y., Szekanecz, Z., 2009b. Effects of rituximab treatment on endothelial dysfunction, carotid atherosclerosis, and lipid profile in rheumatoid arthritis. Clin. Rheumatol. 28, 705–710.

Kerekes, G., Soltesz, P., Nurmohamed, M.T., Gonzalez-Gay, M.A., Turiel, M., Vegh, E., Shoenfeld, Y., Mcinnes, I., Szekanecz, Z., 2012. Validated methods for assessment of subclinical atherosclerosis in rheumatology. Nat. Rev. Rheumatol. 8, 224–234.

Kerekes, G., Soltesz, P., Szucs, G., Szamosi, S., Der, H., Szabo, Z., Csathy, L., Vancsa, A., Szodoray, P., Szegedi, G., Szekanecz, Z., 2011. Effects of adalimumab treatment on vascular disease associated with early rheumatoid arthritis. Isr. Med. Assoc. J. 13, 147–152.

Kerekes, G., Szekanecz, Z., Der, H., Sandor, Z., Lakos, G., Muszbek, L., Csipo, I., Sipka, S., Seres, I., Paragh, G., Kappelmayer, J., Szomjak, E., Veres, K., Szegedi, G., Shoenfeld, Y., Soltesz, P., 2008. Endothelial dysfunction and atherosclerosis in rheumatoid arthritis: a multiparametric analysis using imaging techniques and laboratory markers of inflammation and autoimmunity. J. Rheumatol. 35, 398–406.

Kerr, G., Aujero, M., Richards, J., Sayles, H., Davis, L., Cannon, G., Caplan, L., Michaud, K., Mikuls, T., 2014. Associations of hydroxychloroquine use with lipid profiles in rheumatoid arthritis: pharmacologic implications. Arthritis Care Res. (Hoboken) 66, 1619–1626.

Ketelhuth, D.F., Hansson, G.K., 2015. Modulation of autoimmunity and atherosclerosis - common targets and promising translational approaches against disease. Circ. J. 79, 924–933.

Kim, H.J., Kim, M.J., Lee, C.K., Hong, Y.H., 2015. Effects of methotrexate on carotid intima-media thickness in patients with rheumatoid arthritis. J. Korean Med. Sci. 30, 1589–1596.

Kiortsis, D.N., Mavridis, A.K., Filippatos, T.D., Vasakos, S., Nikas, S.N., Drosos, A.A., 2006. Effects of infliximab treatment on lipoprotein profile in patients with rheumatoid arthritis and ankylosing spondylitis. J. Rheumatol. 33, 921–923.

Kirkham, B.W., Wasko, M.C., Hsia, E.C., Fleischmann, R.M., Genovese, M.C., Matteson, E.L., Liu, H., Rahman, M.U., 2014. Effects of golimumab, an anti-tumour necrosis factor-alpha human monoclonal antibody, on lipids and markers of inflammation. Ann. Rheum. Dis. 73, 161–169.

Klareskog, L., Hamsten, A., 2004. Statins in rheumatoid arthritis—two birds with one stone? Lancet 363, 2011–2012.

Kobezda, T., Ghassemi-Nejad, S., Mikecz, K., Glant, T.T., Szekanecz, Z., 2014. Of mice and men: how animal models advance our understanding of T-cell function in RA. Nat. Rev. Rheumatol. 10, 160–170.

Konijn, N., Van Tuyl, L., Den Uijl, D., Ter Wee, M., Kerstens, P., Voskuyl, A., van Schaardenburg, D., Lems, W., Nurmohamed, M., 2015. Prednisolone causes dose related unfavourable effects on body composition in early rheumatoid arthritis patients during the first year of treatment. Ann. Rheum. Dis. 74, 239.

Kotyla, P.J., Owczarek, A., Rakoczy, J., Lewicki, M., Kucharz, E.J., Emery, P., 2012. Infliximab treatment increases left ventricular ejection fraction in patients with rheumatoid arthritis: assessment of heart function by echocardiography, endothelin 1, interleukin 6, and NT-pro brain natriuretic peptide. J. Rheumatol. 39, 701–706.

Kume, K., Amano, K., Yamada, S., Hatta, K., Ohta, H., Kuwaba, N., 2011. Tocilizumab monotherapy reduces arterial stiffness as effectively as etanercept or adalimumab monotherapy in rheumatoid arthritis: an open-label randomized controlled trial. J. Rheumatol. 38, 2169–2171.

Lachmann, H.J., Kone-Paut, I., Kuemmerle-Deschner, J.B., Leslie, K.S., Hachulla, E., Quartier, P., Gitton, X., Widmer, A., Patel, N., Hawkins, P.N., 2009. Use of canakinumab in the cryopyrin-associated periodic syndrome. N. Engl. J. Med. 360, 2416–2425.

Lazzerini, P.E., Acampa, M., Capecchi, P.L., Fineschi, I., Selvi, E., Moscadelli, V., Zimbone, S., Gentile, D., Galeazzi, M., Laghi-Pasini, F., 2015. Antiarrhythmic potential of anticytokine therapy in rheumatoid arthritis: tocilizumab reduces corrected QT interval by controlling systemic inflammation. Arthritis Care Res. (Hoboken) 67, 332–339.

Lazzerini, P.E., Acampa, M., Capecchi, P.L., Hammoud, M., Maffei, S., Bisogno, S., Barreca, C., Galeazzi, M., Laghi-Pasini, F., 2013. Association between high sensitivity C-reactive protein, heart rate variability and corrected QT interval in patients with chronic inflammatory arthritis. Eur. J. Intern. Med. 24, 368–374.

Lazzerini, P.E., Acampa, M., Hammoud, M., Maffei, S., Capecchi, P.L., Selvi, E., Bisogno, S., Guideri, F., Galeazzi, M., Pasini, F.L., 2008. Arrhythmic risk during acute infusion of infliximab: a prospective, single-blind, placebo-controlled, crossover study in patients with chronic arthritis. J. Rheumatol. 35, 1958–1965.

Lazzerini, P.E., Capecchi, P.L., Bisogno, S., Galeazzi, M., Marcolongo, R., Pasini, F.L., 2003. Reduction in plasma homocysteine level in patients with rheumatoid arthritis given pulsed glucocorticoid treatment. Ann. Rheum. Dis. 62, 694–695.

Li, W.G., Tu, Q., Gu, X.J., 2010. Effect on content of serum inflammatory cytokines of patients with ankylosing spondylitis in early stage treated by long snake moxibustion at Governor Vessel and functional exercise. Zhongguo Zhen Jiu 30, 200–202.

Lima-Martinez, M.M., Campo, E., Salazar, J., Paoli, M., Maldonado, I., Acosta, C., Rodney, M., Contreras, M., Cabrera-Rego, J.O., Iacobellis, G., 2014. Epicardial fat thickness as cardiovascular risk factor and therapeutic target in patients with rheumatoid arthritis treated with biological and nonbiological therapies. Arthritis 2014, 782850.

Lindhardsen, J., Gislason, G.H., Jacobsen, S., Ahlehoff, O., Olsen, A.M., Madsen, O.R., Torp-Pedersen, C., Hansen, P.R., 2013. Non-steroidal anti-inflammatory drugs and risk of cardiovascular disease in patients with rheumatoid arthritis: a nationwide cohort study. Ann. Rheum. Dis. June 8 Epub.

Liu, Y.J., Wang, Z.G., Li, Z.L., Wei, M., Cai, X., Zhou, M., Zhu, J.L., 2010. Effect of arthroscopic debridement for adolescent ankylosing spondylitis with early hip-joint disease. Zhonghua Yi Xue Za Zhi 90, 1048–1050.

Ljung, L., Askling, J., Rantapaa-Dahlqvist, S., Jacobsson, L., Group, A.S., 2014. The risk of acute coronary syndrome in rheumatoid arthritis in relation to tumour necrosis factor inhibitors and the risk in the general population: a national cohort study. Arthritis Res. Ther. 16, R127.

Maki-Petaja, K.M., Booth, A.D., Hall, F.C., Wallace, S.M., Brown, J., Mceniery, C.M., Wilkinson, I.B., 2007. Ezetimibe and simvastatin reduce inflammation, disease activity, and aortic stiffness and improve endothelial function in rheumatoid arthritis. J. Am. Coll. Cardiol. 50, 852–858.

Maki-Petaja, K.M., Hall, F.C., Booth, A.D., Wallace, S.M., Yasmin, Bearcroft, P.W., Harish, S., Furlong, A., Mceniery, C.M., Brown, J., Wilkinson, I.B., 2006. Rheumatoid arthritis is associated with increased aortic pulse-wave velocity, which is reduced by anti-tumor necrosis factor-alpha therapy. Circulation 114, 1185–1192.

Makrilakis, K., Fragiadaki, K., Sfikakis, P.P., Kitas, G.D., 2015a. Chemerin and cardiovascular risk in rheumatoid arthritis after interleukin 6 receptor blockade. J. Rheumatol. 42, 349.

Makrilakis, K., Fragiadaki, K., Smith, J., Sfikakis, P.P., Kitas, G.D., 2015b. Interrelated reduction of chemerin and plasminogen activator inhibitor-1 serum levels in rheumatoid arthritis after interleukin-6 receptor blockade. Clin. Rheumatol. 34, 419–427.

Manfredi, A.A., Baldini, M., Camera, M., Baldissera, E., Brambilla, M., Peretti, G., Maseri, A., Rovere-Querini, P., Tremoli, E., Sabbadini, M.G., Maugeri, N., 2016. Anti-TNFalpha agents curb platelet activation in patients with rheumatoid arthritis. Ann. Rheum. Dis. 75, 1511–1520.

Marcora, S.M., Chester, K.R., Mittal, G., Lemmey, A.B., Maddison, P.J., 2006. Randomized phase 2 trial of anti-tumor necrosis factor therapy for cachexia in patients with early rheumatoid arthritis. Am. J. Clin. Nutr. 84, 1463–1472.

Marks, J.L., Edwards, C.J., 2012. Protective effect of methotrexate in patients with rheumatoid arthritis and cardiovascular comorbidity. Ther. Adv. Musculoskelet. Dis. 4, 149–157.

Martin-Martinez, M.A., Gonzalez-Juanatey, C., Castaneda, S., Llorca, J., Ferraz-Amaro, I., Fernandez-Gutierrez, B., Diaz-Gonzalez, F., Gonzalez-Gay, M.A., 2014. Recommendations for the management of cardiovascular risk in patients with rheumatoid arthritis: scientific evidence and expert opinion. Semin. Arthritis Rheum. 44, 1–8.

Martini, G., Biscaro, F., Boscaro, E., Calabrese, F., Lunardi, F., Facco, M., Agostini, C., Zulian, F., Fadini, G.P., 2015. Reduced levels of circulating progenitor cells in juvenile idiopathic arthritis are counteracted by anti TNF-alpha therapy. BMC Musculoskelet. Disord. 16, 103.

Maxwell, L., Singh, J.A., 2009. Abatacept for rheumatoid arthritis. Cochrane Database Syst. Rev. CD007277.

Maxwell, S.R., Moots, R.J., Kendall, M.J., 1994. Corticosteroids: do they damage the cardiovascular system? Postgrad. Med. J. 70, 863–870.

McCarey, D.W., Mcinnes, I.B., Madhok, R., Hampson, R., Scherbakov, O., Ford, I., Capell, H.A., Sattar, N., 2004. Trial of Atorvastatin in Rheumatoid Arthritis (TARA): double-blind, randomised placebo-controlled trial. Lancet 363, 2015–2021.

McGettigan, P., Henry, D., 2006. Cardiovascular risk and inhibition of cyclooxygenase: a systematic review of the observational studies of selective and nonselective inhibitors of cyclooxygenase 2. JAMA 296, 1633–1644.

McInnes, I.B., Kim, H.Y., Lee, S.H., Mandel, D., Song, Y.W., Connell, C.A., Luo, Z., Brosnan, M.J., Zuckerman, A., Zwillich, S.H., Bradley, J.D., 2014. Open-label tofacitinib and double-blind atorvastatin in rheumatoid arthritis patients: a randomised study. Ann. Rheum. Dis. 73, 124–131.

McInnes, I.B., Thompson, L., Giles, J.T., Bathon, J.M., Salmon, J.E., Beaulieu, A.D., Codding, C.E., Carlson, T.H., Delles, C., Lee, J.S., Sattar, N., 2015. Effect of interleukin-6 receptor blockade on surrogates of vascular risk in rheumatoid arthritis: MEASURE, a randomised, placebo-controlled study. Ann. Rheum. Dis. 74, 694–702.

Metsios, G.S., Stavropoulos-Kalinoglou, A., Douglas, K.M., Koutedakis, Y., Nevill, A.M., Panoulas, V.F., Kita, M., Kitas, G.D., 2007. Blockade of tumour necrosis factor-alpha in rheumatoid arthritis: effects on components of rheumatoid cachexia. Rheumatology (Oxford) 46, 1824–1827.

Micha, R., Imamura, F., Wyler Von Ballmoos, M., Solomon, D.H., Hernan, M.A., Ridker, P.M., Mozaffarian, D., 2011. Systematic review and meta-analysis of methotrexate use and risk of cardiovascular disease. Am. J. Cardiol. 108, 1362–1370.

Minoretti, P., Bruno, A., Di Vito, C., Emanuele, E., 2007. Leflunomide as an antiatherogenic drug. Med. Hypotheses 68, 1175–1176.

Mirjafari, H., Welsh, P., Verstappen, S.M., Wilson, P., Marshall, T., Edlin, H., Bunn, D., Chipping, J., Lunt, M., Symmons, D.P., Sattar, N., Bruce, I.N., 2014. N-terminal pro-brain-type natriuretic peptide (NT-pro-BNP) and mortality risk in early inflammatory polyarthritis: results from the Norfolk Arthritis Registry (NOAR). Ann. Rheum. Dis. 73, 684–690.

Morgan, C.L., Emery, P., Porter, D., Reynolds, A., Young, A., Boyd, H., Poole, C.D., Currie, C.J., 2014. Treatment of rheumatoid arthritis with etanercept with reference to disease-modifying anti-rheumatic drugs: long-term safety and survival using prospective, observational data. Rheumatology (Oxford) 53, 186–194.

Morris, S.J., Wasko, M.C., Antohe, J.L., Sartorius, J.A., Kirchner, H.L., Dancea, S., Bili, A., 2011. Hydroxychloroquine use associated with improvement in lipid profiles in rheumatoid arthritis patients. Arthritis Care Res. (Hoboken) 63, 530–534.

Myasoedova, E., Crowson, C.S., Green, A.B., Matteson, E.L., Gabriel, S.E., 2014. Longterm blood pressure variability in patients with rheumatoid arthritis and its effect on cardiovascular events and all-cause mortality in RA: a population-based comparative cohort study. J. Rheumatol. 41, 1638–1644.

Myasoedova, E., Crowson, C.S., Kremers, H.M., Roger, V.L., Fitz-Gibbon, P.D., Therneau, T.M., Gabriel, S.E., 2011. Lipid paradox in rheumatoid arthritis: the impact of serum lipid measures and systemic inflammation on the risk of cardiovascular disease. Ann. Rheum. Dis. 70, 482–487.

Nakata, H., Steinberg, S.M., Koh, Y., Maeda, K., Takaoka, Y., Tamamura, H., Fujii, N., Mitsuya, H., 2008. Potent synergistic anti-human immunodeficiency virus (HIV) effects using combinations of the CCR5 inhibitor aplaviroc with other anti-HIV drugs. Antimicrob. Agents Chemother. 52, 2111–2119.

Nissen, S.E., Nicholls, S.J., Sipahi, I., Libby, P., Raichlen, J.S., Ballantyne, C.M., Davignon, J., Erbel, R., Fruchart, J.C., Tardif, J.C., Schoenhagen, P., Crowe, T., Cain, V., Wolski, K., Goormastic, M., Tuzcu, E.M., 2006. Effect of very high-intensity statin therapy on regression of coronary atherosclerosis: the ASTEROID trial. JAMA 295, 1556–1565.

Norris, S., White, M., Mankan, A.K., Lawless, M.W., 2010. Highly sensitivity adhesion molecules detection in hereditary haemochromatosis patients reveals altered expression. Int. J. Immunogenet. 37, 125–133.

Novikova, D.S., Popkova, T.V., Lukina, G.V., Luchikhina, E.L., Karateev, D.E., Volkov, A.V., Novikov, A.A., Aleksandrova, E.N., Nasonov, E.L., 2016. The effects of rituximab on lipids, arterial stiffness and carotid intima-media thickness in rheumatoid arthritis. J. Korean Med. Sci. 31, 202–207.

Nurmohamed, M., 2015. EULAR recommendation update on cardiovascular disease in RA. Ann. Rheum. Dis. 74, 9.

Nurmohamed, M., Bao, Y., Signorovitch, J., Trahey, A., Mulani, P., Furst, D.E., 2015. Longer durations of antitumour necrosis factor treatment are associated with reduced risk of cardiovascular events in patients with rheumatoid arthritis. RMD Open 1, e000080.

Nurmohamed, M.T., van Halm, V.P., Dijkmans, B.A., 2002. Cardiovascular risk profile of antirheumatic agents in patients with osteoarthritis and rheumatoid arthritis. Drugs 62, 1599–1609.

Oh, Y.B., Ahn, M., Lee, S.M., Koh, H.W., Lee, S.H., Kim, S.H., Park, B.H., 2013. Inhibition of Janus activated kinase-3 protects against myocardial ischemia and reperfusion injury in mice. Exp. Mol. Med. 45, e23.

Ormseth, M.J., Oeser, A.M., Cunningham, A., Bian, A., Shintani, A., Solus, J., Tanner, S.B., Stein, C.M., 2014. Reversing vascular dysfunction in rheumatoid arthritis: improved augmentation index but not endothelial function with peroxisome proliferator-activated receptor gamma agonist therapy. Arthritis Rheumatol. 66, 2331–2338.

Panoulas, V.F., Toms, T.E., Douglas, K.M., Sandoo, A., Metsios, G.S., Stavropoulos-Kalinoglou, A., Kitas, G.D., 2014. Prolonged QTc interval predicts all-cause mortality in patients with rheumatoid arthritis: an association driven by high inflammatory burden. Rheumatology (Oxford) 53, 131–137.

Patel, A.M., Moreland, L.W., 2010. Interleukin-6 inhibition for treatment of rheumatoid arthritis: a review of tocilizumab therapy. Drug Des. Devel. Ther. 4, 263–278.

Peters, M.J., Nurmohamed, M.T., 2013. Cardiovascular risk management in rheumatoid arthritis: are we still waiting for the first step? Arthritis Res. Ther. 15, 111.

Peters, M.J., Symmons, D.P., Mccarey, D., Dijkmans, B.A., Nicola, P., Kvien, T.K., Mcinnes, I.B., Haentzschel, H., Gonzalez-Gay, M.A., Provan, S., Semb, A., Sidiropoulos, P., Kitas, G., Smulders, Y.M., Soubrier, M., Szekanecz, Z., Sattar, N., Nurmohamed, M.T., 2010a. EULAR evidence-based recommendations for cardiovascular risk management in patients with rheumatoid arthritis and other forms of inflammatory arthritis. Ann. Rheum. Dis. 69, 325–331.

Peters, M.J., van Halm, V.P., Voskuyl, A.E., Smulders, Y.M., Boers, M., Lems, W.F., Visser, M., Stehouwer, C.D., Dekker, J.M., Nijpels, G., Heine, R., Dijkmans, B.A., Nurmohamed, M.T., 2009. Does rheumatoid arthritis equal diabetes mellitus as an independent risk factor for cardiovascular disease? A prospective study. Arthritis Rheum. 61, 1571–1579.

Peters, M.J., Vis, M., van Halm, V.P., Wolbink, G.J., Voskuyl, A.E., Lems, W.F., Dijkmans, B.A., Twisk, J.W., De Koning, M.H., van De Stadt, R.J., Nurmohamed, M.T., 2007. Changes in lipid profile during infliximab and corticosteroid treatment in rheumatoid arthritis. Ann. Rheum. Dis. 66, 958–961.

Peters, M.J., Watt, P., Cherry, L., Welsh, P., Henninger, E., Dijkmans, B.A., Mcinnes, I.B., Nurmohamed, M.T., Sattar, N., 2010b. Lack of effect of TNFalpha blockade therapy on circulating adiponectin levels in patients with autoimmune disease: results from two independent prospective studies. Ann. Rheum. Dis. 69, 1687–1690.

Petri, M., Lakatta, C., Magder, L., Goldman, D., 1994. Effect of prednisone and hydroxychloroquine on coronary artery disease risk factors in systemic lupus erythematosus: a longitudinal data analysis. Am. J. Med. 96, 254–259.

Pham, T., Gossec, L., Constantin, A., Pavy, S., Bruckert, E., Cantagrel, A., Combe, B., Flipo, R.M., Goupille, P., Le Loet, X., Mariette, X., Puechal, X., Schaeverbeke, T., Sibilia, J., Tebib, J., Wendling, D., Dougados, M., 2006. Cardiovascular risk and rheumatoid arthritis: clinical practice guidelines based on published evidence and expert opinion. Jt. Bone Spine 73, 379–387.

Popa, C., Netea, M.G., Radstake, T., van Der Meer, J.W., Stalenhoef, A.F., van Riel, P.L., Barerra, P., 2005. Influence of anti-tumour necrosis factor therapy on cardiovascular risk factors in patients with active rheumatoid arthritis. Ann. Rheum. Dis. 64 303–305.

Popa, C., Netea, M.G., van Riel, P.L., van Der Meer, J.W., Stalenhoef, A.F., 2007a. The role of TNF-alpha in chronic inflammatory conditions, intermediary metabolism, and cardiovascular risk. J. Lipid Res. 48, 751–762.

Popa, C., van den Hoogen, F.H., Radstake, T.R., Netea, M.G., Eijsbouts, A.E., Den Heijer, M., van Der Meer, J.W., van Riel, P.L., Stalenhoef, A.F., Barrera, P., 2007b. Modulation of lipoprotein plasma concentrations during long-term anti-TNF therapy in patients with active rheumatoid arthritis. Ann. Rheum. Dis. 66, 1503–1507.

Protogerou, A.D., Zampeli, E., Fragiadaki, K., Stamatelopoulos, K., Papamichael, C., Sfikakis, P.P., 2011. A pilot study of endothelial dysfunction and aortic stiffness after interleukin-6 receptor inhibition in rheumatoid arthritis. Atherosclerosis 219, 734–736.

Provan, S.A., Berg, I.J., Hammer, H.B., Mathiessen, A., Kvien, T.K., Semb, A.G., 2015. The impact of newer biological disease modifying anti-rheumatic drugs on cardiovascular risk factors: a 12-Month longitudinal study in rheumatoid arthritis patients treated with rituximab, abatacept and tociliziumab. PLoS One 10, e0130709.

Rainsford, K.D., Parke, A.L., Clifford-Rashotte, M., Kean, W.F., 2015. Therapy and pharmacological properties of hydroxychloroquine and chloroquine in treatment of systemic lupus erythematosus, rheumatoid arthritis and related diseases. Inflammopharmacology 23, 231–269.

Rao, V.U., Pavlov, A., Klearman, M., Musselman, D., Giles, J.T., Bathon, J.M., Sattar, N., Lee, J.S., 2015. An evaluation of risk factors for major adverse cardiovascular events during tocilizumab therapy. Arthritis Rheumatol. 67, 372–380.

Raterman, H.G., Levels, H., Voskuyl, A.E., Lems, W.F., Dijkmans, B.A., Nurmohamed, M.T., 2013. HDL protein composition alters from proatherogenic into less atherogenic and proinflammatory in rheumatoid arthritis patients responding to rituximab. Ann. Rheum. Dis. 72, 560–565.

Reiss, A.B., Carsons, S.E., Anwar, K., Rao, S., Edelman, S.D., Zhang, H., Fernandez, P., Cronstein, B.N., Chan, E.S., 2008. Atheroprotective effects of methotrexate on reverse cholesterol transport proteins and foam cell transformation in human THP-1 monocyte/macrophages. Arthritis Rheum. 58, 3675–3683.

Ridker, P.M., 2004. High-sensitivity C-reactive protein, inflammation, and cardiovascular risk: from concept to clinical practice to clinical benefit. Am. Heart J. 148, S19–S26.

Ridker, P.M., 2014. Targeting inflammatory pathways for the treatment of cardiovascular disease. Eur. Heart J. 35, 540–543.

Ridker, P.M., Howard, C.P., Walter, V., Everett, B., Libby, P., Hensen, J., Thuren, T., Group, C.P.I., 2012. Effects of interleukin-1beta inhibition with canakinumab on hemoglobin A1c, lipids, C-reactive protein, interleukin-6, and fibrinogen: a phase IIb randomized, placebo-controlled trial. Circulation 126, 2739–2748.

Ridker, P.M., Luscher, T.F., 2014. Anti-inflammatory therapies for cardiovascular disease. Eur. Heart J. 35, 1782–1791.

Robertson, J., Peters, M.J., Mcinnes, I.B., Sattar, N., 2013. Changes in lipid levels with inflammation and therapy in RA: a maturing paradigm. Nat. Rev. Rheumatol. 9, 513–523.

Rollefstad, S., Ikdahl, E., Hisdal, J., Olsen, I.C., Holme, I., Hammer, H.B., Smerud, K.T., Kitas, G.D., Pedersen, T.R., Kvien, T.K., Semb, A.G., 2015. Rosuvastatin-induced carotid plaque regression in patients with inflammatory joint diseases: the rosuvastatin in rheumatoid arthritis, ankylosing spondylitis and other inflammatory joint diseases study. Arthritis Rheumatol. 67, 1718–1728.

Ronda, N., Favari, E., Borghi, M.O., Ingegnoli, F., Gerosa, M., Chighizola, C., Zimetti, F., Adorni, M.P., Bernini, F., Meroni, P.L., 2014. Impaired serum cholesterol efflux capacity in rheumatoid arthritis and systemic lupus erythematosus. Ann. Rheum. Dis. 73, 609–615.

Ronda, N., Greco, D., Adorni, M.P., Zimetti, F., Favari, E., Hjeltnes, G., Mikkelsen, K., Borghi, M.O., Favalli, E.G., Gatti, R., Hollan, I., Meroni, P.L., Bernini, F., 2015. Newly identified antiatherosclerotic activity of methotrexate and adalimumab: complementary effects on lipoprotein function and macrophage cholesterol metabolism. Arthritis Rheumatol. 67, 1155–1164.

Roos, M.A., Gennero, L., Denysenko, T., Reguzzi, S., Cavallo, G., Pescarmona, G.P., Ponzetto, A., 2010. Microparticles in physiological and in pathological conditions. Cell Biochem. Funct. 28, 539–548.

Ross, R., 1999. Atherosclerosis—an inflammatory disease. N. Engl. J. Med. 340, 115–126.

Roubille, C., Martel-Pelletier, J., Haraoui, B., Tardif, J.C., Pelletier, J.P., 2013. Biologics and the cardiovascular system: a double-edged sword. Antiinflamm. Antiallergy Agents Med. Chem. 12, 68–82.

Roubille, C., Richer, V., Starnino, T., Mccourt, C., Mcfarlane, A., Fleming, P., Siu, S., Kraft, J., Lynde, C., Pope, J., Gulliver, W., Keeling, S., Dutz, J., Bessette, L., Bissonnette, R., Haraoui, B., 2015a. The effects of tumour necrosis factor inhibitors, methotrexate, non-steroidal anti-inflammatory drugs and corticosteroids on cardiovascular events in rheumatoid arthritis, psoriasis and psoriatic arthritis: a systematic review and meta-analysis. Ann. Rheum. Dis. 74, 480–489.

Roubille, C., Richer, V., Starnino, T., Mccourt, C., Mcfarlane, A., Fleming, P., Siu, S., Kraft, J., Lynde, C., Pope, J., Gulliver, W., Keeling, S., Dutz, J., Bessette, L., Bissonnette, R., Haraoui, B., 2015b. Evidence-based recommendations for the management of comorbidities in rheumatoid arthritis, psoriasis, and psoriatic arthritis: expert opinion of the canadian dermatology-rheumatology comorbidity initiative. J. Rheumatol. 42, 1767–1780.

Rozman, B., Praprotnik, S., Logar, D., Tomsic, M., Hojnik, M., Kos-Golja, M., Accetto, R., Dolenc, P., 2002. Leflunomide and hypertension. Ann. Rheum. Dis. 61, 567–569.

Ruiz-Irastorza, G., Ramos-Casals, M., Brito-Zeron, P., Khamashta, M.A., 2010. Clinical efficacy and side effects of antimalarials in systemic lupus erythematosus: a systematic review. Ann. Rheum. Dis. 69, 20–28.

Sarzi-Puttini, P., Atzeni, F., Shoenfeld, Y., Ferraccioli, G., 2005. TNF-alpha, rheumatoid arthritis, and heart failure: a rheumatological dilemma. Autoimmun. Rev. 4, 153–161.

Sattar, N., Crompton, P., Cherry, L., Kane, D., Lowe, G., Mcinnes, I.B., 2007. Effects of tumor necrosis factor blockade on cardiovascular risk factors in psoriatic arthritis: a double-blind, placebo-controlled study. Arthritis Rheum. 56, 831–839.

Schlesinger, N., Alten, R.E., Bardin, T., Schumacher, H.R., Bloch, M., Gimona, A., Krammer, G., Murphy, V., Richard, D., So, A.K., 2012. Canakinumab for acute gouty arthritis in patients with limited treatment options: results from two randomised, multicentre, active-controlled, double-blind trials and their initial extensions. Ann. Rheum. Dis. 71, 1839–1848.

Schroeder, L.L., Tang, X., Wasko, M.C., Bili, A., 2015. Glucocorticoid use is associated with increase in HDL and no change in other lipids in rheumatoid arthritis patients. Rheumatol. Int. 35, 1059–1067.

Schultz, O., Oberhauser, F., Saech, J., Rubbert-Roth, A., Hahn, M., Krone, W., Laudes, M., 2010. Effects of inhibition of interleukin-6 signalling on insulin sensitivity and lipoprotein (a) levels in human subjects with rheumatoid diseases. PLoS One 5, e14328.

Scott, P.A., Kingsley, G.H., Smith, C.M., Choy, E.H., Scott, D.L., 2007. Non-steroidal anti-inflammatory drugs and myocardial infarctions: comparative systematic review of evidence from observational studies and randomised controlled trials. Ann. Rheum. Dis. 66, 1296–1304.

Seriolo, B., Ferrone, C., Cutolo, M., 2008. Longterm anti-tumor necrosis factor-alpha treatment in patients with refractory rheumatoid arthritis: relationship between insulin resistance and disease activity. J. Rheumatol. 35, 355–357.

Seriolo, B., Paolino, S., Sulli, A., Fasciolo, D., Cutolo, M., 2006. Effects of anti-TNF-alpha treatment on lipid profile in patients with active rheumatoid arthritis. Ann. N. Y Acad. Sci. 1069, 414–419.

Sfikakis, P.P., Bournia, V.K., Kitas, G., 2014. Do non-steroidal anti-inflammatory drugs increase or decrease cardiovascular risk in patients with rheumatoid arthritis? Clin. Exp. Rheumatol. 32, S-8–9.

Sherer, Y., Shoenfeld, Y., 2006. Mechanisms of disease: atherosclerosis in autoimmune diseases. Nat. Clin. Pract. Rheumatol. 2, 99–106.

Shoenfeld, Y., Gerli, R., Doria, A., Matsuura, E., Cerinic, M.M., Ronda, N., Jara, L.J., Abu-Shakra, M., Meroni, P.L., Sherer, Y., 2005. Accelerated atherosclerosis in autoimmune rheumatic diseases. Circulation 112, 3337–3347.

Sidiropoulos, P.I., Siakka, P., Pagonidis, K., Raptopoulou, A., Kritikos, H., Tsetis, D., Boumpas, D.T., 2009. Sustained improvement of vascular endothelial function during anti-TNFalpha treatment in rheumatoid arthritis patients. Scand. J. Rheumatol. 38, 6–10.

Simmonds, R.E., Lali, F.V., Smallie, T., Small, P.L., Foxwell, B.M., 2009. Mycolactone inhibits monocyte cytokine production by a posttranscriptional mechanism. J. Immunol. 182, 2194–2202.

Singh, J.A., Wells, G.A., Christensen, R., Tanjong Ghogomu, E., Maxwell, L., Macdonald, J.K., Filippini, G., Skoetz, N., Francis, D., Lopes, L.C., Guyatt, G.H., Schmitt, J., La Mantia, L., Weberschock, T., Roos, J.F., Siebert, H., Hershan, S., Lunn, M.P., Tugwell, P., Buchbinder, R., 2011. Adverse effects of biologics: a network meta-analysis and Cochrane overview. Cochrane Database Syst. Rev. CD008794.

Skoog, T., Dichtl, W., Boquist, S., Skoglund-Andersson, C., Karpe, F., Tang, R., Bond, M.G., De Faire, U., Nilsson, J., Eriksson, P., Hamsten, A., 2002. Plasma tumour necrosis factor-alpha and early carotid atherosclerosis in healthy middle-aged men. Eur. Heart J. 23, 376–383.

Smolen, J.S., Landewe, R., Breedveld, F.C., Buch, M., Burmester, G., Dougados, M., Emery, P., Gaujoux-Viala, C., Gossec, L., Nam, J., Ramiro, S., Winthrop, K., De Wit, M., Aletaha, D., Betteridge, N., Bijlsma, J.W., Boers, M., Buttgereit, F., Combe, B., Cutolo, M., Damjanov, N., Hazes, J.M., Kouloumas, M., Kvien, T.K., Mariette, X., Pavelka, K., van Riel, P.L., Rubbert-Roth, A., Scholte-Voshaar, M., Scott, D.L., Sokka-Isler, T., Wong, J.B., van Der Heijde, D., 2013. EULAR recommendations for the management of rheumatoid arthritis with synthetic and biological disease-modifying antirheumatic drugs: 2013 update. Ann. Rheum. Dis. 73, 492–509.

Soubrier, M., Jouanel, P., Mathieu, S., Poujol, D., Claus, D., Dubost, J.J., Ristori, J.M., 2008. Effects of anti-tumor necrosis factor therapy on lipid profile in patients with rheumatoid arthritis. Jt. Bone Spine 75, 22–24.

Souto, A., Salgado, E., Maneiro, J.R., Mera, A., Carmona, L., Gomez-Reino, J.J., 2015. Lipid profile changes in patients with chronic inflammatory arthritis treated with biologic agents and tofacitinib in randomized clinical trials: a systematic review and meta-analysis. Arthritis Rheumatol. 67, 117–127.

Steiner, G., Urowitz, M.B., 2009. Lipid profiles in patients with rheumatoid arthritis: mechanisms and the impact of treatment. Semin. Arthritis Rheum. 38, 372–381.

Suissa, S., Bernatsky, S., Hudson, M., 2006. Antirheumatic drug use and the risk of acute myocardial infarction. Arthritis Rheum. 55, 531–536.

Szekanecz, Z., 2008. Pro-inflammatory cytokines in atherosclerosis. Isr. Med. Assoc. J. 10, 529–530.

Szekanecz, Z., Besenyei, T., Szentpetery, A., Koch, A.E., 2010. Angiogenesis and vasculogenesis in rheumatoid arthritis. Curr. Opin. Rheumatol. 22, 299–306.

Szekanecz, Z., Kerekes, G., Der, H., Sandor, Z., Szabo, Z., Vegvari, A., Simkovics, E., Soos, L., Szentpetery, A., Besenyei, T., Szucs, G., Szanto, S., Tamasi, L., Szegedi, G., Shoenfeld, Y.,

Soltesz, P., 2007. Accelerated atherosclerosis in rheumatoid arthritis. Ann. N. Y Acad. Sci. 1108, 349–358.

Szekanecz, Z., Kerekes, G., Soltesz, P., 2009. Vascular effects of biologic agents in RA and spondyloarthropathies. Nat. Rev. Rheumatol. 5, 677–684.

Szekanecz, Z., Kerekes, G., Kardos, Z., Baráth, Z., Tamási, L., 2016. Mechanisms of inflammatory atherosclerosis in rheumatoid arthritis. Curr. Immunol. Rev. in press.

Szekanecz, Z., Koch, A.E., 2010. Vasculogenesis in rheumatoid arthritis. Arthritis Res. Ther. 12, 110.

Takacova, M., Nogova, P., Habekova, M., Stanekova, D., 2008. Prevalence of a 32 bp deletion in the gene for human immunodeficiency virus 1 co-receptor ccr5 in slovak population. Acta Virol. 52, 261–264.

Takashima, K., Miyake, H., Kanzaki, N., Tagawa, Y., Wang, X., Sugihara, Y., Iizawa, Y., Baba, M., 2005. Highly potent inhibition of human immunodeficiency virus type 1 replication by TAK-220, an orally bioavailable small-molecule CCR5 antagonist. Antimicrob. Agents Chemother. 49, 3474–3482.

Tam, L.S., Gladman, D.D., Hallett, D.C., Rahman, P., Urowitz, M.B., 2000. Effect of antimalarial agents on the fasting lipid profile in systemic lupus erythematosus. J. Rheumatol. 27, 2142–2145.

Tam, L.S., Kitas, G.D., Gonzalez-Gay, M.A., 2014. Can suppression of inflammation by anti-TNF prevent progression of subclinical atherosclerosis in inflammatory arthritis? Rheumatology (Oxford) 53, 1108–1119.

Tam, L.S., Tomlinson, B., Chu, T.T., Li, T.K., Li, E.K., 2007. Impact of TNF inhibition on insulin resistance and lipids levels in patients with rheumatoid arthritis. Clin. Rheumatol. 26, 1495–1498.

Tanaka, R., Takahashi, Y., Kodama, A., Saito, M., Ansari, A.A., Tanaka, Y., 2010. Suppression of CCR5-tropic HIV type 1 infection by OX40 stimulation via enhanced production of beta-chemokines. AIDS Res. Hum. Retroviruses 26, 1147–1154.

Thornton, C.C., AL-Rashed, F., Calay, D., Birdsey, G.M., Bauer, A., Mylroie, H., Morley, B.J., Randi, A.M., Haskard, D.O., Boyle, J.J., Mason, J.C., 2016. Methotrexate-mediated activation of an AMPK-CREB-dependent pathway: a novel mechanism for vascular protection in chronic systemic inflammation. Ann. Rheum. Dis. 75, 439–448.

Timar, O., Szekanecz, Z., Kerekes, G., Vegh, J., Olah, A.V., Nagy, G., Csiki, Z., Danko, K., Szamosi, S., Nemeth, A., Soltesz, P., Szucs, G., 2013. Rosuvastatin improves impaired endothelial function, lowers high sensitivity CRP, complement and immuncomplex production in patients with systemic sclerosis—a prospective case-series study. Arthritis Res. Ther. 15, R105.

Toms, T.E., Panoulas, V.F., Douglas, K.M., Griffiths, H.R., Kitas, G.D., 2008. Lack of association between glucocorticoid use and presence of the metabolic syndrome in patients with rheumatoid arthritis: a cross-sectional study. Arthritis Res. Ther. 10, R145.

Tournadre, A., Tatar, Z., Pereira, B., Chevreau, M., Gossec, L., Gaudin, P., Soubrier, M., Dougados, M., 2015. Application of the European Society of Cardiology, Adult Treatment Panel III and American College of Cardiology/American Heart Association guidelines for cardiovascular risk management in a French cohort of rheumatoid arthritis. Int. J. Cardiol. 183, 149–154.

Tremblay, C.L., Giguel, F., Chou, T.C., Dong, H., Takashima, K., Hirsch, M.S., 2005. TAK-652, a novel CCR5 inhibitor, has favourable drug interactions with other antiretrovirals in vitro. Antivir. Ther. 10, 967–968.

Tsai, W.C., Ou, T.T., Yen, J.H., Wu, C.C., Tung, Y.C., 2015. Long-term frequent use of non-steroidal anti-inflammatory drugs might protect patients with ankylosing spondylitis from cardiovascular diseases: a nationwide case-control study. PLoS One 10, e0126347.

Turiel, M., Tomasoni, L., Sitia, S., Cicala, S., Gianturco, L., Ricci, C., Atzeni, F., De Gennaro Colonna, V., Longhi, M., Sarzi-Puttini, P., 2010. Effects of long-term disease-modifying antirheumatic drugs on endothelial function in patients with early rheumatoid arthritis. Cardiovasc. Ther. 28, e53–e64.

Tzoulaki, I., Murray, G.D., Lee, A.J., Rumley, A., Lowe, G.D., Fowkes, F.G., 2005. C-reactive protein, interleukin-6, and soluble adhesion molecules as predictors of progressive peripheral atherosclerosis in the general population: Edinburgh artery study. Circulation 112, 976–983.

Uchida, H.A., Nakamura, Y., Kaihara, M., Norii, H., Hanayama, Y., Sugiyama, H., Maeshima, Y., Yamasaki, Y., Makino, H., 2006. Steroid pulse therapy impaired endothelial function while increasing plasma high molecule adiponectin concentration in patients with IgA nephropathy. Nephrol. Dial. Transplant. 21, 3475–3480.

Ursini, F., Naty, S., Grembiale, R.D., 2010. Infliximab and insulin resistance. Autoimmun. Rev. 9, 536–539.

Ursini, F., Russo, E., Letizia Hribal, M., Mauro, D., Savarino, F., Bruno, C., Tripolino, C., Rubino, M., Naty, S., Grembiale, R.D., 2015. Abatacept improves whole-body insulin sensitivity in rheumatoid arthritis: an observational study. Medicine (Baltimore) 94, e888.

van Den Oever, I.A., van Sijl, A.M., Nurmohamed, M.T., 2013. Management of cardiovascular risk in patients with rheumatoid arthritis: evidence and expert opinion. Ther. Adv. Musculoskelet. Dis. 5, 166–181.

van Denderen, J.C., Peters, M.J., van Halm, V.P., Van Der Horst-Bruinsma, I.E., Dijkmans, B.A., Nurmohamed, M.T., 2006. Statin therapy might be beneficial for patients with ankylosing spondylitis. Ann. Rheum. Dis. 65, 695–696.

Van Doornum, S., Jennings, G.L., Wicks, I.P., 2006. Reducing the cardiovascular disease burden in rheumatoid arthritis. Med. J. Aust. 184, 287–290.

Van Doornum, S., Mccoll, G., Wicks, I.P., 2002. Accelerated atherosclerosis: an extraarticular feature of rheumatoid arthritis? Arthritis Rheum. 46, 862–873.

Van Doornum, S., Mccoll, G., Wicks, I.P., 2005. Tumour necrosis factor antagonists improve disease activity but not arterial stiffness in rheumatoid arthritis. Rheumatology (Oxford) 44, 1428–1432.

van Halm, V.P., Nurmohamed, M.T., Twisk, J.W., Dijkmans, B.A., Voskuyl, A.E., 2006. Disease-modifying antirheumatic drugs are associated with a reduced risk for cardiovascular disease in patients with rheumatoid arthritis: a case control study. Arthritis Res. Ther. 8, R151.

van Sijl, A.M., Boers, M., Voskuyl, A.E., Nurmohamed, M.T., 2014. Confounding by indication probably distorts the relationship between steroid use and cardiovascular disease in rheumatoid arthritis: results from a prospective cohort study. PLoS One 9, e87965.

van Sijl, A.M., van Eijk, I.C., Peters, M.J., Serne, E.H., van Der Horst-Bruinsma, I.E., Smulders, Y.M., Nurmohamed, M.T., 2015. Tumour necrosis factor blocking agents and progression of subclinical atherosclerosis in patients with ankylosing spondylitis. Ann. Rheum. Dis. 74, 119–123.

van Vollenhoven, R.F., Fleischmann, R., Cohen, S., Lee, E.B., Garcia Meijide, J.A., Wagner, S., Forejtova, S., Zwillich, S.H., Gruben, D., Koncz, T., Wallenstein, G.V., Krishnaswami, S., Bradley, J.D., Wilkinson, B., Investigators, O.S., 2012. Tofacitinib or adalimumab versus placebo in rheumatoid arthritis. N. Engl. J. Med. 367, 508–519.

van Walsem, A., Pandhi, S., Nixon, R.M., Guyot, P., Karabis, A., Moore, R.A., 2015. Relative benefit-risk comparing diclofenac to other traditional non-steroidal anti-inflammatory drugs and cyclooxygenase-2 inhibitors in patients with osteoarthritis or rheumatoid arthritis: a network meta-analysis. Arthritis Res. Ther. 17, 66.

Vassilopoulos, D., Gravos, A., Vlachopoulos, C., Kandili, A., Ioakeimidis, N., Pectasides, D., Stefanadis, C., 2015. Adalimumab decreases aortic stiffness independently of its effect in disease activity in patients with rheumatoid arthritis. Clin. Rheumatol. 34, 359–364.

Vis, M., Nurmohamed, M.T., Wolbink, G., Voskuyl, A.E., De Koning, M., van De Stadt, R., Twisk, J.W., Dijkmans, B.A., Lems, W.F., 2005. Short term effects of infliximab on the lipid profile in patients with rheumatoid arthritis. J. Rheumatol. 32, 252–255.

Voloshyna, I., Seshadri, S., Anwar, K., Littlefield, M.J., Belilos, E., Carsons, S.E., Reiss, A.B., 2014. Infliximab reverses suppression of cholesterol efflux proteins by TNF-alpha: a possible mechanism for modulation of atherogenesis. Biomed. Res. Int. 2014, 312647.

Vyas, D., O'dell, K.M., Bandy, J.L., Boyce, E.G., 2013. Tofacitinib: the First Janus Kinase (JAK) inhibitor for the treatment of rheumatoid arthritis. Ann. Pharmacother. 47, 1524–1531.

Wanders, A., Heijde, D., Landewe, R., Behier, J.M., Calin, A., Olivieri, I., Zeidler, H., Dougados, M., 2005. Nonsteroidal antiinflammatory drugs reduce radiographic progression in patients with ankylosing spondylitis: a randomized clinical trial. Arthritis Rheum. 52, 1756–1765.

Wasserman, M.J., Weber, D.A., Guthrie, J.A., Bykerk, V.P., Lee, P., Keystone, E.C., 2004. Infusion-related reactions to infliximab in patients with rheumatoid arthritis in a clinical practice setting: relationship to dose, antihistamine pretreatment, and infusion number. J. Rheumatol. 31, 1912–1917.

Weisman, M.H., 2002. What are the risks of biologic therapy in rheumatoid arthritis? An update on safety. J. Rheumatol. Suppl. 65, 33–38.

Westlake, S.L., Colebatch, A.N., Baird, J., Curzen, N., Kiely, P., Quinn, M., Choy, E., Ostor, A.J., Edwards, C.J., 2011. Tumour necrosis factor antagonists and the risk of cardiovascular disease in patients with rheumatoid arthritis: a systematic literature review. Rheumatology (Oxford) 50, 518–531.

Westlake, S.L., Colebatch, A.N., Baird, J., Kiely, P., Quinn, M., Choy, E., Ostor, A.J., Edwards, C.J., 2010. The effect of methotrexate on cardiovascular disease in patients with rheumatoid arthritis: a systematic literature review. Rheumatology (Oxford) 49, 295–307.

Wolfe, F., Michaud, K., 2004. Heart failure in rheumatoid arthritis: rates, predictors, and the effect of anti-tumor necrosis factor therapy. Am. J. Med. 116, 305–311.

Wong, M., Oakley, S.P., Young, L., Jiang, B.Y., Wierzbicki, A., Panayi, G. Chowienczyk, P., Kirkham, B., 2009. Infliximab improves vascular stiffness in patients with rheumatoid arthritis. Ann. Rheum. Dis. 68, 1277–1284.

Wright, K., Crowson, C.S., Gabriel, S.E., 2014. Cardiovascular comorbidity in rheumatic diseases: a focus on heart failure. Heart Fail Clin. 10, 339–352.

Wu, X., Zhao, R., Li, Z., Yao, M., Wang, H., Han, J., Qu, S., Chen, X., Qian, L., Sun, Y., Xu, Y., Gu, J., 2004. A novel small peptide as a targeting ligand for receptor tyrosine kinase Tie2. Biochem. Biophys. Res. Commun. 315, 1004–1010.

Yamaoka, K., Tanaka, Y., 2013. Targeting the Janus kinases in rheumatoid arthritis: focus on tofacitinib. Expert Opin. Pharmacother. 15, 103–113.

Zhang, J., Xie, F., Yun, H., Chen, L., Muntner, P., Levitan, E.B., Safford, M.M., Kent, S.T., Osterman, M.T., Lewis, J.D., Saag, K., Singh, J.A., Curtis, J.R., 2016. Comparative effects of biologics on cardiovascular risk among older patients with rheumatoid arthritis. Ann. Rheum. Dis. 75, 1813–1818.

Zhang, W., Doherty, M., Arden, N., Bannwarth, B., Bijlsma, J., Gunther, K.P., Hauselmann, H.J., Herrero-Beaumont, G., Jordan, K., Kaklamanis, P., Leeb, B., Lequesne, M., Lohmander, S., Mazieres, B., Martin-Mola, E., Pavelka, K., Pendleton, A., Punzi, L., Swoboda, B., Varatojo, R., Verbruggen, G., Zimmermann-Gorska, I., Dougados, M., 2005. EULAR evidence based recommendations for the management of hip osteoarthritis: report of a task force of the EULAR Standing Committee for International Clinical Studies Including Therapeutics (ESCISIT). Ann. Rheum. Dis. 64, 669–681.

Index

'*Note:* Page numbers followed by "f" indicate figures and "t" indicate tables.'

H

I

K

L

M

N

V

W

X

FSC
www.fsc.org
MIX
Papier | Fördert
gute Waldnutzung
FSC® C083411

Kolibri 360 GmbH
Ferdinand-Jühlke-Straße 7
99095 Erfurt, Deutschland
produktsicherheit@kolibri360.de